A GUIDE TO ADULT NEUROPSYCHOLOGICAL DIAGNOSIS

Anthony Y. Stringer, Ph. D.
Associate Professor of Rehabilitation Medicine
Department of Rehabilitation Medicine
Emory University School of Medicine
Atlanta, Georgia

With the assistance of
Robert C. Green, M. D.
Assistant Professor of Neurology
Emory University
Atlanta, Georgia

F. A. DAVIS COMPANY • Philadelphia

F. A. Davis Company
1915 Arch Street
Philadelphia, PA 19103

Printed in the United States of America

Last digit indicates print number: 10 9 8 7 6 5 4 3 2 1

Medical Editor: Robert W. Reinhardt
Developmental Editor: Bernice M. Wissler
Production Editor: Jessica Howie Martin
Cover Designer: Steven Ross Morrone

As new scientific information becomes available through basic and clinical research, recommended treatments and drug therapies undergo changes. The author(s) and publisher have done everything possible to make this book accurate, up to date, and in accord with accepted standards at the time of publication. The authors, editors, and publisher are not responsible for errors or omissions or for consequences from application of the book, and make no warranty, expressed or implied, in regard to the contents of the book. Any practice described in this book should be applied by the reader in accordance with professional standards of care used in regard to the unique circumstances that may apply in each situation. The reader is advised always to check product information (package inserts) for changes and new information regarding dose and contraindications before administering any drug. Caution is especially urged when using new or infrequently ordered drugs.

Library of Congress Cataloging-in-Publication Data

Stringer, Anthony Y.
A guide to adult neuropsychological diagnosis / Anthony Y. Stringer; with the assistance of Robert C. Green.
p. cm.
Includes bibliographical references and indexes.
ISBN 0-8036-0072-0 (pbk.)
1. Neuropsychological tests. 2. Neuropsychiatry. 3. Brain—Diseases—Diagnosis. I. Green, Robert C., 1954- . II. Title.
[DNLM: 1. Neuropsychology—classification—case studies. 2. Mental Disorders—diagnosis—case studies. WL 103.5 S918g 1995]
RC386.6.N48S77 1995
616.8'0475—dc20
DNLM/DLC
for Library of Congress 95-41972

To my parents, Laura and Young, whose love nurtured me.
To my wife, Cathie, whose companionship sustains me.
To my daughter, Ayanna, whose inventiveness inspires me.

PREFACE

The basic impetus for this book was the need for a common frame of reference and a set of operational definitions for the broad range of health care practitioners and researchers concerned with neuropsychological disorders. The absence of such a frame of reference is widely evident. It can be seen in the use by neuropsychologists of vague terms like "visual perceptual deficit," "impaired executive functions," and "problem-solving deficit," which lack a commonly accepted meaning. It can be seen in interdisciplinary conferences, where even terms like "apraxia," which have a specific meaning, are used differently by different professionals. It is perhaps most evident in the common failure to disentangle disorders (e.g., separation of concentration disorders from memory disorders), with such a failure often leading to a focus on the wrong problems during rehabilitation.

The lack of a frame of reference is circumvented in research settings by defining neuropsychological disorders in terms of performance of a specific test or research task. Thus, "problem-solving deficit" may be defined as a certain score on a test that requires the sorting of cards using different strategies. Operationally defining a disorder in this manner leads to greater clarity of terminology but limits the extent to which we can generalize the results for situations in which other tests of the same disorder are used. We often end up learning more about the test than about the underlying disorder it is meant to measure.

A Guide to Adult Neuropsychological Diagnosis is intended to be an initial step toward providing a common frame of reference for the disparate professionals involved in neuropsychological diagnosis. It attempts to operationally define neuropsychological disorders by listing clinical indicators as objectively as possible. In most cases, detecting the appropriate clinical indicators is insufficient to diagnose a disorder. A host of other factors could also account for the presence of a given clinical indicator. Consequently, factors that must be ruled out before making a diagnosis are included for each disorder. More than 140 neuropsychological disorders are defined in this manner, and this number encompasses both rarely seen and common clinical syndromes.

Chapters 2 through 19 of this book provide a descriptive classification of major adult neuropsychological disorders. As described previously, clinical indicators and factors that must be ruled out before making a diagnosis are listed for each disorder. Also listed for each class of disorder are associated descriptive features, lesion locations, etiologies, potential disabling consequences, assessment instruments and procedures, and neuropsychological treatment approaches. Case studies are presented to illustrate the clinical presentation of the major disorders and the common problems that arise in attempting diagnosis. A comprehensive review of the clinical and research literature pertinent to each disorder is beyond the scope of this book. Clinical and research reports documenting the lesion locations associated with each disorder are cited in the references, with a bias toward more recent studies that incorporate neuroradiological localization of lesions.

The book contains separate Anatomical, Etiological, Test, and Behavioral Indexes. Through the use of the appropriate index, the reader can quickly find the disorder or disorders that may arise from damage to a particular brain structure, are associated with a particular disease etiology, or are implied by a particular behavior. Neuropsychological tests and assessment procedures can be located by using the Test Index.

Although this book is not intended as an introductory text, its language is intended to make it accessible to clinicians and students with varying degrees of experience. Behavioral neurologists, neuropsychologists, speech pathologists, and other health care professionals will find this book useful when making diagnostic decisions, interpreting clinical data, or selecting assessment procedures. The references documenting the lesion locations of the various disorders will be useful to clinicians preparing to give depositions or court testimony. It is hoped that this text will make accurate diagnosis easier; facilitate clinical training of students, interns, residents, and post-doctoral fellows; and promote better comprehension of neuropsychological disorders in multidisciplinary clinical and research settings.

I gratefully acknowledge the assistance of Dr. Robert C. Green, whose critical comments were instrumental in reshaping several chapters. Additionally, I wish to thank the editors at F. A. Davis for their patience, support, and willingness to embrace this project. I wish also to acknowledge my many colleagues, whose frequent inquiries about my progress spurred me on to complete this book.

Anthony Y. Stringer, Ph. D.
Atlanta, Georgia

CONTENTS

ADULT NEUROPSYCHOLOGICAL DIAGNOSIS

1

Neuropsychological diagnosis involves the systematic collection of human performance data to aid in drawing conclusions about brain function in patients suspected of having neurological or psychiatric disease. The data used in neuropsychological diagnosis are drawn from the patient's history, from observations of the patient in structured and naturalistic settings, and from the results of standardized procedures and normed tests. Underlying the neuropsychologist's conclusions is a solid foundation of clinical case analysis and empirical research on brain-behavior relationships.

Neuropsychological diagnosis contributes to the diagnosis of neurological and psychiatric disease, the determination of the type and degree of functional disability, and the planning of rehabilitation therapy and vocational training. Consequently, accurate neuropsychological diagnosis is vital in all clinical settings in which brain-damaged patients undergo evaluation and treatment. Accurate diagnosis is not possible, however, when clear, operational definitions of disorders do not exist. This has long been the case for most neuropsychological disorders.

DEFINITION AND CATEGORIZATION OF NEUROPSYCHOLOGICAL DISORDERS

In this book, the term *disorder* refers to any derangement or abnormality in the way a person functions. The term *adult neuropsychological disorder* refers to specific abnormalities of behavior shown by patients as a result of vascular, traumatic, or other forms of brain damage and disease. It is assumed that the brain damage occurred during adulthood and that, before the onset of the damage, examination of the patient would not have revealed any of the behavioral findings that characterize neuropsychological disorders. Neurological disease causes, but is not synonymous with, neuropsychological disorder. This becomes obvious when one considers that a single neurological disease can cause multiple neuropsychological disorders. The disorders described in this book involve disturbances in the way the brain receives, interprets, stores, uses, and responds to information. Thus, neuropsychological disorders are the cognitive, emotional, and behavioral manifestations of disease in the brain.

Regardless of the approach taken, categorization of neuropsychological disorders poses many problems. The syndrome approach to categorization involves clustering neuropsychological signs and symptoms according to the frequency with which they occur together in the same patient. Unfortunately, features considered to be part of a syndrome often occur singly. A good illustration of this is the continuing debate over Gerstmann's syndrome, which consists of a deficit in writing, a deficit in identifying one's own fingers, the inability to distinguish between right and left, and poor mathematical calculation ability. The question is whether Gerstmann's syndrome is really a syndrome at all, because its individual elements often occur singly.

In the anatomical approach to categorization, neuropsychological signs, symptoms, and disorders are grouped by the area of the brain that produces these features when damaged. The problems with this approach include:

1. The same neuropsychological disorder may arise following damage in different brain areas.
2. Brain areas such as the frontal lobes are so large and are involved in such diverse functions that damage to them can result in varying and seemingly contradictory signs in different patients.
3. The relationship between some disorders and the brain is tentative or unknown.
4. The relationship between the brain and behavior varies among individuals because of differences in heredity and developmental history.

Another approach is to categorize disorders based on their underlying cognitive or neurological mechanisms. For example, hemiakinesia, the inability to move an arm or leg spontaneously, could be grouped with hemi-inattention, the failure to notice stimuli on one side of the body, because both may involve a deficit in the brain's arousal system.[1] The difficulty is with the word *may*. Few neuropsychological disorders are understood sufficiently to permit agreement among researchers regarding the underlying cause. Because of the pace with which theories are tested and abandoned in neuropsychology, a system of categorization based on underlying mechanisms would need constant revision.

A descriptive approach to neuropsychological categorization is used in this text. This approach involves categorizing disorders by the type of behavior they produce. The descriptive approach is atheoretical in that no attempt is made to resolve controversies regarding the mechanisms that underlie the various disorders. Although it is hoped that neuroscience will ultimately provide the answers to questions of mechanism and that a theoretically based system will be produced that can evolve, this goal remains distant. Until this goal is reached, a descriptive approach is probably the soundest means of categorizing neuropsychological disorders.

The adult neuropsychological disorders described in this book are grouped into 18 descriptive categories.

1. Disorders of alertness
2. Disorders of concentration
3. Stimulus neglect
4. Stimulus imperception
5. Spatial imperception
6. Disorders of visual-motor integration
7. Disorders of stimulus localization
8. Disorders of stimulus recognition
9. Disorders of interhemispheric transfer
10. Disorders of voluntary cognitive control of movement
11. Disorders of oral language
12. Disorders of written language
13. Disorders of emotional communication
14. Calculation disorders
15. Memory disorders
16. Illusions and hallucinations
17. Neuropsychological disorders of emotion, ideation, and behavior
18. Intellectual decline

In each category, a variable number of disorders are listed and defined. In some instances, the existence of listed disorders is not firmly established. In these cases, the disorders are identified as putative.

Despite the largely descriptive approach taken in this book, some elements of the syndrome and anatomical approaches to categorization are incorporated. In keeping with the syndrome approach, a notation is made when a disorder is considered part of a syndrome, and the label commonly used by researchers and clinicians to identify the syndrome is included. Consistent with the anatomical approach, lesion locations of each disorder are listed, along with documenting references.

NOMENCLATURE

The terms used in the clinical literature to refer to neuropsychological disorders vary from author to author. For example, more than one dozen schemes for classifying aphasia exist, some of which apply the same term to different clinical disorders. To cope with the variability in terminology, I have attempted to choose diagnostic labels that are most descriptive of the disorders in this book. In most cases, terms already in general use are used. In the few instances in which no agreed-upon term is available, I have attempted to provide one appropriate for the disorder in question. Other labels used in the literature to refer to each disorder are parenthetically included.

Some assistance with diagnostic terminology is provided by the official nomenclature of the American Psychiatric Association's *Diagnostic and Statistical*

Manual of Mental Disorders, Fourth Edition (DSM-IV),[2] although as of this writing, the revised third edition (DSM-III-R) continues to be used in some settings.[3] Neuropsychological disorders could be coded only imprecisely using DSM-III-R, and this situation unfortunately changes only partially when using DSM-IV. Table 1–1 summarizes the similarities and differences in coding neuropsychological disorders in DSM-III-R and DSM-IV. As can be seen, DSM-IV contains diagnostic codes applicable to most of the major types of neuropsychological disorders. Significantly, DSM-IV codes are available in areas in which DSM-III-R provided no vi-

Table 1–1. **CODING OF ADULT NEUROPSYCHOLOGICAL DISORDERS IN DSM-III-R AND DSM-IV**

Chapter in This Text	Type of Neuropsychological Disorder	Coding Options in DSM-III-R	Coding Options in DSM-IV
2	Alertness	Delirium Factitious disorder Conversion disorder (Part of) somatization disorder	Same options as DSM-III-R
3	Concentration	No precise options	Attention deficit/hyperactivity disorder NOS Cognitive disorder NOS Mild neurocognitive disorder
4	Stimulus neglect	No precise options	Cognitive disorder NOS Mild neurocognitive disorder
5	Stimulus imperception	No precise options Psychogenic imperception may be coded as: Conversion disorder Malingering Factitious disorder (Part of) somatization disorder	Cognitive disorder NOS Mild neurocognitive disorder Same options as in DSM-III-R for psychogenic imperception
6	Spatial imperception	No precise options	Cognitive disorder NOS Mild neurocognitive disorder
7	Visual-motor integration	(Part of) dementia	Cognitive disorder NOS Mild neurocognitive disorder
8	Stimulus localization	No precise options	Cognitive disorder NOS Mild neurocognitive disorder
9	Stimulus recognition	(Part of) dementia	Cognitive disorder NOS Mild neurocognitive disorder
10	Interhemispheric transfer	No precise options See also codes for the bilateral presentations of these disorders	Cognitive disorder NOS Mild neurocognitive disorder See also codes for the bilateral presentations of these disorders
11	Voluntary cognitive control of movement	(Part of) dementia (Part of) delirium Conversion disorder (Part of) somatization disorder Factitious disorder	(Part of) dementia Catatonic disorder due to a general medical condition Cognitive disorder NOS Mild neurocognitive disorder Conversion disorder

Table 1–1. **CODING OF ADULT NEUROPSYCHOLOGICAL DISORDERS IN DSM-III-R AND DSM-IV** *Continued*

Chapter in This Text	Type of Neuropsychological Disorder	Coding Options in DSM-III-R	Coding Options in DSM-IV
		Malingering	(Part of) somatization disorder Factitious disorder Malingering
12	Oral language	No precise options	Expressive language disorder Mixed receptive-expressive language disorder Communication disorder NOS
13	Written language	No precise options	Reading disorder Disorder of written expression Learning disorder NOS
14	Emotional communication	No precise options	No precise options
15	Calculation	No precise options	Mathematics disorder
16	Memory	Amnestic syndrome/disorder Alcohol amnestic disorder Barbiturate or similarly acting sedative or hypnotic amnestic disorder Other or unspecified substance amnestic disorder Psychogenic amnesia (Part of) multiple personality (Part of) psychogenic fugue Malingering Factitious disorder (Part of) somatization disorder	Amnestic disorder due to a general medical condition Substance-induced persisting amnestic disorder Dissociative amnesia (Part of) dissociative identity disorder (Part of) dissociative fugue Malingering Factitious disorder (Part of) somatization disorder
17	Illusions and hallucinations	(Part of) delirium Organic hallucinosis	Psychotic disorder due to a general medical condition
18	Emotion, ideation, and behavior	Organic delusional syndrome/disorder (Part of) delirium Organic personality syndrome/disorder Organic affective syndrome/disorder (Part of) amnestic syndrome/disorder (Part of) dementia	Personality change due to a general medical condition Mood disorder due to a general medical condition (Part of) dementia (Part of) delirium Impulse control disorder NOS Cognitive disorder NOS Mild neurocognitive disorder
19	Intellectual decline	(Part of) dementia Borderline intellectual functioning	(Part of) dementia Borderline intellectual functioning

Abbreviation: NOS, not otherwise specified.

able coding options.

An advancement in DSM-IV is the provision of some diagnostic codes for use in adults that DSM-III-R reserved for infants, children, and adolescents. For example, an adult with previously normal reading ability who develops a reading deficit as a result of a brain lesion can be given the DSM-IV diagnosis of "Reading Disorder." The corresponding diagnosis in DSM-III-R is "Developmental Reading Disorder," which is reserved for children or adolescents who do not have a neurological disorder. Thus, DSM-IV permits many neuropsychological disorders to be coded for which DSM-III-R made no provision (see Table 1–1).

Another major change in DSM-IV is in the conceptualization of mental disorders that are secondary to medical conditions. DSM-III-R distinguished between organic and functional mental disorders. The former applied to disorders caused by brain dysfunction of known etiology. Functional disorders either lacked an established organic cause or were thought to be a response to psychological or social factors. DSM-IV does not distinguish between organic and functional disorders, because such a distinction implies that functional disorders do not have a biological basis. As a consequence of this change, many DSM-III-R disorders have been renamed, as indicated in Table 1–1. For example, the DSM-III-R diagnosis "Organic Personality Disorder" in DSM-IV has become "Personality Change due to a General Medical Condition," with the condition being specified by the clinician.

As in DSM-III-R, DSM-IV does not permit the level of specificity and precision needed by health care professionals involved in neuropsychological diagnosis. This is most evident in such diagnostic codes as "Cognitive Disorder Not Otherwise Specified" and "Mild Neurocognitive Disorder." These codes are meant as residual diagnoses to be used for patients who do not meet criteria for some other, more precisely defined disorder. Unfortunately, DSM-IV precisely defines so few neuropsychological disorders that these residual codes become wastebasket categories that subsume a broad range of clinical presentations. For example, a patient who fails to notice a tactile stimulus on the left side of his or her body and a patient who perseveres in giving the same answer to different questions could both receive a diagnosis of "Cognitive Disorder Not Otherwise Specified" despite their different presentations and, possibly, different areas of brain dysfunction.

Despite this lack of diagnostic specificity, DSM-IV provides more options for coding neuropsychological disorders and achieves somewhat greater precision than its predecessors. DSM-IV should be considered a working draft because the diagnosis of mental disorders continues to be refined. It is hoped that the trend toward the inclusion of more neuropsychological disorders and the use of precise diagnostic codes will continue with DSM-V.

The *International Classification of Diseases, Ninth Revision, Clinical Modification* (ICD-9-CM)[4] provides many more options for coding neuropsychological disorders than are available in DSM-IV. For example, ICD-9-CM provides codes for neuropsychological disorders such as aphasia, alexia, agnosia, and achromatopsia. Unfortunately, even with its additional coding options, ICD-9-CM falls short of including a majority of the neuropsychological disorders listed in this book. Nonetheless, each chapter in this text includes a discussion of the coding options provided by DSM-IV and ICD-9-CM.

ETIOLOGICAL DIAGNOSIS

A word of caution is warranted concerning the etiology of adult disorders. As previously stated, neurological disease causes, but is not synonymous with, neuropsychological disorder. Knowing that a specific neuropsychological disorder is present can suggest a neurological diagnosis but is rarely sufficient to establish it. Correct neuropsychological diagnosis is only one step toward arriving at a correct neurological diagnosis. The former is well within the province of neuropsychologists, physicians, and speech pathologists. Neurological diagnosis, however, can be accomplished only by the physician. This book is written to aid the process of neuropsychological diagnosis. It is not a manual for diagnosing neurological disease.

For example, a neuropsychologist may determine, based on a thorough examination, that a patient has akinesia. As noted previously, patients with this disorder have difficulty in initiating movement. In addition, the speed with which their movements are carried out is reduced. The neuropsychologist may conclude that the presence of this disorder suggests damage in the basal ganglia, but neurological consultation is required to determine whether the disorder is the result of brain trauma, Parkinson's disease, or some other pathological process.

CLINICAL INDICATORS, FACTORS TO RULE OUT, AND LESION LOCATIONS

I have attempted to provide clear and objective clinical indicators for each of the neuropsychological disorders. Each clinical indicator stands alone. If several indicators are listed, only one must be observed for the clinician to suspect that the disorder is present. Each clinical indicator is demarcated by a unique alphabetical character. Some clinical indicators have two or more parts that must be considered together. This is indicated by subscripting. For example, "a" and "b" denote two independent clinical indicators. Letters with subscripted numbers, such as "a_1" and "a_2," refer to one clinical indicator having two parts that must be considered together.

Also listed for each disorder are associated descriptive features. This information gives the reader a more complete picture of the disorders, but the presence or absence of the associated features does not affect the diagnosis.

Although only a single clinical indicator is needed for a given diagnosis to be considered, all "factors that must be ruled out" listed for the suspected disorder must be taken into account. Failure to rule out even a single factor makes a firm diagnosis impossible. Each lesion location listed for each disorder stands alone. Damage in one, not all, of the listed anatomical areas is sufficient to produce the neuropsychological disorder.

The lesion locations apply to neuropsychological disorders and not to neuropsychological functions or abilities. For example, left thalamic lesions may cause language disorder (aphasia), but this does not mean that language is a function mediated by the left side of the thalamus. A lesion may cause a disorder because it interrupts a fiber pathway connecting other brain areas that mediate a neuropsychological ability. Alternatively, a lesion in one area can cause a disorder by depriving other brain areas of afferent stimulation. In other cases, a lesion may block the output of brain areas that are critical for a given ability and, again, produce a disorder.

Focal lesions also may impair indirectly the functioning of remote brain areas. A lesion in one brain area may, for example, compress other areas through displacement of brain tissue and edema. Focal lesions can also reduce blood flow and metabolic rate in distant brain areas.[5–7] In both of these ways, the functioning of remote brain areas can be impeded, although they themselves do not have a lesion. Consequently, the distinction between disorder and function must be kept in mind when using the lesion locations in this text. In the previous example, the thalamic lesion may cause aphasia because it deprives the left temporal lobe of important afferent input, not because the thalamus is a center for language.

When using the lesion locations, it is also important to bear in mind the mediating role of individual differences. Every individual differs slightly in the way his or her brain is "wired." This variability in brain wiring arises from factors such as differences in heredity, developmental experience, and reorganization of brain function as a result of prior lesions. If the individual differences were great enough, no generalization among patients would be possible. Fortunately, individuals do not vary to this degree, and the known lesion locations of the disorders apply to the majority of patients encountered. Nonetheless, the clinician must be alert to exceptions. I have, for example, encountered a case of left cerebral hypoplasia to which few of the traditional anatomical correlates applied.[8] In addition, most clinicians have seen left-handed individuals with aphasia following a right-hemisphere lesion rather than the more typical left-sided lesion.

To take into account individual variability, I have attempted to include all lesion locations reported in the literature for each neuropsychological disorder, even though some of the locations are based on rare or exceptional cases. The relative frequency of each disorder following left- and right-hemisphere lesions is also reported.

RELIABILITY AND VALIDITY

Although objectivity is the goal of diagnosis, some degree of subjectivity is inevitable when diagnostic decisions are made. The ideal would be to specify exact test-score ranges that could govern the clinician's diagnostic decisions. Unfortunately, this is not possible because of the variety of neuropsychological tests in use and the unavailability of normative data at all age and education levels. Use of the neuropsychological tests listed under each diagnostic category can add to the objectivity and certainty of the clinician's diagnosis. Many of the tests listed include cutoff scores that can be used to distinguish more objectively between brain-damaged and healthy individuals.

In this book, a distinction is made between tests and procedures. The former are generally standardized and normed instruments, although some of the tests included here require further validation. Empirically proven tests are not always available for measuring behaviors of interest to the neuropsychologist. In these instances, the clinician must incorporate various clinical procedures for which experience has demonstrated utility but for which norms and validating data are unavailable. Use of such procedures is a necessity, but they do increase the risk of misdiagnosis. Such procedures should be used only by experienced clinicians and work best when used in conjunction with validated instruments.

To aid the clinician in the selection of appropriate tests and procedures, the reliability and validity of each assessment instrument are discussed, when such information is available. *Reliability* refers to the stability of an assessment instrument. A reliable instrument is one that yields the same result when used in the same patient under similar test conditions. The index used to measure reliability is termed the *reliability coefficient*. Such coefficients vary from 0, indicating that the instrument yields random results, to 1, indicating that the instrument is totally reliable.

The reliability of an instrument can be measured in several different ways that yield different types of reliability coefficients. Several types of reliability are discussed in this text. Inter-rater, inter-judge, and inter-scorer reliability refer to the extent to which different raters obtain the same result from an instrument. The extent to which a single judge obtains the same result when scoring an instrument more than once is termed *intra-judge reliability*. *Parallel-form reliability* refers to the extent to which different forms of the same test yield the same result. *Test-retest reliability* refers to the extent to which a test yields the same result when administered more than once to the same person. *Split-half reliability* splits the test and measures the extent to which the two halves yield the same result. Cronbach's alpha, an index of the internal consistency of a test, is equivalent to the average split-half reliability coefficient for all possible divisions of the test into halves. A detailed discussion of reliability coefficients is beyond the scope of this book but is available elsewhere.[9,10]

Validity refers to the extent to which a test measures the factor it is intended to measure. For the neuropsychological instruments discussed in this book, validity is typically demonstrated by documenting a test's sensitivity to revealing brain damage, documenting its ability to discriminate patients from healthy individuals or to discriminate between patient groups (i.e., *discriminant validity*), or documenting that it correlates with other instruments that measure what the test is designed to measure (i.e., *convergent validity*). A small number of test developers attempt to document *ecological validity* (i.e., the correlation of a test with some aspect of functioning in a person's everyday environment).

Factor analysis, a statistical technique that identifies underlying variables in a large set of measures, can aid in determining the validity of tests. Using factor analysis, the items or components of a test can be grouped into relatively homogeneous sets. Examination of these sets helps to identify what properties are included in and measured by a test. A detailed discussion of test validity is available elsewhere.[9,11]

EXAMINER TRAINING AND TEST CONDITIONS

Although some tests can be administered by a variety of health care professionals, other tests require the specialized training available only in a graduate psychology or neuropsychology program. Such tests are restricted to use by licensed psychologists and, in some instances, speech pathologists. Notation is made of the level of training and experience required for administration of each test. Administration of any listed test by individuals outside of the appropriate health care professions or by health care professionals lacking the appropriate training and experience is unethical and invalidates any result obtained. Objective clinical indicators and standardized instruments are not sufficient to guarantee accurate clinical judgments. Formal training and supervision in neurological or neuropsychological examination procedures are a necessity. The responsibility for arriving at an accurate neuropsychological diagnosis ultimately rests with the individual clinician.

In all instances, patients are assumed to have been examined under optimal conditions. The patients must be cooperative, motivated to try their best, and relatively free of nervousness and tension; otherwise, their performance during a neuropsychological examination could be affected negatively and the results invalidated. In this text, with the exception of patients who have disorders of oral language, it is assumed that test instructions were comprehended by the patients and that the patients were capable of giving verbal responses when required. In addition, except for patients who have disorders of voluntary cognitive control of movement, it is assumed that they were capable of motor responses. Except for patients who have disorders of alertness and concentration, it is assumed that they were paying attention during the examination. Patients are assumed to have been appropriate in their behavior so that valid testing was possible. Although these points are not repeatedly listed as "factors to rule out" under each of the disorders in this book, it is implicitly assumed that the well-trained clinician will have taken them into account before making a diagnostic decision. Failure to take these variables into account invalidates the results of any examination.

EXAMPLES OF CLINICAL USE OF THIS TEXT

The indexes may often be the starting point for clinical use of this book. Specific neuropsychological disorders can be located in the appropriate index by the behavioral abnormalities they produce, by their lesion locations, or by their cause. Health care professionals with backgrounds in neuropsychological or neurological assessment and neuroanatomy will find the behavioral and anatomical indexes the most useful starting points. Examiners who are less familiar with neuropsychological procedures and neurological populations will find the etiologic index more helpful, because it requires only that the user know what neurological condition (e.g., stroke, traumatic brain injury, Parkinson's disease) is occurring in the patient to locate neuropsychological disorders that may be present.

After the neuropsychological disorders of interest are located in the indexes, the user can review clinical indicators, factors that must be ruled out, lesion locations of each disorder, and the variety of tests and procedures that can be used by a trained professional to assess and treat the patient. The user will also have access to information on possible etiologies and disabling consequences of the neuropsychological disorders. Examples of how various users might approach the use of this text follow.

Example 1

While examining a patient, a physician observes that the patient's left hand constantly conflicts with the right hand. The left hand may, for instance, unbutton a shirt just buttoned by the right hand. When the patient's attention is drawn to this behavior, the patient expresses frustration with the uncooperative left hand. Looking under "Hand(s)" in the behavioral index, the physician will find listed "(Acting at) Cross Purposes." There the physician will learn that the behavior is associated with diagonistic apraxia, a disorder caused by a lesion in the corpus callosum. From the information provided in this text, the physician will be able to assess more carefully the presence of this disorder in the patient and to identify disease processes requiring additional medical assessment and intervention.

Example 2

A neuropsychologist is preparing to testify to the presence of brain damage in a patient who sustained a blow to the head that left him dazed but conscious. The patient's computed tomography (CT) scans are normal. Based on the patient's neuropsychological test results, however, the neuropsychologist intends to testify that the patient has sustained frontal lobe damage. This pleases the patient's attorney, but the opposing counsel is expected to question how paper-and-pencil test results can establish the presence of brain damage when CT scans failed to do so. Through the use of this text's behavioral and anatomical indexes, the neuropsychologist can relate test results to neuropsychological disorders that have known lesion locations in the brain. The references listed with the lesion locations provide an empirical basis for the assertion that neuropsychological data are valid for detecting and localizing brain damage, regardless of CT scan results. By citing these references and studies documenting the insensitivity of CT scans to the subtle pathological changes that occur in the brain following minor head trauma,[12] the neuropsychologist can respond authoritatively to the opposing counsel's questions.

Example 3

A speech therapist is preparing to assess a patient referred to her following surgical resection of an anterior communicating artery aneurysm. Not having previously seen a patient with this diagnosis, the therapist is uncertain about what to expect. Neuropsychological disorders likely to be present can be located in the text by looking up "Anterior Communicating Artery" in the anatomical index or by looking up "Aneurysm" in the etiologic index. After these disorders are located, the speech therapist is better able to select assessment procedures that are appropriate for the patient as well as to anticipate the need for consultation with a neuropsychologist to address problem areas that are outside of the speech therapist's expertise.

EXAMPLES OF RESEARCH USE OF THIS TEXT

This book lends itself to a number of research uses. The clinical indicators and factors that must be ruled out for each disorder can be used as inclusion and exclusion criteria for subject selection in studies of specific neuropsychological disorders. A number of research questions are generated by the text itself. Do the lesion locations listed for each disorder, many of which are based on the study of small numbers of patients, remain accurate when larger samples are studied? Is the accuracy of neuropsychological diagnosis improved through the systematic use of this text? Does the breakdown of the major categories of neuropsychological disorders (i.e., the "variety of presentations") in this book adequately describe the variable behaviors seen in clinical populations?

Finally, this book can be a stimulus for the use of epidemiological approaches in the field of neuropsychology. Systematic, large-scale investigations of the pattern and incidence of neuropsychological disorder following various lesions or neurological diseases are lacking for all but a few categories of disorders. A few investigators are beginning to look at gender and racial differences in neuropsychological functioning after brain damage, but virtually no examinations of the comorbidity of various disorders and geographic variation in incidence have taken place.

Knowledge gained from these and other investigations will certainly lead to major revision or perhaps even abandonment of the diagnostic approach taken in this book. Whether this text is the beneficiary or the casualty of future research remains to be seen, but if it plays any role in spurring these investigations, it will have fulfilled a vital function.

REFERENCES

1. Heilman, KM, Watson, RT, and Valenstein, E: Neglect and related disorders. In Heilman, KM and Valenstein, E (eds): Clinical Neuropsychology, Second Edition. Oxford University Press, New York, 1985, p 243.
2. American Psychiatric Association: Diagnostic and Statistical Manual of Mental Disorders, Fourth Edition. American Psychiatric Association, Washington, DC, 1994.
3. American Psychiatric Association: Diagnostic and Statistical Manual of Mental Disorders, Third Edition, Revised. American Psychiatric Association, Washington, DC, 1987.
4. The International Classification of Diseases, Ninth Revision, Clinical Modification. Med-Index Publications, Salt Lake City, 1991.
5. Endo, H, Larsen, B, and Lassen, NA: Regional cerebral blood flow alterations remote from the site of intracranial tumors. J Neurosurg 46:270, 1977.

6. Melamed, E, et al: Correlation between regional cerebral blood flow and EEG frequency in the contralateral hemisphere in acute cerebral infarction. J Neurol Sci 26:21, 1975.
7. Slater, R, et al: Diaschisis with cerebral infarction. Stroke 8:684, 1977.
8. Stringer, AY and Fennell, EB: Hemispheric compensation in a child with left cerebral hypoplasia. Clin Neuropsychol 1:124, 1987.
9. Franzen, MD: Reliability and Validity in Neuropsychological Assessment. Plenum Press, New York, 1989.
10. Magnusson, D: Test Theory. Addison-Wesley, Reading, MA, 1967.
11. Kerlinger, FN: Foundations of Behavioral Research, Second Edition. Holt, Rinehart and Winston, New York, 1973.
12. Shores, A, et al: Neuropsychological assessment and brain imaging technologies in evaluation of the sequelae of blunt head injury. Aust N Z J Psychiatry 24:133, 1990.

DISORDERS OF ALERTNESS

2

DEFINITION

Disorders of alertness involve a failure to maintain a state of wakefulness in which the individual is ready and able to respond to events occurring in the environment. The person fails to remain awake and prepared despite having had adequate rest and sleep. A person's level of alertness can be temporarily altered by drugs; therefore, it must be demonstrated that the patient's change in alertness is not caused by acute intoxication. In addition, the change in alertness must be evident to outside observers and not just subjectively reported by the individual. Psychiatric disorders such as depression and schizophrenia can cause an individual to appear sleepy, apathetic, or unresponsive, and consequently must be ruled out before diagnosing all but one of the disorders included in this category.

The disorders of alertness include lethargy or obtundation, stupor, and psychogenic underresponsiveness or unresponsiveness. Coma, although it is the severest form of alertness disorder, is not discussed in this chapter. Comatose patients have such a severe alertness deficit that they are not amenable to even cursory neuropsychological examination and thus are outside the scope of this book. Patients with ventral pontine lesions may be unable to respond to the environment except through eye blinks because of total quadriplegia (i.e., "locked-in syndrome"). These patients do not have an impairment of alertness and are rarely seen in neuropsychological practices. Consequently, the locked-in syndrome is not included in this text. Thorough coverage of coma and the locked-in syndrome can be found in Plum and Posner.[1]

Akinetic mutism, sometimes termed *persistent vegetative state*, is listed in this chapter because it is typically mentioned in books on alertness disorders. Patients with akinetic mutism appear alert even though they fail to interact with the environment. Because of the apparent preservation of alertness in patients who have akinetic mutism, it is discussed elsewhere in this text. Akinesia is discussed in Chapter 11 and mutism in Chapter 12.

NOMENCLATURE

The terms *lethargy* or *obtundation*, *stupor*, and *psychogenic unresponsiveness* are in common use in neurological literature. In ICD-9-CM,[2] stupor is grouped with coma under the same diagnostic code. Lethargy is included in the ICD-9-CM diagnosis of malaise and fatigue. There is no diagnostic code in DSM-IV[3] that directly corresponds to these disorders. Lethargy or obtundation, as well as stupor, may be seen in some patients given a DSM-IV diagnosis of delirium, but there is no diagnostic code for a patient who is underaroused but lacks the other features of delirium. Delirium itself has been variously referred to as "acute confusional state," "acute brain syndrome," "metabolic encephalopathy," "toxic psychosis," and "psychosis associated with organic brain syndrome" in the neurological and psychiatric literature.

Psychogenic unresponsiveness (or underresponsiveness), depending on the degree of intentional control the patient exerts over the symptoms, would be diagnosed in DSM-IV as a factitious disorder or a conversion disorder. If the condition is part of a larger profile of symptoms having no clear organic basis, psychogenic unresponsiveness would be considered an aspect of the DSM-IV somatization disorder. In addition, as noted later, psychogenic unresponsiveness is often associated with, or caused by, several other mental disorders, including major depression and some forms of schizophrenia.

VARIETY OF PRESENTATION

1. Lethargy or obtundation

Clinical Indicators

a_1. Gradual or rapid drifting off to sleep when not directly stimulated

a_2. Awakening in response to loud noise or vigorous shaking

a_3. Drowsy appearance while awake

Associated Features

a. Waxing and waning of drowsiness over the course of 1 or more days
b. Decreased initiation and speed of spontaneous movement (see Akinesia)
c. Confusion and limited awareness of events going on in the environment (see Ideational Confusion or Disorientation)
d. Restlessness, irritability, and agitation, particularly at night
e. Inability to concentrate on tasks or conversations
f. Frequent loss of train of thought when speaking
g. Tendency to trail off into silence when speaking
h. Assessment of other neuropsychological functions often difficult and of questionable validity

Factors to Rule Out

a. Normal fatigue and sleepiness caused by lack of adequate rest
b. Use of prescribed or recreational drugs that have sedating effects [drugs that the patient is taking should be checked for sedating effects in a current *Physician's Desk Reference* (PDR)][4]
c. Significantly depressed mood (see Chap. 18 for assessment techniques)
d. Prolonged absence of meaningful environmental stimulation caused by vision or hearing loss or prolonged stay in medical settings where there is little that is meaningful or familiar for the patient to focus on (e.g., intensive care)
e. Intentional or unconscious failure to respond to the environment (see Psychogenic Unresponsiveness)
f. Narcolepsy: Recurrent, sudden, transient, and irresistible attacks of sleep, often during sedentary activities and despite adequate sleep at night; can be distinguished from lethargy or obtundation by the suddenness of its onset and the brevity (i.e., a few minutes) of the episodes

RULES FOR DIAGNOSIS

Clinical Indicators: Each is independent (only one must be observed for the disorder to be suspected) *except* when subscripting is used. Subscripted numbers (a_1, a_2) denote an indicator with multiple parts that must be considered together.
Associated Features: These are listed to give a more complete picture of the disorder. The presence or absence of these features does not affect the diagnosis.
Factors to Rule Out: All must be taken into account. Failure to rule out even one of these factors makes a firm diagnosis impossible.
Lesion Locations: Each location stands alone; damage in only one of the listed areas is sufficient to produce the disorder.

g. Catalepsy: Recurrent, sudden attacks of transient paralysis and loss of muscle tone, often precipitated by a pleasant or unpleasant emotional experience; can be distinguished from lethargy or obtundation by the suddenness of its onset, the brevity of the episodes, and the fact that the patient remains alert although unable to move

Lesion Locations

a. Brainstem ascending reticular activating system fibers originating at the level of the pons and mesencephalon[5–7]
b. Reticular activating system projection zones in the diencephalon (nonspecific thalamic nuclei, including the reticular nucleus, interlaminar nucleus, and centrum medianum) and limbic system (hypothalamus)[5,6]
c. Supratentorial masses that invade the diencephalon[1]
d. Supratentorial masses that compress the diencephalon through horizontal displacement of supratentorial tissue[8,9]
e. Upper brainstem compression as a result of herniation of the cingulate gyrus (cingulate herniation), the uncus and hippocampal gyri (uncal herniation), or the cerebral hemispheres and basal ganglia (central transtentorial herniation; Fig. 2–1)[1,10–15]
f. Subtentorial masses or destructive lesions outside the brainstem that compress the reticular activating system directly or through herniation of the superior cerebellar vermis or the cerebellar tonsils (Fig. 2–2)[1]
g. Bilateral, diffuse lesions of the cerebral cortex and underlying white matter[1,16–19]

Lesion Lateralization

a. Incidence is greater following left-sided supratentorial lesions[20,21]

2. Stupor

Clinical Indicators

a_1. Sleeping most of the time when not directly stimulated
a_2. Brief periods of only limited responsiveness (e.g., groaning or restless movement) without meaningful interaction following repeated intense stimulation (e.g., pain, bright light, loud noise, manipulation of the limbs)

Associated Features

a. Restlessness, irritability, agitation, or violent outbursts at night or in response to repeated intense stimulation
b. Valid assessment of other neuropsychological functions not possible

Factors to Rule Out

a. Normal fatigue and sleepiness caused by lack of adequate rest
b. Use of prescribed or recreational drugs that have sedating effects (drugs that the patient is taking should be checked for sedating effects in a current PDR)[4]
c. Catatonic schizophrenia: a mental disorder that can manifest itself as decreased responsivity to environmental stimuli, reduced spontaneous activity, and mutism (see Chap. 18 for assessment techniques)

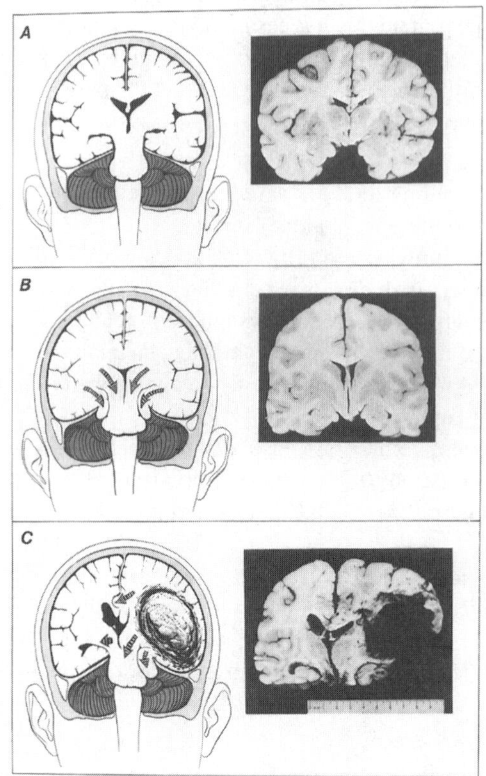

FIGURE 2–1. Upper brainstem compression as a result of supratentorial lesions. (*A*) Normal relationship of the supratentorial and intratentorial compartments. (*B*) Central transtentorial herniation in a patient with multiple cerebral metastases from carcinoma of the lung. The diencephalon is compressed and elongated. (*C*) Uncal herniation in a patient with a massive hemorrhagic infarct. The cingulate gyrus is herniated under the falx cerebri, and the uncus ipsilateral to the lesion is markedly swollen. A degree of central transtentorial herniation is also present. (From Plum and Posner,[1] p 92, with permission.)

d. A severe major depressive episode (see Chap. 18 for assessment techniques)
e. Intentional or unconscious failure to respond to the environment (see Psychogenic Unresponsiveness)
f. Narcolepsy: Recurrent, sudden, transient, and irresistible attacks of sleep, often during sedentary activities and despite adequate sleep at night; can be distinguished from stupor by the suddenness of its onset and the brevity (i.e., a few minutes) of the episodes
g. Catalepsy: Recurrent, sudden attacks of transient paralysis and loss of muscle tone, often precipitated by a pleasant or unpleasant emotional experience; can be distinguished from stupor by the suddenness of its onset, the brevity of the episodes, and the fact that the patient remains alert although unable to move

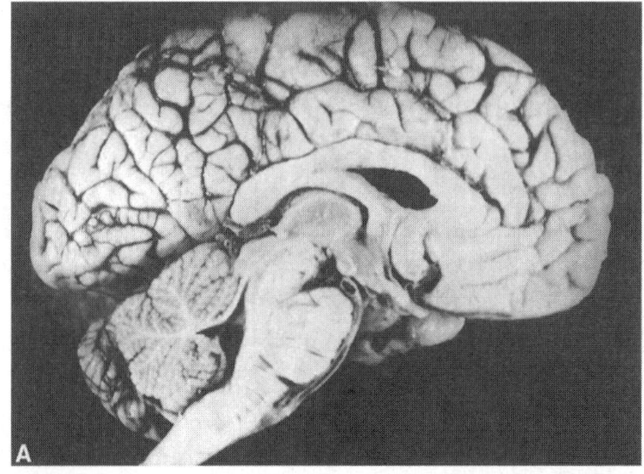

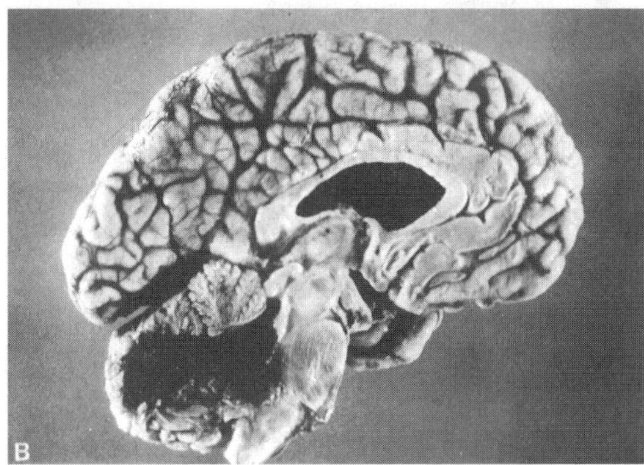

FIGURE 2–2. Compression of the reticular activating system as a result of cerebellar hemorrhage. (*A*) Normal midsagittal brain section. (*B*) Results of a massive cerebellar hemorrhage. Herniation of the cerebellar tonsils and vermis is present, and the diencephalon is swollen because of shifts of supratentorial structures. Swelling is also seen in the pons and midbrain. (From Plum and Posner,[1] p 154, with permission.)

Lesion Locations

a. Brainstem ascending reticular activating system fibers originating at the level of the pons and mesencephalon[5–7]
b. Reticular activating system projection zones in the diencephalon (nonspecific thalamic nuclei, including the reticular nucleus, intralaminar nucleus, and centrum medianum) and limbic system (hypothalamus)[5,6]
c. Supratentorial masses that invade the diencephalon[1]
d. Supratentorial masses that compress the diencephalon through horizontal displacement of supratentorial tissue[8,9]
e. Upper brainstem compression as a result of herniation of the cingulate gyrus (cingulate herniation), the uncus and hippocampal gyri (uncal herniation), or the cerebral hemispheres and basal ganglia (central transtentorial herniation; see Fig. 2–1)[1,10–15]
f. Subtentorial masses or destructive lesions outside of the brainstem that compress the reticular activating system directly or through herniation of the superior cerebellar vermis or the cerebellar tonsils (see Fig. 2–2)[1]
g. Bilateral, diffuse lesions of the cerebral cortex and underlying white matter[1,16–19]

Lesion Lateralization

a. Incidence is greater following left-sided supratentorial lesions[20,21]

3. Psychogenic underresponsiveness or unresponsiveness

Clinical Indicators

a_1. Presence of clinical indicators of either lethargy or obtundation, or stupor (see previous text)

a_2. Palpable resistance of the eyelids to passive opening by the examiner, with rapid closure once they are forced open

b_1. Presence of clinical indicators of either lethargy or obtundation, or stupor (see previous text)

b_2. Avoidance of potential self-injury, even when grossly underaroused and unresponsive (e.g., when the patient's arm is raised above the face and dropped by the examiner, the patient avoids letting the arm strike the face)

c_1. Presence of clinical indicators of either lethargy or obtundation, or stupor (see previous text)

c_2. Rapid change in level of alertness, for better or worse, in response to skeptical comments made in the presence of the patient*

Associated Features

a. Current absence of an etiological factor known to be associated with lethargy or obtundation, or stupor
b. Previous experience of a transient reduction in alertness caused by drug ingestion, head trauma, or other physiological cause
c. Recent experience of an emotionally traumatizing event or situation, including the onset of illness itself
d. Presence of undesirable situations or events that the patient can avoid through his or her symptoms (i.e., "secondary gain")
e. A major depressive episode (see Chap. 18 for assessment techniques)
f. Catatonic schizophrenia, a mental disorder that can manifest itself as decreased responsivity to environmental stimuli, reduced spontaneous activity, and mutism (see Chap. 18 for assessment techniques)

Factors to Rule Out

NOTE: Misclassifying a physiologically based disorder of alertness as psychogenic unresponsiveness can have life-threatening consequences for the patient. It is essential that all of the following factors be ruled out before making a diagnosis. The difficulty of arriving at a correct diagnosis in this instance requires close collaboration between the physician and the neuropsychologist.

a. Normal fatigue and sleepiness caused by lack of adequate rest
b. Use of prescribed or recreational drugs that have sedating effects (drugs that the patient is taking should be checked for sedating effects in a current PDR)[4]
c. Prolonged absence of meaningful environmental stimulation caused by vision

*Any skeptical comments should be made in an objective, clinical manner, with care taken to avoid insulting the patient.

or hearing loss or prolonged stay in medical settings where there is little that is meaningful or familiar for the patient to focus on (e.g., intensive care)

d. Physiologically based underarousal: patient should have an electroencephalographic record that is characteristic of an alert individual and should show normal nystagmus in response to unilateral ice-water irrigation of the ears (normal nystagmus under these conditions consists of quick jerking movements of the eyes away from the ear being irrigated with ice water)
e. Narcolepsy: Recurrent, sudden, transient, and irresistible attacks of sleep, often during sedentary activities and despite adequate sleep at night
f. Catalepsy: Recurrent, sudden attacks of transient paralysis and loss of muscle tone, often precipitated by a pleasant or unpleasant emotional experience

Lesion Locations

Not directly attributable to acquired structural brain damage*

4. Akinetic mutism (see Akinesia, Mutism)

ETIOLOGY

A vast array of pathological conditions can cause reduced alertness. This topic has been extensively covered elsewhere,[1] and is only summarized here.

Brainstem Reticular Activating System Damage

Direct damage to the reticular activating system can drastically and often irreversibly lower arousal and can result from any of the following conditions:

1. Basilar artery occlusion by thrombosis or embolism
2. Pontine hemorrhage
3. Vertebral artery occlusion
4. Rupture of a vertebrobasilar artery aneurysm
5. Hematoma in or around the brainstem following trauma to the rear of the head
6. Brainstem abscess, granuloma, or neoplasm
7. Demyelinating disease (e.g., multiple sclerosis) affecting neurons within the brainstem

Supratentorial and Subtentorial Lesions

An equally diverse number of conditions arising in the supratentorial or subtentorial areas, excluding direct brainstem damage, can lower alertness. These conditions include:

1. Cerebrovascular disease, including carotid artery stenosis or occlusion
2. Increased intracranial pressure

*This does not preclude an association with biochemical, hereditary, or developmental brain abnormalities.

3. Mass lesions, including neoplasms, infection-related abscesses or empyema, infarcts, hemorrhages, foreign bodies embedded in the brain, and pituitary apoplexy[22]
4. Traumatic brain injury resulting in diffuse white matter damage
5. Anoxia of any etiology (e.g., choking, suffocation, strangulation, drowning, gas poisoning, uncontrolled hypertension, pulmonary disease, severe anemia)
6. Infection of the brain or meninges

Reduction in Brain Metabolism

Brain function is highly dependent on a stable metabolism. The following conditions reduce alertness by negatively affecting brain metabolism:

1. Nutritional deficiency, particularly thiamine, nicotinic acid, and folic acid deficiency, caused by either poor diet or genetic defects that prevent utilization of nutrients
2. Electrolyte imbalance from such causes as gastrointestinal obstruction, fistulas, severe and prolonged diarrhea or vomiting, prolonged intravenous fluid injection, excessive diuresis, poison ingestion, dehydration, and water intoxication
3. Organ failure (see later text)

Organ Failure

Organ failure is a common cause of decreased alertness. In many cases, cancer is the etiological factor involved because of its potential to damage multiple organs, including the brain, through metastasis. The following organs and conditions are also commonly implicated in reduced alertness:

1. Liver failure as a result of severe alcoholism
2. Kidney failure and side effects of dialysis
3. Pulmonary disease
4. Pancreatitis[23]
5. Hypoadrenalism (Addison's disease)
6. Hyperadrenalism (Cushing's syndrome)
7. Rare cases of hyperthyroidism or hypothyroidism[24,25]
8. Hypoparathyroidism or hyperparathyroidism
9. Thyroid or adrenal failure as a result of hypopituitarism
10. Reduced cardiac output causing anoxia, as a result of myocardial infarction, heart failure, cardiac arrhythmia, and so forth

Temperature

If body temperature decreases below 32°C (89.6°F) or increases above 42°C (107.6°F), stupor or coma is likely to occur.[26,27] Increased body temperature (hyperthermia) in adults is often the result of heat stroke. The causes of reduced body temperature include:

1. Hypothalamic disorders
2. Myxedema
3. Hypopituitarism
4. Overdoses of alcohol, barbiturates, or phenothiazines
5. Exposure to extreme cold

Seizure Disorder

Reduced alertness may occur at various points during an epileptic seizure. A reduction in alertness precedes the onset of the seizure in some patients. During the seizure itself (i.e., the ictal phase), the reduction in alertness can progress to a coma-like state. Postictal stupor or coma can last for minutes or hours, perhaps because of metabolic depression after the intense neuronal activity of the ictal phase. Multiple or sustained seizures (i.e., status epilepticus) can cause ischemia and subsequent cell damage or death,[28] with an expected deleterious effect on arousal capacity. In some patients, lethargy or obtundation, or stupor can be triggered and maintained by prolonged mild seizure discharge.[29]

Selective Vulnerability

Some populations are more likely than others to develop a disorder of alertness in the presence of the previously described etiological factors. Specifically, traumatically brain-injured, mentally retarded, normal elderly, and demented populations all have a high probability of developing an alertness disorder when some other etiological factor appears and further compromises brain function. These populations are also more likely to develop decreases in alertness in response to sedating medications or lack of sleep. In the absence of other etiological factors, a decline in alertness may be noted in the late stages of Alzheimer's disease.

Mental and Emotional Disorders

Psychogenic unresponsiveness is associated with severe depression and catatonic schizophrenia. Although the emerging consensus is that these mental disorders have a physiological basis in the brain, it is unknown whether any associated reduction in alertness can also be linked to physiological abnormalities.

Psychogenic unresponsiveness may result from a conversion disorder precipitated by the onset of major stress or emotional trauma. Obvious sources of such stress include defective interpersonal relationships or events occurring in the environment. However, it is important not to overlook the stress created by having a major disease itself. Merskey and Buhrich[30] found that 67 percent of patients diagnosed as hysterical (i.e., having conversion disorder) also had an organically based illness, and in nearly one half of these patients, the organic illness was neurological. Thus, conversion disorder may coexist with neurological disease, making determination of the cause of reduced alertness more complicated.

Slater[31] studied a group of patients originally diagnosed as having hysteria.

Subsequently, nearly one half of the patients were found to have an organic illness that could account for the symptoms originally thought to be psychogenic. This high frequency of misdiagnosis is understandable when the initial presentation of Slater's patients is considered. No physical findings in the medical examinations of many of Slater's patients pointed to a clear physical cause of their condition. The patients frequently showed such a large and varied array of symptoms that it appeared unlikely that any organic disease process could account for them. Many of the patients showed signs of significant emotional distress and anxiety, and some even had symptom remission following psychotherapeutic intervention. As Slater aptly points out, in the development of virtually all diseases, there is a symptom-free period. The presence of some psychogenic symptoms in a patient does not mean that all the patient's symptoms are psychogenic, and emotional distress is so prevalent in all stages of life that its occurrence in conjunction with the onset of a symptom does not prove the existence of a conversion disorder.

Successful treatment of a symptom (as with psychotherapy) cannot be interpreted as proof of a particular cause. In uncontrolled clinical settings, symptoms may remit for reasons having nothing to do with treatment. This further underscores the need to rule out definitively all other potential causes of reduced alertness before coming to a diagnosis of psychogenic unresponsiveness. The consequences of misdiagnosis are costly to the patient.

Frank malingering may also underlie psychogenic unresponsiveness. There is no reliable way to distinguish the patient who knowingly and willfully attempts to appear unresponsive from the patient with a conversion disorder who is unresponsive without full awareness and intent. Any individual case of psychogenic unresponsiveness falls on a continuum from full awareness and control of the symptoms to total unawareness and lack of control. Where the case lies on this continuum can be determined only by direct admission by the patient.

DISABLING CONSEQUENCES

If the underlying cause of a disorder of alertness is treatable and can be identified in time, full recovery with no long-term disability may be possible. This is particularly true of psychogenic unresponsiveness, in which the underlying mental disorder may readily respond to pharmacological or psychological intervention. If the cause of an alertness disorder is not identified and treated, the disorder can progress to the point of coma and eventual death.

Persistent cases of mild lethargy or obtundation that are not treatable prevent an individual from driving or working in any job that requires sustained alertness, precision, independent responsibility, compliance with a schedule, or avoidance of hazards. The person is also unable to live without supervision because of the danger that he or she will not remain alert while appliances are on. As a minimum, external structuring of the environment (e.g., preventing unsupervised use of potentially dangerous appliances) is necessary. The person is unable to assume responsibility for others, such as a small child or elderly relative. Individuals with persistent stupor must be considered totally disabled and dependent on relatives and society for their survival and support.

ASSESSMENT INSTRUMENTS

Glasgow Coma Scale

The Glasgow Coma Scale (GCS)[32,33] is the most widely used objective scale for measuring level of alertness. This brief, easy-to-administer test provides a numerical score that indicates level of alertness based on observation of eye opening, motor responses, and verbal behavior. It has been shown to have moderate internal consistency (Cronbach's alpha = .69), and high inter-rater (.95) and test-retest (.85) reliability in a large neurosurgical sample.[34] In this same sample, the GCS correlated moderately (.56) with independent ratings of level of consciousness by nurses and with patient outcome as measured by the Glasgow Outcome Scale (.56). The GCS is suitable for bedside use with comatose or severely obtunded patients and can be administered serially. It requires little training and consequently can be administered by most health care professionals, including physicians, nurses, psychologists, and speech therapists.

Comprehensive Level of Consciousness Scale

The Comprehensive Level of Consciousness Scale (CLOCS)[34] is an eight-item behavioral scale that assesses level of alertness by observing posture, eye position at rest, spontaneous eye opening, general motor functioning, abnormal ocular movements, pupillary light reflexes, general responsiveness, and best communicative effort. It includes a standardized administration that is explained in detail, stimuli that are graded in intensity, and a glossary of technical terms. The test can be administered in 3 to 5 minutes.

In a direct comparison with the GCS in a large neurosurgical sample,[34] the CLOCS had greater internal consistency (Cronbach's alpha = .86), and was comparable to the GCS in its inter-rater (.96) and test-retest (.89) reliability. The CLOCS was superior to the GCS in its correlation with independent ratings of level of consciousness by nurses (.71) and was comparable to the GCS in its correlation (.58) with the Glasgow Outcome Scale. With the exception of inter-rater reliability, all of these indexes improved with the deletion of the items pertaining to eye position at rest (scale 2) from the CLOCS. The CLOCS is suitable for bedside administration and can be administered serially. Although it does require a greater degree of training than the GCS, the CLOCS can nonetheless be administered by a variety of health care professionals, including physicians, nurses, psychologists, and speech therapists.

Rancho Los Amigos Levels of Cognitive Functioning Scale

The Rancho Los Amigos Levels of Cognitive Functioning Scale (Rancho)[35] consists of an eight-category ordinal scale, developed for use with traumatic brain injury populations, that permits categorization of the cognitive level of a patient based on responsiveness to environmental stimuli, level of confusion, level of agitation, and presence of cognitive deficits. Inter-rater (.87 to .94) and test-retest (.82) reliability are high for the Rancho.[36] Its chief disadvantages are that it cannot separate changes in one aspect of behavior (e.g., communication) from another (e.g., level of agitation), and that often patients cannot be precisely classified on the scale because they show attributes of several categories simultaneously. The Rancho is suitable for bedside use with patients of all levels of severity and is in widespread use in rehabilitation settings. It can be administered by physicians, nurses, psychologists, vocational counselors, and speech, occupational, and physical therapists.

Disability Rating Scale

The Disability Rating Scale (DRS)[37] is an eight-item test measuring arousal and awareness, activities of daily living, physical dependence, and employability. The arousal items are a modification of the GCS; numerical values are inverted so that high scores correspond to greater impairment and low scores correspond to lesser impairment. Inter-rater reliability for the entire DRS is high (.97 to .98), and ratings are correlated with evoked brain potential indexes at a statistically significant level (.35 to .78).[38] A study directly comparing the DRS and the Rancho found that inter-rater (.92 to .98) and test-retest (.91 to .95) reliability were higher for the DRS.[36] Ease of administration and brevity make the DRS suitable for bedside use. Like the Rancho, it can be administered by a diverse group of health care professionals.

NEUROPSYCHOLOGICAL TREATMENT

Medical examination and treatment are the essential first steps in dealing with an alertness disorder and should precede any intervention conducted by the neuropsychologist. Depending on the underlying cause, an alertness disorder can progress to coma and death. Thus, early intervention by a physician is mandatory. Even when the underlying cause of the disorder has been treated, the patient's level of alertness may remain low for weeks. Consequently, neuropsychological treatments may be necessary even when a clear medical cause of the alertness disorder has been identified and treated. Neuropsychological interventions can be initiated concurrently with medical interventions.

The neuropsychological approach to treating alertness disorders consists of providing a frequent schedule of meaningful, multisensory environmental stimulation. At minimum, the patient's room should be well lit, with plenty of pictures, a clock, and a calendar on the surrounding walls. Drab room colors are to be avoided. Stimuli familiar to the patient, such as favorite music and pictures of relatives, may be of use in increasing the patient's responsiveness to the environment. Although background music and television programs may be helpful when people are not available, stimulation provided by hospital staff and relatives is likely to be more salient and meaningful to the patient. Stimulation can take the form of talking to the patient (even if the patient is unable to respond), reading to the patient, showing the patient pictures, stimulating the patient with objects of varying texture, or providing various foods for the patient to taste. An effort should be made to make each interaction multisensory, for example, talking about an object that the patient is touching and seeing.

Whenever possible, opportunities should be provided for the patient to initiate activities and to respond in an ongoing and interactive manner. Social activities, because they involve a large degree of initiation and ongoing mutual interaction, can be useful with these patients. Getting the patient more emotionally involved with the activity through exhortation or through setting mutual goals for the activity may also increase the patient's attentiveness and arousal.

Efforts to ensure that the patient has adequate sleep at night help to increase alertness during the day. Patients may also need regularly scheduled rest periods during the day to permit them to stay alert during treatment times. Flexibility in scheduling rest periods is important; some patients may require a 10-minute rest period for every 30 minutes of treatment. Brief treatment periods during which the patient is able to remain alert and interactive are preferable to longer treatment periods during which the patient's alertness is minimal. Treatment sessions should be terminated when the patient's level of alertness wanes. A daily record of the length of treatment sessions should be kept, and the patient should be liberally praised for any increases in the length of treatment that he or she can tolerate.

Patients who have alertness disorders along with agitation and confusion are often less tolerant of this stimulation approach. Briefer and less intense stimulation is more appropriate for these patients. Social stimulation, particularly if it involves several people at once, may be difficult for them to tolerate. Any form of stimulation used with these patients should be well under staff control so that it can be rapidly tapered and withdrawn if the patient's agitation and confusion are exacerbated.

Patients with psychogenic underresponsiveness may show symptomatic improvement when confronted about their motives. Any attempt to confront the patient about the validity of the symptoms should be done in conjunction with providing tangible and immediate rewards for symptom remission. Such rewards may include access to special foods desired by the patient (as a supplement to standard meals automatically provided to maintain the patient's health), opportunities to engage in desirable activities, or simple social praise.

In addition to making rewards available, remission of symptoms should permit the patient to avoid restrictions that are undesirable to him or her. For example, most patients enjoy access to visitors and telephones. With permission from the next of kin, these or other desirable activities can be partially limited until the patient begins to show symptom remission. Care must be taken not to violate the patient's legal rights when imposing restrictions, and written consent and cooperation must always be obtained from responsible family members. Even when restrictions are not imposed, the threat of potential restrictions can be an effective motivator for symptom remission.

Confrontation techniques carry the risk of making the patient more defensive and determined to persist with the symptom presentation. Consequently, symptoms may worsen in psychogenically underresponsive patients following institution of a confrontational approach. With consistency and persistence on the part of staff, however, the patient's resistance may ultimately be worn down. In any event, the patient should feel that at least some staff members are available to listen sympathetically and to offer insightful opinions and advice in a less challenging manner. He or she needs to feel that some staff are "sharing the burden" of the return to a healthier psychological adjustment.

The psychogenically underresponsive patient may progress most when given a treatment program that combines confrontation, environmental stimulation, structured rewards and restrictions, and insight-oriented counseling. As a result, members of the treatment team often assume specialized roles. The physician is often the one who assumes responsibility for confronting the patient. The neuropsychologist plays a more supportive role by providing an opportunity for the patient to talk about his or her underlying motivations and by offering insight and direction. With direction from the neuropsychologist, other staff (e.g., nurses; speech, occupational, and physical therapists) provide a program of environmental stimulation with set performance expectations and appropriate rewards and restrictions.

CASE ILLUSTRATION

CASE 2–1

G.E.-I. was a 79-year-old man who worked as a portrait artist. He was admitted to the hospital following a hemorrhagic infarct in the distribution of the right middle cerebral artery. Computed tomography (CT) scans showed decreased density in both cortical (posterior frontal and parietal) and subcortical (internal capsule, basal ganglia, and thalamus) areas. There was a mass effect causing complete effacement of the frontal horn of the right lateral ventricle and extending up into the body of the ventricle. Old infarcts were visible in the head of the left caudate nucleus, the left occipital lobe, and the right cerebellar hemisphere. All four infarctions were attributed to cardiac emboli. History was positive for coronary atherosclerotic heart disease and coronary artery bypass grafts 2 and 4 years before the current admission. The patient also had a 50-year history of bipolar affective disorder. Current medications included furosemide, dipyridamole, and lithium carbonate. He had previously been treated with warfarin sodium for anticoagulation, but this had been discontinued because of the cerebral hemorrhage.

At admission, G.E.-I. was oriented with cues to person, place, time, and situation. He had a left hemiparesis, a left visual field cut, and impaired memory. On the hospital ward, he was observed to sleep constantly, although he could be aroused by someone loudly calling his name. When he was awake, his concentration was poor. With repeated stimulation, he could maintain concentration for several minutes before returning to sleep. Similar observations were recorded over several days by multiple staff people.

After 11 days in the acute-care hospital, G.E.-I. was transferred to a rehabilitation facility. Warfarin sodium was restarted at this time to decrease the likelihood of additional emboli. For the next 2 weeks, the patient's mental status remained unchanged. He slept when not directly stimulated, became alert when his name was called or when he was gently shaken, and maintained concentration for 15 to 20 minutes. By day 20 of his admission, the patient's motivation for therapy had declined. In recreation therapy, he was asked to attempt a painting. When he failed to paint to his satisfaction, he lost interest and became less alert. In speech therapy, alertness was maintained only when G.E.-I. was performing a task that he found easy. When confronted with more challenging cognitive tasks, his alertness rapidly declined, and the therapist suspected that he was pretending to be asleep. The patient became less arousable in the morning and no longer assisted nurses or occupational therapists with his grooming and dressing. His appetite decreased, and he began losing weight, taking in only 64% of his estimated calorie requirements.

On the morning of the 24th day of his hospitalization, G.E.-I. was difficult to arouse. By noon, he had become even less responsive. He would not open his eyes or respond to any commands. He responded to pain in the form of pressure applied with the side of a pen above the nail bed of his firmly held index finger by moaning and moving his right arm. Table 2–1 shows G.E.-I.'s performance on the GCS, CLOCS, Rancho, and DRS. All four scales place the patient at a fairly low level of function. Furosemide, lithium carbonate, and warfarin sodium were withheld pending determination of the cause of his mental status changes.

Medical examination revealed normal blood pressure and temperature. Laboratory blood analysis showed electrolyte depletion and elevated levels of blood urea nitrogen and lithium. A repeat CT scan showed no new hemorrhages and no extension of the mass effect of the right hemisphere infarction. Dehydration was diagnosed, and the patient was started on intravenous fluids. Over the next 2 days, one spontaneous verbalization and some spontaneous movements of the limbs were noted. After 4 days, G.E.-I. was opening his eyes, moving in bed, and attempting to speak, although he was still incomprehensible. He subsequently became talkative and alert, and began again to participate in therapy. Mental status returned to baseline, with the patient continuing to have difficulty maintaining arousal for periods longer than 30 minutes.

Table 2–1. **G.E.-I.'s PERFORMANCE ON FOUR MEASURES OF ALERTNESS**

Scale	Score	Description
Glasgow Coma Scale	7	Eyes do not open; limb withdraws in response to pain; makes incomprehensible moans
Comprehensive Level of Consciousness Scale (scale 2 omitted)	19	No abnormal posture or tone; eyes do not open; no spontaneous movements; no abnormal ocular movements; normal pupillary light reflexes; gross, disorganized withdrawal from pain; moaning in response to pain
Rancho Los Amigos Levels of Cognitive Functioning Scale	Level II	Inconsistent, purposeless, nonspecific reactions to stimuli; responds to pain
Disability Rating Scale	19	Eyes do not open; incomprehensible verbal response; withdrawing motor responses; no self-care; totally dependent; not employable; extremely severe disability

DISCUSSION

Case 2–1 illustrates how alertness disorders can evolve over time and the multiple etiological factors that are often involved. G.E.-I. initially presented in a lethargic or obtunded state. The large hemorrhagic infarct with subsequent mass effect in an elderly individual with multiple prior cerebrovascular accidents probably accounts for the initial lethargy, but evidence suggests that the patient's frustration and disappointment over his seemingly intractable deficits began to contribute to his condition. The further decrease in arousal in response to difficult tasks and the decreasing participation in self-care activities led to a suspicion of psychogenic underresponsiveness. The history of bipolar affective disorder increased the likelihood of this diagnosis.

A further sharp decline in alertness occurred, with G.E.-I. ultimately becoming stuporous. The electrolyte depletion, elevated blood urea nitrogen and lithium levels, and good response to intravenous fluids provides convincing evidence that dehydration was the important factor in the onset of the stupor. Dehydration probably resulted from a combination of poor fluid intake and the potent diuretic effect of furosemide. Lithium toxicity is a major risk when patients are simultaneously taking a diuretic. Lithium toxicity can cause lethargy, stupor, or coma and was probably a contributing factor in this case. Dipyridamole can cause fainting episodes but not the sustained stupor seen in this patient. Warfarin increases the risk of cerebral hemorrhage, but the negative repeat CT scan results ruled this out as a factor in G.E.-I.'s stupor.

The CLOCS and DRS provided the most detailed descriptions of G.E.-I.'s mental status (see Table 2–1). Unlike the other scales, the DRS contains items related to self-care, degree of dependence, and employability. These items may be irrelevant in situations in which the patient is stuporous, but they can be relevant if the alertness disorder is less severe and the focus of the treatment team is on rehabilitation and reintegration into the community rather than on diagnosis alone.

REFERENCES

1. Plum, F and Posner, J: Diagnosis of Stupor and Coma, Third Edition. FA Davis, Philadelphia, 1980.
2. The International Classification of Diseases, Ninth Revision, Clinical Modification. Med-Index Publications, Salt Lake City, 1991.
3. American Psychiatric Association: Diagnostic and Statistical Manual of Mental Disorders, Fourth Edition. American Psychiatric Association, Washington, DC, 1994.
4. Physician's Desk Reference, 48th Edition. Medical Economics Company, Montvale, NJ, 1994.
5. Mills, RP and Swanson, PD: Vertical oculomotor apraxia and memory loss. Ann Neurol 4:149, 1978.
6. Segarra, JM: Cerebral vascular disease and behavior. I. The syndrome of the mesencephalic artery (basilar artery bifurcation). Arch Neurol 22:408, 1970.
7. Moruzzi, G and Magoun, HW: Brain stem reticular formation and activation of the EEG. Electroencephalogr Clin Neurophysiol 1:455, 1949.
8. Ropper, AH: Lateral displacement of the brain and level of consciousness in patients with an acute hemispheral mass. N Engl J Med 314:953, 1986.
9. Ropper, AH: A preliminary MRI study of the geometry of brain displacement and level of consciousness with acute intracranial masses. Neurology 39:622, 1989.

10. Jefferson, G: The tentorial pressure cone. Arch Neurol Psychiatry 40:857, 1938.
11. McNealy, DE and Plum, F: Brainstem dysfunction with supratentorial mass lesions. Arch Neurol 7:10, 1962.
12. Meyer, A: Herniation of the brain. Arch Neurol Psychiatry 4:387, 1920.
13. Azambuja, N, Lindgren, E, and Sjogren, SE: Tentorial herniations. I. Anatomy. II. Pneumography. III. Angiography. Acta Radiol 46:215, 1956.
14. Schwartz, GA and Rosner, AA: Displacement and herniation of the hippocampal gyrus through the incisura tentorii: A clinicopathologic study. Arch Neurol Psychiatry 46:297, 1941.
15. Sunderland, S: The tentorial notch and complications produced by herniations of the brain through that aperture. Br J Surg 45:422, 1958.
16. Adams, JH: The neuropathology of head injuries. In Vinken, PJ and Bruyn, GW (eds): Handbook of Clinical Neurology, Volume 23, Injuries of the Brain and Skull, Part I. North-Holland, Amsterdam, 1975, p 35.
17. Ommaya, AK and Gennarelli, TA: Cerebral concussion and traumatic unconsciousness: Correlation of experimental and clinical observations on blunt head injuries. Brain 97:633, 1974.
18. Strich, SJ: The pathology of brain damage due to blunt head injuries. In Walker, AE, Caveness, WF, and Critchley, M (eds): The Late Effects of Head Injury. Charles C Thomas, Springfield, IL, 1969.
19. Reyes, MG: Subcortical cerebral infarctions in sickle cell trait. J Neurol Neurosurg Psychiatry 52:516, 1989.
20. Albert, ML, et al: Cerebral dominance for consciousness. Arch Neurol 33:453, 1976.
21. Schwartz, B: Hemisphere dominance and consciousness. Acta Neurol Scand 43:513, 1967.
22. Weisberg, LA: Pituitary apoplexy. Am J Med 63:109, 1977.
23. Sjaastad, O, et al: Chronic relapsing pancreatitis, encephalopathy with disturbance of consciousness, and CSF amino acid aberration. J Neurol 220:83, 1979.
24. Menendez, CE and Rivlin, RS: Thyrotoxic crisis and myxedema coma. Med Clin North Am 57:1463, 1973.
25. Thomas, FB, Mazzaferri, EL, and Skillman, TG: Apathetic thyrotoxicosis: A distinctive clinical and laboratory entity. Ann Intern Med 72:679, 1970.
26. Costrini, AM, et al: Cardiovascular and metabolic manifestations of heat stroke and severe heat exhaustion. Am J Med 66:296, 1979.
27. Reuler, JB: Hypothermia: Pathophysiology, clinical settings, and management. Ann Intern Med 89:519, 1978.
28. Plum, F, Howse, DC, and Duffy, TE: Metabolic effects of seizures. In Plum, F (ed): Brain Dysfunction and Metabolic Disorders. Raven Press, New York, 1974, p 141.
29. Ellis, JM and Lee, SI: Acute prolonged confusion in later life as an ictal state. Epilepsia 19:119, 1978.
30. Merskey, H and Buhrich, NA: Hysteria and organic brain disease. Br J Med Psychol 48:359, 1975.
31. Slater, E: Diagnosis of "hysteria." Br Med J 1:1395, 1965.
32. Teasdale, G and Jennett, B: Assessment of impaired consciousness and coma. Lancet 2:81, 1974.
33. Jennett, B and Teasdale, G: Assessment of impaired consciousness. In Jennett, B and Teasdale, G (eds): Management of Head Injuries. FA Davis, Philadelphia, 1981, p 77.
34. Stanczak, DE, et al: Assessment of level of consciousness following severe neurological insult: Comparison of psychometric qualities of Glasgow Coma Scale and Comprehensive Level of Consciousness Scale. J Neurosurg 60:955, 1984.
35. Hagan, C, Malkmus, D, and Durham, P: Levels of cognitive functions. In Rehabilitation of Head Injured Adult: Comprehensive Physical Management. Professional Staff Association of Rancho Los Amigos Hospital, Downey, CA, 1979.
36. Gouvier, WD, et al: Reliability and validity of the Disability Rating Scale and the Levels of Cognitive Functioning Scale in monitoring recovery from severe head injury. Arch Phys Med Rehab 68:94, 1987.
37. Rappaport, M, et al: Evoked brain potentials and disability in brain-damaged patients. Arch Phys Med Rehab 58:333, 1977.
38. Rappaport, M, et al: Disability Rating Scale for severe head trauma patients: Coma to community. Paper presented at the 42nd Annual Assembly of the American Academy of Physical Medicine and at the 57th Annual Session of the American Congress of Rehabilitation Medicine, Washington, DC, 1980.

DISORDERS OF CONCENTRATION

3

Concentration consists of voluntarily and purposefully directing one's thoughts and actions toward one stimulus or several stimuli. Concentration is narrower in meaning than the concept of attention, which includes not only the direction of a person's thoughts but also the ability to detect and orient to stimuli. Attention is usually conceptualized as consisting of both conscious processes, which are under voluntary control, and unconscious processes, which operate automatically. The voluntary and conscious processes embodied in the concept of concentration can be considered a subset of the larger set of processes that comprise attention.

Many aspects of attention and concentration are under investigation in cognitive and neuropsychology laboratories. Only three aspects of concentration, however, are typically assessed in clinical settings:

1. The amount of information that can be concentrated on simultaneously (i.e., the span of concentration)

2. The efficiency with which two or more tasks can be performed simultaneously compared with the performance of any one of the tasks alone (i.e., divided concentration)
3. The ability to sustain concentration on a set of stimuli small enough to reside within a person's span of concentration while ignoring other potentially distracting internal or external stimuli (i.e., vigilance)

Impairment in these areas can be termed, respectively, *concentration span reduction*, *divided concentration deficiency*, and *distractibility*. These are the three disorders covered in this chapter.

The disorders of alertness discussed in Chapter 2 are related to, but not identical with, disorders of concentration. Concentration depends on a normal level of alertness without which concentration becomes impossible. Concentration deficits, however, are at least partially dissociable from alertness disorders in that the former can occur in patients who have preserved alertness.

The failure to detect, notice, or attend to stimuli (i.e., stimulus neglect) is also conceptually related to the disorders of concentration. Stimulus neglect involves an apparent failure of the automatic attentional processes responsible for monitoring the environment and detecting sensory input. Stimulus neglect is not typically conceptualized as a deficit in the voluntary processes that make up a person's ability to concentrate. Concentration may be normal in patients with stimulus neglect as long as stimuli are placed in a location where they can be detected and perceived. Similarly, patients with no stimulus neglect may be impaired in one or more aspects of their concentration. Stimulus neglect is discussed in Chapter 4.

NOMENCLATURE

The terms *attention* and *concentration* are often used interchangeably by lay persons and some clinicians. These terms are not used interchangeably in this text for both conceptual and practical reasons. As discussed previously, concentration includes only a subset of the processes involved in attention; thus, the two concepts are not identical. The term *attention* is used in the label given to a subtype of stimulus neglect (see Hemi-inattention). In addition, *stimulus neglect* is often described as an attention disorder in the neurology literature. To avoid confusing the concentration disorders with stimulus neglect, only the term *concentration* is used in discussing the disorders in this chapter.

DSM-IV[1] includes the diagnoses "Attention-Deficit/Hyperactivity Disorder Not Otherwise Specified," which can be used to code adult-onset concentration disorders resulting from brain damage. Attention deficit disorder, however, is usually conceptualized as a developmental disorder; therefore, this use of the term can be misleading. The DSM-IV diagnoses "Cognitive Disorder Not Otherwise Specified" and "Mild Neurocognitive Disorder" are less misleading and can be used to code concentration disorders. Unfortunately, these terms are more generic and do not indicate the specific type of problem exhibited by the patient when they are used to code concentration disorders. In this instance, no additional codes are available in ICD-9-CM[2] for the concentration disorders.

Clinical Indicators: Each is independent (only one must be observed for the disorder to be suspected) *except* when subscripting is used. Subscripted numbers (a_1, a_2) denote an indicator with multiple parts that must be considered together.~
Associated Features: These are listed to give a more complete picture of the disorder. The presence or absence of these features does not affect the diagnosis.
Factors to Rule Out: All must be taken into account. Failure to rule out even one of these factors makes a firm diagnosis impossible.
Lesion Locations: Each location stands alone; damage in only one of the listed areas is sufficient to produce the disorder.

VARIETY OF PRESENTATION

1. Concentration span reduction

Clinical Indicators

a_1. Inaccurate immediate reproduction of target information that is divided into equivalent, discrete units

a_2. Relatively preserved immediate reproduction of the target information until the last 1 or 2 units of information are added

Associated Features

a. Varying concentration span for different types of information (e.g., verbal versus nonverbal information)
b. Divided concentration deficiency (see later text)
c. Distractibility (see later text)
d. Confused ideation (see Ideational Disorientation or Confusion)

NOTE: Decreased ability to concentrate in combination with ideational disorientation or confusion is referred to as a confusional state.

e. Presence of any other neuropsychological disorder, including global neuropsychological dysfunction (see Chap. 19)

Factors to Rule Out

a. Normal level of performance for age and education
b. Reduced alertness (see Chap. 2)
c. Distractibility so severe that it impedes focusing on any task, ruled out by documenting preserved reproduction up to the addition of the last 1 or 2 units of information
d. Preoccupation with repetitive thoughts, ideas, or rituals to a point at which nothing else can be focused on (see Chap. 18 for assessment techniques)

e. A constant flow of tangential or loosely related thoughts to a point at which nothing else can be focused on (see Chap. 18 for assessment techniques)
f. Presence of delusional ideas that impede focusing on other tasks (see Chap. 18 for assessment techniques)
g. Presence of ongoing hallucinations or illusions (see Chap. 17) that impede focusing on other tasks (see Chaps. 17 and 18 for assessment techniques)
h. Depression, anxiety, or other intense emotional reactions present during testing of concentration span (see Chap. 18 for assessment techniques)
i. Reduced concentration span before the onset of the brain lesion

Lesion Locations

a. Caudate nucleus lesions[3]
b. Combined basal ganglia and brainstem lesions[4]
c. Hemispheric (frontal, temporal, and parietal) lesions[5]

Lesion Lateralization

a. May follow right- or left-sided lesions

2. Divided concentration deficiency

Clinical Indicators

a_1. Inability to perform two simultaneous tasks accurately
a_2. Relatively preserved performance of either task alone
b_1. A decrement in performance of one task when a second task is added
b_2. Relatively preserved performance of the original task before the addition of the second task

Associated Features

a. Greater impairment of divided concentration produced by tasks that are highly similar to each other (e.g., two verbal tasks) than by tasks that differ substantially (e.g., a verbal and a motor task)
b. Greater impairment of divided concentration produced by tasks whose performance is dependent on the same brain areas than by tasks that depend on different brain areas
c. Differing degree of impairment of divided concentration across tasks or type of information (e.g., verbal versus visuospatial information)
d. Concentration span reduction (see previous text)
e. Distractibility (see later text)
f. Confused ideation (see Ideational Disorientation or Confusion)

NOTE: Decreased ability to concentrate in combination with ideational disorientation or confusion is referred to as a confusional state.

g. Presence of any other neuropsychological disorder, including global neuropsychological dysfunction (see Chap. 19)

Factors to Rule Out

a. Concentration span reduction so severe that it accounts for the deficit in divided concentration, ruled out by documenting preserved single-task performance
b. Distractibility so severe that it accounts for the deficit in divided concentration, ruled out by documenting preserved single-task performance

c. Normal level of performance for age and education
d. Reduced alertness (see Chap. 2)
e. Preoccupation with repetitive thoughts, ideas, or rituals to a point at which divided concentration is impeded (see Chap. 18 for assessment techniques), ruled out by documenting preserved single-task performance
f. A constant flow of tangential or loosely related thoughts to a point at which divided concentration is impeded (see Chap. 18 for assessment techniques), ruled out by documenting preserved single-task performance
g. Presence of delusional ideas that impede divided concentration (see Chap. 18 for assessment techniques), ruled out by documenting preserved single-task performance
h. Presence of ongoing hallucinations or illusions (see Chap. 17) that impede divided concentration (see Chap. 17 and 18 for assessment techniques), ruled out by documenting preserved single-task performance
i. Depression, anxiety, or other intense emotional reactions present during testing of divided concentration (see Chap. 18 for assessment techniques), ruled out by documenting preserved single-task performance
j. Reduced divided concentration before the onset of the brain lesion

Lesion Locations

a. Frontal lobe[6]
b. Parietal lobe[6]
c. Callosal lesions with and without extension into right hemisphere[7,8]
d. Presumed diffuse brain damage[9–11]

Lesion Lateralization

a. Possible greater association with right-sided lesions[6–8]

3. Distractibility

Clinical Indicators

a. Frequent shifting of concentration away from an ongoing task to concentrate on random internal (e.g., thoughts) or external (e.g., background noise) stimuli that are irrelevant to task performance
b_1. Failure to respond to stimuli that occur after relatively long waiting periods
b_2. Preserved response to stimuli that occur after relatively short waiting periods
c_1. Rapid decrement in performance of the same task over time
c_2. Relatively preserved initial performance of the task
d_1. Inaccurate task performance when distractors (e.g., background noise, competing visual stimuli) are present in the environment
d_2. Relatively preserved performance of the same task in environments in which few or no distractors are present

Associated Features

a. Better sustained concentration on tasks that evoke a high degree of personal interest
b. Better sustained concentration when task performance can lead to a tangible reward or the avoidance of an undesirable consequence
c. Poorer sustained concentration as the subjective difficulty of the task increases

d. Concentration span reduction (see previous text)
e. Divided concentration deficiency (see previous text)
f. Confused ideation (see Ideational Disorientation or Confusion)

NOTE: Decreased ability to concentrate in combination with ideational disorientation or confusion is referred to as a confusional state.

g. Presence of any other neuropsychological disorder, including global neuropsychological dysfunction (see Chap. 19)

Factors to Rule Out

a. Concentration span reduction so severe that it accounts for the deficit in divided concentration
b. Normal level of performance for age and education
c. Reduced alertness (see Chap. 2)
d. Preoccupation with repetitive thoughts, ideas, or rituals to a point at which sustained concentration is impeded (see Chap. 18 for assessment techniques)
e. A constant flow of tangential or loosely related thoughts to a point at which sustained concentration is impeded (see Chap. 18 for assessment techniques)
f. Presence of delusional ideas that impede sustained concentration (see Chap. 18 for assessment techniques)
g. Presence of ongoing hallucinations or illusions (see Chap. 17) that impede sustained concentration (see Chaps. 17 and 18 for assessment techniques)
h. Depression, anxiety, or other intense emotional reactions present during testing of sustained concentration (see Chap. 18 for assessment techniques)
i. Reduced sustained concentration before the onset of the brain lesion

Lesion Locations

a. Medial cortical and limbic pathway lesions[12]
b. Callosal lesions with and without extension into right hemisphere[7]
c. Frontal lobe lesions, particularly dorsolateral lesions[13,14]
d. Temporal lobe lesions[15]

Lesion Lateralization

a. A more common association with right-sided lesions in frontal lobe patients[13,14]

ETIOLOGY

Concentration disorders can accompany brain damage of virtually any etiology. They are a core feature of traumatic brain injury but can also be seen in patients who have cerebrovascular disease, central nervous system infections, demyelinating disease, degenerative disease, compromised brain metabolism, electrolyte imbalance, a prolonged history of substance abuse, or exposure to toxic substances.

DISABLING CONSEQUENCES

Concentration disorders produce significant vocational disability. Most jobs require people to sustain performance over extended periods of time, and employees whose concentration wanders are unlikely to perform to the employer's level of expectation. In addition, distracting noise and occasional interruptions are an inevitable part of many jobs and pose major barriers to individuals with deficient concentration.

Jobs that involve physical rather than tedious sedentary activity are easier for concentration-impaired patients to perform. These patients, however, are at grave risk in situations in which they must use potentially dangerous equipment, or even in situations in which they must simply pay attention to what is happening around them to avoid inadvertent hazards. Even when the job is more physical than mental and contains few safety hazards, problems can still arise for patients with concentration deficits. Many such jobs involve rapid performance or production quotas that are particularly hard for these patients to maintain.

Sedentary or intellectually demanding jobs pose the greatest difficulty for patients who have concentration deficits. Being unable to divide concentration, for example, will severely disable a trial attorney who must attend to his or her notes, the responses of witnesses, the reactions of jurors, the objections of opposing counsel, and the procedural rulings of the judge. A secretary who must divide his or her time among typing, answering phone calls, and greeting people who enter the office can also be disabled by even a subtle deficit in dividing concentration. Students, who spend hours in lectures on subjects that may or may not interest them, have obvious potential for being disabled by a concentration disorder.

Less disability is produced by the concentration disorders in the home environment. Potential for injury exists during cooking, and such activities may have to be supervised. Otherwise, patients are usually safe and able to function in familiar domestic settings. Driving, however, places constant demands on the ability to concentrate and is unlikely to be accomplished safely by patients with impairment in this area.

Leisure activities that involve the use of motorized vehicles (e.g, boating) or power tools (e.g., gardening, woodworking) may no longer be safe for the patient. Sedentary leisure activities (e.g., reading, attending the ballet, watching a televised football game) are certainly safer for these patients, but the concentration deficit may lessen enjoyment of the activity.

ASSESSMENT INSTRUMENTS

High Sensitivity Cognitive Screen—Signaling to Numbers

The High Sensitivity Cognitive Screen (HSCS)—Signaling to Numbers,[16] an auditory digit vigilance procedure, is *not commercially available.*

This brief test is part of a larger screening battery used for detecting brain damage. It consists of a random series of single digits read to the patient at a rate of one number per second. The patient is instructed to tap the table whenever an odd number is read. A total of 30 digits are read, and no more than 4 errors of omission (failing to signal to odd numbers) or commission (signaling to an even number) are expected in healthy individuals.

I compare the number of errors made in the first 15 trials of the digit vigilance procedure to the errors made in the final 15 trials, because the patient's concentration can wane over the course of the test. I also employ an audiotaped version of the procedure, using a different sequence of 30 digits, that contains a distracting background conversation. Before administering either version of the procedure, it is useful to verify that the patient knows what odd numbers are by having him or her recite them.

Inter-rater reliability was reported to be high (.97) for the signaling-to-numbers task.[16] Test-retest reliability was artifactually low (.18), because ceiling effects reduced variability in scores in the combined sample of neurologic and normal controls employed in the reliability study. The validity of individual tasks within the HSCS have not been reported.

The signaling-to-numbers procedure provides a simple measure of sustained concentration that does not require the patient to perform other cognitive activities such as mental arithmetic or repetition of digits, functions that can be compromised for reasons other than a concentration disorder. The brevity of the procedure may reduce its sensitivity to subtle concentration deficits that manifest themselves only after the patient has been working at a task for an extended period of time. The validity of the procedure as a measure of sustained concentration has not been empirically demonstrated; consequently, results must be interpreted cautiously.

The signaling-to-numbers procedure can be administered in a laboratory or at bedside and is appropriate for use by neuropsychologists, physicians, speech pathologists, and other individuals trained and experienced in cognitive assessment. Because the validity of the procedure requires further study, the clinician must rely on his or her clinical experience and confirmatory data from other, more established tests and procedures. Consequently, the signaling-to-numbers procedure should be administered only by experienced clinicians as part of a larger battery of tests.

Continuous Performance Test

The Continuous Performance Test (CPT; Vigil) can be obtained from *For Thought, Ltd., 9 Trafalgar Square, Nashua, NH 03063.*

The CPT measures sustained concentration by presenting target stimuli embedded in a larger series of foils to which the patient is required to make some response. No one version of the CPT is in widespread use. Stimuli used by various researchers and clinicians vary from target letters, digits, or shapes to complex sequences of stimuli (e.g., a string of digits repeated twice in a row). The color, size, duration, and interstimulus interval varies from setting to setting. Because the CPT is usually administered by computer, the typical response is a key press. Reaction time, errors of omission, and errors of commission (the latter may also be further subdivided depending on the nature of the task) can all be recorded, and a number of performance indexes can be computed from these results.

The CPT has been used mainly at research institutions, but a proprietary version entitled Vigil is available. Vigil is user-friendly (no programming experience is required) and offers maximum flexibility in stimulus choice, duration, and interstimulus interval. Responses are recorded by the computer, and accuracy and reaction time summary scores are computed and can be printed out in a choice of formats. One unfortunate limitation is that Vigil uses only digits or letter stimuli. No nonverbal stimulus options are included.

Another disadvantage of Vigil, and of CPT in general, is the lack of a standardized and accepted procedure for administering the test. The procedure I favor is based on the first report of a CPT task for use with brain-damaged patients[17] that has been updated for administration by computer.[18] Patients are asked to respond to Xs that follow As. Each block of 100 trials contains 10 Xs preceded by As, 17 As not followed by Xs, 5 Xs not preceded by As, and 68 other random letters. Stimuli are blue with a gray background and measure 1.5 cm wide and 2.2 cm high. Stimuli appear center screen for a duration of 200 msec with a 1.5-second interstimulus interval. I present 200 trials, which take approximately 6 minutes and are not too frustrating for brain-damaged patients.

No general conclusions about the reliability and validity of CPT in brain-damaged populations can be drawn because of the diversity in procedures used across settings. The lack of standardization and demonstrated reliability and validity requires that CPT results be interpreted cautiously. CPT procedures should be administered only by individuals with extensive training and experience in cognitive and neuropsychological assessment. CPT data should be interpreted only in conjunction with more established measures of concentration. CPT tasks are appropriate for office or laboratory use.

Wechsler Adult Intelligence Scale–Revised (WAIS-R) and WAIS-R as a Neuropsychological Instrument (WAIS-R NI) Digit Span

The WAIS-R[19] and WAIS-R NI[20] digit span can be obtained from *The Psychological Corporation, P.O. Box 9954, San Antonio, TX 78204-2498.*

The WAIS-R, which is familiar to all neuropsychologists, neurologists, and psychiatrists, involves presentation of progressively longer sequences of digits, which the patient repeats. A second series of digits is presented for the patient to repeat in reverse order. When the patient fails to report the correct digits in the correct sequence twice within the same trial, testing is discontinued (WAIS-R version).

The digit span test yields a forward digit span score that reflects the amount of material on which a patient can focus at one time. A reversed or backward digit span score is also obtained and is often interpreted as an index of the ability to divide concentration. In the case of a backward digit span, concentration is presumably divided between the task of retaining the original sequence of digits and the task of reversing the order of the digits prior to reporting them. A discrepancy between forward and backward digit span, with the latter being significantly lower, is usually interpreted as a decline in the ability to divide concentration. Standard scoring of the WAIS-R requires the summation of the forward and backward digit span scores, but neuropsychologists often compare the individual scores because of the richer interpretative information such a comparison yields.

The WAIS-R NI digit span procedure differs slightly from the WAIS-R procedure. Items are administered for as long as the patient recalls the correct digits, even if the digits are incorrectly sequenced. This yields a richer set of data for interpretation, including scores reflecting the number of digits recalled in any order and the number of digits correctly recalled and sequenced. The WAIS-R NI manual includes useful tables showing the cumulative percentages of longest digit span and of the difference between forward and backward digit span results for individuals in each age group of the standardization sample.

Test-retest reliability coefficients for the WAIS-R digit span reported in the test manual range from .70 to .89, and stability coefficients were .89 and .82, respectively, for healthy individuals in the two age groups (25 to 34 years and 45 to 54 years) that were tested twice. Most validity studies of the WAIS-R have examined the test as a whole rather than the validity of the individual subtests. A "freedom from distraction" factor usually emerges in factor-analytic studies of the WAIS-R,[21] on which the digit span loads. However, methodological weaknesses and inconsistent findings across factor-analytic studies prevent firm conclusions about the WAIS-R factor structure.[22]

Digit span procedures provide a simple measure of concentration. Although memory is a component of digit span, it is generally not a major confounding factor, even in amnestic populations. As long as the delay between digit presentation and repetition is kept to a minimum, even amnestic subjects can do well on digit span tasks. The WAIS-R digit span is normed on a sample of over 1800 healthy individuals stratified to be representative of the United States population in age, gender, race, geographic residence, occupation, and education, based on 1970 census data. This gives the test a solid normative base not shared by more informal digit span procedures included in mental status examinations. The WAIS-R NI manual provides a wealth of interpretative hypotheses that should be explored when various patterns of digit span performance are obtained.

Administration of the WAIS-R digit span is restricted to individuals trained in psychometric assessment. The test is appropriate for bedside or laboratory use.

Wechsler Memory Scale–Revised Digit Span

The Wechsler Memory Scale–Revised (WMS-R) digit span[23] can be obtained from *The Psychological Corporation, P.O. Box 9954, San Antonio, TX 78204-2498.*

The administration procedure for the WMS-R digit span subtest is essentially the same as that used for the WAIS-R digit span subtest. A useful addition are tables of percentile scores for forward and backward digit span for six age groups, the youngest of which is 25 to 34 years and the oldest of which is 70 to 74 years. In addition, the digit span scores are included in an Attention/Concentration Index that summarizes overall concentration ability. Comparison of the Attention/Concentration Index with the WMS-R General Memory Index provides one means of distinguishing between concentration and memory disorders. A table is provided in the test manual for determining whether a concentration-memory index discrepancy is statistically significant at the 85 percent and 95 percent levels of confidence.

Test-retest stability coefficients reported in the test manual for forward and backward digit span range across age groups from .48 to .82. The digit span subtest appears to have good internal consistency, with split-half coefficients ranging from .76 to .87. An attention-concentration factor emerged in factor-analytic studies conducted on the WMS-R standardization sample. Digit span loaded on this factor. Forward and backward digit span loaded on the same factor, suggesting that they measure the same or closely related variables in normal samples.

The availability of percentile tables is an asset of the WMS-R digit span not possessed by the WAIS-R version of the test. Digit span scores decrease with age, but the percentile tables for each age group in the WMS-R permit this factor to be taken into account. An additional asset of the WMS-R version of digit span is that it is normed on a more recent sample, stratified to represent the United States population in age, gender, race, geographic region, and education using 1980 census data. Occupation was not considered in selecting cases for the normative sample, and the size of the sample (316) is smaller than that of the WAIS-R standardization sample. Education level is positively correlated with the Attention/Concentration Index, but the effect on digit span alone is not reported. A table of means and standard deviations for the Attention/Concentration Index at three education levels is provided, permitting the examiner to take this factor into account when interpreting the scores. A similar table for the individual subtest scores, including digit span, would be desirable, but is not provided.

The WMS-R Attention/Concentration Index is reported in the test manual to distinguish patients with schizophrenia, alcoholism, post-traumatic stress disorder, dementia, Huntington's disease, traumatic brain injury, stroke, and seizure disorder from normal controls at statistically significant levels of confidence. Notably, amnestic Korsakoff's syndrome patients and depressed patients did not differ from normal controls on the Attention/Concentration Index.

Individuals who are competent to administer the WAIS-R digit span subtest are also competent to administer the WMS-R version. The test can be performed at bedside, in the office, or in the laboratory.

Memory Assessment Scale Verbal Span

The Memory Assessment Scale (MAS) verbal span[24] can be obtained from *Psychological Assessment Resources, Inc., P.O. Box 998, Odessa, FL 33556.*

The MAS verbal span test is equivalent in format and administration to the WAIS-R and WMS-R digit span tests. The test yields a verbal span score that combines the results of forward and backward digit span trials. The verbal span score is combined with a visual span score to yield an index of "short-term memory," an unfortunate label, because these tests measure concentration more than memory.

The reliability of the MAS subtests was investigated by retesting a group of 30 normal subjects approximately 6 months after their initial test session. Generalizability coefficients for the verbal span test varied from .78 to .79, depending on which normative database was used to score the test (see later text). Separate factor analyses, computed on normal and neurological disorder samples, are reported in the MAS manual. The factor analysis of the data from normal samples yielded two factors, one of which was interpreted as an attention-concentration factor that had loadings primarily from verbal and visual span. Three factors emerged from the analysis of the neurological sample, one of which was a "short-term memory-concentration factor" with loadings from verbal and visual span. Groups of patients with dementia, traumatic brain injury, and lateralized stroke are all reported to perform significantly ($p < .05$) below normal controls on the verbal span test, but the test failed to differentiate left- from right-hemisphere stroke patients.

The subtests of the MAS are normed on a sample of 843 adults, with a subset of 467 selected to match the United States population in gender and education across four age ranges. Norms are available for a broader age range (i.e., 18 years to more than 70 years) than other versions of digit span. The MAS also includes a table that permits the user to take into account the effect of education on digit span performance. The authors of the MAS include a table listing minimum differences between subtest scores that must be obtained for the difference to be significant at the .05 level of statistical probability. This table is particularly helpful when comparing verbal and visual span performance. Unfortunately, the verbal span score is based on both forward and backward digit span performance, whereas the visual span score (see MAS Visual Span) is based only on forward visual span. The meaning of a difference between MAS verbal and visual span scores is consequently difficult to interpret, because the two tests vary on multiple dimensions.

The MAS should be administered only by individuals trained in standardized cognitive assessment, including psychologists and speech pathologists. It is suitable for bedside, office, or laboratory administration.

WAIS-R NI Spatial Span Subtest

The WAIS-R NI spatial span subtest[20] can be obtained from *The Psychological Corporation, P.O. Box 9954, San Antonio, TX 78204-2498.*

This test consists of 10 cubes randomly affixed to a board. The cubes are numbered on the examiner's side of the board, but are blank on the patient's side. The test is administered by touching the cubes in a specified numerical sequence, which the patient attempts to replicate in forward order. In a later series of trials, the patient must reverse the order demonstrated by the examiner. The test is meant to be a visual analogue of the WAIS-R NI digit span procedure and yields an analogous set of scores permitting the examiner to distinguish reductions in the span of material a patient can focus on from reductions in divided concentration.

Reliability and validity data are not available for this test. The WAIS-R NI manual provides a wealth of interpretative hypotheses that should be explored when various patterns of spatial span performance are obtained. Empirical investigation of the properties of the spatial span test and the establishment of norms are necessary before the test can be considered truly comparable to the digit span.

The WAIS-R NI spatial span subtest results should be interpreted only by experienced neuropsychologists because of the lack of normative data and the many factors that can lower spatial-span performance. The test is suitable for bedside, office, or laboratory administration.

WMS–R Visual Memory Span

The WMS-R Visual Memory Span[23] can be obtained from *The Psychological Corporation, P.O. Box 9954, San Antonio, TX 78204-2498.*

Patients are shown a seemingly random pattern of colored squares on a card. The examiner touches the squares in a predetermined order and requests that the patient touch the squares in the same order. During a second set of trials, patients must touch the squares in reverse order. The test provides a visuospatial equivalent of forward and backward digit span. Percentile scores are available for several age groups, and the visual memory span scores are included in the WMS-R Attention/Concentration Index. "Visual memory span" is an unfortunate name for this test because, like digit span, it is interpreted as a measure of concentration span and of the ability to divide concentration.

Split-half reliability is reported in the test manual to vary among age groups from .57 to .84. For some age groups, visual memory span has less internal consistency reliability than digit span, a point that should be kept in mind when comparing digit and visual span performance. Test-retest reliability ranges from .53 to .68, with coefficients again differing from digit span at some age levels. Validity studies done on the WMS-R have focused on the Attention/Concentration Index rather than on visual memory span alone. The results of these studies were summarized previously (see WMS-R Digit Span).

Administration of visual memory span places considerable demands on the examiner's spatial ability; it is not as easy to administer as the WAIS-R NI spatial span test. However, the normative data available for the WMS-R visual memory span give it an empirical advantage not possessed by the WAIS-R NI version. Neuropsychologists will be interested in comparing digit and visual memory span scores, but must do so with caution because of the differences in the reliability of the two tests. A table permitting the examiner to determine what constitutes a significant difference between digit and visual memory span at various levels of statistical probability would be useful, but is not provided in the WMS-R manual.

Individuals trained and experienced in standardized cognitive testing and interpretation, including psychologists and speech pathologists, can administer the WMS-R visual memory span subtest. The test is appropriate for bedside, office, or laboratory use.

Memory Assessment Scale Visual Span

The MAS Visual Span can be obtained from *Psychological Assessment Resources, Inc., P.O. Box 998, Odessa, FL 33556.*

The MAS version of visual span is equivalent in design and administration to the WMS-R forward visual memory span subtest, with the unfortunate exception that the MAS version does not include a reversed visual span condition that could be used as an index of a patient's ability to divide concentration between two spatial tasks. The MAS visual span score is summed with the verbal memory span subtest score to yield an index of "short-term memory," which might be more aptly labeled a concentration index.

Like digit span, the MAS visual span subtest loads on an attention-concentration factor in factor-analytic studies of normal and neurological disorder populations (see MAS Verbal Memory Span). The visual span subtest distinguished patients with dementia, traumatic brain injury, and lateralized stroke from normal controls ($p < .05$) and, like its verbal counterpart, failed to distinguish patients with left- from right-hemisphere stroke at a statistically significant level.[24] Generalizability coefficients varied from .74 to .76 among normative samples.[24]

The visual span subtest shares the same strengths as the MAS verbal memory span subtest, including a large normative database, a broad range of age norms, and norms for three education levels. Like the WMS-R visual memory span subtest, the MAS version employs a flat stimulus card with no verbal information present on the card itself to cue the examiner as to the correct location to which to point. A key is provided to help the examiner decode the target locations on the stimulus card. This, however, adds another element of difficulty in administration, because the examiner must divide his or her concentration between the key, the stimulus card, and the written sequence of locations to be touched on the card. After the patient begins to respond, the examiner must pay attention to the locations touched by the patient and compare them to the target sequence. With a minimally impaired patient, the examiner may occasionally find that his or her concentration fails before the patient's does. Finally, the absence of a reversed visual span condition is an unfortunate omission that makes the test less comparable to digit span and less useful than the WMS-R and WAIS-R NI versions.

The MAS subtests should be interpreted only by individuals trained in standardized cognitive assessment. They are suitable for bedside, office, or laboratory administration.

Behavioral Monitoring Procedure

The Behavioral Monitoring Procedure is *not commercially available*.

Concentration deficits may be episodic or specific to certain times, locations, or activities. Table 3–1 depicts a form for use in tallying the occurrence of distractibility. The form can be modified to provide room to record events that occurred just before, during, and after the episode of distractibility; this information can be useful when the examiner wishes to identify types of stimuli that trigger distractibility. An essential feature of the form is the definition of the target behavior. The definition should consist entirely of concrete, specific, and observable terms. A bonus of such procedures is that they not only provide a record of the target behavior but may also reduce the frequency of the behavior after patients are aware that they are being monitored.

The reliability of behavioral monitoring can be determined for each use of the procedure. Having two observers keep simultaneous independent tallies of the tar-

Table 3–1. **BEHAVIORAL MONITORING PROCEDURE**

PATIENT:

DATES MONITORED:___ / ___ / ___ to ___ / ___ / ___

TARGET BEHAVIOR: Distractibility—discontinuing an ongoing task to observe, respond to, or talk about something happening in the environment that is unrelated to the ongoing task.

INSTRUCTIONS: Place a mark in the appropriate box for each occurrence of the target behavior.

MONDAY	TUESDAY	WEDNESDAY	THURSDAY	FRIDAY
TOTAL	TOTAL	TOTAL	TOTAL	TOTAL

get behavior for 1 or 2 days provides a good reliability check. When discrepancies occur between the two raters, the definition of the target behavior often needs to be made more objective.

Behavioral monitoring can be performed by virtually any clinical staff person as well as by lay people (e.g., family members), after the purpose and mechanics of the procedure are explained to them. The procedure is suitable for use in any environment in which problem behaviors occur and observers can be present.

NEUROPSYCHOLOGICAL TREATMENT

Treatment of concentration disorders should be initiated simultaneously on three fronts. First, every effort should be made to alter the patient's environment to facilitate concentration. This includes removing potential distractors, eliminating interruptions, simplifying work so that the patient has one and not multiple simultaneous tasks to perform, reducing the length of time the patient must work continuously, and providing incentives to keep the patient focused on his or her task. Such incentives include tangible rewards for sustained work, delivered after relatively brief intervals of time or after a certain level of productivity is reached and maintained. In addition, anything that can be done to make the work intrinsically interesting for the patient can improve concentration. Some patients take a greater interest in tasks after they know the purpose of the task. For other patients, shifting work assignments may be necessary so that they spend most of their time on activities that they enjoy and that are also productive.

The second treatment front consists of establishing a reliable monitoring and feedback system. The patient's level of productivity must be monitored at frequent intervals and feedback given immediately so that the patient can adjust his or her performance. When concentration wanes and productivity diminishes, the patient must be told immediately and cued to direct his or her concentration back to the task.

The third treatment front targets the concentration disorder itself. Paper-and-pencil or computer-based activities that require the patient to sustain concentration, to perform in the presence of distractors, to concentrate on a progressively broader amount of information, and to divide concentration can be a valuable part of the patient's treatment. Computer-based activities permit the alteration of task difficulty in accordance with the patient's success in concentration. Computer-based activities also have the advantage of offering immediate feedback to the patient. Computer exercises, unfortunately, often do not sufficiently resemble everyday activities to gain the patient's interest and may not produce improvement in concentration that generalizes to more realistic vocational, educational, or domestic settings. As long as the previous two treatment fronts are not neglected, this weakness of computer exercises should not limit the patient's progress.

CASE ILLUSTRATIONS

CASE 3–1

O.H. was an unemployed 18-year-old man who suffered a traumatic brain injury in a motor vehicle accident shortly after graduating from high school. The patient was comatose for 3 weeks. When he regained consciousness, he was noted to have left-sided weakness, a seizure disorder, and multiple cognitive deficits including impaired problem solving, word-finding difficulty (see Anomic Aphasia), difficulty concentrating, and episodic aggressive outbursts. He underwent a period of intensive inpatient rehabilitation and was then referred for neuropsychological testing to determine his potential for job training. Before his accident, he had maintained a C average in high school and had been considering going to college to study architecture.

When initially examined, O.H. was alert, relaxed, and cooperative. No psychiatric symptoms, including obsessional thoughts, tangentiality, loosening of associations, delusional ideation, hallucinations, or illusions were elicited during the interview or during subsequent observation while formal testing was under way. He denied depression and was generally free of anxiety, with the exception of evident concern about pleasing the examiner and doing whatever was expected of him.

O.H.'s neuropsychological examination included administration of the verbal and visual span subtests of the MAS. Using age norms, the patient scored below the first percentile on both subtests. He successfully repeated only four digits in forward sequence and two in reverse sequence. His performance was also compared to those of individuals of his age and level of education. His verbal span score remained below the first percentile, but his visual span score rose to the first percentile. Only a single error was made on the digit vigilance procedure, which occurred on the 12th trial out of 30.

DISCUSSION

Case 3–1 illustrates the typical presentation of concentration span reduction in a patient having traumatic brain injury. The examiner should also suspect that divided concentration is impaired, because the patient repeated twice as many digits in forward sequence as he was able to do in reverse sequence. However, O.H.'s attention span was so limited that that deficit alone may account for the poor divided concentration performance. His concentration was worse than that of 99 percent of his age and education peers and is unlikely to have been that low premorbidly, considering that he was able to maintain at least a C average in high school. No psychiatric symptoms were present that could account for his deficit. The patient was not particularly distractible, as evidenced by his normal digit vigilance performance and the absence of behavioral signs of distractibility during a demanding series of cognitive tests.

CASE 3–2

I.B. was a 78-year-old woman who had suffered bilateral cerebellar infarctions. She had a high school education and had worked as a nursing assistant and physical therapy aide until age 65 years. Following her stroke, she was noted to have bilaterally poor gross and fine motor coordination, left-sided motor weakness, and poor speech articulation. She received 4 weeks of inpatient rehabilitation and was then admitted to a day hospital for continued intensive treatment. A neuropsychological examination was conducted because of complaints by therapists that the patient was so distractible that this deficit jeopardized her physical rehabilitation.

I.B. repeated five digits in forward sequence and four in reverse sequence on the WAIS-R digit span subtest, obtaining an age-corrected scaled score of 9. She made six errors on the digit vigilance procedure, one of which occurred within the first 15 trials, whereas the remainder occurred during the last 15 trials. In addition, she was noted by the examiner to discontinue performing tasks in which she was engaged whenever any novel stimulus occurred in the environment. Even an innocuous movement, such as the examiner rubbing his hand across his hair, caused the patient to stop what she was doing and orient to the examiner's hand. She would spontaneously return to her task after being distracted for a moment. She tolerated 4 hours of testing, at no point showing any decline in her level of alertness.

Interview and observation of I.B. during testing and during her rehabilitation therapies established the absence of any significant psychiatric disorders, including depression, anxiety, hallucinations, or delusions. The patient's family was also contacted for information on how she behaved before her stroke. They spontaneously noted that she was now unable to concentrate because she would "get off" what she was doing, and indicated that this had not been characteristic of her before the stroke. She had, for example, successfully handled her own bills and checking account and had been able to talk to one or two people in group social settings without being distracted by conversations around her.

DISCUSSION

The patient in case 3–2 presented with apparent distractibility. The diagnosis is based on her poor digit vigilance performance, which clearly worsened over the course of the procedure. Distractibility was also evident at a behavioral level; the patient frequently oriented to trivial, random stimuli appearing in the environment. I.B.'s concentration span and divided concentration were normal for her age. The effects of age and education have not been studied for the digit vigilance procedure; however, the task is quite easy, and a person with a high school education can be expected to perform it well. The patient was of advanced age, and this is a viable alternative interpretation of the test results. However, the observations made by the patient's family suggest that she changed considerably since her stroke, which would argue against age as the sole determinant of her poor performance. Psychiatric symptoms were not a feature of the patient's presentation.

Based on I.B.'s examination, several recommendations were made to alter the way in which physical and occupational therapy were conducted. It was recommended that the patient be treated by a single therapist, with no aide present to act as a distractor, in a quiet environment where no other patients were simultaneously being treated. Therapists were instructed to cue the patient verbally when they were about to make an unexpected movement or when some other distraction was imminent, and to ask the patient to continue what she was doing despite the distraction. This was done deliberately at intervals during treatment sessions to train the patient to persist in tasks despite changes occurring in the environment. With warning, I.B. was able to persist with her work and ignore things happening around her. Whenever the distractor caught her by surprise, however, she would again stop working and orient to the distraction.

CASE 10–1*

P.H. was a right-handed, 37-year-old man who had completed 2 years of college and worked successfully as a marketing consultant. His job involved making calls to business firms to sell them telemarketing services. He did not have an office, but worked in a large room that was divided into work stations. People were constantly walking around; interruptions were frequent; and the environment was full of noise from computer equipment, ringing phones, and conversations. The room included an area where as many as 100 phone operators placed survey calls.

P.H. was taken to an emergency room one morning after complaining to his wife of a severe headache and subsequently losing consciousness. The initial computed tomography (CT) scans revealed a large subarachnoid hemorrhage whose epicenter appeared to be in the territory of the anterior communicating artery. There was a large collection of blood in the interhemispheric fissure. A collection of blood between the frontal horns measured 1 cm. There was also an intraventricular hemorrhage, primarily in the right lateral ventricle, and hydrocephalus was noted. The

*See Chapter 10 for a more detailed discussion of this case.

patient underwent a ventriculostomy to relieve the hydrocephalus. Subsequent CT scans showed a hematoma in the rostrum of the corpus callosum and the development of an infarct in the left basal ganglia. The aneurysm appeared to seal itself; therefore, no additional surgery was necessary.

P.H. was fully alert at the time of the neuropsychological examination, and no psychiatric symptoms were noted in the interview or in informal observation. The patient's mood was stable and undisturbed. The WMS-R digit and visual span subtests were administered. P.H. scored at the 81st percentile in his forward digit span and at the 3rd percentile in his backward digit span. He was at the 46th percentile in his forward visual span and at the 66th percentile in his backward visual span. No errors were made on the digit vigilance procedure, nor were there any behavioral signs of distractibility.

DISCUSSION

Divided concentration deficiency is clearly evident in this case, and is specific to performance on digit span and presumably other verbal tasks. Reduced concentration span cannot explain the deficit in divided concentration, assuming that the patient is average to above average in basic concentration span. The percentile scores are based on age norms; therefore, the deficit is not attributable to age. Education norms are not available for the WMS-R subtests, but this patient's 2 years of college would not lead the examiner to expect him to perform as poorly as he did in divided concentration tests. The deficit is not likely to have been present before his illness, considering that he was successful at his work in an office in which interruptions were constant and distractors were ubiquitous. No signs of mood disturbance or other psychiatric disorder were present.

REFERENCES

1. American Psychiatric Association: Diagnostic and Statistical Manual of Mental Disorders, Fourth Edition. American Psychiatric Association, Washington, DC, 1994.
2. The International Classification of Diseases, Ninth Revision, Clinical Modification. Med-Index, Salt Lake City, 1991.
3. Mendez, MF, Adams, NL, and Lewandowski, KS: Neurobehavioral changes associated with caudate lesions. Neurology 39:349, 1989.
4. Kimura, D, Hahn, A, and Barnett, HJ: Attentional and perseverative impairment in two cases of familial fatal parkinsonism with cortical sparing. Can J Neurol Sci 14:597, 1987.
5. Berthier, M and Starkstein, S: Acute atypical psychosis following a right hemisphere stroke. Acta Neurol Belg 87:125, 1987.
6. Nestor, PG, et al: Divided attention and metabolic brain dysfunction in mild dementia of the Alzheimer's type. Neuropsychologia 29:379, 1991.
7. Wale, J and Geffen, G: Focused and divided attention in each half of space with disconnected hemispheres. Cortex 25:33, 1989.
8. Wale, J and Geffen, G: Hemispheric specialization and attention effects of complete and partial callosal section and hemispherectomy on dichotic monitoring. Neuropsychologia 24:483, 1986.
9. Stuss, DT, et al: Reaction time after head injury: Fatigue, divided and focused attention, and consistency of performance. J Neurol Neurosurg Psychiatry 52:742, 1989.
10. Kewman, DG, Yanus, B, and Kirsch, N: Assessment of distractibility in auditory comprehension after traumatic brain injury. Brain Inj 2:131, 1988.

11. Stuss, DT, et al: Subtle neuropsychological deficits in patients with good recovery after closed head injury. Neurosurgery 17:41, 1985.
12. Sharpe, MH: Distractibility in early Parkinson's disease. Cortex 26:239, 1990.
13. Belyi, BI: Mental impairment in unilateral frontal tumours: Role of the laterality of the lesion. Int J Neurosci 32:799, 1987.
14. Woods, DL and Knight, RT: Electrophysiologic evidence of increased distractibility after dorsolateral prefrontal lesions. Neurology 36:212, 1986.
15. Lawson, JS, McGhie, A, and Chapman, J: Distractibility in schizophrenia and organic cerebral disease. Br J Psychiatry 113:527, 1967.
16. Faust, D and Fogel, BS: The development and initial validation of a sensitive bedside cognitive screening test. J Nerv Ment Dis 177:25, 1989.
17. Rosvold, HE, et al: A continuous performance test of brain damage. J Consult Clin Psychol 20:343, 1956.
18. Halperin, JM, et al: Assessment of the continuous performance test: Reliability and validity in a nonreferred sample. Psychological Assessment 3:63, 1991.
19. Wechsler, D: WAIS-R Manual. Wechsler Adult Intelligence Scale Revised. The Psychological Corporation, New York, 1981.
20. Kaplan, E, et al: WAIS-R NI Manual. WAIS-R as a Neuropsychological Instrument. The Psychological Corporation, San Antonio, 1991.
21. Parker, K: Factor analysis of the WAIS-R at nine age levels between 16 and 74 years. J Consult Clin Psychol 51:302, 1983.
22. Franzen, MD: Reliability and Validity in Neuropsychological Assessment. Plenum Press, New York, 1989.
23. Wechsler, D: Wechsler Memory Scale–Revised Manual. The Psychological Corporation, San Antonio, 1987.
24. Williams, JM: Memory Assessment Scales. Professional Manual. Psychological Assessment Resources, Odessa, FL, 1991.

STIMULUS NEGLECT

4

Stimulus neglect is failure to notice or detect a stimulus in the absence of a sensory deficit such as blindness or deafness. When sensory deficits are present in a patient suspected of having neglect, it must be demonstrated that the sensory deficits are not sufficiently severe to explain why the patient fails to detect the stimulus. The varieties of neglect include hemi-inattention, in which unilateral stimuli are not detected; sensory extinction, in which unilateral stimuli are not detected when a contralateral stimulus is present; hemispatial neglect, in which attention to and visualization of space is unilaterally distorted; and simultanagnosia, in which the ability to attend to multiple stimuli is diminished. Pseudoneglect, a unique form of the disorder arising after disconnection of the cerebral hemispheres, is discussed in Chapter 10.

NOMENCLATURE

Stimulus neglect is often described as an attention disorder, because the afflicted patient is inattentive to or fails to orient toward stimuli in a particular part of space or on one side of the body. Attention has a broader meaning in psychology, encompassing not only the ability to detect and orient but also the ability to concentrate on a selected number of stimuli while ignoring extraneous input. To avoid confusion with stimulus neglect, the disorders of concentration are discussed separately in Chapter 3.

Stimulus neglect can be coded in DSM-IV[1] under "Cognitive Disorder Not Otherwise Specified" or "Mild Neurocognitive Disorder." ICD-9-CM[2] includes the diagnosis "Psychophysical Visual Disturbances," which can be stretched to include some forms of stimulus neglect but falls short of capturing all presentations of this category of disorders.

Considerable confusion in terminology exists in the stimulus neglect literature. Some authors treat hemi-inattention, extinction, hemispatial neglect, and simultanagnosia as at least partially distinct subtypes of neglect. In other references, these conditions are viewed as points on a continuum, with extinction representing a mild form and inattention a more severe form of neglect. In other sources, the terms *hemi-inattention*, *hemineglect*, and *hemispatial neglect* are used synonymously. Even simultanagnosia is regarded by some clinicians as a bilateral form of inattention rather than as a distinct type of neglect.

In this text, hemi-inattention, extinction, hemispatial neglect, and simultanagnosia are treated as at least partially distinct aspects or subtypes of stimulus neglect. This approach is taken partly because the clinical presentation of each subtype is different. Patients with hemi-inattention fail to respond to the unanticipated presentation of stimuli to one side of the body. Patients with extinction respond to a unilaterally presented stimulus as long as no contralateral stimulus simultaneously competes for their attention. Simultanagnosic patients present an even greater contrast in that they fail to respond to any stimulus outside of the center of their visual attention.

Patients with hemispatial neglect also show a subtle difference in their presentation that contrasts with the other subtypes. The deficit in these patients appears to be tied more to conceptual space (i.e., their internal representation of the world) than to external space. For example, these patients do not simply fail to detect a stimulus in the left visual field, but fail to detect the *left half* of a stimulus that appears entirely in their right visual field. If you change their mental perspective by asking them to mentally picture a scene from a different direction, the part of the scene that is neglected may also change.

Although a common mechanism may underlie all the manifestations of neglect, the previous example illustrates how the clinical presentations of the four subtypes differ. The subtypes also differ in the frequency with which they occur following left- and right-hemisphere lesions in humans. Extinction is often seen after lesions on either side of the brain, whereas hemispatial neglect tends to be more closely associated with right-hemisphere lesions.[3] Simultanagnosia appears only after bilateral lesions.

The four subtypes of neglect also differ in the frequency with which they are observed in clinical settings. Because it requires relatively symmetrical bilateral lesions, simultanagnosia is infrequent. Hemi-inattention is also rare in my experience, and, indeed, few cases have appeared in the literature. Most of the patients labeled as having hemi-inattention in the literature have actually had hemispatial neglect or extinction according to the clinical indicators specified in this chapter.

Because of the many features particular to hemi-inattention, extinction, hemispatial neglect, or simultanagnosia, each is treated separately in this chapter. These terms are not used interchangeably in this text, and the differences in their clinical presentation are highlighted.

RULES FOR DIAGNOSIS

Clinical Indicators: Each is independent (only one must be observed for the disorder to be suspected) *except* when subscripting is used. Subscripted numbers (a_1, a_2) denote an indicator with multiple parts that must be considered together.
Associated Features: These are listed to give a more complete picture of the disorder. The presence or absence of these features does not affect the diagnosis.
Factors to Rule Out: All must be taken into account. Failure to rule out even one of these factors makes a firm diagnosis impossible.
Lesion Locations: Each location stands alone; damage in only one of the listed areas is sufficient to produce the disorder.

VARIETY OF PRESENTATION

1. Hemi-inattention (see also Pseudoneglect)

Clinical Indicators

a_1. Failure to notice a stimulus presented to one side of the body or one side of space

a_2. Improved stimulus detection on the unattended side when attention is specifically directed to that side

a_3. The deficit can occur in one sensory modality or in several sensory modalities simultaneously

Associated Features

a. Failure to detect a stimulus on one side when simultaneously stimulated from the other side (see Sensory extinction)

b. Failure to notice a portion of a stimulus (see Hemispatial neglect)

c. Denial that a limb belongs to oneself or treating the limb as an impersonal object (see Somatoparaphrenia)

d. Denial of deficits resulting from brain damage (see Anosognosia)
e. Difficulty in initiating or rapidly performing movements (see Akinesia)

Factors to Rule Out

a. Sensory loss (e.g., blindness, deafness, decreased sensitivity to touch) in any sensory modality in which hemi-inattention is suspected, ruled out by documenting preserved stimulus detection when attention is directed to the previously unattended side.

Lesion Locations

For tactile inattention:

a. Parietal lobe, particularly angular gyrus and superior parietal lobule[4,5]
b. Frontal and temporal lobes, including the inferior frontal, precentral, postcentral, superior temporal, and supramarginal gyri[6]
c. Thalamus[7]

For visual inattention:

a. Thalamus[6]
b. Cortical and subcortical hemispheric[8]
c. White matter beneath the supramarginal, angular, and cingulate gyri[9]
d. Basal ganglia (caudate nucleus and putamen), with damage often including the internal and external capsules[10,11]
e. Dorsolateral frontal lobe[11]
f. Supplementary motor area, anterior cingulate gyrus, motor strip[11]

For auditory inattention:

a. Thalamus[6]
b. Inferior parietal lobule[12]
c. Cortical and subcortical hemispheric[8]
d. Frontal lobe[11]
e. Supplementary motor area, anterior cingulate gyrus, motor strip[11]

Lesion Lateralization

a. Can occur following right- or left-sided lesions; right-sided lesions more common in reports
b. In most cases, side of the body that is neglected contralateral to the side of the brain that is damaged; however, ipsilateral visual inattention following left basal ganglia damage reported[11]

2. Sensory extinction (also called sensory suppression; see also Pseudoneglect)

Clinical Indicators

a_1. Failure to notice stimuli on the right or left sides when simultaneously stimulated from both sides (i.e., double or bilateral simultaneous stimulation)

a_2. Deficit still more pronounced on one side when sensory extinction occurs on both sides

a_3. Relatively preserved ability to detect stimuli on either side when stimulated from only one side

a_4. Deficit occurring in one sensory modality or in several sensory modalities simultaneously

b_1. Failure to notice stimuli above or below the horizontal midline of one visual field when simultaneously stimulated from above and below (i.e., *altitudinal extinction*)
b_2. Relatively preserved detection above or below the horizontal midline when stimulated in only one portion (i.e., upper or lower) of the visual field
c_1. Failure to report or inaccurate reporting of verbal stimuli presented to the left ear when a different verbal stimulus is simultaneously presented to the right ear (i.e., verbal dichotic stimulation)*
c_2. Relatively preserved report of verbal stimuli presented to either ear alone
NOTE: This pattern of performance is termed unilateral verbal dichotic extinction.

Associated Features

a. A recent history of hemi-inattention (see previous text)
b. Failure to notice a portion of a stimulus (see Hemispatial neglect)
c. Denial that a limb belongs to oneself or treating the limb as an impersonal object (see Somatoparaphrenia)
d. Denial of deficits resulting from brain damage (see Anosognosia)
e. Difficulty in initiating or rapidly performing movements (see Akinesia)
f. Inability to perceive more than one stimulus simultaneously (see Simultanagnosia)
g. Impaired visual guidance of movement (see Optic ataxia)
h. Inability to control eye movement on demand (see Oculomotor apraxia)

NOTE: When simultanagnosia, optic ataxia, and oculomotor apraxia occur together, the entire complex is referred to as Balint's syndrome.

i. Disorders of interhemispheric transfer (see Chap. 10) in patients showing unilateral verbal dichotic extinction

Factors to Rule Out

a. Sensory loss in the area in which extinction occurs, ruled out by documenting accurate response to unilateral stimulation or, in the case of altitudinal extinction, documenting accurate response to a single stimulus above or below the midline
b. Normal individual variation in task performance, left-hemisphere language-dominant healthy individuals showing more frequent or more accurate reporting of verbal stimuli presented to the right ear during verbal dichotic stimulation

Lesion Locations

For tactile extinction:

a. Parietal lobe, particularly the inferior parietal lobule, or the combined lesions of the parietal and occipital lobes[13,14]
b. Frontal lobe, particularly the cingulate gyrus[12,13,15]

*The left hemisphere is presumed to be dominant for language when the patient is right-handed. The pattern of left- and right-sided indicators are reversed in left-handed patients with right-hemisphere language dominance. Patients with other dominance patterns have less predictable clinical findings.

c. Anterior thalamus[16,17]
d. Basal ganglia (lenticular, caudate, and putamen)—internal capsule with occasional extension to the centrum ovale, corona radiata, and temporal lobe [10,18,19]
e. Internal capsule, with or without periventricular white matter involvement[19,20]

For visual extinction:

a. Parietal lobe, particularly the inferior parietal lobule, with or without frontal or occipital involvement[12,21,22]
b. Frontal lobe, particularly the dorsolateral area[12,15]
c. Thalamus[17]
d. Basal ganglia (putamen)—posterior internal capsule with occasional extension to the centrum ovale, corona radiata, and temporal lobe[18]
e. Periventricular white matter, with or without involvement of the posterior internal capsule[19]
f. Pons—mesencephalon[23]

For altitudinal extinction (reported only in visual modality):

a. Combined lesions of the parietal and occipital lobes[24]

For auditory extinction:

a. Parietal lobe, particularly the inferior parietal lobule, with or without frontal or occipital lobe involvement[12,14,22]
b. Frontal lobe[12]
c. Basal ganglia, particularly the caudate and lenticular areas—periventricular white matter lesions, with or without involvement of the internal capsule[19]

For unilateral verbal dichotic extinction:

a. Corpus callosum, particularly the anterior two thirds or posterior trunk[25–30]
b. Deep posterior intersection of the parietal and occipital lobes near the lateral wall of the lateral ventricle at the level of the trigone[31]
c. Temporal lobe, sometimes extending to occipital lobe[31,32]
d. Internal capsule (anterior limb more frequently than posterior limb) or external capsule[33]

Lesion Lateralization

a. Equally likely following right- or left-sided lesions[3,34]
b. Stimulus opposite the side of the brain lesion usually extinguished during bilateral simultaneous stimulation; however, ipsilateral extinction and ipsilateral verbal dichotic extinction reported following left-sided lesions[13,31]

3. Hemispatial neglect (includes dressing apraxia; see also Pseudoneglect)

Clinical Indicators

a_1. Failure to notice and explore either the right or left sides of an object or other stimulus that is seen or touched
a_2. Deficit still greatest on either the right or left sides of the stimulus when the left, center, and right portions of a stimulus are all incompletely perceived or explored
b. Failure to notice and explore either the top or bottom portions of an object or other stimulus that is seen or touched (i.e., *altitudinal neglect*)

c_1. Omission of details from either the right or left sides of a stimulus that is recalled from memory, as evidenced by any of the following errors:
   1) Verbally reporting details from only one side of an object, scene, or other stimulus that is being recalled
   2) Drawing only one side of an object, scene, or other stimulus that is being recalled
   3) Crowding all details into one side of an object, scene, or other stimulus that is being drawn from memory

c_2. Dependence of the side of the stimulus that is omitted on the direction from which the stimulus is imagined (e.g., patient with left hemispatial neglect consistently omitting whatever is to the left from his or her imagined point of view)

c_3. Deficit still much more severe on one side when details are omitted from both the right and left sides of the stimulus being recalled

d. Failure to dress either the right or left side of the body, but not both (i.e., dressing apraxia)

Associated Features

a. Failure to detect a stimulus on one side when simultaneously stimulated from the other side (see Sensory extinction)
b. Denial that a limb belongs to oneself or treating the limb as an impersonal object (see Somatoparaphrenia)
c. Denial of deficits resulting from brain damage (see Anosognosia)
d. Difficulty in initiating or rapidly performing movements (see Akinesia)
e. Loss of acuity in one visual half-field (i.e., homonymous hemianopsia)

Factors to Rule Out

a. Sensory loss on the neglected side of the body severe enough to account for the failure to notice stimuli on that side
b. Muscle weakness on the neglected side of the body that prevents full movement of the eyes or limbs during exploration of a stimulus
c. Weakness of the muscles of the arms or hands sufficient to prevent dressing in cases of suspected dressing apraxia
d. Impaired coordination of the muscles of the arms or hands sufficient to prevent dressing in cases of suspected dressing apraxia
e. Impaired ability to initiate arm or hand movements (see Akinesia) sufficient to prevent dressing in cases of suspected dressing apraxia
f. Impaired ability to persist with ongoing arm or hand movements (see Motor impersistence) sufficient to prevent dressing in cases of suspected dressing apraxia
g. Impaired ability to terminate ongoing arm or hand movements (see Motor perseveration) sufficient to prevent dressing in cases of suspected dressing apraxia

Lesion Locations

a. Parietal lobe, particularly the inferior parietal lobule and angular gyrus–intraparietal sulcus, with or without extension to the frontal, temporal, or occipital lobes[3,4,7,14,21–23,35–42]

b. Frontal lobe, including the superior, inferior, prefrontal, dorsolateral, supplementary motor, and anterior cingulate areas[11,21,39,40]
c. Thalamus[6,17,37,42,43]
d. Basal ganglia (globus pallidus, putamen, caudate), with or without involvement of the anterior and posterior limbs of the internal capsule or periventricular white matter, with occasional extension to the centrum ovale, corona radiata, and temporal lobe[11,18,19,44,45]
e. Internal capsule[20,46]

Lesion Lateralization

a. More common and more severe following right-sided lesions[3,36,42,45]
b. Side of space that is neglected opposite the side of the brain that contains the lesion; ipsilateral neglect may occur and may be more severe than contralateral neglect following left hemisphere damage[47]

4. **Simultanagnosia**

Clinical Indicators

a. Inability to perceive more than one stimulus at a time
b. Inability to perceive more than one aspect or portion of an object or scene at a time

Associated Features

a. Impaired visual guidance of movement (see Optic ataxia)
b. Inability to control eye movement upon demand (see Oculomotor apraxia)

NOTE: When simultanagnosia occurs with oculomotor apraxia and optic ataxia, the entire complex is referred to as Balint's syndrome.

c. Impaired visual recognition of objects (see Visual object agnosia)
d. Impaired recognition of formerly familiar faces (see Prosopagnosia)
e. Impaired perception of colors (see Achromatopsia)
f. Markedly restricted scanning of visual stimuli

Factors to Rule Out

a. A decrease in the acuity of vision sufficient to prevent the patient from clearly seeing stimuli regardless of where the stimuli are placed in the visual field

Lesion Locations

a. Occipital lobe or combined lesions of the occipital and parietal lobes[24,48–51]

Lesion Lateralization

a. Occurs only after bilateral lesions

5. **Pseudoneglect (see Chap. 10)**

ETIOLOGY

The most common cause of stimulus neglect is cerebrovascular accident. The neglect patients reported by Ferro, Kertesz, and Black[19] had subcortical strokes involving the lateral lenticulostriate branches of the middle cerebral artery, the medial lenticulostriate arteries, and the anterior choroidal arteries. Strokes of the anterior thalamo-subthalamic paramedian artery (originating from the posterior communicating artery) or the posterior thalamo-subthalamic paramedian artery (originating from the posterior cerebral artery) were implicated in the subcortical lesions that produced neglect in the patients reported by Bogousslavsky, Regli, and Assal.[17] The middle cerebral artery is usually implicated in cortical strokes that result in neglect.

Unilateral verbal dichotic suppression may follow callosal transection for the treatment of intractable seizures. Naturally occurring cases may follow aneurysms of the pericallosal artery[25] or occlusion of the posterior cerebral artery.[32] Bilateral watershed infarcts in the zone between the middle and posterior cerebral arteries may lead to simultanagnosia. Other conditions that bilaterally compromise brain function, including hypoxia and degenerative disease, can result in simultanagnosia.

Neglect also may result from brain tumors, usually rapidly growing, cancerous varieties. Traumatic brain injury, particularly if there is subsequent bleeding into the brain, can cause stimulus neglect. Heilman and Howell[14] reported a patient whose seizures produced transient neglect. Electroconvulsive therapy for the treatment of psychiatric disorders can also produce transient neglect.[52] Graff-Radford and Rizzo[9] have documented the presence of stimulus neglect in a multiple sclerosis patient.

DISABLING CONSEQUENCES

Depending on the severity of the neglect syndrome, the resulting disability can be devastating. A patient with neglect is potentially unable to perform jobs involving attention to visual detail (e.g., photography, copy editing, construction, assembly line work), drawing (e.g., drafting, architecture, graphic art), auditory perception (e.g., sound studio work), or the use of vision or touch to guide the activity of the hands (e.g., hairdressing, equipment operation, carpentry). Many basic everyday activities may be restricted, including the ability to dress, apply makeup, groom hair, cook, or perform housework. Walking may be risky because of a tendency to bump into objects on the neglected side of space. A high potential exists for injury to the neglected side of the body as a result of accidents during cooking or walking. Driving is typically impossible. Leisure activities are often severely restricted, including sports participation, reading, watching television or movies, or enjoying music.

ASSESSMENT INSTRUMENTS

Halstead-Reitan Battery Sensory-Perceptual Examination

The Halstead-Reitan Battery (HRB) Sensory-Perceptual Examination (SPE) is available from *Reitan Neuropsychological Laboratory, 1338 East Edison Street, Tucson, AZ 85719.*

This examination includes tests of visual fields; extinction to bilateral simultaneous stimulation in the visual, auditory, and tactile modalities; and other tests of tactile stimulus perception. The procedures for examining visual fields and sensory extinction are brief, easily administered at bedside, and appropriate for any health care professional trained in neurological or neuropsychological assessment. Specific training in administration and interpretation of the HRB is required for some of the other tactile tests included in the examination.

The procedures included in the SPE for assessing neglect are standardizations of accepted, time-honored parts of the neurological examination and thus are supported by many decades of clinical experience. In addition to this support, a large amount of literature specifically addresses the reliability and validity of the HRB. A full discussion of this literature is provided by Lezak[53] and Franzen.[54]

Unfortunately, many of the reliability and validity studies that have been done on the HRB did not include the SPE. When the SPE tests are included in the evaluation, they emerge as highly useful measures. Goldstein and Shelly,[55] in a frequently cited study, found that the tactile extinction variable correctly classified 64.6 percent of right- and left-brain–damaged patients. Auditory extinction tests correctly classified 62.5 percent, and visual extinction correctly classified 68.8 percent of these patients. These percentages of correct classification are equal to or better than any other individual test in the HRB.

Goldstein and Shelly[55] did a factor analysis of their data and found that all three measures of extinction from the SPE loaded together on a single factor, which they labeled the suppression factor. Other than a tactile recognition factor derived from other tests included in the SPE, the suppression factor was the only factor from the HRB that discriminated right- and left-brain–damaged patients at a statistically significant level. A multivariate procedure (step-wise discriminant function) led to a higher percentage of correct classifications in the Goldstein and Shelly study than did the above univariate procedures. However, the authors noted that tactile suppression was the first factor to emerge in the discriminant function analysis, indicating that it is the variable producing the greatest separation between the groups of patients.

The SPE does not include procedures for specifically detecting hemi-inattention, although failure to detect unilateral stimulation should raise the examiner's suspicion. When unilateral stimulation errors occur, I include a series of trials in which the patient is informed of the side of the body that will be stimulated, and asked only to report when the stimuli occur. If the patient no longer makes errors in unilateral stimulation under this new set of instructions, it is likely that the previous errors were the result of hemi-inattention rather than sensory loss.

Dichotic Listening Test

The Dichotic Listening Test[56] is *not commercially available.*

In the Dichotic Listening Test, pairs of digits are presented simultaneously by means of audiotape and stereo headphones, with each member of a pair presented to a different ear. Digits are presented at a rate of 2 per second, with a 10-second interval between trials. Six pairs of digits are presented on each trial; this number of pairs was chosen to maximize ear advantages. Digits fall between the numbers 1 and 20, excluding 7, 11, and 17 because of their similar phonology. Digits are randomly assigned to trials but are not repeated within a trial. Digit pairs are random with the exception that they are required to be of equal syllable length.

The original tape was constructed manually and contained random asynchronies, requiring that headphones be reversed after every sixth trial. Additionally, only 12 trials were recorded, so that the tape must be rewound between the three blocks of trials shown in Table 4–1. Greater synchrony can be achieved between digit pairs using computerized recording techniques, and it is recommended that all 36 trials be recorded. Table 4–1 presents the complete set of digit pairs used in the test.

Table 4–1. **DICHOTIC LISTENING TEST STIMULI**

Examples

a.	**R 1 13 3 12 6 5**	**b. R 12 4 8 18 8 1**	**c. R 3 14 8 13 9 2**
	L 4 15 9 2 8 10	**L 3 5 9 14 2 6**	**L 5 16 12 20 10 4**

Free Recall*	**Right Ear First**	**Left Ear First**
Trial 1	*Trial 13*	*Trial 25*
R 5 6 2 3 13 1	R 10 8 12 9 15 4	R 10 8 12 9 15 4
L 10 8 12 9 15 4	L 5 6 2 3 13 1	L 5 6 2 3 13 1
Trial 2	*Trial 14*	*Trial 26*
R 1 8 14 10 4 12	R 6 2 18 9 5 3	R 6 2 18 9 5 3
L 6 2 18 9 5 3	L 1 8 14 10 4 12	L 1 8 14 10 4 12
Trial 3	*Trial 15*	*Trial 27*
R 2 9 20 8 14 3	R 4 10 13 12 16 5	R 4 10 13 12 16 5
L 4 10 13 12 16 5	L 2 9 20 8 14 3	L 2 9 20 8 14 3
Trial 4	*Trial 16*	*Trial 28*
R 15 10 12 14 16 6	R 19 1 3 13 18 9	R 19 1 3 13 18 9
L 19 1 3 13 18 9	L 15 10 12 14 16 6	L 15 10 12 14 16 6
Trial 5	*Trial 17*	*Trial 29*
R 16 18 20 3 2 5	R 19 13 15 6 8 4	R 19 13 15 6 8 4
L 19 13 15 6 8 4	L 16 18 20 3 2 5	L 16 18 20 3 2 5
Trial 6	*Trial 18*	*Trial 30*
R 3 5 13 15 2 16	R 8 12 14 18 4 19	R 8 12 14 18 4 19
L 8 12 14 18 4 19	L 3 5 13 15 2 16	L 3 5 13 15 2 16
Trial 7	*Trial 19*	*Trial 31*
R 3 6 19 1 13 12	R 10 8 20 4 16 5	R 10 8 20 4 16 5
L 10 8 20 4 16 5	L 3 6 19 1 13 12	L 3 6 19 1 13 12
Trial 8	*Trial 20*	*Trial 32*
R 1 15 16 14 10 8	R 9 19 20 18 4 6	R 9 19 20 18 4 6
L 9 19 20 18 4 6	L 1 15 16 14 10 8	L 1 15 16 14 10 8
Trial 9	*Trial 21*	*Trial 33*
R 6 20 5 2 15 9	R 8 14 4 1 13 10	R 8 14 4 1 13 10
L 8 14 4 1 13 10	L 6 20 5 2 15 9	L 6 20 5 2 15 9

Table 4–1. **DICHOTIC LISTENING TEST STIMULI** *(Continued)*

Free Recall*							**Right Ear First**							**Left Ear First**						
Trial 10							*Trial 22*							*Trial 34*						
R	1	18	5	10	3	20	R	9	19	12	6	2	15	R	9	19	12	6	2	15
L	9	19	12	6	2	15	L	1	18	5	10	3	20	L	1	18	5	10	3	20
Trial 11							*Trial 23*							*Trial 35*						
R	14	20	2	16	8	5	R	19	15	1	18	9	12	R	19	15	1	18	9	12
L	19	15	1	18	9	12	L	14	20	2	16	8	5	L	14	20	2	16	8	5
Trial 12							*Trial 24*							*Trial 36*						
R	20	16	2	4	3	1	R	19	18	10	13	4	6	R	19	18	10	13	4	6
L	19	18	10	13	4	6	L	20	16	2	14	3	1	L	20	16	2	14	3	1
_____% R ear							_____% R ear							_____% R ear						
_____% L ear							_____% L ear							_____% L ear						

*During trials 1 through 12, patients recall digits in any order they wish. During trials 13 through 24 and 25 through 36, the examiner specifies which ear should be reported on first.

Three "example" trials are administered before the start of the test to facilitate the patient's understanding of the task. On Example and Test Trials 1 through 12, patients are asked to report as many digits as they can during the intertrial interval. Ear preferences may emerge on these trials, reflected in a higher percentage of digits accurately recalled from a particular ear. Such ear preferences do not necessarily reflect left- or right-hemisphere language dominance, because response strategies chosen by the patient (e.g., reporting digits from the right ear first) heavily influence dichotic listening test results.

On trials 13 through 24, patients are instructed to report digits from the right ear first, effectively shifting their focus to that ear. Patients are asked to report digits from the left ear first on trials 25 through 36. These last two trial blocks permit an assessment of how flexibly patients can shift from giving priority to one ear over another when reporting dichotic digits.

In dichotic listening procedures such as the Dichotic Listening Test, the similar input to each ear places processing demands on the same brain regions. In this manner, the input from the two ears competes for access to areas of the brain appropriate for processing the information, resulting in a procedure that can be highly sensitive to auditory extinction. Extinction-like effects can be produced in normal persons, in whom an ear advantage emerges for selected types of information. Generally, the right ear is 10 to 15 percent more accurate than the left ear for verbal dichotic information in left-hemisphere language-dominant normal people.[57] The ear advantage must exceed this level before it can be considered a possible indication of brain damage. Such ear advantages can be eliminated in normal persons and in some patient populations by directing attention to the extinguished side. The format of the Dichotic Listening Test permits an assessment of the effect of directing attention to a specified ear.

Reliability and validity data are not available for the Dichotic Listening Test, nor have extensive normative data been reported. At present, the test is most useful for intraperson comparisons, and valid interpretation depends on the emergence of large ear differences. The test is recommended for use only by experienced neuropsychologists because of the absence of normative data to guide interpretation. Caution is recommended in using the test in elderly populations, because the effects of advanced age on performance are unknown. The Dichotic Listening Test is appropriate for office or laboratory administration. Although it is not commercially available, it can be constructed from the information provided with the aid of an audiovisual laboratory.

Test of Visual Neglect

The Test of Visual Neglect is *not commercially available, but can be constructed from a diagram provided by Albert.*[47]

The Test of Visual Neglect consists of a 20- by 26-cm page containing 40 lines 2.5 cm in length. On casual inspection, the lines appear to be placed randomly on the page. In actuality, the page contains a column of four lines in the center, with three columns of six lines each to the left and right of center. Patients are instructed to cross out all lines on the page. The numbers of uncrossed lines on the left, center, and right sides of the page are tallied separately. Reliability data were not reported for this instrument by Albert.[47] The test separated brain-damaged from non brain-damaged controls with 100 percent accuracy and was correlated with measures of stimulus perception, recognition, and perceptual-motor integration. The test can be administered at bedside and is suitable for use by virtually all health care professionals.

Line Bisection Test

The Line Bisection Test is *not commercially available, but can be constructed from a diagram provided by Schenkenberg, Bradford, and Ajax.*[58]

The test consists of a sheet of 21.5- by 28-cm paper containing 20 horizontal lines of varying length. Eighteen of the lines are grouped in columns of six lines each, respectively oriented on the page so that they lie mostly to the left of center, in the center, or mostly to the right of center (see Fig. 4–3). Two additional lines are placed at the top center and bottom center of the page for demonstration purposes. Rotating the page 180 degrees yields an alternate form comparable to the original.

Patients are instructed to make a single mark through the center of each line, cutting it in halves. They are asked not to omit any lines and are not permitted to move the page. Line omissions are noted, and patients are subsequently shown the omitted lines and asked to bisect them. Scores consist of the number of lines omitted and the average deviation from the true center of the line [Percent deviation = (sum of measured left halves − sum of true halves)/sum of true halves × 100]. Positive percent deviation scores indicate left neglect, and negative scores indicate right neglect. All scores can be computed for the test as a whole or separately for each column of lines. The test is relatively brief and can be administered at bedside.

Reliability of measurement of the left halves of the lines is high (.99), as would be expected. Test-retest reliability varied from .84 to .93 across groups of patients with lateralized, diffuse, or no brain damage in the original standardization sample. Validity data are limited. The number of line omissions on the test correlated moderately, but at a statistically significant level (r = .548), with the presence of neglect in patient drawings. The test successfully discriminated right-brain-damaged patients from left-, diffuse-, and nonbrain-damaged controls, but only when the right hand was used to bisect the lines and only when the left-of-center lines were considered. The test is best used in conjunction with other measures of neglect. It should be administered only by professionals trained in neurological or neuropsychological assessment and interpretation, because the test results often need to be considered in conjunction with other test data.

Quality Extinction Test

The Quality Extinction Test (QET)[13] is *not commercially available*.

The QET consists of an assortment of materials differing in texture (i.e., carpeting, sandpaper, velvet, wire screen, foam rubber, and a paint roller). These materials are shown to the patient and then used to stimulate the palms of the hands with the patient's eyes occluded either unilaterally or bilaterally. The patient is asked to name or otherwise identify the materials felt. During the simultaneous bilateral trials, either the same or different materials are used to stimulate each palm, although the patient is never told that the materials felt on each palm could be different. If the patient fails to detect spontaneously that a different material is being used on each palm or cannot identify the materials, this is counted as an extinction. Thus, this procedure adds an element of complexity not found in most tests of tactile extinction.

No data on the reliability of the QET were reported by its designers. Validity data are also limited. The QET was found to be more sensitive to the presence of brain damage than traditional tactile extinction testing (e.g., as done on the HRB SPE). The QET had a false-negative rate of only 3 percent, compared with a false-negative rate of 44 percent for traditional tactile extinction testing. A small percentage of normal persons also show extinctions on the QET.

The QET is brief and can be done at bedside as well as in an office or laboratory setting. Additional research on the QET is necessary to establish clearly its reliability and validity and to identify a precise cut-off score that separates normal persons from brain-damaged patients (the authors of the test provide a tentative cut-off score). The sensitivity of the QET when other tactile tests fail to reveal tactile neglect suggests that it may be a very useful instrument if validated further. The QET is appropriate for use by health care professionals trained in neurological or neuropsychological assessment and should be used in conjunction with other tests of neglect until it is validated further.

Rey-Osterrieth Complex Figure Test

The Rey-Osterrieth Complex Figure Test is *not commercially available, but can be constructed from a diagram provided by Lezak.*[53]

In this test, patients copy a complex geometric figure and subsequently attempt to reproduce it from memory. Evidence of stimulus neglect may appear as a failure to draw or omission of detail from lateral portions of the figure. This may occur during the initial copying of the figure or during its reproduction from memory. The reliability and validity of this instrument are discussed in Chapters 7 and 16.

Visual Search and Attention Test

The Visual Search and Attention Test (VSAT)[59] can be obtained from *Psychological Assessment Resources, Incorporated, P.O. Box 998, Odessa, FL 33556.*

The VSAT consists of four visual cancellation tasks using letters and symbols. The task is to cross out the letters or symbols that match a specified target stimulus. The test is brief and can be administered at bedside or in a laboratory setting. Normative data are provided for groups ranging from ages 18 to older than 60 years. Test-retest reliability (average retest interval of 2 months) is reported in the test manual to be .95. The VSAT successfully discriminated 84 to 86 percent of brain-damaged and normal subjects in validity studies. The instrument is appropriate for use by health care professionals trained in neurological or neuropsychological assessment and interpretation.

Tactual Performance Test

The Tactual Performance Test (TPT) can be obtained from *Reitan Neuropsychological Laboratory, 1338 E. Edison Street, Tucson, AZ 85719.*

In the TPT, patients explore a board containing grooves into which various wooden shapes can be placed. Each of the wooden shapes must be placed into the correct groove within a 10-minute time limit. The test is performed while the patient is blindfolded, using each hand separately and then both hands together. Following this portion of the test, patients attempt to draw as many shapes as they can recall in their proper location relative to the other shapes on the board. The reliability and validity of this test are discussed in Chapter 5.

Although it is not designed as a measure of neglect, the TPT may nonetheless yield evidence of a neglect disorder. Patients with neglect may fail to explore one half of the form board and thus not place the forms that fit on the neglected side of the board. Additionally, they may not recall forms from one half of the board when attempting to draw them from memory. The disadvantage of the test is that it is cumbersome and can be administered only in an office or laboratory setting. The test is also time-consuming and can be highly frustrating for many patients. It is appropriate for use only by a neuropsychologist trained in the administration of the HRB.

Behavioral Inattention Test

The Behavioral Inattention Test (BIT)[60] can be obtained from *Thames Valley Test Company, 34/36 High Street, Titchfield Fareham, Hants PO14 4AF, England.*

The BIT is a comprehensive battery of tests that includes measures of line crossing, letter cancellation, star cancellation, figure copying, line bisection, drawing, picture scanning, telephone dialing, reading, telling and setting the time, coin sorting, writing, map navigation, and card sorting. A form parallel to the original is available. A unique feature of the BIT is that it includes both conventional clinical subtests (e.g., line bisection) and "behavioral" subtests consisting of stimuli drawn from the everyday environment (e.g., telephone dialing). The "behavioral" subtests provide an opportunity to observe the degree of disability a patient shows when confronted with natural and realistic challenges. Consequently, the BIT is particularly useful in rehabilitation and forensic settings, in which a precise determination of the level of patient disability is essential.

Inter-rater reliability of the BIT was reported in the manual to be .99 based on 13 subjects scored by two raters. Parallel form reliability was .91 based on 10 subjects. Test-retest reliability was .99 based on 10 subjects. In a group of 80 left-sided and right-sided cerebrovascular accident patients, BIT "behavioral" scores correlated .67 with independent therapist evaluations of the patients. Normative data reported in the BIT manual are limited to 50 non-brain-damaged controls.

The BIT is a relatively new instrument and requires further normative study; nonetheless, it is promising. Portions of the BIT can be readily administered at bedside. This test is suitable for administration only by health care professionals trained and experienced in neuropsychological assessment.

Tactile Mazes

Tactile Mazes[61] are *not commercially available.*

The stimuli for this test are two 50- by 40-cm boards each containing a four-armed maze (2-cm-wide maze alleys cut into the board at a depth of 2 cm). Although the overall shapes of the mazes differ, one of each of the four arms of each maze terminates in the upper left, upper right, lower left, and lower right corners of the boards. The patient never sees the mazes; his or her hand is run along the boards to acquaint the patient with their dimensions. A marble is put in one of the four corners, and the patient's forefinger is placed in the center of the maze. The patient is told to search the maze alleys until the marble is found. The maximum time limit is 90 seconds, and the score on each trial is the number of seconds taken to find the marble, up to the maximum. The mazes are alternated for eight trials, with the marble placed at the end of each maze arm in a random order.

Validity and reliability of the task have not been sufficiently demonstrated. In the initial study,[61] 121 patients with lateralized brain damage with and without visual field defects were compared to 30 healthy controls. Patients with visual field deficits performed significantly worse than the controls. Additionally, right-brain-damaged patients with visual field cuts failed to find the marble more often than the other patient groups (result was statistically significant, $p < .001$), possibly because they had hemispatial neglect. This test is not commercially available, but the authors give sufficient instructions for the examiner to construct at least one of the mazes. Further validation of this instrument is required, but given the few available tactile measures for assessing hemispatial neglect, use of this instrument in conjunction with more established measures of neglect is justified. The test should be administered only by health care professionals trained and experienced in neuropsychological assessment. It is suitable for office or laboratory use.

Saccadic Eye Movement Tests

The Saccadic Eye Movement Tests are two procedures, originally presented by Meienberg,[62] that are useful for distinguishing visual field deficits from visual neglect. The examiner faces the patient at a nose-to-nose distance of 50 cm. The patient holds his or her head steady by cradling it in the hands, wrists beneath the chin and the arms bent at the elbows and pressed to the chest. The examiner's hands are held at the patient's eye level with the index fingers raised at one half the nose-to-nose distance to the patient.

In test 1, the examiner's fingers are approximately 50 cm apart. The patient is asked to fixate first on the finger in the intact visual field for 2 to 3 seconds and then to shift his or her eyes to the finger held in the blind visual field. The patient with a visual field deficit does not know initially where the finger is in the blind field, and typically fails to find it after the initial saccadic movement. He or she then makes a second correction saccade to the actual finger position, producing a staircase pattern of eye movements. After several trials of alternately shifting the eyes from one finger to another, the patient learns the position of the finger in the blind field and is able to shift the eyes to it in a single direct saccade. The examiner then moves the finger in the blind field inward to approximately 15 cm from the other finger while the patient is fixated on the opposite finger, taking care not to cue the patient that movement has occurred. The patient then overshoots the finger in the blind hemifield and has to make a correction saccade back to the finger's actual position. After several more trials, the patient with a visual field deficit learns the new finger position and can again move to it directly.

In contrast to the patient with visual field deficits alone, the patient with hemineglect, with or without a visual field deficit, fails to learn the position of the finger in the blind or neglected visual field. The patient constantly undershoots the actual finger location and often gives up searching for it before it is found. It is usually not possible to proceed to the second phase of the test, because the patient never consistently finds the finger in its initial position.

Test 2 is essentially the same as test 1, except that the examiner's fingers are initially 15 cm apart, and once both fingers can be smoothly located by the patient, the finger in the blind visual field is moved to approximately 50 cm from the other finger. Most patients can be tested with both eyes open, but patients having bitemporal visual field deficits should be tested one eye at a time.

As originally described, all patients with visual neglect (6 of 23 patients) could be differentiated from patients having only visual field deficits. The procedure also is useful for determining the degree to which a patient learned to compensate for a long-standing visual field deficit by automatically making larger saccades in the blind direction. Additionally, the procedure can help differentiate patients who are malingering or hysterical from patients who have genuine visual field deficits, because the various patterns of eye movement are not known to the general public. However, the reliability and validity of the procedure have not been directly addressed. The two tests can yield useful qualitative information that should be interpreted only by individuals skilled and trained in neurological, neuropsychological, or ophthalmological examination. The tests are appropriate for bedside, office, or laboratory administration.

Simultaneous Perception Procedure

This procedure was developed by me for detecting simultanagnosia. Stimuli for the procedure (Fig. 4–1) consist of shapes formed by square dots, multipart geometric figures, and letters with light and dark areas. The patient is shown one stimulus at a time and asked to identify it. In the case of the dot patterns, the patient is asked to count the dots if he or she fails to identify the overall pattern.

Each stimulus used in the Simultaneous Perception Procedure consists of discrete parts that may capture the simultanagnosic's visual attention so that he or she fails to perceive the entire configuration. This effect is heightened when the stimulus parts in themselves can be labeled, as is the case with most of the geometric and

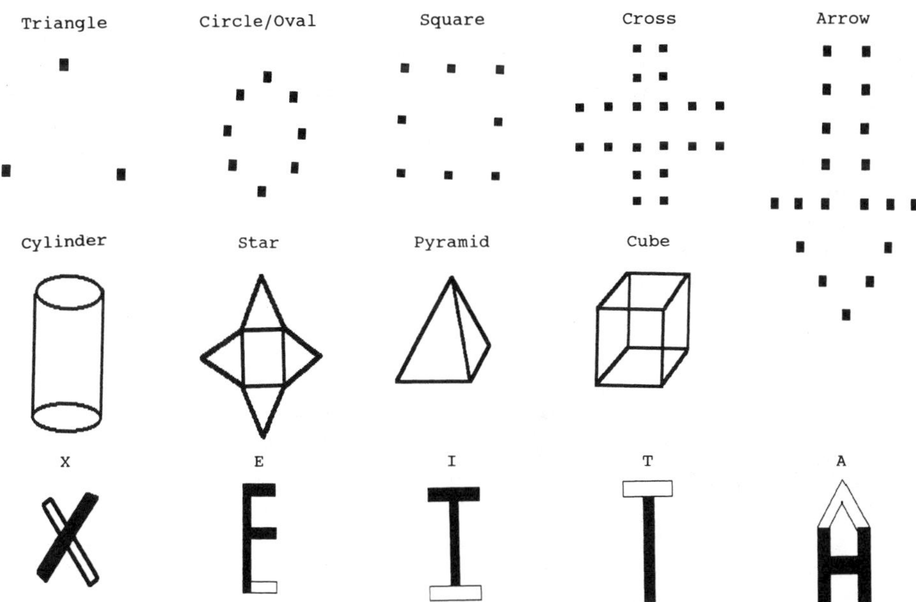

FIGURE 4–1. Simultaneous perception procedure stimuli, which in testing are presented one at a time without identifying labels.

letter stimuli in Figure 4–1. In the case of the dot patterns, simultanagnosic patients may fail to identify any pattern at all or may describe all patterns as squares because of the shape of the dots.

Normative data are not available for this procedure. My clinical experience suggests that healthy individuals have little difficulty in perceiving and identifying all of the stimuli. The Simultaneous Perception Procedure should be administered only by experienced clinicians because of its lack of empirical validation and should be used in conjunction with other tests for neglect.

NEUROPSYCHOLOGICAL TREATMENT

The approach to the patient with stimulus neglect depends on the treatment objective. If it is desirable to have the patient perform tests at his or her maximum level of efficiency, then tasks should be presented in the preserved portions of the patient's visual field. Thus, a patient with left hemispatial neglect may show better reading comprehension if the reading material is placed on the right side. The same patient is more apt to pay attention during a conversation if the other person is to his or her right. The patient with left hemispatial neglect may stop eating after the right half of the plate is empty, even though the left half of the plate is full. Rotating the plate to bring the remaining food into the intact visual field may lead to greater food consumption.

In other circumstances, the treatment objective may be to increase the patient's attention to the neglected side of space. In this instance, tasks may be deliberately placed on the neglected side to give the patient practice in paying attention to this side of space. Performance is likely to be facilitated if the patient is continuously cued to pay attention to the neglected side. The patient should be told to look in the neglected direction and to scan farther in this direction than he or she may think is necessary. In some cases, simply telling the patient to explore the neglected side of space is sufficient, but in other cases, a specific target may be needed to let the patient know when he or she has scanned far enough on the neglected side. For example, a bright red border may be placed in the margin of a page on the patient's neglected side. When reading, the patient can be told to scan until that border comes into view; then he or she will know that the entire line of print has been seen.

A variety of stimulus parameters can be manipulated to lessen the impact of neglect on performance. Increasing the size of print and decreasing the number of stimuli on a page may facilitate reading. Increasing the loudness of auditory stimuli on the neglected side may be beneficial. Using an intact sensory modality to compensate for a neglected one can be an effective technique. For example, a wheelchair-bound patient with left tactile hemi-inattention may frequently hang his or her arm over the side of the wheelchair in a position that makes it prone to injury and swelling. An auditory cue to reposition the left arm may be provided by a bell attached to a flexible plastic stick on the left side of the wheelchair that the patient's arm bumps when it slides off the arm rest.

Virtually any activity that involves scanning, exploring, or manipulating materials in the patient's neglected areas of space can be a useful therapeutic task for patients with stimulus neglect. The range of activities that can be used varies from simple paper-and-pencil letter or shape cancellation tasks to sophisticated computer programs that require the patient to respond rapidly to stimuli occurring in randomly determined positions on the computer monitor. Both extremes of technological sophistication can be effective, and lack of technology need not be a barrier to treatment.

CASE ILLUSTRATIONS

CASE 4–1

F.C. was a 43-year-old woman with a history of poorly managed diabetes. While being treated for an abscess on her left thigh, she suffered a right-hemisphere cerebrovascular accident, resulting in a left hemiparesis. Motor functioning was fully intact on the patient's right. Computed tomographic (CT) scans showed an old lacunar infarct in the left hemisphere and a recent, probably thrombotic infarct in the distribution of the right middle cerebral artery involving the centrum semiovale. Her initial neuropsychological examination revealed full visual fields and no difficulty in detecting stimuli in either visual field during bilateral simultaneous stimulation. She made no errors when asked to identify colors, pictures of objects, and faces of six recent United States presidents. She was also able to obtain a normal score on a test requiring her to match and discriminate among faces shown from different angles in black-and-white photographs. Despite F.C.'s good performance on these visual tasks, she had extreme difficulty in bisecting lines with her right hand. Figure 4–2 shows F.C.'s performance on the Line Bisection Test. She failed to detect four of six lines oriented to the left side of the page, but missed none of the lines oriented to the center or right of the page. Considering only the lines that were detected, F.C. showed a clear tendency to bisect to the right of center.

CASE 4–2

M.E. was a 74-year-old woman who presented with a right-sided embolic cerebrovascular accident. CT scans revealed infarction of the right caudate head of the basal ganglia with involvement of the anterior limb of the internal capsule. Neurological and neuropsychological examinations demonstrated a left hemiparesis (motor functions were normal on the patient's right side), reduced memory, borderline intellectual functioning, and severely impaired problem-solving skills. The patient had the full range of eye movement. No errors in unilateral auditory stimulation occurred, but left-sided auditory extinction (four extinctions in four trials) was identified on the HRB SPE. Extinction could not be assessed in other sensory modalities because of the occurrence of errors in response to unilateral left-sided stimulation that did not decrease when attention was directed to that side.

Figure 4–3 shows M.E.'s attempts to bisect lines with her right hand. A percent deviation score of +40.9 was obtained; omitted lines were not included

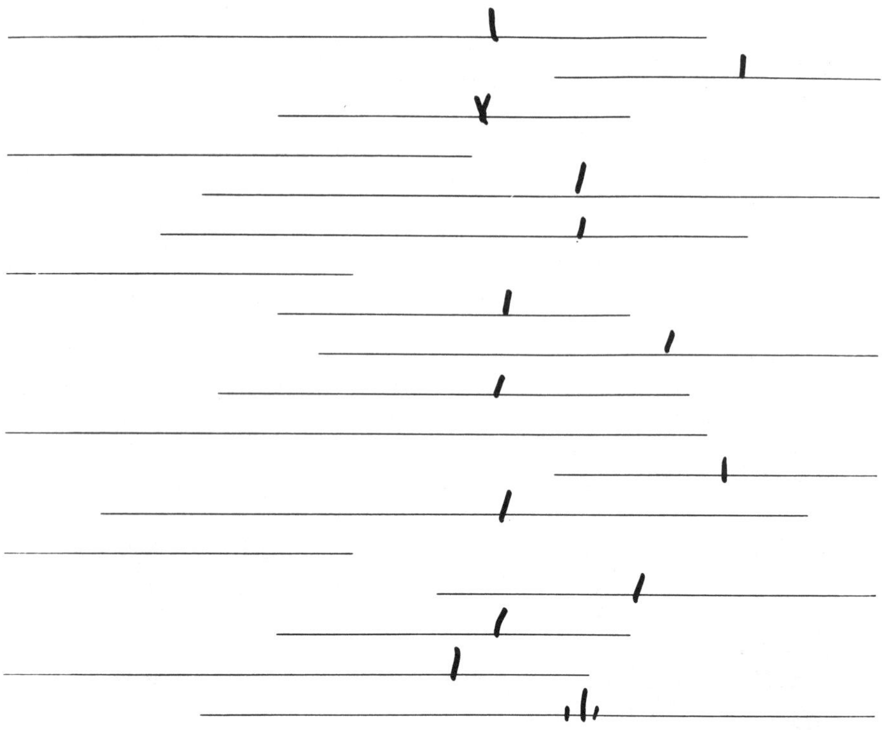

FIGURE 4–2. Line bisection test results in Case 4–1 (F.C.). The demonstration line marked by the examiner is not shown.

when calculating this index. Also notable was the omission of four lines oriented to the left and four lines oriented to the center of the page. One omission occurred on the right side.

CASE 4–3

J.B. was a 22-year-old man who suffered a traumatic brain injury as a result of a bicycle accident. CT scans showed bilateral frontal contusions, hemorrhage in the interhemispheric fissure, and hemorrhage in the right temporal and parietal areas. The patient subsequently hemorrhaged into the genu of the corpus callosum and frontal lobes from a ruptured pericallosal artery aneurysm.

A variety of neuropsychological disorders were evident in this young man, including left-sided visual extinction on 11 of 12 bilateral simultaneous stimulation trials on the HRB SPE. When unilateral visual stimulation alone was presented, no failures to detect the stimulus occurred on the right side, and only two failures occurred on the left. Notably, visual fields were full during confrontation testing. A trend in the same direction was evident in the tactile (four left-sided suppressions) and auditory (one left-sided suppression) modalities, although the results were not as strong. Figure 4–4 shows J.B.'s attempts to draw a flower from a model, and

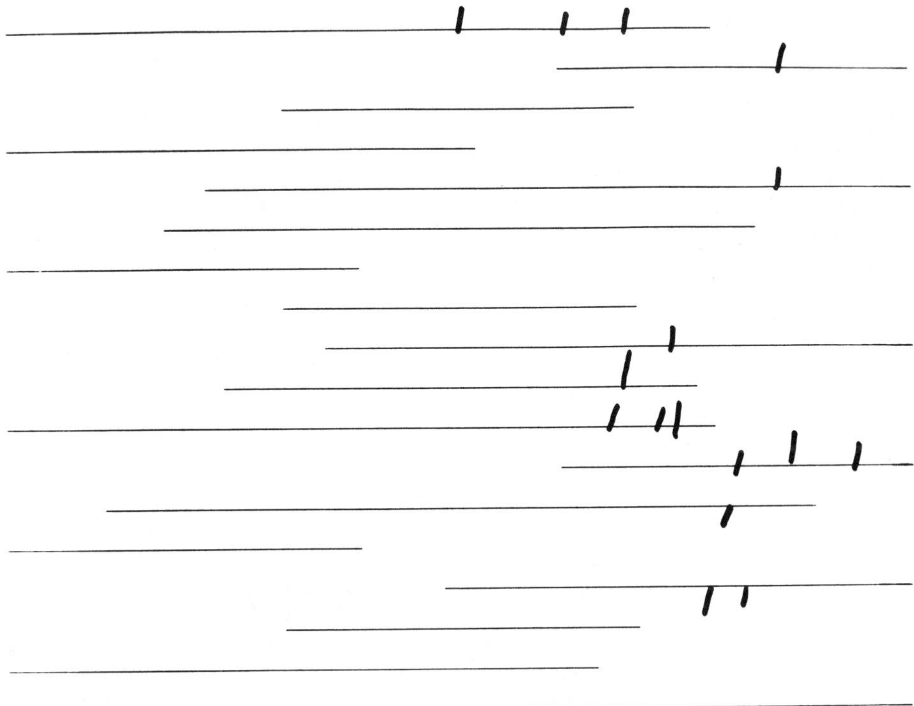

FIGURE 4–3. Line bisection test results in Case 4–2 (M.E.). The demonstration line marked by the examiner is not shown. Multiple marks were placed on some lines by M.E. when she failed to notice her own previous marks.

Figure 4–5 shows J.B.'s rendition of a clock drawn from memory. Both drawings notably lack detail on the left side and show J.B.'s attempt to crowd all details into the right side of the drawings.

DISCUSSION

All three of these patients exhibited hemispatial neglect. The disorder was more severe and was accompanied by sensory extinction in Cases 4–2 and 4–3. Line bisection results varied among the cases. In Case 4–1, errors were made only in the left side of space. However, Case 4–2 demonstrated errors in the left, center, and right portions of the Line Bisection Test. With errors predominating in the left and center, a diagnosis of left hemispatial neglect remains valid. Case 4–3 showed hemispatial neglect in drawings done from memory and with a model present. In all three patients, a brain lesion compromised functioning in brain areas known to be implicated in neglect.

CASE 4–4

L.R. was a 71-year-old retired airline pilot. He suffered a right-hemisphere cerebrovascular accident, which resulted in left-homonymous hemianopsia and left

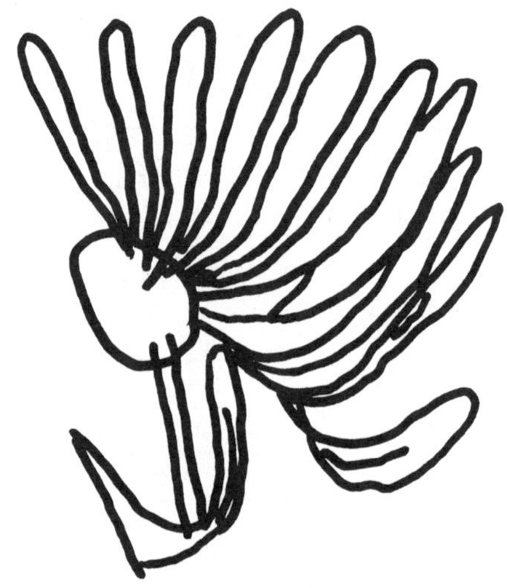

FIGURE 4–4. Drawing of a flower from the model shown on the left by the patient in Case 4–3 (J.B.).

hemiparesis. The patient made a single error in unilateral visual stimulation with both eyes open and no errors in unilateral tactile stimulation on the HRB SPE. In contrast, L.R. failed to respond to left-sided unilateral auditory stimulation; one error was also made on the right. When questioned, he denied any hearing deficit.

Eight additional trials of unilateral auditory stimulation were given in each ear. Left-sided errors occurred in four trials, and no errors occurred on the right. The patient was then instructed to pay attention to his left ear and to indicate whenever

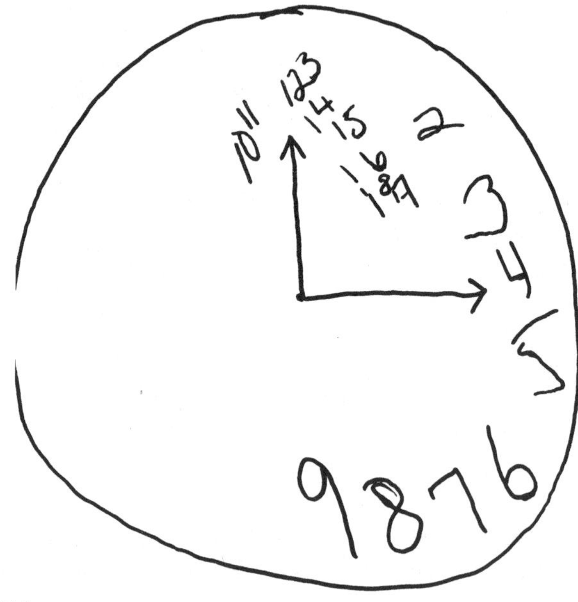

FIGURE 4–5. Rendition of a clock from memory by the patient in Case 4–3 (J.B.).

he heard the stimulus. Eight more trials were given to the left ear only, and the interval between trials varied randomly. The patient reliably detected the onset of the stimulus on each trial, responding within 2 to 3 seconds after presentation.

DISCUSSION

Hemi-inattention in the auditory modality was present in this patient. It is evident that the problem was not caused by a hearing deficit because performance markedly improved when attention was directed to the left side during testing.

CASE 4–5

R.M. was a 50-year-old man with a high school education. After triple coronary artery bypass grafting, he developed atrial fibrillation and an anoxic encephalopathy. Magnetic resonance imaging revealed bilateral watershed area infarctions (i.e., C-shaped infarctions extending from the frontal to the occipital poles), with greater damage evident in the right hemisphere.

R.M. had full visual fields, but visual acuity could not be assessed because of his inability to discriminate even the largest letters on the Snellen chart. Acuity was sufficient for the patient to reliably identify colors, line drawings, and people seen from distances of up to 20 feet. R.M.'s gaze tended to shift to the right when nothing held his attention. He was unable to move his eyes reliably in any direction on demand when his eyes were open. He could move his gaze from side to side, upward, and downward when his eyelids were held shut by the examiner. R.M. was unable to point accurately to positions in space with his right hand, despite having only a mild degree of weakness on this side. Pointing with the left hand was impossible because of severe hemiparesis. R.M. also had difficulty in determining the position of visual, auditory, and left-sided tactile stimuli when reaching was not involved (see Stimulus mislocalization). He produced only meaningless scribbles on even simple drawing or writing tasks, and when he was asked to bisect lines, his performance was grossly distorted and uninterpretable.

When shown photographs of scenes from the BIT, R.M. was able to identify most parts of the pictures. When shown drawings of scenes, however, R.M. initially saw only isolated details to the right of the scene. With encouragement to further explore the drawings, he perceived more details of the scene. R.M. was able to identify only one of five shapes formed by dot patterns, although he was able to count the dots. He successfully identified multipart shapes such as a pyramid and a cylinder, but again had difficulty in integrating black-and-white patterns to perceive letters (three of five correct). His errors on the latter task consisted of ignoring the white portions of the letters and basing his identification of the letters solely on the black portions. R.M. ignored the white portions of the letters even when they were in the center or to the right of the black portions that he perceived correctly.

DISCUSSION

Case 4–5 presented a diagnostic challenge. Left hemispatial neglect was suspected because the patient tended to perceive details from only the right side of complex drawings. However, no such deficit was evident when he viewed comparably complex photographs, and the combination of motor weakness, drawing difficulty, and problems with visual acuity precluded use of line bisection and drawing tasks to detect hemispatial neglect.

The patient showed difficulty in detecting shapes formed by dot patterns, and some difficulty in simultaneously perceiving differently colored portions of letters. These findings suggest at least mild simultanagnosia. Despite the difficulty in assessing visual acuity, the patient saw the stimuli clearly, because he was able to count the dots in each pattern and could identify the portions of the letter stimuli that were in one color. His difficulty in pointing to targets (see Optic ataxia) and inability to shift his gaze on demand (see Oculomotor apraxia) lend support to, but do not confirm, the diagnosis of simultanagnosia, because these three disorders together comprise Balint's syndrome. (See Chap. 7 for a further discussion of this patient's pointing deficit.) The patient's bilateral watershed infarcts are also consistent with this diagnosis.

REFERENCES

1. American Psychiatric Association: Diagnostic and Statistical Manual of Mental Disorders, Fourth Edition. American Psychiatric Association, Washington, DC, 1994.
2. The International Classification of Diseases, Ninth Revision, Clinical Modification. Med-Index, Salt Lake City, 1991.
3. De Renzi, E: Disorders of Space Exploration and Cognition. John Wiley and Sons, New York, 1982.
4. Barbut, D, and Gazzaniga, MS: Disturbances in conceptual space involving language and speech. Brain 110:1487, 1987.
5. Pierrot-Deseilligny, C, Gray, F, and Brunet, P: Infarcts of both inferior parietal lobules with impairment of visually guided eye movements, peripheral visual inattention and optic ataxia. Brain 109:81, 1986.
6. Costlett, HB, et al: Directional hypokinesia and hemispatial inattention in neglect. Brain 113:475, 1990.
7. Heilman, KM: Thalamic neglect. Neurology 29:690, 1979.
8. Cappa, S, et al: Remission of hemineglect and anosognosia during vestibular stimulation. Neuropsychologia 25:775, 1987.
9. Graff-Radford, NR, and Rizzo, M: Neglect in a patient with multiple sclerosis. Eur Neurol 26:100, 1987.
10. Healton, EB, et al: Subcortical neglect. Neurology 32:776, 1982.
11. Damasio, AR, Damasio, H, and Chang Chui, H: Neglect following damage to frontal lobe or basal ganglia. Neuropsychologia 18:123, 1980.
12. Heilman, KM, and Valenstein, E: Auditory neglect in man. Arch Neurol 26:32, 1972.
13. Schwartz, AS, Marchok, PL, and Flynn, RE: A sensitive test for tactile extinction: Results in patients with parietal and frontal lobe disease. J Neurol Neurosurg Psychiatry 40:228, 1977.
14. Heilman, KM, and Howell, GJ: Seizure-induced neglect. J Neurol Neurosurg Psychiatry 43:1035, 1980.
15. Heilman, KM, and Valenstein, E: Frontal lobe neglect in man. Neurology 22:660, 1972.
16. Henderson, VW, Alexander, MP, and Naeser, MA: Right thalamic injury, impaired visuospatial perception, and alexia. Neurology 32:235, 1982.
17. Bogousslavsky, J, Regli, F, and Assal, G: The syndrome of unilateral tuberothalamic artery territory infarction. Stroke 17:434, 1986.
18. Chamorro, A, et al: Visual hemineglect and hemihallucinations in a patient with a subcortical infarction. Neurology 40:1463, 1990.
19. Ferro, JM, Kertesz, A, and Black, SE: Subcortical neglect: Quantitation, anatomy, and recovery. Neurology 37:1487, 1987.

20. Bogousslavsky, J, et al: Subcortical neglect: Neuropsychological, SPECT, and neuropathological correlations with anterior choroidal artery territory infarction. Ann Neurol 23:448, 1988.
21. Weintraub, S, and Mesulam, MM: Visual hemispatial inattention: Stimulus parameters and exploratory strategies. J Neurol Neurosurg Psychiatry 51:1481, 1988.
22. Rapcsak, SZ, Watson, RT, and Heilman, KM: Hemispace-visual field interactions in visual extinction. J Neurol Neurosurg Psychiatry 50:1117, 1987.
23. Rosselli, M, et al: Topography of the hemi-inattention syndrome. Int J Neurosci 27:165, 1985.
24. Rapcsak, SZ, Cimino, CR, Heilman, KM: Altitudinal neglect. Neurology 38:277, 1988.
25. Tanaka, Y, Iwasa, H, and Obayashi, T: Right hand agraphia and left hand apraxia following callosal damage in a right-hander. Cortex 26:665, 1990.
26. Musiek, FE, et al: The dichotic rhyme task: Results in split-brain patients. Ear Hear 10:33, 1989.
27. Corballis, MC, and Ogden, JA: Dichotic listening in commissurotomized and hemispherectomized subjects. Neuropsychologia 26:565, 1988.
28. Alexander, MP, and Warren, RL: Localization of callosal auditory pathways: A CT case study. Neurology 38:802, 1988.
29. Musiek, FE, Reeves, AG, and Baran, JA: Release from central auditory competition in the split-brain patient. Neurology 35:983, 1985.
30. Springer, SP, and Gazzaniga, MS: Dichotic testing of partial and complete split brain subjects. Neuropsychologia 13:341, 1975.
31. Damasio, H, and Damasio, A: "Paradoxic" ear extinction in dichotic listening: Possible anatomic significance. Neurology 29:644, 1979.
32. Damasio, H, et al: Dichotic listening pattern in relation to interhemispheric disconnexion. Neuropsychologia 14:247, 1976.
33. Arboix, A, et al: Auditory ear extinction in lacunar syndromes. Acta Neurol Scand 81:507, 1990.
34. Schwartz, AS, et al: The asymmetric lateralization of tactile extinction in patients with unilateral cerebral dysfunction. Brain 102:669, 1979.
35. Heilman, KM, and Valenstein, E: Mechanisms underlying hemispatial neglect. Ann Neurol 5:166, 1979.
36. Chedru, F, Leblanc, M, and Lhermitte, F: Visual searching in normal and brain-damaged subjects (contribution to the study of unilateral inattention). Cortex 9:94, 1973.
37. Rapcsak, SZ, et al: Selective attention in hemispatial neglect. Arch Neurol 46:178, 1989.
38. Meinberg, O, Harrer, M, and Wehren, C: Oculographic diagnosis of hemineglect in patients with homonymous hemianopia. J Neurol 233:97, 1986.
39. Rubens, AB: Caloric stimulation and unilateral visual neglect. Neurology 35:1019, 1985.
40. Heilman, KM, et al: Directional hypokinesia: Prolonged reaction times for leftward movements in patients with right hemisphere lesions and neglect. Neurology 35:855, 1985.
41. Heilman, KM, Bowers, D, and Watson, RT: Performance on hemispatial pointing task by patients with neglect syndrome. Neurology 33:661, 1983.
42. Colombo, A, De Renzi, E, and Gentilini, M: The time course of visual hemi-inattention. Arch Psychiatr Nervenkr 231:539, 1982.
43. Henderson, VW, Alexander, MP, and Naeser, MA: Right thalamic injury, impaired visuospatial perception, and alexia. Neurology 32:235, 1982.
44. Karnath, HO, and Hartje, W: Residual information processing in the neglected visual half-field. J Neurol 234:180, 1987.
45. Ogden, JA: Anterior-posterior interhemispheric differences in the loci of lesions producing visual hemineglect. Brain Cogn 4:59, 1985.
46. Ferro, JM, and Kertesz, A: Posterior internal capsule infarction associated with neglect. Arch Neurol 41:422, 1984.
47. Albert, ML: A simple test of visual neglect. Neurology 23:658, 1973.
48. Luria, AR: Disorders of simultaneous perception in a case of bilateral occipitoparietal brain injury. Brain 82:437, 1959.
49. Rizzo, M, and Robin, DA: Simultanagnosia: A defect of sustained attention yields insights on visual information processing. Neurology 40:447, 1990.
50. Rizzo, M, and Hurtig, R: Looking but not seeing: Attention, perception, and eye movements in simultanagnosia. Neurology 37:1642, 1987.
51. Trobe, JR, and Bauer, RM: Seeing but not recognizing. Surv Ophthalmol 30:328, 1986.
52. Heilman, KM, Watson, RT, and Valenstein, E: Neglect and related disorders. In Heilman, KM, and Valenstein, E (eds): Clinical Neuropsychology, Second Edition. Oxford University Press, New York, 1985, p 243.

53. Lezak, M: Neuropsychological Assessment, Second Edition. Oxford University Press, New York, 1983.
54. Franzen, MD: Reliability and Validity in Neuropsychological Assessment. Plenum Press, New York, 1989.
55. Goldstein, G, and Shelly, CH: Univariate vs. multivariate analysis in neuropsychological test assessment of lateralized brain damage. Cortex 9:204, 1973.
56. Freides, D: Do dichotic listening procedures measure lateralization of information processing or retrieval strategy? Perception and Psychophysics 21:259, 1977.
57. Rao, SM, et al: Cerebral disconnection in multiple sclerosis. Relationship to atrophy of the corpus callosum. Arch Neurol 46:918, 1989.
58. Schenkenberg, T, Bradford, DC, and Ajax, ET: Line bisection and unilateral visual neglect in patients with neurologic impairment. Neurology 30:509, 1980.
59. Trenerry, MR, et al: Visual Search and Attention Test Professional Manual. Psychological Assessment Resources, Odessa, FL, 1990.
60. Wilson, B, Cockburn, J, and Halligan, P: Behavioural Inattention Test. Thames Valley Test Company, England, 1987.
61. De Renzi, E, Faglioni, P, and Scotti, G: Hemispheric contribution to exploration of space through the visual and tactile modality. Cortex 6:191, 1970.
62. Meienberg, O: Clinical examination of saccadic eye movements in hemianopia. Neurology 33:1311, 1983.

STIMULUS IMPERCEPTION

5

Stimulus imperception is an inability to perceive visual, auditory, or tactual stimuli accurately. In patients with diffuse or bilateral posterior brain damage, stimulus imperception can be so severe that it prevents the recognition of common objects and other stimuli. Stimulus imperception following unilateral brain damage typically spares recognition of stimuli, but the patient is unable to discriminate between subtly dissimilar stimuli.

Reduced sensation impairs the perception of complex stimuli. In patients with elementary sensory loss, the assessment of the ability to discern more complex stimuli adds little to the neuropsychological examination. Not all clinicians discriminate between sensory impairment and impairment of more complex perceptual tasks. When both types of impairment are present, the latter is simply attributed to the former. Unfortunately, when this is done, the clinician has no way of knowing where in the neural circuit between the peripheral receptor and the cortex the lesion has occurred. In this text, the stimulus imperception subtypes are defined in a manner that excludes deficits in more basic sensory perception. This lowers the potential number of lesion sites and maximizes the usefulness of including an assessment of stimulus imperception in the neuropsychological examination.

Impaired perception of spatial information (see Chap. 6) often accompanies stimulus imperception. When present, spatial imperception doubtlessly contributes to the impaired discrimination of stimuli. In some cases of tactile form imperception, the discrimination deficit may be accounted for largely by a spatial factor.[1] Stimulus and spatial imperception are, however, dissociable in the visual modality.[2] Although stimulus and spatial imperception are discussed separately in this text, it is acknowledged that, in the tactile sensory modality, this separation is arbitrary.

Illusions and hallucinations (see Chap. 17) may also accompany stimulus imperception and can impair perception when they are present. Unlike the disorders listed in this chapter, illusions and hallucinations cannot be documented by objective tests or reliably elicited by a stimulus or task that is under the control of the examiner. Consequently, Chapter 17 is devoted to the diagnosis of illusions and hallucinations.

Stimulus imperception includes the subtypes listed under "Variety of Presentation" in the chapter outline. Three general issues concerning the subtyping of stimulus imperception are briefly addressed.

The separation of visual form and facial imperception into two subtypes is questionable, because both involve the perception of visual stimuli, and there is substantial overlap in the lesions that produce these two disorders (see later text). Some theoretical reasons exist for separating the two disorders into two subtypes. Faces occur in a patient's natural environment, and discrimination among faces is vital in human life. In contrast, the abstract shapes used in the clinic to assess visual form perception have no counterpart in nature and play no role in everyday life. Considering the importance of facial discrimination in human life, specialized neural mechanisms for the discrimination among faces may have evolved. No such evolutionary mechanism is likely to exist for discrimination mechanisms tailored to abstract visual forms. Consequently, it is possible that visual form and facial discrimination tasks may be measuring somewhat different, albeit overlapping, discrimination abilities.

I know of no studies that have systematically documented the comorbidity of facial and visual form imperception. I have chosen to list the disorders separately until data on their comorbidity become available. It is hoped that listing these subtypes separately will spur epidemiological study of these disorders.

Another issue centers on the relation between stimulus imperception and agnosia. According to strict definitions, agnosia is an impairment in the ability to recognize certain types of stimuli (e.g., objects, faces) in the absence of sensory or perceptual impairment.[3] However, most published cases of agnosia have some degree of sensory impairment, perceptual impairment, or both. In addition, some authors regard patients with bilateral posterior lesions who have severe sensory and perceptual impairment and who fail to recognize stimuli as having a special category of agnosia commonly referred to as "apperceptive agnosia." Although it was proposed decades ago, the concept of apperceptive agnosia is still controversial and does not fit the strict definition of agnosia as a failure of stimulus recognition in the absence of other perceptual impairments.

The controversy over apperceptive agnosia is likely to continue until more is known about the cognitive and neural processes involved in normal stimulus recognition. At a conceptual level, pure agnosia (i.e., agnosia not caused by sensory or perceptual deficits) can be distinguished from apperceptive agnosia and stimulus imperception. Perception is presumably impaired in the latter two conditions, as evidenced by an inability to match and discriminate among stimuli. In pure agnosia, perceptual impairment may be present but is insufficient to account for the recognition failure. No clear conceptual or clinical division can be made between apperceptive agnosia and stimulus imperception, because both consist of an impairment in basic perceptual ability.

In this book, stimulus imperception and apperceptive agnosia are not distinguished from each other; they are treated as synonymous disorders of perception that can be so severe that they result in failed stimulus recognition. Pure or "associative" agnosia is defined as a disorder of recognition in the absence of sensory and perceptual deficits. Associative agnosia is discussed further in Chapter 9.

Another issue concerns auditory pattern imperception. I have subsumed a small set of perceptual deficits related to the perception of sound and music under this term. Many more deficits in music perception and production may be seen following cortical lesions in professional and amateur musicians, including impairment in reading and writing musical notation (i.e., musical alexia and agraphia), impairment in the oral and instrumental expression of music (i.e., oral expressive and instrumental amusia), and impaired recognition of previously familiar songs.

Musical training is less common in the lay population of the United States than in some European countries, and relatively few North American neuropsychologists include a comprehensive assessment of musical ability in their examinations. In the United States lay population, an extensive assessment of musical ability may yield little interpretable data because of the relative absence of premorbid musical skill and training. Consequently, I have chosen to focus only on those aspects of musical ability that are minimally dependent on premorbid training when characterizing auditory pattern imperception (see later). More comprehensive systems of subtyping music-related deficits have been proposed.[4] Neuropsychologists involved in the assessment of professional and well-trained amateur musicians may wish to use a more comprehensive classification than that provided in this book.

NOMENCLATURE

The specific forms of stimulus imperception have various names in the neurology and neuropsychology literature. Color imperception is also called "achromatopsia" or "dyschromatopsia," "apperceptive color agnosia," and "color amnesia." Color imperception is sometimes confused with color anomia, which is a disorder of oral language rather than a purely perceptual disorder (see Chap. 12).

Tactual form imperception, depending on how it is assessed, has been termed "agraphesthesia," "haptic imperception," and "tactual imperception." Tactual form imperception is sometimes grouped with deficits in tactual recognition under the single label "astereognosis." This clustering is predicated on the belief that deficits in tactual recognition result from deficits in tactual perception. However, cases of impaired tactual recognition with preserved tactual perception have been reported, suggesting that they are distinct entities.[5–7] Consistent with this finding, the term *astereognosis* is reserved in this text for impaired tactual recognition in the absence of tactual form imperception. Astereognosis is discussed in Chapter 9.

The other stimulus imperception disorders are often discussed in the literature in terms of the specific task used to elicit them. Thus, if the task is to discriminate between complex visual designs, the term *visual discrimination* may be used. If the patient is asked to find forms hidden within larger designs, the clinician may speak of "embedded figure performance" or "figure-ground discrimination." If the patient is asked to identify incomplete or blurry figures, the term *closure* may be used. Perceptual deficits involving auditory stimuli may be described as problems in *auditory discrimination*, *rhythm perception*, or *tonal perception*. The terms *facial identification*, *facial perception*, and *facial discrimination* are used in describing facial imperception.

The problem with discussing perceptual disorders in terms of specific diagnostic tasks is that the number of possible tasks is limited only by the imagination of the clinician or researcher. Thus, scores of slightly different terms can be used for the same basic deficit. For practicality, the terms *visual form*, *facial*, *tactual form*, and *auditory pattern imperception* are used in this text to refer to deficits in the performance of these various diagnostic tasks.

Each permutation of a basic visual, facial, tactual, or auditory perception task makes slightly different demands on the brain; consequently, the lesion loci producing impairment in performing the various tasks can vary. The major types of perceptual tasks in use were considered when formulating the clinical indicators and lesion locations for the disorders in this chapter. What these tasks are should be clear after reading the clinical indicators and assessment instruments listed in subsequent text. If the clinician decides to use highly dissimilar tests, the lesion locations for the stimulus imperception disorders may no longer apply.

DSM-IV[8] does not include a diagnostic category specific to stimulus imperception. The nonspecific diagnoses "Cognitive Disorder Not Otherwise Specified" and "Mild Neurocognitive Disorder" may be used for stimulus imperception as a result of brain damage. Psychogenic imperception is coded in DSM-IV as "Conversion Disorder" if the deficit is unconsciously produced by the patient. Deliberate faking or exaggeration of imperception to obtain a material goal is diagnosed as "Malingering" in DSM-IV. If the goal is simply the assumption of a dependent patient role, the code for "Factitious Disorder" can be used. Finally, if psychogenic imperception is part of a long history of multiple somatic complaints having no physiological basis, then the DSM-IV diagnosis "Somatization Disorder" may be appropriate.

Additional ICD-9-CM[9] codes for the stimulus imperception subtypes are difficult to identify. Facial and visual form imperception may be coded as "Unspecified Subjective Visual Disturbances," "Unspecified Visual Disturbance," or "Other Specified Visual Disturbances." Unfortunately, much of the precision of neuropsychological diagnosis is lost when these rather vague terms are used. In addition, inclusion of the word *subjective* in diagnostic codes implies that the diagnosis is based on patient complaints rather than on objective testing. This is not the case in the neuropsychological examination that uses objective performance measures.

Tactual form imperception may be coded in ICD-9-CM as a "Disturbance of Skin Sensation," although this term is only marginally appropriate because it includes symptoms such as numbness, tingling, and burning sensations rather than being restricted to discrimination deficits. ICD-9-CM includes the diagnostic code "Impairment of Auditory Discrimination," which can be used for auditory pattern imperception.

RULES FOR DIAGNOSIS

Clinical Indicators: Each is independent (only one must be observed for the disorder to be suspected) *except* when subscripting is used. Subscripted numbers (a_1, a_2) denote an indicator with multiple parts that must be considered together.

Associated Features: These are listed to give a more complete picture of the disorders. The presence or absence of these features does not affect the diagnosis.

Factors to Rule Out: All must be taken into account. Failure to rule out even one of these factors makes a firm diagnosis impossible.

Lesion Locations: Each location stands alone; damage in only one of the listed areas is sufficient to produce the disorder.

VARIETY OF PRESENTATION

1. **Color imperception (also called "achromatopsia" or "dyschromatopsia," "apperceptive color agnosia," "and color amnesia"; see also Color anomia)**

Clinical Indicators

a. Inaccurate sorting of colors by hue
b. Inaccurate matching of colors
c. Inaccurate detection of colored stimuli embedded in distractingly colored backgrounds

Associated Features

a. Loss of color vision or all colors appearing to be the same reported by patient
b. Color imperception occurring in all or only a portion of the visual field (e.g., hemiachromatopsia, or color imperception in one visual half-field)
c. Impairment of spatial perception (see Chap. 6)
d. Impaired recognition of previously familiar faces (see Prosopagnosia)
e. Presence of homonymous hemianopsia (loss of acuity in one visual half-field) or quadrantanopsia (loss of acuity in one quadrant of the visual field of each eye)
f. Impaired oral language (see Chap. 12)
g. Impaired written language (see Chap. 13)

Factors to Rule Out

a. Loss of visual acuity so severe that the patient fails to see color stimuli regardless of where they are presented in the visual field.
b. Impaired oral or written language sufficient to prevent responses on color perception tests. If language is impaired, color perception tests that do not require language comprehension or verbal responses should be used.
c. A history of premorbid deficits in color perception.

Lesion Locations

a. Inferior temporal and occipital lobes, fusiform and lingual gyri[10–18]

Lesion Lateralization

a. Occurrence following right- or left-sided lesions
b. Unilateral lesions causing color imperception in the contralateral visual field

2. **Visual form imperception**

Clinical Indicators

a. Inaccurate matching or discrimination of complex visual stimuli, excluding faces
b. Inaccurate detection of visual forms embedded in complex backgrounds (i.e., impaired figure-ground discrimination)
c_1. Inaccurate determination of the identity of visual stimuli that are partially obscured, shown from unusual angles, or lack salient details
c_2. Preservation of ability to identify the same stimuli presented clearly and in full detail

Associated Features

a. Preservation of ability to discriminate stimuli based on size, length, or other elementary physical properties
b. Presence of homonymous hemianopsia (i.e., loss of acuity in one visual half-field)
c. Impaired oral language (see Chap. 12)

Factors to Rule Out

a. Loss of visual acuity so severe that the patient fails to see stimuli regardless of where in the visual field they are presented
b. Failure to detect portions of visual stimuli as a result of stimulus neglect (see Chap. 4)
c. Impaired concentration (see Chap. 3) during lengthy testing of perceptual ability

Lesion Locations

a. Cerebral hemisphere, especially posterior to the central sulcus[19–23]
b. Temporal lobe[24,25]
c. Intersection of temporal, parietal, and occipital lobes[26]

Lesion Lateralization

a. More frequent and more severe following right-sided lesions[19,20,24–26]

3. Facial imperception

Clinical Indicator

a. Inaccurate matching or discrimination of faces based on their visual details

Associated Features

a. Presence of homonymous hemianopsia (i.e., loss of acuity in one visual half-field)
b. Impaired oral language (see Chap. 12)

Factors to Rule Out

a. Loss of visual acuity so severe that the patient fails to see stimuli regardless of where in the visual field they are presented
b. Failure to detect portions of visual stimuli as a result of stimulus neglect (see Chap. 4)
c. Impaired concentration (see Chap. 3) during lengthy testing of perceptual ability

Lesion Locations

a. Cerebral hemisphere, particularly posterior to the central sulcus[27–30]
b. Combined cerebral hemisphere and brainstem[31]
c. Temporal lobe[32]

Lesion Lateralization

a. More frequent and more severe following right-sided lesions[27–30,32]

4. Tactual form imperception

Clinical Indicators

a_1. Agraphesthesia, or inaccurate matching or discrimination of forms (e.g., letters, numbers, shapes) traced on the skin, usually of the fingertips or palms, while vision is occluded

a_2. Occurrence of deficit on one or both sides of the body

b_1. Inaccurate matching or discrimination of three-dimensional shapes or objects by touch while vision is occluded

b_2. Occurrence of deficit on one or both sides of the body

Associated Features

a. Impaired ability to determine the position of the limbs, fingers, or toes (i.e., proprioception) on one or both sides of the body when vision is occluded
b. Impaired ability to determine the location of tactile stimuli when vision is occluded (see Stimulus mislocalization)
c. Decreased tactile sensation on one or both sides of the body

Factors to Rule Out

a. Loss of tactile sensation so severe that the patient does not feel the tactual form stimulus
b. Inability to palpate three-dimensional stimuli because of weakness or poor coordination of the hand muscles

Lesion Locations

a. Cerebral hemisphere, particularly posterior to the central sulcus in some reports[33–36]

Lesion Lateralization

a. More frequent, more severe, or both following right-sided lesions[33–36]
b. Left-sided lesions tending to produce contralateral impairment, whereas right-sided lesions tend to produce bilateral impairment[33–35]

5. Auditory pattern imperception (also called "amusia")

Clinical Indicators

a. Inaccurate matching or discrimination of nonmeaningful, pronounceable combinations of consonant and vowel sounds (i.e., consonant and vowel combinations that do not spell words)
b. Inaccurate matching or discrimination of patterns or sequences of sound that vary in pitch
c. Inaccurate matching or discrimination of patterns or sequences of sound that vary in intensity
d. Inaccurate matching or discrimination of patterns or sequences of sound that vary in timbre
e. Inaccurate matching or discrimination of patterns or sequences of sound that vary in rhythm
f. Inaccurate matching or discrimination of patterns or sequences of sound that vary in harmony

Associated Features

a. Impaired oral language, particularly pure word deafness (see Chap. 12)
b. Normal or near-normal hearing of pure tones and speech during audiologic examination
c. Impaired localization of sounds in space when vision is occluded (see Stimulus mislocalization)

d. Recent history of partial or total deafness following cortical lesions
e. Impaired recognition of familiar music and environmental sounds (see Auditory agnosia)

Factors to Rule Out

a. Loss of hearing in both ears so severe that it prevents the patient from detecting and responding to sounds
b. Impaired concentration (see Chap. 3) during lengthy testing of perceptual ability

Lesion Locations

a. Cerebral hemisphere[37–39]
b. Temporal lobe, particularly the superior temporal gyrus, including Heschl's gyrus and the auditory radiation, and the combined temporal and parietal lobes, particularly the supramarginal and angular gyri[40–43]

Lesion Lateralization

a. May follow right, left, or bilateral lesions
b. Right-sided lesions impairing melodic aspects of music differentially, whereas left-sided lesions may impair rhythmic aspects of music differentially[38]

6. Psychogenic imperception

Clinical Indicators

a_1. Severity of perceptual or spatial impairment exceeding the known extent of the illness or brain lesion

a_2. Atypical course or presentation of the perceptual or spatial impairment as evidenced by any of the following signs:
1) Absence of a clear precipitating illness or brain lesion
2) An unaccountable period between the onset of illness or lesion and the onset of the perceptual or spatial impairment
3) Inconsistent perceptual or spatial performance among equivalent examinations
4) Inconsistent perceptual or spatial performance among equivalent situations (e.g., situations that place equal demands on perceptual or spatial ability and that are equally likely to facilitate perceptual or spatial performance)

a_3. Motivational factors contributing to the presence of the perceptual or spatial impairment, as evidenced by any of the following signs:
1) Failure to exert the effort required to perform perceptual or spatial tasks
2) Perceptual or spatial impairment permitting avoidance of unpleasant consequences or responsibilities
3) Perceptual or spatial impairment leading to or expected to produce emotional benefits or material compensation

Associated Features

a. Some degree of impaired perceptual or spatial performance caused by neurological illness or brain lesion

b. Depressed mood or major depressive disorder
c. Fear or anxiety
d. Hysterical conversion disorder: A mental disorder characterized by the unconscious expression of mental and emotional conflicts and stress through physical symptoms
e. Post-traumatic stress disorder: A mental disorder arising after the experience of intense emotional or physical trauma and stress, characterized by panic, a tendency to reexperience the source of trauma in dreams or waking flashbacks, and reenactment of behavior shown at the time of the original trauma
f. Malingering: Deliberate feigning of symptoms to reach a goal
g. Factitious disorder: A mental disorder characterized by the intentional feigning of symptoms because of a need to assume the role of a sick person
h. Somatization disorder: A mental disorder characterized by a history of multiple physical complaints of uncertain etiology

Factors to Rule Out

a. Neurological illness or a brain lesion of sufficient extent to account for the perceptual or spatial impairment, ruled out by documenting the excessiveness of the perceptual or spatial impairment and an atypical pattern or course of impairment

Lesion Locations

Not associated with structural brain damage

ETIOLOGY

As with most neuropsychological disorders, cerebrovascular disease is the most common cause of stimulus imperception. Traumatic brain injury, particularly when the posterior cerebral hemispheres are involved, can also cause stimulus imperception. Neoplasm is a less common cause. The severest cases of stimulus imperception result from bilateral posterior damage. In these cases, multiple bilateral strokes may have occurred. Basilar artery occlusion impairs functioning in both posterior hemispheres and is common in severe cases of imperception. Degenerative diseases can lead to atrophy and dysfunction in both cerebral hemispheres and can consequently lead to imperception. Any disease process that diffusely affects brain functioning is a potential cause of stimulus imperception. This includes anoxia as a result of cardiac arrest and metabolic compromise of the brain as a result of poisoning or intoxication. Carbon monoxide and mercury poisoning, in particular, have been documented as causes in cases of stimulus imperception. Alcoholism and other forms of substance abuse can reduce the level of performance on perceptual tasks, particularly in middle-aged and older individuals.

DISABLING CONSEQUENCES

The severity of stimulus imperception varies widely among patients. Patients who have circumscribed, unilateral lesions may have mild degrees of deficit that are demonstrable in the clinic but go unnoticed in daily life. For example, a patient who is unable to distinguish colors in the superior right quadrant of his or her visual field may be unaware of the deficit and is unlikely to experience disability.

As the severity of the disorder increases, so does the resulting disability. A patient with severe visual form imperception may suffer the same degree of disability as a blind individual. He or she may be able to avoid obstacles when not distracted, but may have extreme difficulty in crowded, noisy environments. Crossing the street or using public transportation is hazardous at best, and driving is impossible in these individuals. Jobs that require the use of vision (and there are few that do not) are beyond the patient's capacity without significant modification of work duties.

With training and a flexible and sympathetic employer, blind individuals can successfully perform many jobs that are traditionally held by sighted individuals. However, patients with visual form imperception are more disadvantaged by the reception of distorted visual information. It is difficult to ignore visual input when it is available. Even after training, a patient with visual form imperception may base decisions and actions on distorted visual input and make errors in discrimination as a consequence.

Facial imperception is primarily socially disabling. The patient risks offending others and embarrassing himself or herself by misperceiving other individuals. In severe cases, recognition of even familiar people is impaired because their faces are poorly perceived. In less severe cases, recent acquaintances pose the greatest perceptual challenge. With increasing familiarity, the patient may learn to distinguish people based on voice, clothing style, or some easily perceived physical characteristic. Advancement in some business and professional occupations depends on social contact and interaction. Facial imperception places the patient at a competitive disadvantage in these occupations.

Color imperception tends to be less disabling because it is compensated for more easily. Driving ability may initially be impaired because the patient cannot distinguish red and green traffic lights. However, most patients can learn quickly to tell one signal from another based on the position of the light, and thus are able to drive safely. Occupations in which color perception is essential are not possible for the patient with color imperception. Thus, careers in fashion, interior decorating, and the visual arts are impractical in these persons. Some color-blind patients see the world entirely as varying shades of gray. These patients may not be able to distinguish dirty from clean and may therefore be unable to function in cleaning occupations.

Western society places proportionately less emphasis on the senses of touch and hearing than it does on vision. Consequently, tactual form and auditory pattern imperception may produce less disability. The patient with auditory imperception is unlikely to be successful in music-related careers. Music is also a major form of entertainment in most societies, and leisure-time enjoyment may decline in patients with auditory pattern imperception. Tactual form imperception may cause some decline in the ability to perform jobs requiring fine motor coordination, particularly when the patient is unable to monitor their hands visually. Such situations may arise in machine repair fields, in which the patient must work in tight spaces with parts that are small and hard to see and reach. In most instances, however, visual guidance of the hands substitutes well for an acute sense of tactual form. If the patient has little loss of actual tactile sensation, disability may be minimal.

ASSESSMENT INSTRUMENTS

Rosenbaum Pocket Vision Screener

The Rosenbaum Pocket Vision Screener is available from *Medi-Source Incorporated, 50 Gordon Drive, Syosset, NY 11791.*

This test consists of a 3.5- by 7-inch card containing stimuli from the standard Snellen chart reduced in size so that visual acuity can be tested at the bedside or in office settings. The standard Snellen chart requires 20 feet of space, whereas the Rosenbaum Pocket Vision Screener needs to be held only 14 inches from the patient's eyes in good lighting. Stimuli include numbers printed in different sizes that yield a distance equivalent varying from what the normal person can see at 20 feet to what can be seen at 800 feet. The test can be used to detect visual acuities varying from 20/20 (normal) to 20/800. A visual acuity of 20/800 indicates that a patient can see at 20 feet only what a person with normal 20/20 vision can see at 800 feet.

The Rosenbaum Pocket Vision Screener also includes Es oriented in varying directions and X-and-O sequences that can be used to assess acuity in patients who cannot read or verbally report numbers. Patients need only point in the directions where the E's are oriented or report the X and O sequences. Visual acuity is assessed in each eye separately, with and without glasses.

The Rosenbaum Pocket Vision Screener can be interpreted by most experienced clinicians. When significant declines in visual acuity are detected that have not previously been noted, the patient should be referred to an ophthalmologist or optometrist for diagnosis and treatment.

Ishihara's Test for Color Blindness

Ishihara's Test for Color Blindness is available from *Kanehara and Company, Limited, P.O. Box Number 1, Hongo P.O., Tokyo 113-91, Japan.*

This test consists of 24 plates containing multicolored dots that form a background and a contrastingly colored foreground. The foreground dots form a number, which the patient is asked to identify. On seven plates, the foreground dots form a trail, which the patient is asked to trace. These latter plates are useful for patients who cannot read or verbally report numbers. Incorrect responses include misperception of or complete failure to perceive the foreground pattern or trail. Specific types of errors are made on each plate by patients with specific subtypes of color blindness; error patterns are detailed in the accompanying manual. Care must be taken to record the exact type of error made. A screening version of the test using only six plates can also be used, but if errors are detected, the full test should be administered.

Ishihara's Test for Color Blindness can detect the most common forms of congenital color blindness, as well as color blindness acquired as a result of cerebral lesions. This test does not detect certain rare forms of congenital color blindness, but these are not usually a focus of neuropsychological assessment. The test can be administered at bedside or in an office or laboratory setting, assuming the presence of adequate lighting. Interpretation is fairly straightforward in distinguishing normal from abnormal performance, and the test consequently is appropriate for use by most clinicians familiar with neurological populations. When an abnormal performance is detected and congenital color blindness is suspected, referral to an ophthalmologist or optometrist is recommended.

Benton Visual Form Discrimination

The Benton Visual Form Discrimination[44] is available from *Oxford University Press, Incorporated, 200 Madison Avenue, New York, NY 10016.*

This test requires patients to match visual forms, distinguishing each correct choice from an incorrect choice in which a major element is rotated and from an incorrect choice in which a major element is distorted. The correct choice appears in all four locations on the response card an equal number of times, making it possible to detect a simple failure to notice stimuli in a particular location. Analysis of the types of errors made makes it possible to distinguish patients who have difficulty with the spatial aspects of the test (e.g., errors that involve a failure to perceive the rotation of major or peripheral elements) from patients who have actual form perception deficits (e.g., errors that involve a failure to perceive the distortion of a major element).

Normative data are based on a sample of 85 healthy individuals and non-neurological patients. Reliability coefficients are not reported. Age, gender, and education are reported to be unrelated to test performance. The test is highly sensitive to the presence of brain damage, and the authors of the test note that performance in a given patient may be lowered for a variety of reasons.

The Benton Visual Form Discrimination test provides a quick measure of form and spatial perception. Its sensitivity to multiple deficits requires that close attention be paid to the type of errors made by patients. The results of the Benton Visual Form Discrimination Test are meaningful only in the context of a comprehensive neuropsychological examination. Interpretation should be attempted only by experienced neuropsychologists or behavioral neurologists. The test is suitable for bedside, office, or laboratory administration.

Benton Facial Recognition Test

The Benton Facial Recognition Test[44] is available from *Oxford University Press, Incorporated, 200 Madison Avenue, New York, NY 10016.*

This test measures the ability to discriminate among unfamiliar faces and is available in both a short and long form. Items require three kinds of discrimination: between front-view photographs, between front-view and three-quarter-view photographs, and between front-view photographs taken under different lighting conditions. Norms are based on a sample of 286 non-neurological patients and healthy volunteers ranging in age from 16 to 74 years. Age and education are reported in the manual to be significantly related to test performance, and a correction factor is incorporated into the scoring procedure. Short-form scores are reported in the clinical manual to correlate highly with long-form scores in both brain-damaged (r = .92) and control (r = .88) samples. No other reliability coefficients are reported.

The Benton Facial Recognition Test is sensitive to lateralized lesions.[29] When aphasic patients are excluded from the data analysis, a high proportion of right-hemisphere-damaged patients show defective test performance. Within the sub-group of right-hemisphere-damaged patients, those with posterior lesions are more often impaired than those with anterior lesions. The presence or absence of visual field deficits does not appear to affect test performance. Test performance is also not significantly lowered in psychiatric populations.[45]

Although many tests of visual form perception exist, the Benton Facial Recognition Test provides one of the few standardized measures of facial perception. Although the test was originally conceived as a measure of facial agnosia (see Prosopagnosia), its authors quickly discovered that it was not useful in this capacity and instead developed it as a measure of perception. The test is appropriate for office, bedside, or laboratory administration and can be interpreted by clinicians with experience in the diagnosis of visual perceptual disorders.

Visual Object and Space Perception Battery

The Visual Object and Space Perception Battery (VOSP)[46] is available from *Thames Valley Test Company, 7–9 The Green, Flempton, Bury St. Edmunds, Suffolk, IP 28 6EL, England.*

The VOSP consists of eight tests of object and spatial perception. Each test measures one conceptual component of perception. Object perception is measured using incomplete (degraded) letters, silhouettes of objects rotated 90 degrees from the lateral view and shown progressively rotated back to the lateral view in steps of 1.5 degrees until the patient can identify the object, and silhouettes of real objects that must be discriminated from nonsensical shapes.

Spatial perception is measured using tasks such as dot counting, position discrimination (i.e., determining which of two dots is centered within a square), spatial localization (i.e., identifying a number within a frame that corresponds to the position of a dot within another frame), and spatial estimation (i.e., determining the number of cubes present based on the spatial configuration of a drawing). Also included is a shape detection screening task, which the patient must pass before proceeding with other VOSP tests. The screening task requires patients to detect an X embedded in a distracting background pattern.

Reliability coefficients are not reported in the VOSP manual. Normative and validation studies used patients with right- and left-hemisphere lesions and control patients admitted to the British National Hospital for Neurology and Neurosurgery for "extra-cerebral neurological conditions."[46] The effect of age on VOSP performance was negligible up to age 50 years, after which a decrement in performance was observed. Separate cut-off scores were established for patients younger than and older than 50 years of age. Of the normal controls in each age group, 5 percent or fewer fell below the cut-off scores.

Differences in the mean scores obtained by brain-damaged and control patients across the VOSP tests are quite small. However, a series of chi-square analyses documented that a higher percentage of right-hemisphere than left-hemisphere patients fell below the cut-off scores established for each test. More left-hemisphere patients scored below the cut-off on the silhouette and dot-counting subtests than expected by chance. No statistically significant differences between brain-damaged and control groups are reported for the shape detection screening test.

The VOSP is a new instrument that requires further study, particularly in the area of reliability. The VOSP includes tests that are not available elsewhere in a standardized and normed format. The unusual object perception tasks have the potential to detect fairly subtle object perception deficits. The battery places minimal demand on language abilities and can thus be used to test perception in patients with partially compromised oral communication. Comprehension of verbal instructions, however, is required.

The VOSP can be administered at bedside or in office or laboratory settings. No purchase restrictions apply to the battery; therefore, it can be used by neuropsychologists, neurologists, speech pathologists, and other health care professionals experienced with neurological populations. Care must be exercised when interpreting test results because of the battery's unknown reliability. Only clinicians who are highly experienced in the diagnosis of perceptual disorders should attempt to interpret VOSP results.

Whisper Procedure

Neuropsychologists are principally concerned with hearing loss sufficient to interfere with testing of cognitive functions. The patient is usually aware of and able to report such hearing difficulties. In other cases, the patient's behavior betrays the hearing loss (e.g., frequent requests for the examiner to speak up or repeat information). Some patients are embarrassed by their hearing loss and deny or attempt to mask it.

The examiner's suspicions about a loss of hearing can be verified by asking the patient to repeat a series of letters, digits, or words whispered by the examiner. The patient's vision should be occluded to prevent the patient from being aided by the examiner's facial movements. Stimuli that were repeated successfully when they were spoken at a conversational volume should be used, and the whispered stimuli should be delivered from the same distance and spatial location as the conversational volume stimuli. Care must be taken to ensure that the whisper is not so soft that even a person with confirmed normal hearing could not perceive it. Practice in whispering stimuli to a person with normal hearing will help the examiner to calibrate the volume of his or her voice.

A large discrepancy between what the patient can hear at a conversational volume and what he or she can hear at a lower volume justifies a strong suspicion of hearing impairment. The patient should then be referred to an audiologist for a formal hearing assessment. The whisper procedure cannot be used in aphasic patients who have documented speech repetition deficits. These patients require audiologic examination for documentation of hearing impairment. The whisper procedure is appropriate for use in any test setting where background noise can be kept to a minimum. The procedure can be interpreted by any clinician experienced with neurological, elderly, or hearing-impaired populations.

Phoneme Discrimination Test

The Phoneme Discrimination Test[44] is available from *Oxford University Press, Incorporated, 200 Madison Avenue, New York, NY 10016.*

This test consists of 30 pairs of tape-recorded pseudowords, which the patient identifies as being either the same or different. In 15 of the pairs, the pseudowords differ in one phonemic feature. Normative data are based on 30 non-neurological patients. Reliability coefficients are not reported in the clinical manual, and the effects of age, gender, and education on test performance are unknown. The test is sensitive to phonemic discrimination deficits in left-hemisphere-damaged aphasic patients, whereas nonaphasic patients with right-hemisphere damage have relatively little difficulty in performing the test. Studies comparing nonaphasic patients with left- versus right-hemisphere-damaged patients are not available. Data are available on a live-voice presentation format administered to non-neurological controls. This procedure greatly increases the difficulty of the test and may decrease its sensitivity to subtle phonemic discrimination deficits.[44] When a tape is not available, the examiner may consider live-voice administration with the patient's vision occluded.

The major weakness of the Phoneme Discrimination Test is the lack of normative data. Further study of its reliability and validity is necessary. The relative ease with which right-hemisphere-damaged patients perform the test suggests that concentration may be less of a factor in patient performance than is the case in other auditory discrimination tests (see Seashore Rhythm Test). The Phoneme Discrimination Test is most easily administered in office and laboratory settings. If a portable tape player is available and background noise can be minimized, the test can also be administered at bedside. Interpretation of the test should be attempted only by experienced speech pathologists, neuropsychologists, and neurologists because of its limited normative database.

Speech–Sounds Perception Test

The Speech-Sounds Perception Test is available from *Reitan Neuropsychological Laboratory, 1338 East Edison Street, Tucson, AZ 85719.*

Pseudowords are presented on tape, and the patient attempts to identify them from a set of printed multiple-choice options. Corrections for the effects of age, gender, and education on test performance are available.[47] Test-retest reliability has varied from .49 to .77,[48,49] and one study reported a coefficient alpha of .89.[50]

The Speech-Sounds Perception Test has successfully discriminated between normal and moderately to severely impaired brain-damaged patients[51] and psychiatric and neurological patients,[52] but not normal and mildly impaired hypoxic patients.[53] A recent investigation found that the Speech-Sounds Perception Test is a good general indicator of brain damage anywhere in the brain, but cannot be used to infer a right- or left-sided lesion lateralization.[54] The Speech-Sounds Perception Test is administered as a part of the Halstead-Reitan Battery. Unfortunately, it does not appear to improve the ability of the battery to differentiate neurological from "pseudoneurological" patients, leading to the proposal that it be dropped.[54]

Part of the success of the Speech-Sounds Perception Test as a general index of brain damage may be a result of the multiple skills required for successful performance. The test is long and requires the capacity to sustain concentration and effort. Not only does it assess auditory perception, but it also requires phonological analysis of pseudowords. This makes it a sensitive test but complicates interpretation of results. The test has high sensitivity but low specificity. Novice users of the test must guard against misinterpretation of test scores.

The Speech-Sounds Perception Test is appropriate for office or laboratory administration. If a portable tape player is available, the test may be administered at bedside; however, extraneous noise or unexpected interruptions may affect patient performance negatively. If these factors cannot be eliminated, the test should not be attempted at bedside. Interpretation should be restricted to neuropsychologists with specific training in the Halstead-Reitan Battery.

Seashore Rhythm Test

The Seashore Rhythm Test is available from *Reitan Neuropsychological Laboratory, 1338 East Edison Street, Tucson, AZ 85719.*

In this test, patients judge whether pairs of rhythmic beats, presented by a tape recording, are the same or different. Corrections for the effects of age, gender, and education on test performance are available.[47] Test-retest reliability has varied from .37 to .57.[48,49] One study obtained a coefficient alpha of .78 for the Seashore Rhythm Test in a combined sample of normal and brain-damaged individuals.[50]

The Seashore Rhythm Test has successfully discriminated moderately to severely impaired brain-damaged samples from normal controls,[51,55] but it may not be sensitive to subtle or mild neuropsychological deficits.[53] The test failed to discriminate cerebral dysfunction of varied causes from non-brain-damaged psychiatric patients in another study.[52] Another investigation found that the Seashore Rhythm Test is a good general indicator of damage anywhere in the brain, but cannot be used to infer right- or left-sided lesion lateralization.[54] The Seashore Rhythm Test is administered as a part of the Halstead-Reitan Battery. Unfortunately, the test does not appear to improve the ability of the battery to differentiate neurological from "pseudoneurological" patients, leading to the proposal that the test be dropped.[54]

The Seashore Rhythm Test is appropriate for office or laboratory administration. If a portable tape player is available, the test may be used at bedside; however, extraneous noise or unexpected interruptions may affect patient performance negatively. If these factors cannot be eliminated, the test should not be attempted at bedside. Interpretation should be restricted to neuropsychologists with specific training in the Halstead-Reitan Battery.

Comprehensive Ability Battery, Auditory Ability Subtests

The Comprehensive Ability Battery (CAB), Auditory Ability Subtests[56] are available from *Institute for Personality and Ability Testing, Incorporated, P.O. Box 188, Champaign, IL 61820.*

The CAB is a broad battery of relatively short tests intended to measure the primary mental abilities comprising human intelligence. The Auditory Ability Subtests measure pitch discrimination (part I) and tonal memory (part II). In part I, pairs of tones are presented using audiotape, and the patient is asked to specify whether the second tone is higher, lower, or equivalent in pitch. In part II, pairs of four- and five-tone sequences are presented. The two tonal sequences are identical, except that one tone in the second sequence is of a different pitch than the corresponding tone in the first sequence. The patient must identify the ordinal position of the discrepant tone in the second sequence.

Although the Auditory Ability Subtests measure abilities that may be dissociable in some neurological patients, the scores from parts I and II are added together. Neuropsychologists may wish to consider the scores on parts I and II separately. The test manual reports split-half reliability coefficients for the Auditory Ability Subtests total score that vary from .71 to .82 among various samples. Two factor-analytic studies support the contention that the Auditory Ability Subtests measure a factor that is distinct from what the other CAB subtests measure.[56]

Most of the reliability and validity studies conducted on the CAB have been in normal adolescent (i.e., high school) samples in the United States and Canada. Norms are available for high school, college, and prison samples. The CAB has not been used with any sizeable samples of brain-damaged patients. This is unfortunate, because several of the CAB subtests lend themselves to inclusion in neuropsychological examinations. The format of the CAB is most suited for group testing and must be adapted for use with individual neurological patients (e.g., substituting a verbal response recorded by the examiner for the written CAB machine-scored forms).

The CAB Auditory Ability Subtests should be administered only in settings where background noise is at a minimum. Typically, these are office or laboratory settings. The subtests may be used at bedside if a portable tape player is available and background noise can be eliminated. Test results from neurological patients should be interpreted only by an experienced neuropsychologist because of the lack of demonstrated reliability and validity in neurological populations. Caution must be exercised when interpreting results because of the absence of empirical guidelines.

Tactual Sensitivity Screen

The Tactual Sensitivity Screen is *not commercially available.*

Neuropsychologists are typically concerned with tactual sensory deficits, because they can alter interpretation or completely invalidate certain perceptual tests. I use the following procedures, not to calibrate the degree of tactual impairment, but to rule out the confounding effects of tactual sensation loss on tests of finger localization (see Finger mislocalization), graphesthesia, and stereognosis.

1. While his or her vision is occluded, the patient's fingers are touched lightly on the nail or palm side, depending on where the touch will be delivered during finger localization testing. The interval between touches varies randomly among 5, 10, and 15 seconds. The patient is asked only to report when he or she feels the touch and does not have to identify which finger was touched. Each finger should be touched at least twice.

2. The palms or palm sides of the fingertips are touched with the sharp and dull ends of a pin in a randomly alternating order. The patient is asked to identify which end of the pin was used. The procedure should be repeated at least 10 times.

3. With a stylus, three straight lines are traced across the patient's palm while the patient observes. The first line is drawn from the midpoint of the wrist to the base of the middle finger and is described to the patient as "a line down your palm from your wrist to your fingers." The second line travels across the middle of the palm from the thumb side to the fifth-finger side and is described as "a line across the middle of your palm." The third line travels from the base of the thumb to the base of the fifth finger and is described as "a diagonal line from the base of your thumb to the base of your little finger." These lines are then traced with the patient's vision occluded, and the patient is asked to identify the direction of the lines verbally, by pointing or by retracing the line across the palm with a finger from the opposite hand. Both palms are tested, and each line is traced at least three times in random order.

In all three procedures, patients should be correct in 90 to 100 percent of the trials. If this criterion is not met, the examiner should not conclude that tactile sensory deficits have been fully ruled out.

Halstead-Reitan Battery Sensory-Perceptual Examination, Fingertip Number-Writing and Tactile Form Recognition Subtests

The Halstead-Reitan Battery (HRB) Sensory-Perceptual Examination (SPE), Fingertip Number-Writing, and Tactile Form Recognition Subtests are available from *Reitan Neuropsychological Laboratory, 1338 East Edison Street, Tucson, AZ 85719.*

In the Fingertip Number-Writing Subtest, the numbers 3, 4, 5, and 6 are traced in random order on each fingertip, and the patient is asked to identify the numbers verbally. The Tactile Form Recognition Subtest involves palpation of flat, plastic shapes (i.e., circle, square, triangle, and cross) behind a screen and identification of the shapes by pointing to their corresponding visual representations. Other SPE subtests include an assessment of visual fields, attention to unilateral and bilateral stimulation, localization of stimuli applied to the fingers, and identification of coins by touch.

Various indices can be calculated from the SPE, including scores on each individual test, scores for each side of the body, and various combinations of subtest scores. Age, education, and gender corrections are available for some SPE combination scores,[47] but most examiners also look at scores from each side of the body on individual subtests.

The SPE is assumed to be a reliable and valid measure, because it is derived from procedures that have been used by neurologists for a long time. Unfortunately, empirical demonstration of its reliability and validity is lacking. A tactual recognition factor derived from the SPE was found to be one of only two factors from the HRB that discriminated right- from left-hemisphere brain-damaged patients in one study.[57]

Specific training in the HRB is required for use and interpretation of the Fingertip Number-Writing and Tactile Form Recognition Subtests. Tactile Form Recognition is appropriate for office or laboratory administration but is too cumbersome for bedside administration without changing the administration format. The Fingertip Number-Writing subtest can be administered readily in any setting.

Tactile Form Perception Test

The Tactile Form Perception Test[44] is available from *Oxford University Press, Incorporated, 200 Madison Avenue, New York, NY 10016.*

In this test, patients attempt to match geometric figures felt with either hand while their vision is occluded to visually presented line drawings. Two forms (A and B) of equivalent difficulty are available, one of which may be administered to each hand. Normative data are based on 90 healthy individuals ranging in age from 15 to 70 years and an additional 25 normal elderly volunteers ranging from 71 to 80 years of age. Age appears to be only slightly related to test performance, with elderly volunteers scoring an average of 1 point lower in each hand than younger individuals.[44]

Reliability coefficients are not reported, but data presented in the test manual suggest that parallel form reliability is high (i.e., the two forms yield virtually equivalent scores). The test is sensitive to hemispheric damage causing decreases in tactile sensation, tactile perception, and spatial perception. Care must be taken to distinguish sensory from higher-level perceptual deficits when interpreting the test.

The Tactile Form Perception Test may be administered at bedside, in the office, or in the laboratory. It is brief and causes patients only minimal frustration. The test should be interpreted only by experienced clinicians such as neuropsychologists, neurologists, physiatrists, and occupational therapists, because many factors can affect performance of this measure.

Rey Skin-Writing Procedure

The Rey Skin-Writing Procedure[58] is *not commercially available.*

In this test, a series of numbers and letters is traced in the dominant and nondominant palms using a stylus. In one block of trials, the stimuli are traced on the forearm; in another condition, the palms are held close together and the stimuli are traced larger, so that portions of each stimulus fall on both palms. Cut-off scores are based on relatively small samples of manual laborers, skilled technicians, and people holding a baccalaureate degree. Data on 14 elderly people aged 68 to 83 years are also available.[58] Inspection of the normative data reveals that the elderly group performed slightly worse than the other, presumably younger groups. More extensive norms across the decades of life are clearly necessary. The current norms should be considered tentative and provisional. Results of the procedure must be interpreted cautiously in elderly persons.

Similar tests of graphesthesia are included in most neurological examinations. The Rey Skin-Writing Procedure standardizes the neurological assessment of graphesthesia and provides at least a provisional normative database on which to base interpretation of the results. The procedure can be administered at bedside, in the office, or in the laboratory. Interpretation is not always straightforward, because factors other than agraphesthesia can lower the level of the patient's performance. These factors include sensory deficits and difficulty in interpreting or identifying linguistic stimuli. The procedure should be interpreted only by a neurologist or neuropsychologist because of the many factors that can affect patient performance.

Tactual Performance Test

The Tactual Performance Test (TPT) is available from *Reitan Neuropsychological Laboratory, 1338 East Edison Street, Tucson, AZ 85719.*

In this test, patients attempt to fit variously shaped blocks into slots on a board while blindfolded. The test is administered to each hand separately and then to both hands together. After completion of this portion of the test, the board and blindfold are removed, and the patient attempts to draw a representation of the shapes in their correct spatial locations on the board. Scores are based on the time required to place blocks into the board, the number of blocks correctly drawn (TPT memory score), and the number of drawn blocks placed in the correct spatial location (TPT location score). The test measures not only tactile perception but also memory for tactual and tactual-spatial information. Corrections are available for the impact of age, gender, and education on TPT performance.[47]

As an integral part of the HRB, the TPT has long been in use, and a substantial normative database has accumulated.[47,59–61] The reliability and validity of the TPT have often been studied and reviewed.[58,62,63] The TPT has been demonstrated to have acceptable split-half and test-retest reliability in a variety of samples, although reliability coefficients vary considerably among studies.[49,50,64] Various scores derived from the TPT have successfully discriminated non-neurological control subjects from brain-damaged patients.[52–55] Reduced performance may be the result of impaired tactile discrimination, although other factors can also lower performance because of the complexity of the test. The TPT is sensitive to deficits in planning, organization, concentration, motor speed, coordination, memory, and so forth.

The TPT is appropriate only for office or laboratory administration. It can be extremely time-consuming and frustrating for the patient, and one reviewer questioned its clinical utility.[58] A shortened, six-hole version of the TPT is available that can decrease both the time needed to administer the test and the patient's level of frustration.[65] Interpretation of the TPT should be attempted only by experienced neuropsychologists who have had specific training in administering and interpreting the results of HRB.

Dichotomous Forced-Choice Symptom Validity Test of Sensory Perception

The Dichotomous Forced-Choice Symptom Validity Test of Sensory Perception is *not commercially available.*

This test provides a means of detecting malingered sensory perceptual deficits. A stimulus is presented in the impaired sensory modality, and the patient is asked to make a dichotomous decision concerning the stimulus. In cases of suspected malingered sensory impairment, the patient can be asked to report the presence or absence of a visual stimulus or to make a two-choice perceptual discrimination.

This technique has been used to diagnose malingering in a patient who presented with agraphesthesia.[66] The patient was asked to discriminate 3 from 4 (easy version) and G from O (hard version) traced on the skin surface. In a case reported later, I asked a patient suspected of malingering visual symptoms to discriminate Q from O presented visually. In the auditory modality, patients can be asked to report the presence or absence of tones or to discriminate between two different tones.

Symptom validity testing requires the presentation of a large number of trials so that the patient's performance can be compared to results expected from chance alone. I usually administer 100 trials. Borderline cases may require 200 trials before a definitive diagnosis can be made. The level of performance expected by chance can be determined using the z-approximation to the binomial distribution.[67] Patients performing significantly below chance are likely to be malingering or exaggerating their perceptual symptoms. On a 100-item test, a result of 59 errors (41 correct) is significantly different from chance at the .05 level of statistical confidence, and a result of 63 errors (37 correct) is significant at the .01 level of statistical confidence.

The Dichotomous Forced-Choice Symptom Validity Test can be administered at bedside, in the office, or in the laboratory. It is recommended for use only by physicians and psychologists because of the serious consequences to the patient of being labeled a malingerer. In any diagnostic decision, the possibility of clinician error exists. The advantage of a probability-based decision is the known likelihood that the clinician is in error.

NEUROPSYCHOLOGICAL TREATMENT

Treatment options for stimulus imperception are limited. In most cases, no treatment is offered. In many clinics, perceptual disorders are sometimes identified in the driving evaluation done by the occupational therapy department. Rather than receiving treatment, the patient is often simply told to return in 6 months to see if he or she has improved sufficiently to pass the driving test.

When treatment is offered, it usually consists of practice in the area of deficiency. Patients are given increasingly challenging perceptual tasks to perform, with reinforcement offered for successes at these tasks. These activities may be administered using paper and pencil or, with increasing frequency, a computer. Popular video games marketed for home entertainment provide excellent practice of perceptual skills in a format that is exciting and appealing to the patient, although the difficulty level of such games may exceed the maximal capacity of many stimulus-imperception patients.

Fortunately, computer-based cognitive remediation programs have multiplied, offering many options for practice of perceptual skills at a level of difficulty appropriate for each patient. The limitations of these programs are the lack of research showing their effectiveness and the dissimilarity of the perceptual tasks to everyday life. When remediation tasks diverge from tasks performed in everyday life, there may be little generalization of treatment effects beyond the clinic. Just as video games do not prepare a person for a career in computer programming, computerized perceptual training programs may not prepare a patient for the perceptual demands of driving.

CASE ILLUSTRATIONS

CASE 5–1

J.V. was a 46-year-old Army veteran who last worked as a gas station attendant in 1984. He suffered a motor vehicle accident that year that left him a paraplegic (injury was to the 11th thoracic spinal segment), and he was unable to continue his work. He was healthy until 1991, when he suffered a right thalamic hemorrhage with hydrocephalus. Left upper extremity weakness resulted, and he was admitted to a rehabilitation hospital for a comprehensive treatment program.

At the time of admission, J.V.'s mental status was judged by his physician to be normal. Neuropsychological examination was requested to further assess the patient's cognitive status. The patient showed no deficits in concentration. His visual fields were full, and visual acuity was 20/20 in each eye. J.V. correctly identified colors, objects, and the faces of recent United States presidents. There was no evidence of stimulus neglect during unilateral stimulation, double simultaneous stimulation, line bisection, or drawing. Judgment of the spatial orientation of lines was intact for his age using the Benton Line Orientation Test. In contrast, the patient obtained a score in the severely impaired range on the Benton Facial Recognition Test.

J.V.'s intellectual functioning was in the average range. No errors were made on the HRB Aphasia Screening Test, suggesting that he had grossly intact language functions. Memory for both paragraphs and visual designs was above average on the Wechsler Memory Scale–Revised.

This patient had severe left-sided tactile sensory loss and was unable to detect which of his fingers the examiner touched when his eyes were closed. He also could not determine the direction of movement of a line traced with a dull point on his left palm, reporting only that he felt a tickle. In the right hand, J.V. was accurate in localizing the fingers that were stimulated and could clearly perceive the presence of a dull point, as well as the direction of movement of lines traced in the palm. He matched tactual forms to visual forms without error. In contrast, he was below the cut-off score for manual laborers in the number of errors he made in the right palm on the Rey Skin-Writing Procedure.

DISCUSSION

J.V. presented with facial and tactual form imperception. The diagnosis of the former is relatively unambiguous, considering the patient's impaired matching and discrimination of faces on the Benton Facial Recognition Test with preserved visual acuity and concentration and the absence of any deficits in detecting stimuli in the environment. The diagnosis of tactual form imperception is based on the presence of agraphesthesia in the right hand, even though the patient could accurately match tactual shapes placed in the right hand to visual representations. The left hand may also have been impaired, but valid assessment of tactual form perception could not be conducted in this patient's left hand because of its decreased sensation.

CASE 5–2

W.S. was a 45-year-old man who had completed 2 years of college and worked as a sales manager. He had been in good health until he was struck on the forehead, nose, and left ear by a plate glass door that fell from its hinges at a hotel. He subsequently fell and hit the rear of his head on the ground. There was no loss of consciousness, although the patient was dazed and bled from his left ear and nose. Immediate medical attention was not sought.

Over the next 2 to 3 months, the patient developed pain in his left ear in response to high-pitched noise, blurred vision, and seizure-like episodes during which he suffered occipital pain, fell, felt cold, was unable to see, and became frightened and confused for several minutes. He also reported being more forgetful, quick-tempered, and depressed. He also stated that he was now "dyslexic," because he reversed the orientation of letters when writing. W.S. believed that his work as a sales manager had suffered as a result of the changes in his mental functioning, and he engaged an attorney to sue the hotel where he was injured. The attorney arranged for the patient's evaluation.

A neurological examination, which included a computed tomographic (CT) scan, an electroencephalogram (EEG), a visual evoked potential study, and a glucose tolerance test, failed to reveal any evidence of neurological illness. An examination conducted by a clinical psychologist revealed signs of depression, preoccupation with bodily function, and possible signs of organic brain damage. More comprehensive neuropsychological testing was recommended.

In an interview with the neuropsychologist, W.S. denied any loss of memory for events preceding the accident. However, he was inconsistent in his report of what his mental functioning was like in the hours after the accident. On one occasion, he denied having experienced any confusion or memory lapses and was able to describe his activities following the accident. During a subsequent interview, the examiner told him that most people experience confusion and amnesia following head trauma. W.S. then stated that his wife had told him that he actually had not carried out any of the activities he thought he had in the hours after the accident, and concluded that he must have been confused.

Formal neuropsychological testing revealed overall intellectual functioning to be in the low average range, with the patient having difficulty on tests that required careful attention to visual details, construction of designs and puzzles, perceptual judgment, and rapid motor performance. Memory appeared to be severely impaired.

The most striking findings occurred on visual tests. The patient showed a restriction of both the temporal and nasal portions of his visual field in each eye, so that he reported seeing stimuli only in the center of his visual field. Notably, in the previous neurological examination, visual fields were found to be full. Visual acuity was corrected to 20/30 in each eye with glasses. The patient recognized colors, line drawings of objects, and photographs of recent United States presidents without error. When copying simple geometric figures or complex designs, W.S. spatially distorted the figures (e.g., placed details in an incorrect spatial position, failed to keep proper proportions among the parts of figures) but included all important details. He was completely unable to perform the Benton Facial Recognition and Visual Form Discrimination Tests. When presented with a random sequence of two letters to discriminate (i.e., O and Q), W.S. was correct on only 44 out of 100 trials. Performance was no better on a second set of 100 trials.

DISCUSSION

This patient was unable to match and discriminate visual forms and faces despite having adequate visual acuity. This led to suspicion of visual form and facial imperception. However, a number of inconsistencies are present in his performance. His initial accident appeared quite minor, with a decline in function occurring over several months rather than being immediately apparent. The patient's condition worsened over time rather than improving or remaining the same. His report of his deficits changed in accordance with what he thought was typical of traumatically brain-injured individuals. His deficits changed from one examination to the next, with visual fields appearing full when examined by a neurologist but subsequently appearing markedly restricted during the neuropsychological examination.

The inconsistencies in this patient's performance led to additional testing to determine if his visual perceptual problems were caused by malingering. The patient performed at a level worse than chance on a simple two-choice discrimination task, suggesting that he was deliberately attempting to respond incorrectly. This same result was obtained when the test was repeated for verification. Although deficits in visual perception may have been present, assessment could not be performed validly because of the patient's bias in the direction of poor performance. A diagnosis of psychogenic imperception was made. When independent psychiatric examination supported this diagnosis, the patient's attorney persuaded him to drop the lawsuit and to enter psychotherapy.

CASE 5–3

J.S. was a 49-year-old woman with an 11th-grade education who had worked as a retail manager before suffering cardiac arrest caused by coronary atherosclerotic heart disease. Mild anoxic encephalopathy resulted from her cardiac arrest, and she developed right-sided weakness, lethargy, and slurred speech. She complained of a subjective decrease in her vision, although visual evoked potential tests were normal, and she was able to recognize objects and maneuver around barriers in the environment.

Neuro-ophthalmological examination revealed an area of decreased vision (i.e., a scotoma) in the right superior temporal quadrant of her visual field, which was thought to be consistent with a left inferior occipital lesion. Vertical upward gaze was restricted, and this was considered to be a hysterical symptom. Psychiatric consultation was recommended. A neurologist noted impaired visual guidance of reaching movements (see Optic ataxia), inability to shift gaze on demand (see Oculomotor apraxia), and "visual bewilderment" (the precise behaviors referred to by the latter term were not specified). Balint's syndrome (see Chaps. 4, 7, and 11) was diagnosed. Subsequent magnetic resonance imaging (MRI) scans revealed periventricular white-matter disease and possible bilateral watershed-area infarcts. An EEG was consistent with a diffuse encephalopathy involving the gray matter.

Neuropsychological consultation was not requested until several weeks later, after J.S. was transferred to a rehabilitation hospital. At that time, she was able to reach for targets accurately and could readily shift her gaze in any direction on demand. J.S. was severely impaired on virtually all visual perceptual tests administered to her, although validity of testing could not be completely established because of her limited visual acuity (20/400 in each eye). Performance fell below the cut-off score on Ishihara's Test; the patient's pattern of responses was suggestive of total color blindness. She was impaired even on plates that required her simply to trace a colored pattern. No spontaneous reports of difficulty in seeing color were offered by the patient, although she acknowledged her difficulty after viewing the colored plates.

DISCUSSION

This case was a diagnostic challenge. A neuro-ophthalmologist mistakenly attributed the patient's initial inability to shift gaze to psychological factors, even though this deficit is known to follow bilateral watershed infarcts and diffuse damage extending to the combined parietal and occipital areas (see Oculomotor apraxia). It is probable the patient initially presented with Balint's syndrome, which consists of oculomotor apraxia, optic ataxia (see Chap. 11), and simultanagnosia (see Chap. 4). However, simultanagnosia was not clearly documented, although it may account for the vague notation of "visual bewilderment." An additional problem in making a diagnosis of Balint's syndrome is the patient's reduced visual acuity. Documenting normal visual evoked potentials is not tantamount to documenting normal visual acuity, and although questions remain about the patient's visual acuity, the diagnosis of Balint's syndrome and of any of the stimulus perception disorders remains uncertain.

Despite these remarks, it appears likely that this patient had color imperception. Ishihara's Test was used to assess her color vision. The stimuli for this test are more than twice the size of the stimuli the patient must have seen accurately to have a visual acuity of 20/400; therefore, decreased visual acuity does not adequately account for her poor performance in color perception tests.

Although the patient had a scotoma in one quadrant of her visual field, it is highly improbable that all portions of Ishihara's Test fell within the area of her scotoma or even within one quadrant of her visual field. In addition, the patient had recovered from her oculomotor apraxia sufficiently that her eye movements were noted to be unrestricted at the time of testing. Her spontaneous eye movements would have more than compensated for any loss of perception as a result of a scotoma.

Most of the plates in Ishihara's Test require the reading of numbers, which could have been selectively impaired. However, she was required to read numbers during testing of visual acuity, and did so successfully until the stimuli became too small for her to see. In addition, the patient was impaired even on plates that merely required her to trace a colored pattern. Optic ataxia could impair visual tracing; however, the patient had become accurate in her ability to visually guide her hands to targets, suggesting that she had recovered from her optic ataxia by the time color perception was tested.

REFERENCES

1. Semmes, J: A non-tactual factor in astereognosis. Neuropsychologia 3:295, 1965.
2. Benton, A: Visuoperceptual, visuospatial, and visuoconstructive disorders. In Heilman, KM, and Valenstein, E (eds): Clinical Neuropsychology, Second Edition. Oxford University Press, New York, 1985, p 151.
3. Bauer, RM, and Rubens, AB: Agnosia. In Heilman, KM, and Valenstein, E (eds): Clinical Neuropsychology, Second Edition. Oxford University Press, New York, 1985, p 187.
4. Critchley, M, and Henson, RA: Music and the Brain. Heinemann, London, 1977.
5. Hecaen, H, and David, M: Syndrome parietale traumatique: Asymbolie tactile et hemiasomatognosie paroxystique et douloureuse. Rev Neurol 77:113, 1945.
6. Hecaen, H: Introduction à la Neuropsychologie. Larousse, Paris, 1972.
7. Delay, J: Les Astereognosies. Pathologie du Toucher. Clinique, Physiologie, Topographie. Masson, Paris, 1935.
8. American Psychiatric Association: Diagnostic and Statistical Manual of Mental Disorders, Fourth Edition. American Psychiatric Association, Washington, DC, 1994.
9. The International Classification of Diseases, Ninth Revision, Clinical Modification. Med-Index Publications, Salt Lake City, 1991.
10. Zeki, S: A century of cerebral achromatopsia. Brain 113:1721, 1990.
11. Aldrich, MS, et al: Ictal cortical blindness with permanent visual loss. Epilepsia 30:116, 1989.
12. Kolmel, HW: Pure homonymous hemiachromatopsia. Findings with neuro-ophthalmologic examination and imaging procedures. Eur Arch Psychiatry Neurol Sci 237:237, 1988.

13. Heywood, CA, Wilson, B, and Cowey, A: A case study of cortical colour "blindness" with relatively intact achromatic discrimination. J Neurol Neurosurg Psychiatry 50:22, 1987.
14. Levine, DN, Warach, J, and Farah, M: Two visual systems in mental imagery: Dissociation of "what" and "where" in imagery disorders due to bilateral posterior cerebral lesions. Neurology 35:1010, 1985.
15. Damasio, AR, and Damasio, H: The anatomic basis of pure alexia. Neurology 33:1573, 1983.
16. Brazis, PW, Biller, J, and Fine, M: Central achromatopsia. Neurology 31:920, 1981.
17. Young, RS, and Fishman, GA: Loss of color vision and Stiles' II1 mechanism in a patient with cerebral infarction. J Ophthalmol Soc Am 70:1301, 1980.
18. Green, GJ, and Lessell, S: Acquired cerebral dyschromatopsia. Arch Ophthalmol 95:121, 1977.
19. Bisiach, E, Nichelli, P, and Spinnler, H: Hemispheric functional asymmetry in visual discrimination between univariate stimuli: An analysis of sensitivity and response criterion. Neuropsychologia 14:335, 1976.
20. Dee, HL: Visuoconstructive and visuoperceptive deficits in patients with unilateral cerebral lesions. Neuropsychologia 8:305, 1970.
21. Russo, M, and Vignolo, LA: Visual figure-ground discrimination in patients with unilateral cerebral disease. Cortex 3:113, 1967.
22. Varney, NR: Letter recognition and visual form discrimination in aphasic alexia. Neuropsychologia 19:795, 1981.
23. Teuber, HL, and Weinstein, S: Ability to discover hidden figures after cerebral lesions. Arch Neurol Psychiatr 76:369, 1954.
24. Lansdell, HC: Effect of extent of temporal lobe ablations on two lateralized deficits. Physiol Behav 3:271, 1968.
25. Meier, MJ, and French, LA: Lateralized deficits in complex visual discrimination and bilateral transfer of reminiscence following unilateral temporal lobectomy. Neuropsychologia 3:261, 1965.
26. Newcombe, F, and Russell, WR: Dissociated visual perceptual and spatial deficits in focal lesions of the right hemisphere. J Neurol Neurosurg Psychiatry 32:73, 1969.
27. Benton, AL, and Van Allen, MW: Impairment in facial recognition in patients with cerebral disease. Cortex 4:344, 1968.
28. De Renzi, E, Faglioni, P, and Spinnler, H: The performance of patients with unilateral brain damage on facial recognition tasks. Cortex 4:17, 1968.
29. Hamsher, K, Levin, HS, and Benton, AL: Facial recognition in patients with focal brain lesions. Arch Neurol 36:837, 1979.
30. Bruyer, R, and Vulge, V: Unilateral cerebral lesion and disturbance of face perception. Specificity of the deficit? Acta Neurol Belg 81:321, 1981.
31. Levin, HS, Grossman, RG, and Kelly, PJ: Impairment of facial recognition after closed head injuries of varying severity. Cortex 13:119, 1977.
32. Young, AW, de Haan, EH, and Newcombe, F: Unawareness of impaired face perception. Brain Cogn 14:1, 1990.
33. Boll, TJ: Right and left cerebral hemisphere damage and tactile perception: Performance of the ipsilateral and contralateral sides of the body. Neuropsychologia 12:235, 1974.
34. Fontenot, DJ, and Benton, AL: Tactile perception of direction in relation to hemispheric locus of lesion. Neuropsychologia 9:83, 1971.
35. Carmon, A, and Benton, AL: Tactile perception of direction and number in patients with unilateral cerebral disease. Neurology 19:525, 1969.
36. De Renzi, E, and Scotti, G: The influence of spatial disorders in impairing tactual discrimination of shapes. Cortex 5:53, 1969.
37. Sidtis, JJ, and Feldman, E: Transient ischemic attacks presenting with a loss of pitch perception. Cortex 26:469, 1990.
38. Peretz, I: Hemispheric asymmetry in amusia. Rev Neurol 141:169, 1985.
39. Mavlov, L: Amusia due to rhythm agnosia in a musician with left hemisphere damage: A non-auditory supramodal defect. Cortex 16:331, 1980.
40. Mendez, MF, and Geehan Jr, GR: Cortical auditory disorders: Clinical and psychoacoustic features. J Neurol Neurosurg Psychiatry 51:1, 1988.
41. Tanaka, Y, Yamadori, A, and Mori, E: Pure word deafness following bilateral lesions. A psychophysical analysis. Brain 110:381, 1987.
42. Assal, G, and Buttet, J: Agraphia and preservation of music writing in a bilingual piano teacher. Rev Neurol (Paris) 139:569, 1983.
43. Milner, B: Laterality effects in audition. In Mountcastle, VB (ed): Interhemispheric Relations and Cerebral Dominance. Johns Hopkins University Press, Baltimore, 1962, p 177.

44. Benton, AL, et al: Contributions to Neuropsychological Assessment. A Clinical Manual. Oxford University Press, New York, 1983.
45. Levin, HS, and Benton, AL: Facial recognition in "pseudoneurological" patients. J Nerv Mental Dis 164:135, 1977.
46. Warrington, EK, and James, M: The Visual Object and Space Perception Battery Manual. Thames Valley Test Company, Bury St. Edmunds, England, 1991.
47. Heaton, RK, Grant, I, and Matthews, CG: Comprehensive Norms for an Expanded Halstead-Reitan Battery. Demographic Corrections, Research Findings, and Clinical Applications. Psychological Assessment Resources, Odessa, FL, 1991.
48. Matarazzo, JD, et al: Psychometric and clinical test-retest reliability of the Halstead Impairment Index in a sample of healthy, young, normal men. J Nerv Ment Dis 158:37, 1974.
49. Goldstein, G, and Watson, JR: Test-retest reliability of the Halstead-Reitan Battery and the WAIS in a neuropsychiatric population. Clin Neuropsychol 3:265, 1989.
50. Charter, RA, et al: Reliability of the WAIS, WMS, and Reitan Battery: Raw scores and standardized scores corrected for age and education. Int J Clin Neuropsychol 9:28, 1987.
51. Bigler, ED, and Tucker, DM: Comparison of verbal IQ, Tactual Performance, Seashore Rhythm and Finger Oscillation Tests in the blind and brain-damaged. J Clin Psychol 37:849, 1981.
52. Barnes, GW, and Lucas, GJ: Cerebral dysfunction vs. psychogenesis in Halstead-Reitan tests. J Nerv Ment Dis 158:50, 1974.
53. Prigatano, GP, et al: Neuropsychological test performance in mildly hypoxic patients with chronic obstructive pulmonary disease. J Consult Clin Psychol 51:108, 1983.
54. Sherer, M: Clinical validity of the Speech-Sounds Perception Test and the Seashore Rhythm Test. J Clin Exp Neuropsychol 13:741, 1991.
55. O'Donnell, JP, et al: Neuropsychological test findings for normal, learning disabled and brain damaged young adults. J Consult Clin Psychol 51:726, 1983.
56. Hakstian, AR, Cattell, RB, and IPAT Staff: Manual for the Comprehensive Ability Battery (CAB). Institute for Personality and Ability Testing, Champaign, IL, 1982.
57. Goldstein, G, and Shelly, CH: Univariate vs. multivariate analysis in neuropsychological test assessment of lateralized brain damage. Cortex 9:204, 1973.
58. Lezak, MD: Neuropsychological Assessment, Second Edition. Oxford University Press, New York, 1983.
59. Russell, EW, Neuringer, C, and Goldstein, G: Assessment of Brain Damage. John Wiley and Sons, New York, 1970.
60. Klove, H: Validation studies in adult clinical neuropsychology. In Reitan, RM, and Davison, LA (eds): Clinical Neuropsychology: Current Status and Applications. John Wiley and Sons, New York, 1974, p 211.
61. Reitan, RM, and Wolfson, D: The Halstead-Reitan Neuropsychological Test Battery. Neuropsychology Press, Tucson, 1985.
62. Spreen, O, and Strauss, E: A Compendium of Neuropsychological Tests. Administration, Norms, and Commentary. Oxford University Press, New York, 1991.
63. Franzen, MD: Reliability and Validity in Neuropsychological Assessment. Plenum Press, New York, 1989.
64. Schludermann, EH, and Schludermann, SM: Halstead's studies in the neuropsychology of aging. Archives of Gerontology and Geriatrics 2:49, 1983.
65. Russell, E: Comparison of the TPT 10 and 6-hole form board. J Clin Psychol 41:68, 1985.
66. Binder, LM: Forced choice testing provides evidence of malingering. Arch Phys Med Rehabil 73:377, 1992.
67. Hays, WL: Statistics for the Social Sciences, Second Edition. Holt, Rinehart and Winston, New York, 1973.

SPATIAL IMPERCEPTION

6

Spatial imperception involves deficits in the ability to determine the position, orientation, and direction of stimuli in space. Spatial imperception can also manifest itself as a deficit in imagining the spatial configuration of stimuli that are only partially visible or in imagining a stimulus from a different perspective or orientation. The subtypes of spatial imperception listed in the chapter outline are discussed in this chapter.

Local and global astereopsis are disorders of depth perception. Their assessment and diagnosis require the use of a stereoscope. A stereoscope is a viewing instrument containing two eyepieces, each of which shows the same scene from a slightly different position. The disparity between what the two eyes see creates the impression of depth. The two views of the scene are merged by the brain into a single image that appears to have depth.

Images shown in a stereoscope may be representations of actual objects or random patterns of dots or letters. When actual objects are used, depth can be determined based on binocular disparity and the information provided by form, contour, and shading. However, this information is absent when random patterns of dots or letters are used. Consequently, when random pattern images are used, depth can be judged only on the basis of binocular disparity.

Local stereopsis, also called "stereoacuity," is the ability to perceive depth when actual forms are viewed in a stereoscope. Local stereopsis involves the determination of depth from the information provided by form, contour, and shading cues, as well as from the information provided by binocular disparity. Global stereopsis is the ability to perceive depth when random patterns are viewed in a stereoscope. Global stereopsis makes use of the information provided by binocular disparity to determine depth; no form, contour, or shading cues are present to aid in depth perception.

In spatial disorientation, the ability to determine the orientation of stimuli in space is defective. Patients with spatial inflexibility are unable to mentally rotate or manipulate stimuli. Spatial misestimation involves a deficit in making estimates about quantity based on limited spatial information. Topographical disorientation is an impairment in directional sense.

Limiting this chapter to the disorders listed may seem arbitrary because many disorders discussed elsewhere in this text involve an element of spatial perception. However, inclusion of every disorder in which spatial perception plays even a minor role would have made this chapter hopelessly unwieldy. The disorders in which spatial perception plays a primary role are discussed in this chapter. Other disorders in which spatial skill is involved to lesser or varying degrees are listed for completeness (see page 115), but their clinical descriptions can be found in other chapters of this text.

Spatial perception contributes to the general perception of visual and tactual stimuli and to the assignment of meaning (recognition) to these stimuli. Stimulus imperception is discussed in Chapter 5, and disorders of stimulus recognition are discussed in Chapter 9.

NOMENCLATURE

The terms *local stereopsis* and *global stereopsis* are in use in the perceptual and neurology literature, and the inability to perceive depth is sometimes called "stereoblindness." Stereoblindness implies the presence of a severe disability and may not be the ideal term for mild depth perception impairment. The term *astereopsis* is used in this text to refer to the full range of possible impairment in stereopsis. I am unaware of any prior use of this term.

No single term exists to describe impairment in judging spatial orientation.

Typically, the deficit is described in terms of the specific task used to elicit the deficient response. For example, if patients are deficient in judging the angle of lines, they may be described as having line orientation impairment. If the task eliciting the deficit involves judging the orientation of designs, the patient is said to have impairment of design orientation. The term *spatial disorientation* is used in this text to refer to deficient perception of spatial orientation, regardless of the task used to demonstrate this deficit.

A similar situation exists with impairments in the ability to mentally transform the spatial perspective or orientation of stimuli; the deficit is labeled according to the task used to elicit the deficient response. Thus, terms such as *spatial visualization, mental rotation, perspective taking,* and *spatial transformation* may be employed by various researchers and clinicians to describe the same condition. The term *spatial inflexibility* is used in this text to describe all impairments related to mentally manipulating stimuli in space.

Various tasks have been used by neuropsychologists to assess the ability to estimate quantity based on spatial information. One type of task involves presenting a drawing that shows configurations of stacked blocks. The drawing is done so that only a portion of the blocks is visible. The presence of the remainder of the blocks is inferred by the way in which the visible blocks are stacked. The task is to determine how many total blocks must be present (seen and unseen) to make the spatial configuration possible. Another type of task involves presenting an array of dots or letters for brief periods of time using a computer or tachistoscope. The stimuli are not presented long enough for the individual dots or letters to be counted. The number of dots or letters must be determined, instead, from the overall spatial configuration of the array. Performance of these tasks may be referred to as "number" or "block estimation." The term *spatial misestimation* is used in this text to refer to impairment in performing this type of task.

In contrast to the previously described terms, *topographical disorientation* is too frequently used in the clinical literature. This term has been used to describe a patient's inability to recognize his or her room, home, or other familiar building or environment; a tendency to become lost when traveling a previously familiar route; an inability to learn new routes; an inability to describe how to get from one location to another; a failure to locate places accurately on a map; and impairment in sense of direction.

This text restricts the term *topographical disorientation* to impairment of direction sense. The failure to recognize previously familiar environments is called *topographical agnosia* and is discussed in Chapter 9. A person may become lost when traveling a familiar route for any number of reasons; this behavior alone does not imply a particular diagnosis. The inability to learn a new route or describe how to get from one place to another may indicate the presence of a memory disorder, assuming all other explanations have been ruled out. If the memory impairment is specific to routes, the term *topographical amnesia* can be used. Amnesias are discussed in Chapter 16. Performance of map location tasks is heavily influenced by prior knowledge and the presence of stimulus neglect (see Chap. 4) or other perceptual disorders (see Chap. 5). Thus, defective map location abilities also are a nonspecific diagnostic sign.

ICD-9-CM[1] provides several options for diagnostic coding of spatial imperception. Local and global astereopsis may be coded as "Fusion with Defective Stereopsis" under "Disorders of Binocular Vision." Visual spatial disorientation, spatial inflexibility, spatial misestimation, and topographical disorientation may be coded as "Psychophysical Visual Disturbances," "Unspecified Subjective Visual Disturbances," "Unspecified Visual Disturbance," or "Other Visual Disturbance." All of these terms are vague, and none precisely fits the spatial imperception disorders. Consequently, it is difficult to recommend one diagnostic code over another. "Subjective Visual Disturbance" may not be the preferred code because diagnosis of spatial imperception is based on objective testing and not just on subjective complaints made by the patient.

DSM-IV[2] does not include a specific diagnostic code for spatial imperception. The nonspecific diagnoses "Cognitive Disorder Not Otherwise Specified" and "Mild Neurocognitive Disorder" can be used to code spatial imperception.

RULES FOR DIAGNOSIS

Clinical Indicators: Each is independent (only one must be observed for the disorder to be suspected) *except* when subscripting is used. Subscripted numbers (a_1, a_2) denote an indicator with multiple parts that must be considered together.
Associated Features: These are listed to give a more complete picture of the disorders. The presence or absence of these features does not affect the diagnosis.
Factors to Rule Out: All must be taken into account. Failure to rule out even one of these factors makes a firm diagnosis impossible.
Lesion Locations: Each location stands alone; damage in only one of the listed areas is sufficient to produce the disorder.

VARIETY OF PRESENTATION

1. **Local astereopsis**

   Clinical Indicator

   a. Inaccurate perception of depth when viewing objects under stereoscopic conditions

   Associated Features

   a. The presence of global astereopsis (see later text)
   b. Patient awareness or nonawareness of a decline in depth perception

   Factors to Rule Out

   a. Loss of visual acuity in either eye sufficient to prevent stereoscopic viewing

b. Failure to detect visual stimuli on one or both sides of space caused by stimulus neglect (see Chap. 4)

Lesion Locations

a. Cerebral hemisphere[3–6]
b. Posterior to the central sulcus, particularly the parietal lobe and the junction of the parietal, temporal, and occipital lobes[7–9]

Lesion Lateralization

a. More frequent and more severe following right-sided lesions,[3,8] but greater severity after left-sided lesions[9] or no difference in severity between sides of lesions reported by some investigators.[5,6]

2. Global astereopsis

Clinical Indicator

a. Inaccurate perception of depth when viewing patterns of random dots or letters under stereoscopic conditions

Associated Features

a. The presence of local astereopsis (see previous text)
b. Patient awareness or nonawareness of a decline in depth perception

Factors to Rule Out

a. Loss of visual acuity in either eye sufficient to prevent stereoscopic viewing
b. Failure to detect visual stimuli on one or both sides of space as a result of stimulus neglect (see Chap. 4)

Lesion Locations

a. Cerebral hemisphere[4,5,10,11]
b. Posterior to the central sulcus, particularly the parietal lobe and the junction of the parietal, temporal, and occipital lobes[7,8]
c. Temporal lobe[12]

Lesion Lateralization

a. More frequent and more severe following right-sided lesions[5,8,10,11]

3. Spatial disorientation

Clinical Indicator

a. Inaccurate judgment of orientation in space of visually or tactually presented stimuli

Associated Features

a. Homonymous hemianopsia: Loss of acuity in one visual half-field

Factors to Rule Out

a. Loss of visual acuity sufficient to prevent test stimuli from being seen clearly regardless of where in the visual field they are presented
b. Failure to detect visual or tactile stimuli on one or both sides of space as a result of stimulus neglect (see Chap. 4)
c. Loss of tactile sensation sufficient to prevent the patient from feeling a stimulus when tactile orientation tests are used

d. Weakness of the arm or hand muscles sufficient to prevent responses when orientation tests that require manual manipulation are used
e. Poor coordination of the arm or hand muscles sufficient to prevent responses when orientation tests that require manual manipulation are used
f. Impaired initiation of arm or hand movements (see Akinesia) sufficient to prevent responses when orientation tests that require manual manipulation are used
g. Impaired maintenance of ongoing arm or hand movements (see Motor impersistence) sufficient to prevent responses when orientation tests that require manual manipulation are used
h. Perseveration of arm or hand movements (see Motor perseveration) sufficient to prevent responses when orientation tests that require manual manipulation are used

Lesion Locations

a. Cerebral hemisphere[13]
b. Posterior to the central sulcus[14–16]
c. Anterior to the central sulcus[15]

Lesion Lateralization

a. Researchers uncertain whether the disorder is more frequent and more severe following left-sided[13] or right-sided[15,16] lesions.

4. Spatial inflexibility

Clinical Indicators

a. Inaccuracy in mentally rotating or otherwise imagining the movement of stimuli in space
b. Inaccuracy in mentally altering the shape of a stimulus (e.g., imagining the stimulus as it would appear when bent, twisted, or folded)
c. Inaccuracy in mentally combining individual fragments to picture a whole object
d. Inaccuracy in picturing how an object or scene looks from a different angle or direction

Associated Features

a. Homonymous hemianopsia: Loss of acuity in one visual half-field

Factors to Rule Out

a. Loss of visual acuity sufficient to prevent test stimuli from being seen clearly regardless of where in the visual field they are presented
b. Failure to detect or remember visual stimuli on one or both sides of space as a result of stimulus neglect (see Chap. 4)
c. Impaired ability to sustain concentration or divide concentration among several mental activities (see Chap. 3) (even mild concentration deficits can invalidate testing of spatial flexibility)

Lesion Locations

a. Cerebral hemisphere[13,17]
b. Posterior to central sulcus, particularly the parietal and temporal-parietal areas and Wernicke's area[14,15,18–22]
c. Frontal lobe, particularly the prefrontal area[15,21]

Lesion Lateralization

a. Researchers differ regarding whether the disorder is more frequent and severe following left-sided[13,14,18] or right-sided[15,18,21] lesions. Other investigators document little effect of lesion laterality.[17,22]

5. Spatial misestimation

Clinical Indicator

a. Inaccurate estimation of the number of individual elements in an array of dots, letters, blocks, or the like based on the spatial configuration of the array (direct counting of the individual elements in the array must be prevented by presenting the stimulus only briefly or by presenting a drawing of the array that shows the overall spatial configuration while hiding some of the individual elements)

Associated Features

a. Misestimation of briefly presented stimuli that can occur in the left, right, or both visual fields

Factors to Rule Out

a. Loss of visual acuity sufficient to prevent test stimuli from being seen clearly regardless of where in the visual field they are presented
b. Failure to detect or remember visual stimuli on one or both sides of space as a result of stimulus neglect (see Chap. 4)
c. Impaired ability to sustain concentration or divide concentration among several mental activities (see Chap. 3) (even mild concentration deficits can invalidate testing of spatial estimation ability)

Lesion Locations

a. Temporal lobe[23,24]
b. Parietal lobe[23]

Lesion Lateralization

a. Right-sided lesions[23,24]
b. Misestimation of briefly presented stimuli likely to occur only in the contralateral visual field in patients who have parietal lobe lesions[23]
c. Misestimation of briefly presented stimuli can occur in all portions of the visual field in patients who have temporal lobe lesions[23]

6. Topographical disorientation (see also Right-left disorientation)

Clinical Indicators

a. Inaccuracy in following nonverbal maps (i.e., drawings of a route that exclude specific verbal directions, although landmarks may be verbally labeled) when attempting to travel a route
b. Inaccuracy in indicating the directions being traveled (north/south/east/west or left/right) when traversing an actual route or tracing a path on a map

Associated Features

a. Impaired oral language (see Chap. 12)
b. Decreased tactile sensation

c. Impaired ability to draw figures or construct models (see Constructional disability)
d. The presence of dressing apraxia: Failure to dress one half of the body (see Hemispatial neglect)
e. Homonymous hemianopsia: Loss of acuity in one visual half-field
f. Impaired recognition of familiar landmarks (see Topographical agnosia)
g. Impaired memory for routes (see Topographical amnesia)

Factors to Rule Out

a. Loss of visual acuity sufficient to prevent test stimuli from being seen clearly regardless of where in the visual field they are presented
b. Failure to detect visual or tactile stimuli on one or both sides of space as a result of stimulus neglect (see Chap. 4)

Lesion Locations

a. Posterior hemisphere[25,26]
b. Posterior limb of internal capsule with reduced blood perfusion of the parietal lobe[27]
c. Splenium of corpus callosum with extension to the paramedian area of the right temporal lobe and the left hippocampus[28]

Lesion Lateralization

a. More frequently reported following right-sided lesions[26,27] but can also occur following left-sided lesions[25]

7. **Hemispatial neglect (see Chap. 4)**
8. **Pseudoneglect (see Chap. 10)**
9. **Spatial acalculia (see Chap. 15)**
10. **Spatial agraphia (see Chap. 13)**
11. **Optic ataxia (see Chap. 7)**
12. **Constructional disability (see Chap. 7)**
13. **Unilateral constructional disability (see Chap. 10)**
14. **Stimulus mislocalization (see Chap. 8)**
15. **Finger mislocalization (see Chap. 8)**
16. **Right-left disorientation (see Chap. 8)**

ETIOLOGY

Cerebrovascular accident is the primary cause reported in cases of spatial perception disorder. Other common causes include traumatic brain injury and brain neoplasm. Any disease process resulting in posterior cerebral damage can produce impairment of spatial functions. Spatial perception can be decreased in degenerative diseases (e.g., Alzheimer's disease) and in demyelinating diseases (e.g., multiple sclerosis). Alcoholism or abuse of other substances can impair spatial perception, particularly in middle-aged or older individuals.

DISABLING CONSEQUENCES

Ambulation and driving are the two main activities involving spatial perception that virtually all adult members of Western society perform. Impaired spatial perception can make walking hazardous and driving impossible. In severe cases of astereopsis, the patient may misjudge the steepness of curbs, steps, or inclines, creating the potential for a fall. Depth perception must be intact for patients to judge safe driving distances and to decide when to brake. Astereopsis can be sufficient grounds for recommending revocation of a patient's driver's license.

Spatial misestimation can also pose a driving hazard, although alone, it may not be a sufficient reason for recommending that the patient's driver's license be revoked. Spatial misestimation can cause a patient to misjudge how much space is needed to park the car, resulting in potential property damage. It can also pose a hazard when driving in tight spaces (e.g., a narrow street with oncoming traffic and some parked vehicles), in which an estimate must be made of how much room is needed for the car.

Patients with topographical disorientation are prone to become confused about directions or lost. This is frustrating for the patient when walking; when he or she is driving, it can be a source of distraction and stress that edges a marginally safe driver into the hazardous driver category. Generally, patients who have severe topographical disorientation need someone to supervise and help them when they travel by foot or motor vehicle. Depending on the severity of the disorder, supervision may be needed only for unfamiliar routes.

Professional cab, bus, and truck drivers; fork-lift operators; and any other individuals in occupations requiring the operation of a vehicle are unable to work in their chosen field if they develop astereopsis, spatial misestimation, or topographical disorientation. Pilots and air traffic controllers are also likely to be disabled by spatial disorientation. Engineers, architects, carpenters, draftsmen, and visual artists, among others, experience major loss of work capacity as a result of any of the spatial perception disorders. Certain fields of medicine, including surgery and radiology, require good spatial skills, and any of the spatial perception disorders can greatly impede performance in these fields. Professional dancers and choreographers also depend on their spatial abilities, as do virtually all athletes. Participation in any of these or related professions can be curtailed by spatial impairment.

Most active adults make greater use of their spatial abilities during leisure time. Thus, the spatial perception disorders can limit leisure choices. Recreational activities such as visual art, photography, boating, recreational sports, hunting, fly fishing, and target shooting may no longer be possible for people who have spatial perception disorders. Even simple activities such as playing a video game or flying a kite can place demands on spatial skills that the spatially impaired patient cannot meet.

ASSESSMENT INSTRUMENTS

Stereo Test and Randot Stereotest

The Stereo Test and Randot Stereotest are available from *Stereo Optical Company, Incorporated, 3539 North Kenton Avenue, Chicago, IL 60641.*

The Stereo Test employs three-dimensional vectographs of a housefly, a series of circles, and animals to measure local stereopsis. The Randot Stereotest uses random dot patterns to measure the patient's ability to differentiate a form from a homogeneous background without the aid of monocularly visible contours. The Randot Stereotest provides a measure of global stereopsis. Both tests use polarized viewers, which may be worn over prescription glasses, if necessary. In both tests, the most precise measure of depth perception is obtained using the circle stimuli. The Stereo Test permits measurement of stereoacuity from 40 to 800 arc seconds. The Randot Stereotest measures stereoacuity from 20 to 400 arc seconds.

The two stereoscopic vision tests are inexpensive and can be administered at bedside, in the office, or in the laboratory. Interpretation is straightforward, and the tests are appropriate for use by a broad range of clinicians. Patients with significantly impaired depth perception should be referred for ophthalmologic or optometric examination.

Visual Object and Space Perception Battery

See Chapter 5.

Benton Judgment of Line Orientation Test

The Benton Judgment of Line Orientation Test[29] is available from *Oxford University Press, Incorporated, 200 Madison Avenue, New York, NY 10016.*

The patient must match line segments with a set of longer lines on a response card based on the spatial orientation of the lines. Two forms (H and V) of the test are available, each of which employs the same items presented in a slightly different order. On both forms, item difficulty increases as the test progresses. The clinical manual reports split-half reliability for form H ($r = .94$) and V ($r = .91$). A test-retest reliability coefficient of .90 is reported over an interval ranging from 6 hours to 21 days.

Normative data are reported in the clinical manual on a sample of 137 healthy volunteers and non-neurological patients. Age and gender were found to moderate Line Orientation Test performance, and correction factors have been developed to take this into account. Education level appears to interact with age and gender in its impact on performance. No correction factor is available for education, and the test authors note that further investigation of the relation between education and Line Orientation Test performance is necessary. Data reported in the clinical manual support the sensitivity of the Line Orientation Test to lateralized lesions. A higher proportion of right-hemisphere-damaged patients obtained below-normal scores compared with left-hemisphere-damaged patients. In the right-hemisphere group, virtually all impaired patients had posterior lesions, excluding those with indeterminant lesion locations within the right hemisphere.

The chief disadvantage of the Benton Judgment of Line Orientation Test is its length. It can be frustrating for more impaired patients. Practice items are available that help to eliminate patients who are too severely impaired to realistically attempt the test. These patients are considered to be severely impaired in their judgment of line orientation and should be distinguished from patients who cannot perform the test because of poor language comprehension or other factors. The Line Orientation Test can be administered at bedside, in the office, or in the laboratory and can be interpreted by behavioral neurologists and neuropsychologists experienced in the diagnosis of perceptual disorders.

Luria's Neuropsychological Investigation, Section G—Block Estimation and Mental Rotation

Luria's Neuropsychological Investigation,[30,31] Section G—Block Estimation (cards 29–32) and Mental Rotation (card 33) is available from *Spectrum Publications, Incorporated, 86–19 Sancho Street, Holliswood, NY 11423.*

Section G of Luria's Neuropsychological Investigation assesses "higher visual functions"; see Chapter 19 for a full description of Luria's Neuropsychological Investigation. The Block Estimation task requires the patient to estimate the number of blocks shown in a drawing based on its spatial configuration.

In the Mental Rotation task, patients view a parallelogram containing a circle in one corner. One side of the parallelogram is darker than the others and is identified as the base. The base can be any side of the original parallelogram. To the right of the original object are two more parallelograms without circles. The base of these figures is a solid black line upon which each object rests. The patient is asked to put a circle in the right place in one of the two parallelograms so that it will match the original parallelogram. To accomplish this, the original parallelogram must be rotated mentally until its base is at the bottom and it can be compared to the two empty parallelograms to see which one it matches.

These two tasks are relatively quick to administer. The first item of each task is simpler than the items that follow. If the patient fails to pass the first item, the examiner can inform the patient of the correct answer and discuss how the answer was arrived at to make sure the patient comprehends what the tasks require.

Luria's Neuropsychological Investigation does not include normative data or empirical demonstrations of reliability and validity. At the core of Luria's Neuropsychological Investigation is the systematic analysis of qualitative changes in behavior following focal lesions. Luria's method does not lend itself to quantification and norming (see discussion of the Luria-Nebraska Neuropsychological Battery in Chap. 19). The Block Estimation and Mental Rotation tasks should be interpreted only by experienced neurologists and neuropsychologists. Interpretation should be attempted only in the context of a broad and comprehensive battery of tests. Both tasks are suitable for bedside, office, and laboratory administration.

Extrapersonal Orientation Test

The Extrapersonal Orientation Test (EOT)[25] is *not commercially available.*

The EOT consists of five maps made up of nine evenly spaced dots that correspond to nine evenly spaced dots on the floor; dots are spaced several paces apart so that the patient can comfortably walk from one dot to another. Paths along the dot maps are shown by a heavy black line originating at one large dot and traveling from one dot to another before terminating in an arrow at the final dot. The paths shown on all five maps combined involve a total of 35 turns. The top edge of the map is designated north, and the patient is instructed to hold this edge farthest away from his or her body. One wall of the room is also designated north to orient the patient. The patient is required to traverse each path shown on the maps without changing the orientation of the map relative to his or her body.

The reliability of the EOT has not been studied. The EOT successfully discriminated chronic brain-injured (penetrating missile wounds) Korean war veterans from veterans who received peripheral nerve injuries ($p < .01$).[25] The test was particularly sensitive to posterior left-hemisphere lesions, although patients with bilateral posterior lesions showed the greatest impairment.

Although it is not commercially available, the EOT can be constructed from published descriptions and examples.[25] The test results must be interpreted cautiously because the effects of age and education on performance in normal populations are unknown and the reliability of the test is unestablished. Interpretation should be attempted only by experienced neuropsychologists and behavioral neurologists. The floor space required by the EOT makes it suitable only for laboratory and large office settings.

NEUROPSYCHOLOGICAL TREATMENT

The principle underlying the treatment of patients with spatial disorders is to provide practice in their deficient areas. Practice exercises should be graded in difficulty so that they challenge the patient while maintaining a high probability of success. For example, when working with patients who have deficits in depth perception, the task is to first determine at what relative distance the patient can reliably distinguish the depth of two stimuli. The distance between stimuli can then be decreased slightly while the patient continues to determine on each trial which of two stimuli is closer. If the patient's error rate increases, the distance between stimuli can be increased until performance improves, and then gradually decreased again. In this manner, the patient's ability to judge depth may improve over a large series of trials.

Spatial disorientation can be approached in a similar manner. When one is treating spatial disorientation, the objective is to require the patient to make increasingly difficult orientation judgments. Tasks typically involve presenting a target stimulus and then requiring the patient to either duplicate its spatial orientation or select another stimulus with a matching orientation from several choices. Such tasks are easier when the target stimulus is at or close to 0 degrees (i.e., horizontal) or 90 degrees (i.e., vertical). The farther away from horizontal or vertical the spatial orientation, the more difficult the orientation judgment.

The technique of progressively difficult practice trials also can be applied to spatial inflexibility and misestimation. The difficulty level of spatial flexibility tasks (e.g., duplicating the rotation of a target stimulus or selecting a stimulus that matches the target rotation) can be controlled by manipulating the degree of rotation in any given plane, by increasing the number of planes in which rotation occurs (e.g., rotating the stimulus horizontally and vertically), or by increasing the spatial complexity of the stimuli so that more features must be considered when judging the rotation. Varying the spatial complexity or density (i.e., the number of elements) of a spatial array permits the therapist to control the difficulty of spatial estimation tasks.

Compensatory techniques have not been widely used in the treatment of spatial disorders, but a compensatory approach is appropriate when treating topographical disorientation. The therapist can provide written directions for routes, emphasizing the landmarks to look for along the way. If the patient cannot follow even simple left-right directions, the patient can instead be instructed to turn in the direction of a specific landmark. Pictures of salient landmarks can be provided in addition to written directions. It is important to provide instructions for both traveling to and returning from a destination. The patient cannot be expected to spontaneously reverse the original directions to return to the point of origin.

There is a tendency to panic when one becomes lost. For adults, there also can be feelings of embarrassment associated with not knowing where one is and how to get to one's destination. Teaching the patient to relax when lost and to seek orienting landmarks or assistance from others is as important as providing written directions. After the patient has gained some confidence, it can be therapeutic to deliberately get the patient lost and then instruct him or her to find the way back or to get appropriate help. The therapist must, of course, remain in attendance during such trials.

Compensatory techniques also should be exploited when treating other spatial disorders. Patients can be instructed to use brightness, size, and other cues to make depth determinations. Using a ruler or protractor can improve performance on spatial orientation and flexibility tasks. Learning to appropriately multiply the visible units (e.g., blocks or dots) in a spatial array can enhance spatial estimation.

In treating any of the spatial disorders, the patient's motivation to improve is a key factor in the effectiveness of the treatment. Patients who do not work in spatial occupations may see no reason to improve their spatial skills. It can also be difficult to convince patients that their spatial deficits impede their driving. Success or failure in linking the spatial tasks performed in the clinic with an everyday activity that is important to the patient often determines whether the patient will agree to work on his or her spatial skills. Having the patient attempt and fail at the spatial tasks important in his or her life may be necessary to convince him or her that treatment of the disorder is required. Thus, a trial return to spatial work or a simulated driving experience, with care to ensure the patient's safety, may be necessary before formal treatment can begin.

CASE ILLUSTRATIONS

CASE 6–1

W.K. was a 55-year-old man who had completed 2 years of college and worked as a traffic policeman in a small Southern community following his retirement from the United States Air Force. He suffered a left-hemisphere ischemic cerebrovascular accident following carotid endarterectomy. W.K. presented with a right hemiparesis, deficits in the performance of skilled movements on demand (see Apraxia), a mild Broca's aphasia (see Chap. 12), and preserved visual fields with good acuity premorbidly and no current complaints of visual impairment. The patient made no errors when asked to identify colors, drawings of objects, and faces of recent United States presidents. He bisected lines accurately and made no errors with unilateral or bilateral simultaneous stimulation. Memory was low average (scores below the 25th percentile) for orally presented paragraphs and solidly average (scores above the 40th percentile) for geometric figures.

W.K.'s performance on the Benton Judgment of Line Orientation Test was in the moderately impaired range. In contrast, he scored in the normal range on the Benton Facial Recognition Test, which measures the ability to make fine facial discriminations. He was not distractible during testing; his attention never wandered from the task, and he never required redirection.

CASE 6–2

M.N. was a 35-year-old Korean-American woman who had completed high school in Korea and worked as a homemaker and part-time fashion model. She suffered an episode of acute right upper extremity weakness that resolved over a period of 2 weeks and for which she did not seek medical attention. Several weeks later, she became obtunded (see Lethargy or obtundation) and unable to speak, and suffered a recurrence of the right upper extremity weakness, this time to the point where the arm was flaccid. In the emergency department, she gradually became more alert, and further examination revealed blindness in her left eye. Acuity was preserved in her right eye.

M.N.'s computed tomographic (CT) scan showed an area of hyperdensity in the left middle cerebral artery territory underlying the junction of gray and white matter in the posterior part of the frontal-temporal region. Cerebral arteriography showed a filling defect in an anterior branch of the left middle cerebral artery consistent with a partial embolic occlusion. M.N.'s blindness was attributed to an ischemic lesion involving the left ophthalmic artery. An echocardiogram showed a left atrial mass, which was thought responsible for the two episodes of embolization. The mass was excised, and anticoagulants were administered to the patient.

After being referred for comprehensive physical and cognitive rehabilitation, M.N. participated in formal neuropsychological testing. No errors were made during unilateral or bilateral simultaneous stimulation in any sensory modality, although she remained blind in the left eye. She identified colors, objects, and faces of United States presidents with good accuracy. Her line bisection revealed mild neglect (see Chap. 4) of right-sided visual stimuli. The patient was attentive throughout the examination, although her digit span scores were low (five digits in forward sequence, three in reverse sequence). Memory of paragraphs and designs was significantly impaired, although language impairment contributed to her poor performance with paragraphs. M.N. understood oral and written commands and could repeat phrases accurately but showed minimal spontaneous speech (see Transcortical motor aphasia). Her response to questions consisted of brief phrases or single words, regardless of whether she spoke in English or Korean.

Despite M.N.'s unilateral blindness and mild neglect, she obtained a normal score when attempting to make visual discriminations on the Benton Facial Recognition Test. Severe impairment was seen in the Benton Judgment of Line Orientation Test.

CASE 6–3

M.P. was a 63-year-old homemaker who had a high-school education. She suffered a right middle cerebral artery hemorrhage; her CT scan revealed right parietal lobe damage. A subdural hematoma was removed before she began rehabilitation. M.P. was alert and attentive with a forward digit span score of six and reverse digit span score of four. She showed a dense, left-sided, homonymous hemianopsia, with good acuity in the intact portions of her visual field. No errors were made to unilateral or bilateral stimulation in the auditory and tactile modalities. Line bisection test results were accurate, and there were no signs of hemispatial neglect (see Chap. 4) in her drawings. Memory was in the average range for both paragraphs and designs, and her intellectual functioning was high average. M.P. accurately identified colors, objects, and familiar faces. She had no motor or tactual perception deficits. The only areas of impairment were facial discrimination and judgment of spatial orientation; she was severely impaired on the Benton Facial Recognition and Judgment of Line Orientation Tests.

DISCUSSION

Cases 6–1, 6–2, and 6–3 are discussed together because of the similarities in their presentations. All three patients presented with moderate to severe spatial disorientation. Performance was assessed with the Benton Judgment of Line Orientation Test, which places minimal demands on tactual or motor ability. Thus, deficits in these areas probably did not play a role in the patients' spatial orientation performances. As discussed in Chapter 1, the experienced clinician always considers the impact of language and concentration deficits on neuropsychological test performance, even though these deficits are not specifically listed as factors to rule out for every disorder in this text. All three patients were able to sustain concentration and did not show signs of being distractible. Concentration span and divided concentration ability may have been reduced to some degree in all three patients. Two of the patients showed mild language impairment; however, the Benton Judgment of Line Orientation Test places minimal demands on language ability beyond the verbal instructions the patient must comprehend. Neither of the mildly aphasic patients had significant difficulty comprehending any of the test instructions.

A more significant issue in these cases is the possible impact of visual impairments on spatial orientation performance. The patient in Case 6–1 had full visual fields, had no history of visual impairment, voiced no difficulty in seeing any test stimuli, had no evidence of visual stimulus neglect, and performed normally on a variety of visually demanding tests. The patient in Case 6–2 was blind in the left eye and had mild, right-sided, visual stimulus neglect but showed normal acuity in the right eye. The patient in Case 6–3 had a left homonymous hemianopsia but no stimulus neglect and preserved acuity in the intact portions of her visual field. Despite their visual deficits, the patients in Cases 6–2 and 6–3 performed normally on visually demanding stimulus recognition, drawing, and discrimination (Case 6–2 only) tasks.

Thus, all three patients appeared to have sufficient visual capacity to attempt the Benton Judgment of Line Orientation Test in the intact portions of their visual fields. Because these patients did well on visually demanding tests that did not include a spatial orientation factor, visual sensory impairment alone is unlikely to account for their deficient judgment of line orientation. The diagnosis of spatial disorientation appears to be justified in these patients.

CASE 6–4

J.B. was a 17-year-old boy who was a senior in high school. A high fever at age 1 year was thought to have resulted in brain damage, necessitating 1 to 2 years of speech therapy. J.B. attended special education classes throughout school. He developed a seizure disorder, slurred speech, mild right-sided weakness, and difficulty in controlling his temper following a traumatic brain injury at age 17 years. The injury occurred when he was struck by a car while crossing the street. J.B. was unconscious for an undetermined period of time and spent 2 weeks in an intensive care department. There was no retrograde amnesia, but there was a global anterograde amnesia that remained severe for approximately 1 week (see Chap. 16).

J.B. experienced good recovery in strength and articulation; at the time of neuropsychological examination, speech was intelligible and he ambulated without difficulty. He also had good use of both upper extremities. Intellectual functioning was low average, problem-solving ability was preserved, and memory for paragraphs remained severely impaired. Memory of visual designs was only mildly reduced. J.B. was intact on the items comprising the HRB Aphasia Screening Test, with the exception of making written and oral spelling errors. His forward digit span score was seven, and his reversed digit span score was four. He showed no difficulty concentrating during the examination.

There were no indications of stimulus neglect (see Chap. 4) or impaired stimulus recognition (see Chap. 9). Testing of vision-dependent skills was hampered by the patient's difficulty in seeing, a problem he spontaneously reported. He usually wore glasses, but failed to bring them to the test session. Visual acuity was 20/50 in the right eye and 20/100 in the left eye without glasses. He was normal in his ability to do the detailed facial discriminations of the Benton Facial Recognition Test but was severely impaired on the Benton Judgment of Line Orientation Test. One trial of the Extrapersonal Orientation Test was administered, requiring 11 topographical decisions. J.B. initially made only 4 correct turns. On a repeat trial, he made 6 correct turns. Further assessment of this patient was planned when his glasses were available, but he failed to appear at future appointments.

DISCUSSION

This patient presented with possible spatial disorientation. Unfortunately, during the examination, he did not have the prescription glasses that he normally wore, and voiced difficulty in seeing test stimuli. Formal assessment of visual acuity revealed a decrease in his vision. Although a diagnosis of spatial disorientation is a possibility, the impact of decreased visual acuity has not been completely ruled out. He also performed poorly on the Extrapersonal Orientation Test, suggesting possible topographical disorientation. Visual acuity was less of a problem on the Extrapersonal Orientation Test because of the large size of the stimulus materials. No other perceptual or motor deficits were present to detract from the diagnosis of topographical disorientation.

A final point of interest is the etiology of the neuropsychological disorders seen in this patient. The possible occurrence of brain damage during early infancy and the history of special education classes raise the issue of whether deficits were present before the adolescent brain injury. This issue could be resolved in two ways. School records could be examined to determine whether indications of spatial imperception were present before the accident. It is likely that standardized testing was done and that scores were included in the school records, considering the patient's special education placement. Follow-up testing in 6 to 12 months could be done to determine whether there was improvement in spatial ability over time. Although a stable level of performance over this period of time will not help in determining the cause of his deficits, significant improvement would support an interpretation of the spatial deficits as a result of recent brain trauma from which the patient was recovering.

CASE 6–5

A.S. was a 76-year-old retired grade school teacher. She suffered an embolic right-hemisphere cerebrovascular accident secondary to atrial fibrillation. Neuropsychological assessment was requested at the time of admission to an inpatient rehabilitation program. The patient was alert and attentive. No errors were made when she was asked to signal whenever she heard an odd number, suggesting that her ability to sustain concentration was grossly intact. No errors were made on tests of color, object, and familiar face recognition. A.S. was incorrect on all block estimation trials in Section G of Luria's Neuropsychological Investigation. On the first two trials, she underestimated the number of blocks needed to make the configurations and simply counted the blocks that were visible. On the last two trials, the patient overestimated, appearing to make a rough guess about the number of invisible blocks. Further testing had to be discontinued because the patient became dizzy and nauseated.

DISCUSSION

Only a partial examination of this patient was conducted because of her discomfort during the session. The partial results suggest a diagnosis of spatial misestimation. The fact that she succeeded in counting the visible elements of the spatial stimuli suggests she had no difficulty seeing the materials. Her deficit emerged only when she was asked to estimate or infer the number of unseen elements based on the spatial configuration of the stimuli.

REFERENCES

1. The International Classification of Diseases, Ninth Revision, Clinical Modification. Med-Index Publications, Salt Lake City, 1991.
2. American Psychiatric Association: Diagnostic and Statistical Manual of Mental Disorders, Fourth Edition. American Psychiatric Association, Washington, DC, 1994.
3. Danta, G, Hilton, RC, and O'Boyle, DJ: Hemisphere function and binocular depth perception. Brain 101:569, 1978.
4. Hamsher, KD: Stereopsis and the perception of anomalous contours. Neuropsychologia 16:453, 1978.
5. Hamsher, KD: Stereopsis and unilateral brain disease. Invest Ophthalmol Vis Sci 17:336, 1978.
6. Lehmann, D, and Walchli, P: Depth perception and location of brain lesions. J Neurol 209:157, 1975.
7. Vaina, LM, et al: Intact "biological motion" and "structure from motion" perception in a patient with impaired motion mechanisms: A case study. Vis Neurosci 5:353, 1990.
8. Shuare, M: Disturbance of visual-spatial thinking in patients suffering local brain lesions. Neurosci Behav Physiol 12:133, 1982.
9. Rothstein, TB, and Sacks, JG: Defective stereopsis in lesions of the parietal lobe. Am J Ophthalmol 73:281, 1972.
10. Carmon, A, and Bechtoldt, HP: Dominance of the right cerebral hemisphere for stereopsis. Neuropsychologia 7:29, 1969.
11. Benton, AL, and Hecaen, H: Stereoscopic vision in patients with unilateral cerebral disease. Neurology 20:1084, 1970.
12. Ptito, A, et al: Stereopsis after unilateral anterior temporal lobectomy. Dissociation between local and global measures. Brain 114:1323, 1991.
13. Mehta, Z, Newcombe, F, and Damasio, H: A left hemisphere contribution to visuospatial processing. Cortex 23:447, 1987.
14. Mehta, Z, and Newcombe, F: A role for the left hemisphere in spatial processing. Cortex 27:153, 1991.
15. Kim, Y, et al: Visuoperceptual and visuomotor abilities and locus of lesion. Neuropsychologia 22:177, 1984.
16. Meerwaldt, JD, and van-Harskamp, F: Spatial disorientation in right-hemisphere infarction. J Neurol Neurosurg Psychiatry 45:586, 1982.
17. Goldenberg, G: The ability of patients with brain damage to generate mental visual images. Brain 112:305, 1989.
18. Ditunno, PL, and Mann, VA: Right hemisphere specialization for mental rotation in normals and brain damaged subjects. Cortex 26:177, 1990.
19. Dahmen, W, et al: Disorders of calculation in aphasic patients—spatial and verbal components. Neuropsychologia 20:145, 1982.

20. Ratcliff, G: Spatial thought, mental rotation and the right cerebral hemisphere. Neuropsychologia 17:49, 1979.
21. Meier, MJ: Effects of focal cerebral lesions on contralateral visuomotor adaptation to reversal and inversion of visual feedback. Neuropsychologia 8:269, 1970.
22. Butters, N, Barton, M, and Brody, BA: Role of the right parietal lobe in the mediation of cross-modal associations and reversible operations in space. Cortex 6:174, 1970.
23. Warrington, EK, and James, M: Tachistoscopic number estimation in patients with unilateral cerebral lesions. J Neurol Neurosurg Psychiatry 30:468, 1967.
24. Kimura, D: Right temporal lobe damage: Perception of unfamiliar stimuli after damage. Arch Neurol 8:264, 1963.
25. Semmes, J, et al: Correlates of impaired orientation in personal and extrapersonal space. Brain 86:747, 1963.
26. Aimard, G, et al: Spatial disorientation. Report of 5 cases. Rev Neurol 137:97, 1981.
27. Hublet, C, and Demeurisse, G: Pure topographical disorientation due to a deep-seated lesion with cortical remote effects. Cortex 28:123, 1992.
28. Bottini, G, et al: Topographic disorientation—a case report. Neuropsychologia 28:309, 1990.
29. Benton, AL, et al: Contributions to Neuropsychological Assessment. A Clinical Manual. Oxford University Press, New York, 1983.
30. Christensen, AL: Luria's Neuropsychological Investigation Manual. Spectrum Publications, New York, 1975.
31. Christensen, AL: Luria's Neuropsychological Investigation Text. Spectrum Publications, New York, 1975.

DISORDERS OF VISUAL-MOTOR INTEGRATION

7

The disorders of visual-motor integration involve a deficit in the ability to guide motor performance using visual information. Visual input in sighted individuals dominates the guidance of hand performance. Blind individuals must rely on auditory and tactile information. Sighted individuals rely on auditory and tactile information only in unusual or contrived situations. For example, in the clinic, an examiner can blindfold a sighted person and then ask him or her to reach for the source of a sound or to perform a fine motor coordination task. The literature on auditory-motor and tactile-motor integration is sparse, perhaps because auditory and tactile guidance of hand movement rarely occurs in the everyday environment. Consequently, this chapter is limited to visual-motor integration disorders.

A variety of factors must be ruled out before diagnosing a visual-motor integration disorder. Visual acuity must be sufficient for the patient to see the stimuli accurately. The patient also must be able to detect and explore all portions of the visual environment. Visual discrimination and spatial deficits (see Chaps. 5 and 6) can contribute to the patient's failure on visual-motor tasks. However, perceptual impairment alone must not account for the impaired visual-motor performance.

A variety of motor disorders must be ruled out before visual-motor integration deficits can be diagnosed. If motor weakness or poor coordination is present, it must not be severe enough to account for the impaired visual-motor performance. Similarly, poor visual-motor performance must not be the result of an inability to initiate (see Akinesia), sustain (see Motor impersistence), or terminate (see Motor perseveration) movement. The patient's ability to perform skilled movements on command must be preserved.

Because of the many factors that must be ruled out, diagnosis of a pure visual-motor integration disorder is difficult. Often, the clinician can only infer that the disorder exists by noting that the patient's performance on visual tasks deteriorates when a motor component is added. Even in this situation, care must be taken to ensure that the hand being used to perform the task is free of motor deficits.

The variety of presentation of visual-motor integration disorder includes the subtypes listed in the chapter outline.

Only the first two subtypes are discussed in this chapter. Unilateral constructional disability is discussed in Chapter 10 with other disorders of interhemispheric transfer. Spatial agraphia is discussed in Chapter 13 with other disorders of written language.

NOMENCLATURE

The DSM-IV[1] diagnoses of "Cognitive Disorder Not Otherwise Specified" or "Mild Neurocognitive Disorder" can be used to code the visual-motor integration disorders. Several additional coding options are available in ICD-9-CM[2] for visual-motor integration disorders. Optic ataxia may be coded as "Cerebral Ataxia" in ICD-9-CM.

In the neurological literature, constructional disability is sometimes referred to as *constructional apraxia,* although not all researchers agree that a skilled-movement deficit accounts for constructional problems. The more neutral term, *constructional disability,* is used in this text. The clinician wishing to use an ICD-9-CM code has no recourse but to link constructional disability with apraxia, because the only available code is "Other Symbolic Dysfunction," which includes constructional disability and the apraxias.

VARIETY OF PRESENTATION

1. Optic ataxia

Clinical Indicators

a_1. Inaccuracy in reaching for or pointing to a visual target

a_2. Possibility that the deficit may occur on one or both sides of space

a_3. Possibility that the deficit may occur in one or both hands.

RULES FOR DIAGNOSIS

Clinical Indicators: Each is independent (only one must be observed for the disorder to be suspected) *except* when subscripting is used. Subscripted numbers (a_1, a_2) denote an indicator with multiple parts that must be considered together.
Associated Features: These are listed to give a more complete picture of the disorder. The presence or absence of these features does not affect the diagnosis.
Factors to Rule Out: All must be taken into account. Failure to rule out even one of these factors makes a firm diagnosis impossible.
Lesion Locations: Each location stands alone; damage in only one of the listed areas is sufficient to produce the disorder.

Associated Features

a. Inability to move the eyes on demand (see Oculomotor apraxia)
b. Inability to perceive more than one stimulus at a time (see Simultanagnosia)

NOTE: When optic ataxia occurs with oculomotor apraxia and simultanagnosia, the entire complex is referred to as Balint's syndrome.

c. Impaired visual recognition of objects (see Visual object agnosia)
d. Impaired recognition of previously familiar faces (see Prosopagnosia)
e. Impaired perception of colors (see Achromatopsia)

Factors to Rule Out

a. Loss of visual acuity in both eyes sufficient to prevent a target from being seen
b. Failure to detect a visual target as a result of stimulus neglect (see Chap. 4)
c. Inaccuracy in determining the spatial location of a visual target (see Stimulus mislocalization)
d. Weakness of the muscles of the arm or hand sufficient to prevent reaching for a target
e. Impaired coordination of the muscles of the arm or hand sufficient to prevent accurate reaching for a target
f. Impaired ability to initiate arm or hand movements involved in reaching (see Akinesia)
g. Severe impairment of the ability to persist with ongoing hand or arm movements (see Motor impersistence)
h. Severe impairment of the ability to perform skilled movements, including reaching, on demand (see Ideomotor apraxia)

i. Severe impairment of the ability to terminate an ongoing movement (see Motor perseveration)

Lesion Locations

a. Parietal lobe, particularly the intraparietal sulcus, inferior parietal lobule, superior parietal lobule, and angular gyrus, presumed to cause interruption of direct pathways, crossed pathways, or both connecting the occipital and frontal lobes[3–6]
b. Occipital lobe with white-matter (underlying insular cortex) involvement[7] or extension of the lesion to the temporal lobe[8]
c. Combined parietal and occipital lobe involvement[9–14]

Lesion Lateralization

a. Can occur following unilateral (i.e., left or right) or bilateral lesions.
b. Bilateral lesions typically cause bilateral optic ataxia.
c. Unilateral lesions typically cause contralateral optic ataxia but can cause bilateral optic ataxia if both interhemispheric and intrahemispheric (callosal) occipital-frontal pathways are interrupted.[5,11]

2. **Constructional disability (also called constructional apraxia and visuoconstructive disability; see also Unilateral constructional disability)**

Clinical Indicators

a_1. Inaccuracy in making a drawing of a model, as indicated by any of the following signs:
   1) The drawing is a simplified version of the model with individual parts or details omitted.
   2) The individual parts of the drawing are misaligned or otherwise incorrectly placed relative to each other.
   3) The proportionate size of the parts of the drawing do not match the corresponding parts of the model.
   4) The three-dimensional perspective present in a model is lost in the drawing.
   5) Part or all of the drawing is rotated so that its orientation on the page does not match that of the model.

a_2. Preserved ability to detect and point out error or inaccuracy in the drawing

a_3. Inability to produce a substantially better drawing despite awareness of the inaccuracy of the original attempted drawing

a_4. The deficit is present regardless of which hand is used, although different types of drawing errors may be made with each hand

b_1. Inaccuracy in constructing a three-dimensional representation of a model as evidenced by any of the following signs:
   1) The construction is a simplified version of the model with individual parts omitted.
   2) The individual parts of the construction are misaligned or otherwise incorrectly placed relative to each other.

3) The overall spatial configuration or design of the model is lost in the attempted construction so that it no longer resembles the model in its overall shape.
4) Part or all of the construction is rotated so that its orientation on the table does not match that of the model.

b_2. Preserved ability to detect and point out error or inaccuracy in the construction

b_3. Inability to produce a substantially more accurate construction despite awareness of the inaccuracy of the original attempted construction

b_4. Deficit present regardless of which hand is used, although different types of construction errors may be made with each hand

Associated Features

a. Impaired oral language (see Chap. 12)
b. Impaired recognition of the fingers of the hand (see Finger agnosia)
c. Impaired localization of stimulation to the fingers (see Finger mislocalization)
d. Confusion of the right and left sides of the body or space (see Right-left disorientation)
e. Impaired perception of visual stimuli (see Chap. 5)
f. Impaired spatial perception (see Chap. 6)

Factors to Rule Out

a. Loss of visual acuity in both eyes sufficient to prevent a model from being seen
b. Visual stimulus imperception (see Chap. 5) so severe that it prevents accurate perception of the model, ruled out by demonstrating preserved ability to detect and point out errors in the attempted drawing or construction
c. Spatial imperception (see Chap. 6) so severe that it prevents accurate perception of the model, ruled out by demonstrating preserved ability to detect and point out errors in the attempted drawing or construction
d. Weakness of the muscles of the arm or hand sufficient to prevent drawing or construction
e. Impaired coordination of the muscles of the arm or hand sufficient to prevent drawing or construction
f. Impaired ability to initiate arm or hand movements (see Akinesia)
g. Impaired ability to persist with ongoing arm or hand movements (see Motor impersistence)
h. Impaired ability to perform skilled movements on demand (see Ideomotor apraxia)
i. Impaired ability to terminate ongoing movements (see Motor perseveration)

Lesion Locations

a. Cerebral hemisphere, especially posterior to the central sulcus, but can also occur after lesions anterior to central sulcus[15–20]
b. Parietal lobe, with or without associated temporal or occipital involvement[21–27]

c. Frontal lobe[23]
d. Combined temporal and occipital lobes[28]
e. Basal ganglia[29]
f. Thalamus[29]

Lesion Lateralization

a. Possible occurrence after left-sided lesions but tends to be more frequent and more severe after right-sided lesions[17,20,21,23]
b. No difference reported by some investigators in frequency and severity attributable to side of lesion[18,19,29]
c. Possibility that left-sided lesions can lead to misalignment or incorrect placement of parts in drawings and constructions with preservation of the overall spatial configuration
d. Possibility that right-sided lesions can lead to loss of the overall spatial configuration of drawings and constructions with preserved alignment and placement of parts

3. **Unilateral constructional disability (see Chap. 10)**
4. **Spatial agraphia (see Chap. 13)**

ETIOLOGY

Optic ataxia and constructional disability follow disease or injury of the cerebral cortex, particularly when posterior brain areas are involved. Cerebrovascular diseases, traumatic brain injury, degenerative diseases, demyelinating diseases, cerebral infections, and neoplasms can all lead to defective visual-motor integration. Constructional disability also is associated with substance abuse, particularly in middle-aged or elderly individuals. Disruption of brain metabolism and electrolyte imbalance can also produce constructional disability.

DISABLING CONSEQUENCES

Depending on its severity, optic ataxia can be merely a nuisance or severely disabling. Minor misreaching can usually be compensated for after the patient realizes that he or she has a problem in this area. However, if the disorder is severe, compensation may not be possible, and there is great potential for harm. The patient may be unable to accurately retrieve objects from cabinets and may knock over objects in the process. When cooking, the patient may reach in the wrong direction and inadvertently be burned. Thus, these patients may not be safe in the kitchen.

Operating motor vehicles also can be difficult for the patient with optic ataxia. The patient may be unable to reach accurately for controls and may fail to steer the vehicle in the desired direction. Occupations that require careful visual guidance of the hands may be beyond the capacity of the patient. Dentists, surgeons, carpenters, sculptors, drafters, and pilots, among others, who have persistent and severe optic ataxia would be considered totally disabled.

Constructional disability affects a smaller segment of the population than does optic ataxia because daily life in most Western societies does not require drawing or building. Constructional disability, however, is devastating to anyone who works in the building trades or the visual arts. Professions such as architecture or medical illustration are beyond the capacity of patients with this disorder. Jobs involving assembly or repair of equipment (e.g., cameras), machines (e.g., automobiles, computers), or other commercial items (e.g., furniture) cannot be performed adequately by these patients. The average person, on occasion, performs assembly or repair work in the home (e.g., fixing a leaky faucet, assembling a new lawnmower); therefore, some potential for impaired domestic functioning must be acknowledged. However, help is usually available for domestic assembly and repair chores, so that domestic life may not be severely impeded by constructional deficits.

ASSESSMENT INSTRUMENTS

Visuospatial Integration Procedure

The Visuospatial Integration Procedure is *not commercially available.*

Twelve circles are arranged in a semirandom order on a poster board measuring 3 feet by 2 feet. The circles are approximately 1/2 inch in diameter and are arranged so that six lie to the left and six to the right of the center of the board. The circles are of four colors (red, green, blue, and yellow), and each contains a number (1 through 12). The pairing of circles and numbers is random, so that consecutive numbers do not necessarily appear adjacent to each other on the poster. The pairing of circles with colors is also random, so that the colors are scattered across the poster.

The poster is held with the long edge parallel to the table and the numbers in the upright position within reaching distance of the patient. The center of the poster is aligned with the patient's midline. The patient is instructed to find the circle containing a specified number, to identify the color of the circle (to make sure that the patient has correctly located it), and to reach and touch the circle with his or her right index finger. A second set of 12 trials is performed with the left index finger.

When patients successfully guide their fingers to the specified circle, a "+" (plus) is recorded for that trial. When a circle is missed, a "−" (minus) is recorded, and the approximate location touched by the patient is marked on an answer sheet containing a scale drawing of the board. The examiner is allowed to cue the patient on any trial in which the patient cannot find the specified circle or fails to report the correct color. Cuing may include pointing to the target circle or even putting the patient's finger on the target momentarily until the patient verifies that he or she sees it. Scores derived from the procedure include total number correct, number correct in each quadrant of the poster, number correct for each hand, and number correct for each hand within each quadrant. Additional data of interest are the number of incorrect pointing responses that fall to the left of the target circle and the number of incorrect pointing responses that fall to the right of the target circle.

Empirical demonstration of the reliability and validity of the procedure is unavailable. I have used the procedure as part of my clinical examination and found that virtually all patients perform the test flawlessly with the exception of patients having diagnoses of Balint's syndrome (see Optic ataxia, Oculomotor apraxia, and Simultanagnosia) or visual allesthesia (see Stimulus mislocalization). The Visuospatial Integration Procedure should be employed only by neuropsychologists, behavioral neurologists, physiatrists, and occupational therapists with extensive experience in the diagnosis of visual-motor disorders because of the lack of an empirical database to guide interpretation. The procedure is appropriate for office or laboratory administration.

Audiospatial Integration and Localization Procedure

See discussion of the Audiospatial Integration and Localization Procedure in Chapter 8.

Halstead-Reitan Battery Aphasia Screening Test, Spatial Relations Items

See discussion of the Halstead-Reitan Battery (HRB) Aphasia Screening Test (AST), Spatial Relations Items, in Chapter 12.

Benton Visual Retention Test, Administration C, Form E

The Benton Visual Retention Test (BVRT)[30] can be obtained from *The Psychological Corporation, P.O. Box 9954, San Antonio, TX 78204-0954.*

In this test, the patient copies 10 designs of varying complexity. Each design remains in view through the entire test. A shorter, eight-design version can be administered, but this version saves only 1 to 2 minutes compared with the full version. Normative data for the 10-design version are based on 200 patients without neurological problems. The eight-design version is normed on 100 control patients. The two versions correlate .97 with each other and produce no discrepancies in patient classification.

Inter-rater reliability coefficients for the BVRT, Administration C, Form E vary from .94 to .97 among studies.[30] In factor-analytic studies, this test tends to load on visuospatial and perceptual-motor factors. The test correlates more highly with other graphic tests of constructional ability than it does with tests requiring two- and three-dimensional assembly.[31] Administration C, Form E of the BVRT is sensitive to right-hemisphere and bilateral brain damage.[30]

The BVRT, Administration C, Form E can be administered at bedside, in the office, or in laboratory settings. Interpretation is restricted to psychologists who are trained in psychometric assessment and who have experience with patients having neurological deficits.

Boston Spatial-Quantitative Battery, Constructional Deficits Subtest

The Boston Spatial-Quantitative Battery (BSQB), formerly the Boston Parietal Lobe Battery, Constructional Deficits Subtest,[32] is *not commercially available.*

Items for this test can be constructed from the information provided in the test manual. Items include drawings (i.e., clock, daisy, elephant, cross, cube, and house), which the patient copies and draws to command without a model; stick constructions, which the patient copies and reproduces from memory; and three-dimensional block constructions, which the patient reproduces from photographs and from block models. Reliability coefficients are not reported for the BSQB. Normative data are available on 137 neurologically normal men stratified by age (25 to 85 years) and education.[33]

Factor analysis of the BSQB in a sample of 242 patients with aphasia revealed that the constructional tasks loaded on a spatial-quantitative factor.[32] The BSQB Constructional Deficits Subtest is appropriate for office or laboratory administration. Many factors that can influence interpretation of the results may not be evident to inexperienced clinicians; thus, this subtest is recommended for use only by neuropsychologists, behavioral neurologists, and speech pathologists experienced in the diagnosis of constructional deficits.

Beery Development Test of Visual-Motor Integration

The Beery Development Test of Visual-Motor Integration[34] can be obtained from *Psychological Assessment Resources, P.O. Box 998, Odessa, FL 33556.*

In this test, patients attempt to copy 24 designs that increase in difficulty; testing can be discontinued after three successive failures. Test-retest, inter-rater, and split-half reliability studies using the Beery test have been reviewed[35] and have generally reported acceptable to high reliability coefficients. Normative data are available for individuals up to 14 years and 11 months of age, but the test author contends that the norms for 13- to 14-year-old patients are appropriate for older age groups. Validity studies are not available for brain-damaged populations.

The Beery test is an attractive test because of the number of designs included and the grading of difficulty level. The assumption that the test can be used with age groups older than those included in the last standardization sample may hold for young-adult to middle-aged individuals; however, it should not be assumed that norms derived from 13- and 14-year-old persons can be applied to normal elderly populations. The Beery test requires further validation and study in older age groups.

The Beery test can be administered at bedside, in the office, or in laboratory settings. It can be used by a variety of professionals, including grade-school teachers, in child populations. It is recommended that only neuropsychologists and behavioral neurologists attempt interpretation of Beery test results in neurological and elderly populations because of the lack of empirical validation and interpretive guidelines in these populations.

Taylor Complex Figure, Revised Administration

See discussion of the Taylor Complex Figure, Revised Administration (Copy Trial) in Chapter 16.

Wechsler Adult Intelligence Scale-Revised and WAIS-R as a Neuropsychological Instrument, Block Design Subtest

See discussion of the WAIS-R and WAIS-R NI Block Design Subtest in Chapter 19.

Three-Dimensional Block Construction

The Three-Dimensional Block Construction[36] can be obtained from *Oxford University Press, Incorporated, 200 Madison Avenue, New York, NY 10016.*

In this test, patients are presented with three block models of increasing complexity and asked to reproduce them with a set of loose blocks using the models as a guide. Equivalent forms of the test (i.e., forms A and B) are available; empirical investigation has demonstrated that these forms produce virtually identical scores when taken by the same patient.[36] Two other versions that use photographs instead of three-dimensional models are also available. Scoring of the test is based on the number of blocks correctly placed. Errors are also recorded and can include omission of blocks, addition of extra blocks, substitution of incorrect blocks, and displacement (e.g., angular rotation) of blocks.

Normative data for the block model versions are based on 100 patients without brain damage ranging in age from 16 to 63 years. An additional 100 patients without brain damage provided normative data for the photographic model versions; age range was not reported in the clinical manual. The photographic versions are notably more difficult than the block model versions.

No clear gender differences have been documented with Three-Dimensional Block Construction, although the manual reports that women as a group are more variable in their performance on the photographic versions. Subsequent research reported in the clinical manual suggests that block construction ability declines with advancing age and is positively correlated with education. Unfortunately, neither correction factors nor stratified normative tables are included in the manual. The manual reports data that confirm the sensitivity of the block model and photographic versions to unilateral and bilateral cerebral lesions. In general, block construction deficits were more frequent and more severe following right-hemisphere lesions.[36]

Three-Dimensional Block Construction is appropriate for office and laboratory administration. Interpretation should be attempted only by neuropsychologists and neurologists experienced in the diagnosis of visual-motor disorders.

NEUROPSYCHOLOGICAL TREATMENT

As mentioned previously, patients who have optic ataxia can sometimes learn to compensate for their deficit in reaching for targets. In part, this is accomplished by their reaching slowly and carefully and by making one or more correcting movements when their first movement fails to reach the target. This process can be facilitated by providing opportunities for practicing reaching skills. If the patient is consistently off-target in a particular direction or by a certain distance, this information can be given to the patient to aid him or her in planning subsequent movements. Progressively smaller and more distant targets can be used as the patient improves. The patient can eventually be asked to touch slowly moving targets, because this provides an even greater challenge.

Constructional disability is also addressed by providing opportunities for the patient to practice deficient skills. Practice proceeds from simple drawings and models to increasingly complex constructions. Patients may also benefit from explicit training in how to draw and build. For example, patients can be taught to approach complex figures by first sketching the overall shape, then sketching the major internal divisions of the figure, and filling in the details last.

Patients who have difficulty with two-dimensional model building tasks sometimes can be aided by plastic overlays with lines sketched on them that help to segment the model into reproducible units. For example, I use plastic overlays containing 2-by-2 and 3-by-3 grids to segment block designs that are similar to those contained in the Wechsler Adult Intelligence Scale–Revised. The segmented blocks are also numbered consecutively, beginning in the upper left-hand corner and proceeding from left to right until the final block in the lower right-hand corner is reached. By following the numbers, patients learn to construct the block designs in an efficient and systematic manner. As patients progress, the grid and number cues can be removed one line at a time until the designs can be constructed unaided.

Three-dimensional model construction tasks can be approached in a similar manner: by providing successive pictures that show how the model can be constructed in steps. The steps shown in each picture must be sufficiently simple that patients can accomplish them. By learning to follow a sequence of steps beginning with constructing the base of the model and working upward until the entire construction is complete, patients become increasingly systematic and efficient in their approach. As patients progress, progressively more steps of the sequence can be omitted, so that the patients are shown initial pictures in which considerable portions of the model are already completed. This method requires patients to draw on their own resources to complete the initial construction steps.

When pictures of a three-dimensional model are unavailable or fail to work, the therapist can use an extra set of constructional materials to assemble the model while the patient observes. Pausing regularly to let the patient imitate the therapist with his or her own set of materials allows the patient to learn the constructional sequence.

Therapists should not use two- and three-dimensional models that are included in standardized test batteries. Models that do not overlap with those included in test batteries must be constructed by the therapist for use in treatment sessions. Use of standardized test items as treatment exercises invalidates the test for future assessment with the patient.

As with any neuropsychological treatment, generalization to the external environment is a critical issue. Practicing with block designs and abstract three-dimensional models may not benefit a mechanic who has constructional disability and needs to be able to take apart and reassemble carburetors. It is incumbent on the resourceful therapist to seek occupation-specific tools, equipment, and models for use with patients who have special needs. Often, this is accomplished by taking the patient to his or her former place of employment and arranging for supervised practice of relevant constructional skills.

CASE ILLUSTRATIONS

CASE 4–5

R.M. was a 50-year-old man with a high-school education. After triple coronary artery bypass grafting, he developed atrial fibrillation and an anoxic encephalopathy. Magnetic resonance imaging (MRI) scans revealed bilateral watershed-area infarctions (i.e., C-shaped infarctions extending from the frontal to the occipital poles), with greater damage evident in the right hemisphere.

Results of R.M.'s neuropsychological assessment are presented in Chapter 4. Only selected findings are discussed here. The patient had full visual fields, but visual acuity could not be assessed because of his inability to discriminate even the largest letters on the Snellen chart. Acuity was sufficient for the patient to reliably identify colors, line drawings, and people seen from distances of up to 20 feet. He accomplished this despite a probable left hemispatial neglect (see Chap. 4). R.M. was unable to move his eyes reliably in any direction on demand. He identified only one of five shapes formed by dot patterns, although he was able to count the dots. He successfully identified multipart shapes such as a pyramid and a cylinder but had difficulty integrating black-and-white patterns to perceive letters (three of five correct).

R.M. had severe hemiparesis in his left hand but only a mild degree of weakness in his dominant right hand. He was somewhat clumsy in manipulating small objects; however, he readily accomplished gross movements with the right hand and arm and showed no perseveration, initiation deficits, or impersistence. He did show a deficit in performing skilled movements on demand (see Apraxia) but easily succeeded in pointing to positions touched or named on the right side of his body using his right hand. When asked to point to positions on the left side of his body, he pointed to the corresponding positions on the right side.

R.M. was asked to reach for numbered and colored circles on a poster board (i.e., the Visuospatial Integration Procedure) with his right hand. He succeeded in touching only 2 of 12 targets. Most of his other responses were displaced to the right of the actual stimulus location; one response was displaced below the target circle. His errors were greatest for circles appearing on the left side of the board; he pointed to the right side of the board on all trials in which the target was actually oriented to the left. When pointing to targets on the right side of the board, his responses continued to be displaced farther to the right, but they were closer to the actual target position. His two correct responses were to targets located on the right side of the board. Whenever he made an incorrect response, R.M. was asked to identify the color of the target (four possible choices), and in each instance, he was correct.

The Number Location Subtest from the Visual Object and Space Perception Battery (see Chap. 5) was administered. R.M. was correct on only two trials, which is far below the cut-off score for normal persons, suggesting that he had significant difficulty in determining the position of visual stimuli in space. When blindfolded and asked to point to locations where he heard sounds, R.M. was correct on only 4 of 12 trials (see Audiospatial Integration and Localization Procedure). During a second set of 12 trials, the blindfold was removed after a sound had been made, and he was shown a diagram of the possible positions around his head in which the sound could occur. He verbally identified the correct location only 4 of 12 times.

DISCUSSION

The patient in Case 4–5 exhibited inaccurate reaching for targets on both sides of space, with the deficit worse on the patient's left. It is likely that the deficit is present in both hands, given the patient's bilateral lesions, but weakness prevented assessment of the left hand. A diagnosis of optic ataxia is tenable in this case. The patient exhibited many additional features associated with this diagnosis, including an inability to shift gaze on demand (oculomotor apraxia) and a deficit in perceiving multiple stimuli or multipart objects simultaneously (simultanagnosia). Together, these deficits constitute Balint's syndrome.

However, the interpretation of this case was hampered by many confounding factors. The patient's undocumented level of visual acuity impeded the attainment of diagnostic certainty. It should be noted, however, that although the patient did poorly on standard acuity charts, he showed considerable functional sight. The patient's absolute level of acuity remains uncertain, but the fact that he could correctly report the color of all targets he was asked to reach for during the Visuospatial Integration Procedure suggests that his acuity was sufficient for him to detect the target stimuli on this task. The same argument can be made with regard to this patient's probable left hemispatial neglect. Despite this deficit, he clearly detected all stimuli prior to reaching for them.

Muscle weakness prevented assessment of reaching with the left arm; however, the patient had no difficulty reaching the board with the right arm. Impaired coordination, akinesia, perseveration, motor impersistence, or apraxia cannot account for his reaching deficit, because he successfully reached the board (touching the wrong positions) and accurately reached for target positions on his body. The patient clearly had sufficiently preserved movement in the right arm to accomplish reaching tasks.

An additional confounding disorder cannot be ruled out. When asked to touch positions on the left side of his body, the patient touched the corresponding points on his right side. When reaching for visual targets, he erred by touching too far to the right of the actual target. When he was asked to identify verbally the location of visual and auditory targets, he was as inaccurate as when he was reaching for the targets. A disorder involving deficient determination of the spatial location of stimuli (see Stimulus mislocalization) cannot be ruled out in this patient. Consequently, optic ataxia remains a suspected rather than a firm diagnosis.

CASE 7–1

M.M. was a 59-year-old woman with a high-school education. She suffered bilateral intracerebral hemorrhages in the parietal and occipital lobes. Her neuropsychological deficits included impaired discrimination of right from left (see Right-left disorientation) and poor ability to match and discriminate faces (see Facial imperception), despite having 20-20 visual acuity in each eye. She was able to identify correctly all of the drawings in the Halstead-Reitan Battery Aphasia Screening Test and pictures of six recent presidents. Strength, coordination, speed of initiation, and perseverance during movement were intact in both upper extremities. The patient readily pantomimed skilled movements and had no difficulty in using objects. The one motor deficit evident was severe perseveration when she was asked to copy a triple loop.

M.M.'s copy (using the right hand) of the first six and the last six line drawings of the Beery Development Test of Visual-Motor Integration are shown in Figure 7–1. She drew accurate vertical, horizontal, and oblique lines. Some minor difficulty was encountered when she drew a circle (her starting and ending points were not contiguous), and there was a superfluous line in her square. However, these errors were not sufficient for her to fail any of the first six trials.

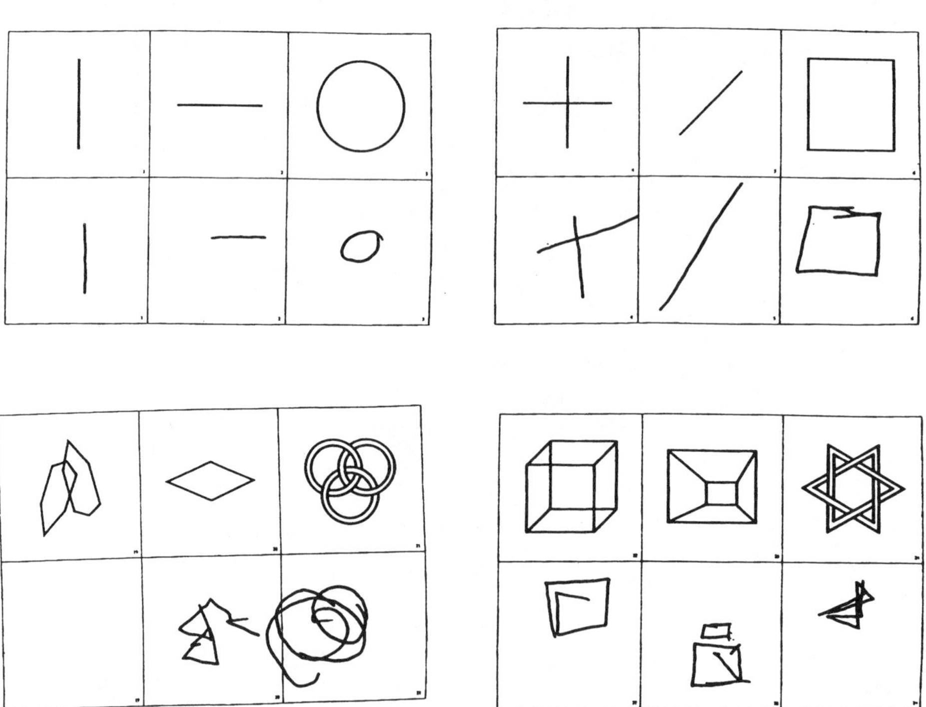

FIGURE 7–1. The first six and final six drawings of the Beery Developmental Test of Visual Motor Integration, as attempted by the patient in Case 7–1.

The patient's performance on the final six trials of the Beery test was contrastingly poor. She refused even to attempt trial 19. The spatial relations of the model parts were grossly distorted on the trials the patient did attempt. She could not maintain the three-dimensional perspective of the model on trial 22, the cube. Using the discontinuation criterion of three consecutive failures, M.M. achieved a scaled score of less than 1 using norms for persons 13 years of age and older. There was no evidence of perseveration in any of the patient's drawings, including the ones she failed to draw correctly.

M.M. was aware of the incorrectness of her drawings to the point that she expressed embarrassment about them. When asked to describe what was wrong, she stated simply that she couldn't finish the drawings because she "didn't know how to make the lines go the right way." Despite her awareness of her errors, she was unable to correct any of her drawings. The patient's performance with her left hand (not shown) was worse, even on the simple drawings. She refused to attempt the entire Beery test using the left hand.

DISCUSSION

Case 7–1 presents a clearer diagnostic picture than does Case 4–5. Constructional disability is indicated by the patient's inability to align the parts of complex drawings and her loss of three-dimensional perspective. She was aware of and able to describe her errors in general terms, but this had no impact on her production. Her associated features included right-left disorientation and impaired matching and discrimination of facial stimuli. Her visual acuity was preserved, and her visual and spatial perception were sufficient for her to detect her constructional errors. No motor deficits were present in the patient with the exception of perseveration. However, perseveration was not evident in any of her drawings and cannot account for her drawing failures. Perhaps the best proof that she had the motor capacity to accomplish drawing was her preserved drawing of the simpler models at the beginning of the Beery test. Only when complex spatial alignment of the parts of the model was required did the patient begin to show a deficit.

REFERENCES

1. American Psychiatric Association: Diagnostic and Statistical Manual of Mental Disorders, Fourth Edition. American Psychiatric Association, Washington, DC, 1994.
2. The International Classification of Diseases, Ninth Revision, Clinical Modification. Med-Index Publications, Salt Lake City, 1991.
3. Perenin, MT, and Vighetto, A: Optic ataxia: A specific disruption in visuomotor mechanisms. I. Different aspects of the deficit in reaching for objects. Brain 111:643, 1988.
4. Pierrot-Deseilligny, C, Gray, F, and Brunet, P: Infarcts of both inferior parietal lobules with impairment of visually guided eye movements, peripheral visual inattention and optic ataxia. Brain 109:81, 1986.
5. Ferro, JM: Transient inaccuracy in reaching caused by a posterior parietal lobe lesion. J Neurol Neurosurg Psychiatry 47:1016, 1984.
6. Auerbach, SH, and Alexander, MP: Pure agraphia and unilateral optic ataxia associated with a left superior parietal lobule lesion. J Neurol Neurosurg Psychiatry 44:430, 1981.

7. Girotti, F, et al: Oculomotor disturbances in Balint's syndrome: Anatomoclinical findings and electrooculographic analysis in a case. Cortex 18:603, 1982.
8. Damasio, AR, and Damasio, H: The anatomic basis of pure alexia. Neurology 33:1573, 1983.
9. Jakobson, LS, et al: A kinematic analysis of reaching and grasping movements in a patient recovering from optic ataxia. Neuropsychologia 29:803, 1991.
10. Ando, S, and Moritake, K: Pure optic ataxia associated with a right parieto-occipital tumour. J Neurol Neurosurg Psychiatry 53:805, 1990.
11. Ferro, JM, et al: Crossed optic ataxia: Possible role of the dorsal splenium. J Neurol Neurosurg Psychiatry 46:533, 1983.
12. Damasio, AR, and Benton, AL: Impairment of hand movements under visual guidance. Neurology 29:170, 1979.
13. Boller, F, et al: Optic ataxia: Clinical-radiological correlations with the EMI scan. J Neurol Neurosurg Psychiatry 38:954, 1975.
14. Gardner-Thorpe, C, et al: Loffler's eosinophilic endocarditis with Balint's syndrome (optic ataxia and paralysis of visual fixation). Q J Med 40:249, 1971.
15. Benowitz, LI, Moya, KL, and Levine, DN: Impaired verbal reasoning and constructional apraxia in subjects with right hemisphere damage. Neuropsychologia 28:231, 1990.
16. Moya, KL, et al: Covariant defects in visuospatial abilities and recall of verbal narrative after right hemisphere stroke. Cortex 22:381, 1986.
17. Mack, JL, and Levine, RN: The basis of visual constructional disability in patients with unilateral cerebral lesions. Cortex 17:515, 1981.
18. Arena, R, and Gainotti, G: Constructional apraxia and visuoperceptive disabilities in relation to laterality of cerebral lesions. Cortex 14:463, 1978.
19. Colombo, A, DeRenzi, E, and Faglioni, P: The occurrence of visual neglect in patients with unilateral cerebral disease. Cortex 12:221, 1976.
20. Black, FW, and Strub, RL: Constructional apraxia in patients with discrete missile wounds of the brain. Cortex 12:212, 1976.
21. Ruessmann, K, Sondag, HD, and Beneicke, U: On the cerebral localization of constructional apraxia. Int J Neurosci 42:59, 1988.
22. Marsh, GG, and Philwin, B: Unilateral neglect and constructional apraxia in a right-handed artist with a left posterior lesion. Cortex 23:149, 1987.
23. Villa, G, Gainotti, G, and DeBonis, C: Constructive disabilities in focal brain-damaged patients. Influence of hemispheric side, locus of lesion and coexistent mental deterioration. Neuropsychologia 24:497, 1986.
24. Matsuoka, H, et al: Impairment of parietal cortical functions associated with episodic prolonged spike-and-wave discharges. Epilepsia 27:432, 1986.
25. Marinkovic, SV, Kovacevic, MS, and Kostic, VS: The isolated occlusion of the angular gyri artery. A correlative neurological and anatomical study—case report. Stroke 15:366, 1984.
26. Hier, DB, Mondlock, J, and Caplan, LR: Behavioral abnormalities after right hemisphere stroke. Neurology 33:337, 1983.
27. Rengachary, SS, Amini, J, and Batnitzky, S: Reversible constructional apraxia from a floating bone flap. Neurosurgery 5:365, 1979.
28. Grossi, D, et al: Visuoimaginal constructional apraxia: On a case of selective deficit of imagery. Brain Cogn 5:255, 1986.
29. Agostoni, E, et al: Apraxia in deep cerebral lesions. J Neurol Neurosurg Psychiatry 46:804, 1983.
30. Sivian, AB: The Benton Visual Retention Test, Fifth Edition. The Psychological Corporation, San Antonio, 1992.
31. Benton, AL: Constructional apraxia and the minor hemisphere. Confinia Neurologica 29:1, 1967.
32. Goodglass, H, and Kaplan, E: The Assessment of Aphasia and Related Disorders, Second Edition. Lea & Febiger, Philadelphia, 1983.
33. Borod, J, Goodglass, H, and Kaplan, E: Normative data on the Boston Diagnostic Aphasia Examination, Parietal Lobe Battery and Boston Naming Test. J Clin Neuropsychol 2:209, 1980.
34. Beery, KE: Revised Administration, Scoring, and Teaching Manual for the Developmental Test of Visual-Motor Integration. Modern Curriculum Press, Cleveland, 1989.
35. Spreen, O, and Strauss, E: A Compendium of Neuropsychological Tests. Administration, Norms, and Commentary. Oxford University Press, New York, 1991.
36. Benton, AL, et al: Contributions to Neuropsychological Assessment. A Clinical Manual. Oxford University Press, New York, 1983.

DISORDERS OF STIMULUS LOCALIZATION

8

The disorders of stimulus localization involve an inability to determine the position of visual, auditory, or tactile stimuli. The variety of presentation includes the subtypes listed in the chapter outline.

In stimulus mislocalization, the position of elementary stimuli cannot be determined by the patient. In finger mislocalization, the patient fails to localize a stimulus to one of his or her fingers, as if the fingers cannot be spatially distinguished. In autotopagnosia, the patient fails to locate his or her body parts that correspond to those that the examiner names or indicates on a model. Patients who have right-left disorientation cannot distinguish the right from the left side of their body, of space, or both.

All of the disorders of stimulus localization are closely related to spatial imperception (see Chap. 6). Before diagnosing the stimulus localization disorders, it must be shown that the patient does not have a sensory deficit that could account for the failure to localize the target stimulus. Additionally, the patient must have sufficient language comprehension to make testing of stimulus localization valid. This is often difficult because of the high incidence of aphasia (see Chap. 12) in patients who have stimulus localization disorders.

NOMENCLATURE

Autotopagnosia and *right-left disorientation* are commonly used terms in the neurology and neuropsychology literature. Although the phenomenon embodied in the term *stimulus mislocalization* has often been described, the term itself is not in common use. When stimulated on the side that is contralateral to their lesioned hemisphere, some patients look instead to the ipsilateral side. This type of lateral mislocalization of a stimulus is called "allesthesia" or "allochiria" in the clinical literature. In the research literature, stimulus mislocalization is often described by referring to the particular task used in a study. For example, a group of patients may be described as having impaired "dot localization," because this type of task was employed in assessing the patients. The more generic term, *stimulus mislocalization,* is used in this text to refer to allesthesia and all other deficits in the judgment of the position of stimuli.

The term *finger mislocalization* also is not in use in the clinical literature. The concept of "finger agnosia" includes both impaired identification of tactually stimulated fingers and impaired recognition of the fingers themselves. These deficits differ considerably from each other. The former is a mislocalization of the fingers

RULES FOR DIAGNOSIS

Clinical Indicators: Each is independent (only one must be observed for the disorder to be suspected) *except* when subscripting is used. Subscripted numbers (a_1, a_2) denote an indicator with multiple parts that must be considered together.
Associated Features: These are listed to give a more complete picture of the disorder. The presence or absence of these features does not affect the diagnosis.
Factors to Rule Out: All must be taken into account. Failure to rule out even one of these factors makes a firm diagnosis impossible.
Lesion Locations: Each location stands alone; damage in only one of the listed areas is sufficient to produce the disorder.

(i.e., the patient knows that a finger was stimulated but cannot determine which one), whereas the latter is a failure to appreciate the meaning of fingers as visual stimuli. Clustering these deficits together appears to be inappropriate because they probably arise from lesions in different parts of the brain. The failure to localize the stimulated finger is discussed in this chapter using the term *finger mislocalization*. Impaired finger recognition (i.e., finger agnosia) is discussed in Chapter 9.

The nonspecific DSM-IV[1] diagnoses of "Cognitive Disorder Not Otherwise Specified" and "Mild Neurocognitive Disorder" can be used to code the stimulus localization disorders. In ICD-9-CM,[2] stimulus mislocalization can be coded as a "Disturbance of Skin Sensation," "Other Abnormal Auditory Perception," or "Psychophysical Visual Disturbance," depending on the sensory modality involved. Finger mislocalization can also be coded as a disturbance of skin sensation. No code approximating autotopagnosia or right-left disorientation is available.

VARIETY OF PRESENTATION

1. Stimulus mislocalization (also called allesthesia and allochiria; see also Finger mislocalization)

Clinical Indicators

a. Inaccuracy in locating the position of visual stimuli in the environment
b. Inaccuracy in locating the position of auditory stimuli in the environment
c. Inaccuracy in locating the position of a tactile stimulus on the body (excluding the fingers)

Associated Features

a. Stimuli possibly perceived as occurring on the side of the body or the side of space opposite to their actual position
b. Stimuli possibly perceived as displaced from their actual position and closer to the midline of the body
c. A recent history of, or concurrent impairment in, the ability to notice or detect stimuli (see Stimulus neglect)

Factors to Rule Out

a. Complete failure to detect the presence of stimuli as a result of loss of visual, auditory, or tactile sensation
b. Complete failure to detect the presence of stimuli as a result of stimulus neglect (see Chap. 4)
c. Normal human error of estimation when attempting to locate the position of a stimulus
d. Intentional or unintentional faking of the deficit (see Psychogenic imperception)

Lesion Locations

For auditory mislocalization

a. Temporal lobe, often in conjunction with the parietal lobe[3–8]
b. Parietal lobe[8]
c. Frontal lobe[8]

d. Occipital lobe[8]

For visual mislocalization

a. Cerebral hemisphere (without further localization)[9,10]
b. Parietal lobe, alone or in conjunction with the temporal and occipital lobes[11–13]
c. Temporal lobe, in conjunction with the frontal, parietal, or occipital lobes[11–13]
d. Occipital lobe, alone or in conjunction with the temporal and parietal lobes[11–13]

For tactual mislocalization

a. Parietal and occipital lobes[14]

Lesion Lateralization

a. Auditory mislocalization possibly following lesions in either hemisphere, with the deficit being greatest contralateral to the lesion, although unilateral lesions may produce bilateral mislocalization[7,8]
b. Visual mislocalization possibly following lesions in either hemisphere but more frequently reported after right-sided lesions[9,10,12,13]
c. Tactual mislocalization, more commonly reported following right-sided lesions

2. Finger mislocalization (see also Finger agnosia)

Clinical Indicators

a_1. Inaccurate identification (by pointing to or moving) of fingers touched by the examiner while vision is occluded

a_2. Deficit occurring in one or both hands

Associated Features

a. Impaired ability to match and discriminate stimuli (see Stimulus imperception)
b. Impaired ability to draw or to construct two- and three-dimensional puzzles (see Constructional disability)
c. Global neuropsychological dysfunction (see Chap. 19)

Factors to Rule Out

a. Tactile sensory loss sufficient to prevent detection of finger stimulation
b. Failure to detect finger stimulation as a result of stimulus neglect (see Chap. 4)

Lesion Locations

a. Cerebral hemisphere (without further localization), including diffuse lesions[15,16]
b. Parietal lobe, alone or in conjunction with the frontal or temporal lobes[17–19]
c. Combined frontal and temporal lobes[19]

Lesion Lateralization

a. Following either left- or right-sided lesions
b. Deficit typically appearing contralateral to the lesion, but both left- and right-sided lesions can produce bilateral finger mislocalization[18,19]

3. Autotopagnosia

Clinical Indicators

a_1. Inaccuracy in locating body parts named by the examiner (body parts used to test location may be on the examiner's body, the patient's body, or on a scale model)

a_2. Relatively preserved recognition of body parts as indicated by any of the following signs:

1) Relatively accurate naming of body parts pointed to by the examiner
2) Relatively accurate multiple-choice identification of body parts pointed to by the examiner
3) Relatively accurate ability to indicate how various body parts are used, by verbal description or by pointing to pictures

b_1. Inaccuracy in locating parts of an actual body (the patient's or the examiner's) corresponding to body parts indicated by the examiner on a scale model

b_2. Relatively preserved ability to match and discriminate pictures of body parts

Associated Features

a. Body parts that cannot be located on command can be located when performing activities involving the body part (e.g., putting on glasses when the eyes could previously not be located)
b. Impaired ability to describe the relative positions of body parts verbally (e.g., where the nose is in relation to the mouth and eyes)
c. Inaccuracy in finding the parts of inanimate objects under test conditions analogous to those used to assess autotopagnosia

Factors to Rule Out

a. Failure to comprehend the names of body parts as a result of impaired oral language (see Chap. 12) when testing involves use of names for body parts
b. Decreased visual acuity sufficient to prevent seeing the part of the body indicated by the examiner when visual models are used
c. Failure to detect the part of the body indicated by the examiner as a result of stimulus neglect (see Chap. 4) when visual models are used
d. Impaired ability to distinguish right from left when testing involves pointing to body parts on a specific side
e. Weakness of the arm or hand sufficient to prevent pointing to body parts
f. Impaired coordination of the arm or hand sufficient to prevent pointing to body parts
g. Impaired ability to initiate movements of the arm or hand (see Akinesia) sufficient to prevent pointing to body parts
h. Impaired ability to persist with ongoing movements of the arm or hand (see Motor impersistence) sufficient to prevent pointing to body parts
i. Impaired ability to terminate ongoing movements of the arm or hand (see Motor perseveration) sufficient to prevent accurate pointing to body parts

j. Severely impaired ability to execute skilled movements of the arm or hand on command (see Ideomotor apraxia)

Lesion Locations

a. Parietal lobe (cortical or subcortical)[20–22]

Lesion Lateralization

a. Left hemisphere

4. Right-left disorientation

Clinical Indicators

a. Inaccuracy in distinguishing the right and left sides of the body, of space, or both from the patient's own frame of reference
b. Inaccuracy in distinguishing the right and left sides of the body, of space, or both, from the frame of reference of a person facing the patient

Associated Features

a. Impaired recognition of the fingers of the hand (see Finger agnosia)
b. Impaired calculation ability (see Acalculia)
c. Impaired ability to write (see Agraphia)

Note: When right-left disorientation occurs in conjunction with finger agnosia, acalculia, and agraphia, the entire complex is referred to as Gerstmann's syndrome.

d. Impaired oral language (see Chap. 12)
e. Global neuropsychological dysfunction (see Chap. 19)

Factors to Rule Out

a. Oral language impairment (see Chap. 12) so severe that the patient is unable to respond accurately during testing of right-left orientation
b. Impaired ability to locate body parts (see Autotopagnosia) when testing of right-left orientation involves pointing to body parts

Lesion Locations

a. Diffuse cerebral hemisphere (without further localization)[16,23]
b. Parietal lobe, including the superior angular gyrus, posterior supramarginal gyrus, and superior parietal lobule[17,24]
c. Thalamus[25]

Lesion Lateralization

a. Left-sided or bilateral lesions[16,23–25]

ETIOLOGY

Any condition capable of causing lateralized or diffuse cerebral dysfunction can lead to the appearance of stimulus localization disorders. Cerebrovascular accidents involving the middle cerebral artery, demyelinating disease, brain trauma, tumors, and degeneration of brain tissue (e.g., Alzheimer's disease) are common causes of these disorders.

DISABLING CONSEQUENCES

Finger mislocalization and autotopagnosia typically do not impede everyday domestic and vocational activities. The patient who has one or both of these disorders may experience no real loss of independence. However, these conditions are often accompanied by other disorders (e.g., aphasia), which do disable the patient.

Stimulus mislocalization can have great impact on the patient's quality of life. Visual stimulus mislocalization may prevent the patient from cooking, cleaning, and performing other household chores. Driving is unsafe, and even walking can be hazardous, particularly if barriers must be avoided. Any vocational activity requiring attention to and use of visual, auditory, or tactile information can be compromised if a patient mislocalizes in the required sensory modality. Construction, repair, or engineering work may be impossible. The patient is unlikely to meet standards in occupations in which there are safety hazards. Jobs in the music industry may be beyond the capabilities of some patients.

Similarly, right-left disorientation compromises performance in occupations involving construction, repair, or engineering skills. Jobs that involve design, reading diagrams or maps, or independent travel (e.g., sales, trucking, delivery) may be impossible. Independence in the home and community are affected less severely, although the patient may need assistance with directions and travel, even in relatively familiar neighborhood settings.

ASSESSMENT INSTRUMENTS

Halstead-Reitan Battery Sensory Perceptual Examination, Unilateral Stimulation Trials

The Halstead-Reitan Battery (HRB) Sensory Perceptual Examination (SPE), Unilateral Stimulation Trials can be obtained from *Reitan Neuropsychological Laboratory, 1338 East Edison Street, Tucson, AZ 85719.*

The HRB-SPE includes trials in which unilateral visual, auditory, and tactile stimuli are delivered; see Chapter 4 for a description of these procedures. Although they are not intended as tests of stimulus mislocalization, these procedures provide an opportunity to observe perceived displacements of unilateral stimuli. The examiner must be alert not only to the occurrence of errors as required by the standard HRB administration, but also to the qualitative nature of the errors, to detect stimulus mislocalization. This disorder may manifest itself during unilateral stimulation trials as a consistent tendency to indicate the wrong side when one side of the body is stimulated.

No investigation of the SPE as a measure of stimulus mislocalization has been conducted. Because of the absence of an empirical foundation on which to base interpretation of mislocalization errors on the SPE, only experienced neuropsychologists and behavioral neurologists should attempt to interpret such errors. In my experience, mislocalization of stimuli to the contralateral side of the body or of space is virtually nonexistent in normal populations; therefore, the occurrence of even a few errors of this type can be regarded as clinically significant. SPE unilateral stimulation trials can be administered at bedside, in the office, or in the laboratory.

Visual Object and Space Perception Battery, Position Discrimination and Number Location Subtests

See discussion of the Visual Object and Space Perception Battery (VOSP) in Chapter 5.

Audiospatial Integration and Localization Procedure

The Audiospatial Integration and Localization Procedure is *not commercially available*.

The audiospatial integration and localization procedure is an expansion of previously published techniques for assessing the ability to locate auditory stimuli.[6] The assessment is conducted in three stages. In stage 1, the patient is asked to report when he or she hears a sound. This is done to verify that the patient has adequate auditory acuity before proceeding with further testing. In stage 2, the patient is asked to reach out with his or her index finger and point to the spot where a sound occurred while his or her vision is occluded. In stage 3, the patient is asked to indicate on a diagram (Fig. 8–1) where a sound occurred; vision is occluded during sound administration. Sounds are made at the locations shown in Figure 8–1 for all

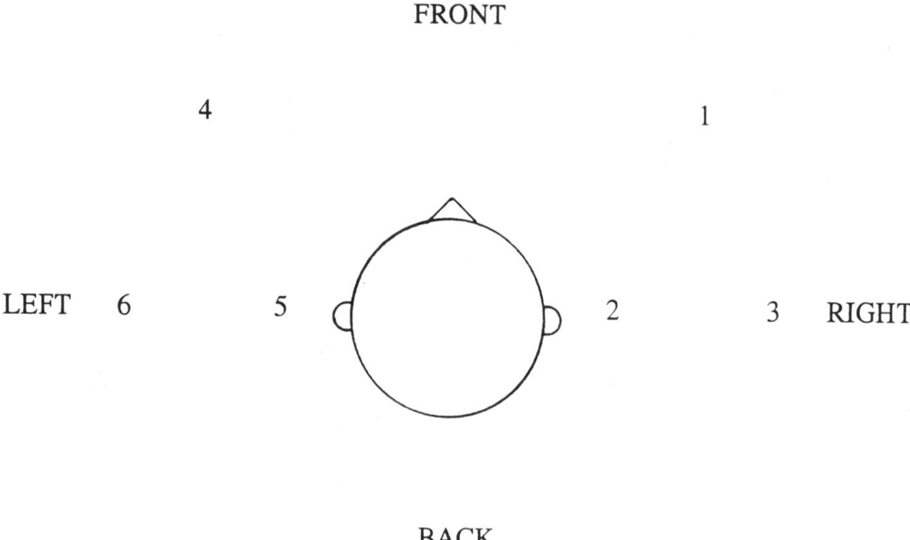

FIGURE 8–1. Auditory stimulation points for the audiospatial integration and localization procedure. (Adapted from Sanchez-Longo, Forster, and Auth,[6] p 655.)

three stages of testing. In stage 1, one sound is delivered in each location. In stages 2 and 3, sounds are delivered twice at each location in a random order for a total of 12 trials in each stage. The sound is made by the examiner rubbing his or her thumb and index finger together. If the patient cannot hear this sound, a louder noise can be made by snapping the fingers.

Reliability and validity data are not available for this procedure. I have used the Audiospatial Integration and Localization Procedure with selected patients having Balint's syndrome (see Optic ataxia, Oculomotor apraxia, and Simultanagnosia) and found the test to be sensitive to both deficits in reaching for and judging the location of sounds. In a series of 50 patients with focal lesions, including cases representing damage to every lobe in each hemisphere, only 6 cases of auditory stimulus mislocalization were identified.[6] The fact that 44 of the patients showed no deficit suggests that audiospatial integration procedures measure a highly specific cognitive deficit.

The Audiospatial Localization Procedure has the advantages of requiring no specialized equipment and of separating judgment of sound position from reaching for the source of a sound. It can be administered in office or laboratory settings. Bedside administration is difficult, because the examiner must walk around the patient's bed to deliver sounds, producing extraneous noise that may cue the patient as to the side on which a target sound will be administered. Interpretation should be attempted only by experienced neuropsychologists and neurologists, because of the limited empirical investigation of the procedure.

Halstead-Reitan Battery Sensory Perceptual Examination, Finger "Agnosia" Subtest

The Halstead-Reitan Battery (HRB) Sensory Perceptual Examination (SPE), Finger "Agnosia" Subtest can be obtained from *Reitan Neuropsychological Laboratory, 1338 East Edison Street, Tucson, AZ 85719.*

Although it is labeled a test of finger agnosia, this HRB-SPE subtest is useful for detecting finger mislocalization as defined in this text. A light touch is delivered to each finger in a random order, and the patient is asked to identify the finger touched. A number system is used to facilitate finger identification, although some patients may have difficulty remembering which numbers go with which fingers. Such patients can be allowed to use an alternative means of identifying the fingers (e.g., pointing, wiggling).

The finger agnosia subtest standardizes a procedure sometimes incorporated in neurological examinations. Scores on this subtest are sometimes combined with scores from other HRB-SPE subtests (see Chaps. 4 and 5). Thorough investigation of the finger agnosia subtest is lacking, but it has substantial support from its long history of use in neurological examinations. The Finger Agnosia Subtest is appropriate for bedside, office, or laboratory administration and can be interpreted by experienced neuropsychologists and neurologists. Although appropriate for use as a measure of finger mislocalization, this subtest should not be used to diagnose finger agnosia (see Chap. 9) as defined in this text.

Benton Finger Localization

The Benton Finger Localization[26] can be obtained from *Oxford University Press, Incorporated, 200 Madison Avenue, New York, NY 10016.*

This test measures the ability to localize fingers stimulated by the examiner. In part A, the patient's fingers are touched with his or her hand visible. In part B, the patient's hand is hidden when his or her fingers are touched. In part C, the patient's hand is hidden, and pairs of his or her fingers are touched simultaneously. The patient can identify the fingers touched by naming them, pointing to them on a drawing of a hand, or calling out a number associated with the stimulated finger.

Normative data are based on 104 patients without neurological problems. Age, gender, and education are reported in the clinical manual to be unrelated to test performance. Defective performance on the test can be categorized into 12 patterns, depending on the severity of impairment, whether one or both hands are assessed, whether performance is unilaterally or bilaterally impaired, and whether the performance of the two hands is symmetrical or nonsymmetrical. Reliability coefficients are not reported in the manual. Data presented in the manual suggest that parts B and C of the test discriminate patients with brain damage from patients without neurological problems. Part A, which permits the patient to use both visual and tactual cues, does not discriminate between brain-damaged and non-neurological samples because even the former group shows a ceiling effect on the test.

The Finger Localization Test is appropriate for bedside, office, or laboratory use and has a relatively straightforward interpretation, making it an appropriate instrument for use by a broad range of clinicians. Results should not automatically be interpreted as indicative of stimulus mislocalization, because tactual sensory impairment can also lower performance levels. This test should be supplemented with additional measures of elementary tactual sensation. The Finger Localization Test should not be used to diagnose finger agnosia (see Chap. 9) as defined in this book.

Boston Spatial-Quantitative Battery, Finger Agnosia Subtest

The Boston Spatial-Quantitative Battery (BSQB), formerly the Boston Parietal Lobe Battery, Finger Agnosia Subtest,[27] is *not commercially available.*

The BSQB Finger Agnosia Test can be constructed from information and illustrations provided by Goodglass and Kaplan.[27] Patients are asked to indicate fingers on drawings as they are named by the examiner. A second set of trials requires the patient to match pairs of his or her fingers to finger pairs indicated on a drawing and to hold up pairs of fingers identical to those held up by the examiner. A third set of trials requires the patient to match fingers touched by the examiner while the patient's vision is occluded to fingers on a drawing. This last set of trials can be used to diagnose stimulus mislocalization. The other trials are useful for diagnosing finger agnosia (see Chap. 9) as defined in this book.

Reliability coefficients are not reported for the BSQB. Normative data are available for 147 neurologically normal men stratified by age (25 through 85 years) and education.[28] Factor analysis of the BSQB in a sample of 242 aphasic patients revealed that portions of the Finger Agnosia Subtest loaded on a finger identification factor.[27] The structure of the Finger Agnosia Subtest facilitates ruling out confounding factors that could alter interpretation of the results. This subtest is most appropriate for office or laboratory administration and is recommended for use by neurologists, neuropsychologists, and speech pathologists.

Personal Orientation Test

The Personal Orientation Test (POT)[29] is *not commercially available.*

The POT consists of five human body diagrams, each showing a ventral and dorsal view. Various locations on the body are numbered in each diagram, and the patient is asked to touch the corresponding locations on his or her body. The reliability of the POT has not been studied. The POT successfully discriminated Korean War veterans with chronic brain injury who had penetrating missile wounds from veterans who had received peripheral nerve injuries ($p < .001$).[29] The POT test is sensitive to anterior left-, posterior left-, and anterior right-hemisphere lesions. Paradoxically, patients with bilateral frontal lobe lesions were less impaired than patients with unilateral anterior lesions. This finding may have been an artifact of the particular subjects in the study and requires further investigation.

Although it is not commercially available, the POT can be constructed from published descriptions and examples.[29] The test must be interpreted cautiously, because the effects of age and education on performance are unknown, and the reliability of the test has not been established. Interpretation should be attempted only by experienced neuropsychologists and neurologists. The POT is appropriate for bedside, office, or laboratory administration.

Boston Spatial-Quantitative Battery, Right-Left Orientation

The Boston Spatial-Quantitative Battery (BSQB), Right-Left Orientation, is *not commercially available.*

This test can be constructed from information provided by Goodglass and Kaplan.[27] Patients are asked to indicate lateral locations on their body and the examiner's body, with and without using a specified hand. Reliability coefficients are not reported for the BSQB. Normative data are available for 147 neurologically normal men stratified by age (25 through 85 years) and education.[28] Interpretation of test results is relatively straightforward, provided that care has been taken to ensure that the patient does not have an oral language comprehension deficit. The subtest is appropriate for bedside, office, or laboratory administration and can be employed by physicians, psychologists, speech pathologists, and occupational therapists.

Benton Right-Left Orientation Test

The Benton Right-Left Orientation Test[26] can be obtained from *Oxford University Press, Incorporated, 200 Madison Avenue, New York, NY 10016.*

In this test, patients are given commands requiring each of the following actions:

a. Pointing to lateral parts of their bodies with either hand
b. Pointing to lateral parts of their bodies with the ipsilateral hand
c. Pointing to lateral parts of their bodies with the contralateral hand
d. Pointing to lateral parts of the examiner's body (requiring a reversal of left-right perspective) with either hand
e. Pointing to lateral parts of the examiner's body with a specified hand (requiring simultaneous appreciation of own and another's left-right perspective)

In addition to the standard version of the test (Form A), a mirror-image alternate form (Form B), a form for use with right hemiplegic patients (Form R), and a form for left hemiplegic patients (Form L) are available. Normative data are reported for Forms A and B in Benton's manual,[26] based on a sample of 234 healthy individuals and non-brain-damaged patients ranging in age from 16 to 64 years. Age, education, and gender did not significantly affect test performance. Data reported in the manual suggest that the test is sensitive to right-left disorientation in patients with both right- and left-hemisphere lesions. Among patients with left-hemisphere damage, a higher proportion of those who had aphasia also showed right-left disorientation. Patients with right-hemisphere damage were impaired only on items requiring them to discriminate left from right from the perspective of someone facing them. The manual does not report reliability coefficients for the test.

The Benton Right-Left Orientation Test can be administered at bedside, in the office, or in the laboratory. Its interpretation is straightforward, and the test is appropriate for administration by psychologists, physicians, speech pathologists, and occupational therapists.

NEUROPSYCHOLOGICAL TREATMENT

Because the disorders of stimulus localization are associated with aphasia, treatment is often rendered by speech therapists. Treatment generally consists of practice and corrective feedback. A patient with stimulus mislocalization may be stimulated in the impaired sensory modality and then asked to determine where the stimulus occurred. Increasing the intensity of the stimulus may facilitate performance. Another strategy involves pairing a stimulus in an intact sensory modality with a stimulus in an impaired modality. For example, if the patient mislocalizes visual but not auditory stimuli, an auditory stimulus occurring on the same side as the visual stimulus may facilitate localization of the visual stimulus. Immediate feedback and rewards for correct responses (e.g., praise, tokens to be exchanged for other rewards, points that are later graphed for the patient to see) enhance motivation and performance. The use of such aids can be decreased gradually as the patient recovers.

Carrying the treatment of stimulus mislocalization into everyday settings and activities promotes generalization of the improvement seen in the clinic. This can be accomplished through homework assignments done with the supervision of relatives or through the use of a job coach in the patient's vocational setting. Cooking, cleaning, or vocational tasks that involve the use of impaired stimulus modalities should be incorporated into the treatment.

Finger mislocalization and autotopagnosia are treated mainly through stimulation and feedback techniques. Having the patient verbalize a strategy for finding the body part that he or she is looking for may be of value. For example, a patient might learn to say, "I am searching for my nose which is on my face above my mouth," as he or she reaches for it. It also may help to verbalize objects and activities associated with the body part (e.g., "I wear my glasses on my nose," "I hitchhike with my thumb"). Visual cues from a mirror or from watching the therapist point to the target body part on his or her own body may also facilitate performance. It may be beneficial to alternate trials in which the patient carries out an activity involving the body part with trials in which the patient simply tries to find the body part. For example, the patient can be asked to put on a wristwatch. If this is accomplished successfully, the patient can subsequently be asked to point to his or her wrist, using the wristwatch as a cue when necessary.

Right-left disorientation can be treated with paper-and-pencil tasks (e.g., maps with varying right and left turns), with practice indicating right and left parts of the body from different perspectives, and with practice making right and left turns on command while walking. The patient's attention should be drawn to cues that help with right and left discriminations. For example, a patient can be cued to think about the hand he or she writes with and to use this as a cue for which is the right or left side. If such natural cues are not effective, the patient can be given a wristband to wear on his or her right arm. If the band is always worn on the right, it can become a reliable cue for use during right-left discrimination tasks.

CASE ILLUSTRATIONS

Both patients presented in this section have complex and challenging clinical presentations, hence the inclusion of one of these cases in several chapters in this book. Both patients are also notable for their interest in and tolerance of extensive neuropsychological examination. In neither patient was there any evidence of effort to fake or exaggerate symptoms. Both patients exerted good effort throughout their examinations and were as eager as the examiner to discover what they could and could not do.

CASE 8–1

J.S. was a 49-year-old woman with an 11th-grade education who worked as a retail manager. She suffered a cardiac arrest, which resulted in a mild anoxic encephalopathy. Her initial neurological examination revealed full visual fields but decreased visual acuity (20/400 in each eye), impaired speech articulation, decreased memory for new information, and mild right-sided weakness with no significant restriction in range of movement of the right arm. There was no loss of hearing nor loss of tactile sensation. J.S.'s magnetic resonance imaging (MRI) scans showed bilateral combined parietal and occipital lobe infarctions and periventricular white-matter degeneration.

Neuropsychological examination revealed some additional cognitive deficits. J.S. was severely impaired in her ability to do detailed visual discriminations and to judge spatial relations. Fine motor coordination was also severely impaired. Her bisection of lines was accurate, however, and she unerringly detected unilateral and bilateral simultaneous stimulation in all sensory modalities. She was able to recognize drawings of objects, colors, and familiar faces. Memory for verbal information was average for her age, but she showed severe impairment when asked to recall new visuospatial information. Intellectual functioning was in the average range, and problem-solving skills were well preserved.

J.S. accurately discriminated between the right and left sides of her body and of space. She correctly localized stimulation to different fingers, but was significantly impaired on the Personal Orientation Test. Her errors included touching locations on the wrong side of her body (e.g., she touched her right inner elbow instead of her left), but more typically, she touched incorrect body parts (e.g., she touched the top of her head instead of her left ear and her thigh instead of her knee). In contrast, she made no errors when asked to match and discriminate locations on duplicates of the Personal Orientation Test body diagrams. Trials in which the patient failed to respond correctly were repeated, with the examiner first touching the correct body location on the patient while the patient's eyes were occluded and then asking the patient to touch the same position. No errors were made by the patient under these conditions.

Despite her accuracy in pointing to positions in space (10 correct responses in 12 trials on the Visuospatial Integration Procedure, described in Chap. 7), J.S. had difficulty in finding corresponding positions in space (3 correct responses in 10 trials on the VOSP Number Location Subtest) and discriminating positions in space (3 correct responses in 10 trials on the VOSP Position Discrimination Subtest). There was no pattern to her errors that would suggest that she was consistently perceiving stimuli as displaced to the right or left of their true location.

J.S. had some difficulty in performing the Audiospatial Localization Procedure, making only 7 correct responses in 12 trials. Again, in no case did she perceive the stimulus as occurring on the wrong side of space. All of her errors consisted of placing the stimulus in the wrong position on the same side of space.

DISCUSSION

A diagnosis of autotopagnosia can be made in Case 8–1. The patient was unable to locate body parts corresponding to locations on a diagram of the human body, despite being able to match the body parts. Although some of her errors suggested a diagnosis of stimulus mislocalization (e.g., she touched her right elbow instead of her left), most of her errors involved confusion in the location of body parts. In addition, she had no difficulty in finding body parts that were touched by the examiner, a skill that would not be preserved if she had tactile stimulus mislocalization. Her errors cannot be explained by failure to see or detect the body parts on the model, because she had no difficulty matching or discriminating them, even with visual acuity of only 20/400. Her success in pointing in response to tactile stimulation rules out a motor explanation of her impairment.

Evidence for a diagnosis of visual stimulus mislocalization can be found in J.R.'s poor performance on the VOSP subtests. Because these tests are normed procedures, the deficit cannot be attributed to normal human error of estimation; the patient is far below the cut-off scores for the normal population. The patient did not have stimulus neglect, but she did have decreased visual acuity. It is possible that her acuity was not sufficient to accomplish the VOSP subtests; therefore, a firm diagnosis of visual stimulus mislocalization cannot be made.

The patient also had difficulty with auditory stimulus localization. In this case, sensory loss is not a viable explanation of the deficit, because the patient's hearing is unimpeded. Although normal human error may contribute to her performance on the Audiospatial Localization Procedure, both my experience and published reports of use of this procedure in clinical populations suggest that this patient has more difficulty than would be expected in a normal person.

CASE 4–5

R.M. was a 50-year-old man with a high-school education. Following triple coronary artery bypass grafting, he developed atrial fibrillation and an anoxic encephalopathy. MRI scans revealed bilateral watershed-area infarctions (C-shaped infarctions extending from the frontal to the occipital poles), with greater damage evident in the right hemisphere.

Results of R.M.'s neuropsychological assessment are presented in Chapters 4 and 7. Only selected findings are discussed here. R.M. had full visual fields, but visual acuity could not be assessed because of the patient's inability to discriminate even the largest letters on the Snellen chart. Acuity was sufficient for the patient to reliably identify colors, line drawings, and people seen from distances of up to 20 feet. He accomplished this despite having probable left hemispatial neglect and evidence of simultanagnosia (see Chap. 4). Tactile sensitivity was also reduced in the left hand.

R.M. had severe weakness in his left hand but only a mild degree of weakness in his dominant right hand. R.M. was somewhat clumsy in manipulating small objects, but he readily accomplished gross movements with the right hand and arm and showed no perseveration, initiation deficits, or impersistence. He did, however, show a deficit in performing skilled movements on demand (see Apraxia) and was inaccurate in reaching for visual and auditory targets.

The Benton Right-Left Orientation Test, Form L, was administered. Although R.M. could not accurately reach for targets, he was able to bring his hand close enough to large, widely spaced targets to make it possible to determine what he was aiming for, even though he did not always smoothly guide his hand to the target. On trials that required touching a particular body location, R.M. would grope with his hand until it reached what he was aiming for.

In his characteristic groping manner, R.M. was able to indicate the right and left parts of the examiner's body specified on the Benton test without error. In contrast, he was correct on only 6 of 12 trials when pointing to right and left parts of his own body. Analysis of his errors revealed that he consistently failed to point to locations on the left side of his body when commanded, pointing instead to the corresponding location on the right side of his body.

Each location that R.M. missed on command on the Benton test was then touched by the examiner while the patient's eyes were occluded. Under this new condition, R.M. was able to locate two of the left-sided positions, but continued to make errors with the other four. In each case, he erred by pointing to a place to the right of the position touched by the examiner, although he did not always point to the corresponding contralateral body part. For example, when the examiner touched his left hand, R.M. indicated a point on the right side of his chest.

R.M. was also asked to identify fingers touched by the examiner while his vision was occluded (Section B of the Benton Finger Localization Test). He was correct in 4 of 10 trials with the right hand and in 2 of 10 trials with the left hand. The patient detected all stimuli administered (i.e., he correctly noted the occurrence of each stimulus), even when he failed to locate the finger stimulated.

The VOSP Number Location Subtest was administered. R.M. was correct on only 2 trials, far below the cut-off score for normals. Most of his errors consisted of his perceiving the stimulus as being farther to the right than its actual location. However, it was not always possible to determine whether R.M. perceived all of his response options because of his deficits in detecting visual stimuli. Consequently, the Visuospatial Integration Procedure (see Chap. 7) was administered, and R.M. was asked to identify the colors of all stimuli that he failed to point to. R.M. correctly pointed to only 2 of 12 targets, but correctly identified the colors of all targets. Notably, all but one of his errors involved reaching for a point to the right of the actual target location.

The Audiospatial Localization Procedure was administered, and R.M. was correct on only 4 of the 12 trials. He detected every auditory stimulus regardless of the side it occurred on. All but one of his errors consisted of identifying the stimulus as having occurred on the wrong side of space. Notably, the errors occurred in both directions: left-sided stimuli were thought to be on the right and right-sided stimuli were thought to be on the left.

DISCUSSION

A diagnosis of right-left disorientation could be considered in Case 4–5 as a consequence of his performance on the Benton Right-Left Orientation Test. However, the pattern of errors is less consistent with this diagnosis than they are with stimulus mislocalization. This impression is confirmed by the fact that the patient continued to make significant errors even in response to tactile stimulation. The errors characteristically involved touching the corresponding body location on the wrong side of the body or displacement of perception of the tactile stimulus toward the wrong side of the body. The patient similarly made errors in response to visual and auditory stimulation.

The errors made by this patient clearly fall outside the realm of normal human error of estimation. The normal population does not confuse the side of space stimuli occur on, particularly not under the conditions employed in the test procedures. Diagnosis of stimulus mislocalization in Case 4–5, however, is complicated by the presence of decreased visual and tactual sensation and probable left hemispatial neglect. The fact that the patient detected all the visual, auditory, and tactile stimuli presented and was inaccurate only in the location in which he perceived the stimuli occurring argues against dismissing his performance as simply a failure to detect stimuli. Thus, despite having some sensory and stimulus detection deficits, the test data suggest that the patient is also impaired in stimulus localization.

A diagnosis of autotopagnosia cannot be made in this patient because he is able to accurately locate positions on the right side of his body. However, he does show bilateral finger mislocalization. Sensation was preserved in the right hand, and loss of sensation or stimulus neglect in the left hand cannot account for the deficit because the patient again succeeded in detecting all stimuli administered.

REFERENCES

1. American Psychiatric Association: Diagnostic and Statistical Manual of Mental Disorders, Fourth Edition. American Psychiatric Association, Washington, DC, 1994.
2. The International Classification of Diseases, Ninth Revision, Clinical Modification. Med-Index Publications, Salt Lake City, 1991.
3. Pinek, B, et al: Audio-spatial deficits in humans: Differential effects associated with left versus right hemisphere parietal damage. Cortex 25:175, 1989.
4. Cornelisse, LE, and Kelly, JB: The effect of cerebrovascular accident on the ability to localize sounds under conditions of the precedence effect. Neuropsychologia 25:449, 1987.
5. Altman, JA, Rosenblum, AS, and Lvova, VG: Lateralization of a moving auditory image in patients with focal damage of the brain hemispheres. Neuropsychologia 25:435, 1987.
6. Sanchez-Longo, LP, Forster, FM, Auth, TL: A clinical test for sound localization and its applications. Neurology 7:655, 1957.
7. Sanchez-Longo, LP, and Forster, FM: Clinical significance of impairment of sound localization. Neurology 8:119, 1950.
8. Klingon, GH, and Bontecou, DC: Localization in auditory space. Neurology 16:879, 1966.
9. Tartaglione, A, et al: Point localization in patients with unilateral brain damage. J Neurol Neurosurg Psychiatry 44:935, 1981.
10. Hannay, HJ, Varney, NR, and Benton, AL: Visual localization in patients with unilateral brain disease. J Neurol Neurosurg Psychiatry 39:307, 1976.
11. Joanette, Y, and Brouchon, M: Visual allesthesia in manual pointing: Some evidence for a sensorimotor cerebral organization. Brain Cogn 3:152, 1984.
12. Jacobs, L: Visual allesthesia. Neurology 30:1059, 1980.
13. Corin, MS, and Bender, MB: Mislocalization in visual space. With reference to the midline at the boundary of a homonymous hemianopia. Arch Neurol 27:252, 1972.
14. Young, RR, and Benson, DF: Where is the lesion in allochiria? Arch Neurol 49:348, 1992.
15. Gainotti, G, and Tiacci, C: The unilateral forms of finger agnosia. An experimental study. Confinia Neurologica 35:271, 1973.
16. Strub, R, and Geschwind, N: Gerstmann syndrome without aphasia. Cortex 10:378, 1974.
17. Matsuoka, H, et al: Impairment of parietal cortical functions associated with episodic prolonged spike-and-wave discharges. Epilepsia 27:432, 1986.

18. Caltagirone, C, Gainotti, G, and Miteli, G: Agnosie digitale et lesions du lobe parietal. Schweiz Arch Neurol Neurochir Psychiatr 118:231, 1976.
19. Kinsbourne, M, and Warrington, EK: A study of finger agnosia. Brain 85:47, 1962.
20. Ogden, JA: Autotopagnosia. Occurrence in a patient without nominal aphasia and with an intact ability to point to parts of animals and objects. Brain 108:1009, 1985.
21. Cambier, J, et al: Right hemiasomatognosia and sensation of amputation caused by left subcortical lesion. Rev Neurol 140:256, 1984.
22. DeRenzi, E, and Scotti, G: Autotopagnosia: Fiction or reality? Report of a case. Arch Neurol 23:221, 1970.
23. Fischer, P, Marterer, A, and Danielczyk, W: Right-left disorientation in dementia of the Alzheimer type. Neurology 40:1619, 1990.
24. Roeltgen, DP, Sevush, S, and Heilman, KM: Pure Gerstmann's syndrome from a focal lesion. Arch Neurol 40:46, 1983.
25. Demeurisse, G, et al: Study of two cases of aphasia by infarction of the left thalamus, without cortical lesion. Acta Neurol Belg 79:450, 1979.
26. Benton, AL, et al: Contributions to Neuropsychological Assessment. A Clinical Manual. Oxford University Press, New York, 1983.
27. Goodglass, H, and Kaplan, E: The Assessment of Aphasia and Related Disorders, Second Edition. Lea & Febiger, Philadelphia, 1983.
28. Borod, J, Goodglass, H, and Kaplan, E: Normative Data on the Boston Diagnostic Aphasia Examination, Parietal Lobe Battery and Naming Test. J Clin Neuropsychol 2:209, 1980.
29. Semmes, J, et al: Correlates of impaired orientation in personal and extrapersonal space. Brain 86:747, 1963.

DISORDERS OF STIMULUS RECOGNITION (ASSOCIATIVE AGNOSIA)

9

The associative agnosias involve a failure to recognize visual, auditory, or tactile stimuli despite adequate perception of the stimuli. The patient is no longer able to appreciate the meaning and significance of certain objects. Although they are normally perceived, the objects appear to be stripped of their meaning. The objects no longer evoke the memories that would normally be associated with them; therefore, the patient fails to identify or behave appropriately toward the objects.

The examiner must not conclude that a patient has an associative agnosia until the following three criteria are satisfied:

1. The patient consistently fails to recognize stimuli with which he or she was previously familiar.
2. The patient is able to match and discriminate among the stimuli that he or she fails to recognize.
3. All alternative means of demonstrating stimulus recognition have failed.

A variety of disorders can impair stimulus recognition by impairing stimulus perception. Associative agnosia impairs recognition only; perception remains intact. In this way, associative agnosia differs from elementary sensory loss (e.g., blindness, deafness, loss of tactile sensitivity), the failure to detect portions of a stimulus (see Stimulus neglect), and impaired perception of the form and features of stimuli (see Stimulus imperception). Each of these disorders must be ruled out or be shown not to be present in sufficient severity to account for stimulus recognition failure. The primary means of accomplishing the latter is to document that patients successfully match and discriminate stimuli they fail to recognize. In many cases, this criterion cannot be satisfied, and the diagnosis of agnosia cannot proceed beyond suspicion.

Table 9–1 summarizes the alternative approaches that should be used to assess recognition ability. Successfully naming a stimulus demonstrates that recognition has occurred. However, patients who have anomic aphasia, an oral language disorder in which naming is impaired (see Chap. 12), may recognize stimuli that they fail to name. Patients with anomic aphasia may be able to demonstrate recognition of a face, a piece of music, or a landmark by providing a description that uniquely fits the target stimulus. For example, when shown a photograph of United States President John F. Kennedy, the patient with anomia may not be able to retrieve the name, but may haltingly respond, "That is the one who was shot." When listening to the melody of "Jingle Bells," the anomic may sing some lyrics, or identify the tune as

Table 9–1. **ALTERNATIVE APPROACHES TO DEMONSTRATING STIMULUS RECOGNITION**

	Name Stimulus	Describe Identity	Describe Use	Multiple Choice	Show Use
Object colors	+	–	–	+	–
Faces	+	+	–	+	–
Visual objects	+	–	+	+	+
Tactile objects	+	–	+	+	+
Fingers	+	–	–	+	+/–
Object sounds	+	–	+	+	+
Music	+	+	–	+	–
Landmarks	+	+	–	+	–

\+ = Appropriate means of demonstrating recognition.
– = Inappropriate means of demonstrating recognition.
+/– = Partially appropriate means of demonstrating recognition.

one sung at Christmas. When shown a picture of the Sphinx, the patient with anomia may respond, "That was built long ago, in the place with the long river." These responses suggest that recognition has occurred.

When a patient is unable to name visually or tactually presented objects, recognition should be assessed further by asking him or her to describe how the objects are used. In the case of sounds, the patient can be asked to describe how the object that produces the sound is used. Unfortunately, many patients with oral language disorders are unable to name or describe stimuli that they may recognize. In these cases, several options should be presented from which the patient must choose the target stimulus. Depending on the abilities of the patient, the options can be presented verbally, visually, or tactually. The patient can make verbal or manual responses (e.g., head nodding, pointing, grasping). For example, the color recognition ability of a patient with aphasia can be assessed by showing the patient drawings of objects and offering several crayon colors, one of which is the correct color for the object, from which the patient can choose to color the drawing. Demonstrating the correct color choices for several drawings often is necessary before the patient comprehends the task.

When a multiple-choice format fails to elicit accurate recognition of stimuli, patients should be asked to pantomime the use of the stimulus. This technique works for visual and tactual objects, for object sounds, and for fingers that have a characteristic function (e.g., the ring finger holds rings, the index finger points, the thumb is used for hitchhiking).

Successful diagnosis of associative agnosia is rare. The lesions that impair stimulus recognition often impair perception, cause language disorders, and impede the patient's ability to execute skilled movements. When multiple disorders are present in the same patient, diagnosis of a specific impairment in recognition may become impossible. Associative agnosia includes the subtypes listed in the chapter outline.

The existence of color agnosia is unproven. Few patients with color agnosia who are entirely free of other disorders that could account for their apparent recognition failure exist in the clinical literature. However, one case that does appear to satisfy all criteria is discussed later in this chapter. The term *auditory affective agnosia* is sometimes used to refer to impaired recognition of emotional prosody. Impaired prosody recognition is a part of sensory aprosodia, a disorder discussed in Chapter 14; consequently, auditory affective agnosia is not included in this chapter.

NOMENCLATURE

The term *agnosia,* as used in the neurology and neuropsychology literature, refers both to disorders of recognition (associative agnosia) and severe disorders of perception (apperceptive agnosia). Only the associative agnosias meet the strict definition of *agnosia* as a disorder of recognition in the absence of impaired perception. Perceptual disorders can lead to impaired recognition, but in these cases, impaired recognition occurs because the stimulus is never adequately analyzed and perceived by the brain. The term *stimulus imperception* is used in this text to refer to the perceptual disorders, including the so-called apperceptive agnosias. The term *agnosia* is reserved for disorders that meet the strict definition of a recognition disorder.

The confusion in the literature between perceptual disorders and recognition disorders is most apparent with respect to finger agnosia and astereognosis. The failure to discriminate between recognition and perceptual components has led to contradictory anatomical findings with respect to these disorders. For consistency and to decrease confusion regarding these disorders, the terms *finger agnosia* and *astereognosis* are restricted to failed recognition of fingers and of tactile objects, respectively, in the absence of perceptual impairment sufficient to account for the deficient performance. Impaired perception of the fingers usually is the result of sensory loss or the failure to localize the finger stimulated by the examiner; both of these deficits are discussed in Chapter 8. Impaired perception of tactile objects is discussed in Chapter 5.

The term *spatial agnosia* is sometimes used to describe patients with stimulus neglect or spatial imperception. This usage also departs from the classic definition of *agnosia*. Spatial and perceptual deficits should be excluded from the concept of agnosia to adhere to the strict definition of the term. Accordingly, spatial agnosia is not listed in this chapter. Stimulus neglect is discussed in Chapter 4 and spatial imperception in Chapter 6.

Agnosia can be coded in DSM-IV[1] as "Cognitive Disorder Not Otherwise Specified" or "Mild Neurocognitive Disorder." ICD-9-CM[2] includes agnosia involving visual stimuli under the code "Psychophysical Visual Disturbance." All other agnosias are subsumed under "Other Symbolic Dysfunction."

RULES FOR DIAGNOSIS

Clinical Indicators: Each is independent (only one must be observed for the disorder to be suspected) *except* when subscripting is used. Subscripted numbers (a_1, a_2) denote an indicator with multiple parts that must be considered together.
Associated Features: These are listed to give a more complete picture of the disorder. The presence or absence of these features does not affect the diagnosis.
Factors to Rule Out: All must be taken into account. Failure to rule out even one of these factors makes a firm diagnosis impossible.
Lesion Locations: Each location stands alone; damage in only one of the listed areas is sufficient to produce the disorder.

VARIETY OF PRESENTATION

1. Color agnosia* (see also Color imperception and stimulus-specific aphasia)

Clinical Indicators

a_1. Failure to identify the characteristic colors of familiar objects

a_2. Relatively preserved ability to match and discriminate among colors when the assessment of color agnosia involves visual presentation of colors

a_3. Failure of all means of demonstrating object color recognition (see Table 9–1)

Associated Features

a. Impaired oral language (see Chap. 12)
b. Unilateral (usually right-sided) muscle weakness (i.e., hemiparesis)
c. The presence of homonymous hemianopsia: loss of visual acuity in one (usually the right) visual half-field

Factors to Rule Out

a. Impaired matching and discrimination of colors (only when tests of object color recognition employ visual stimuli) as a result of any of the following disorders:
   1) Loss of visual acuity so severe that it prevents colored stimuli from being seen regardless of where in the visual field they are presented
   2) Color imperception (see Chap. 5)
   3) Failure to detect portions of visual stimuli as a result of stimulus neglect (see Chap. 4)
b. Inability to demonstrate color recognition through language as a result of oral language impairment, particularly stimulus-specific aphasia (see Chap. 12)

Lesion Locations

a. Occipital lobe[3]
b. Left temporal and occipital lobes in conjunction with right parietal and occipital lobes[4]

Lesion Lateralization

a. Bilateral lesions in all reported cases

2. Prosopagnosia (also called facial agnosia; see also Facial imperception)

Clinical Indicators

a_1. Failure to recognize previously familiar faces

a_2. Relatively preserved matching and discrimination of faces

a_3. Failure of all means of demonstrating facial recognition (see Table 9–1)

Associated Features

a. Failure to recognize one's own face when seeing it in a photograph or reflective surface

---

*The existence of color agnosia is putative; clear demonstrations of this condition have not appeared in the clinical literature.

b. Recognition of people based on nonfacial features (e.g., hairstyle, height, weight, characteristic clothing, voice characteristics, mannerisms)
c. Visual recognition of specific members within a class may also be impaired (e.g., patient unable to tell his or her car from other cars of the same make, model, and color)
d. Impaired recognition of landmarks (see Topographical agnosia)
e. Presence of homonymous hemianopsia (loss of visual acuity in one visual half-field, usually the right) or quandrantanopsia (loss of acuity in one quadrant of the visual field of each eye, usually the right superior quadrant)

Factors to Rule Out

a. Impaired matching and discrimination of faces as a result of any of the following disorders:
   1) Loss of visual acuity so severe that it prevents faces from being seen regardless of where in the visual field they are presented
   2) Facial imperception (see Chap. 5)
   3) Failure to detect portions of visual stimuli as a result of stimulus neglect (see Chap. 4)
b. Unfamiliarity with the faces before the onset of the brain lesion when faces of famous people are used during testing; faces of relatives should be substituted in these instances
c. The delusion that familiar people have been replaced by impostors (see Reduplication)
d. Inability to demonstrate facial recognition through language as a result of oral language impairment (see Chap. 12)

Lesion Locations

a. Temporal (cortical, subcortical, anterior, medial, or inferior) lobe, including parahippocampal, fusiform, and superior temporal gyri and interruption of inferior longitudinal fasciculus, alone or in combination with the occipital or parietal lobes[5–18]
b. Occipital (cortical, subcortical, medial, or inferior) lobe, including interruption of the inferior longitudinal fasciculus, alone or in combination with the temporal or parietal lobes[6,8,10–13,17–19]
c. Parietal (medial) lobe, alone or in combination with the temporal or occipital lobes[9,18]

Lesion Lateralization

a. Although many reported cases have bilateral lesions, the consensus among researchers is that a right-sided lesion is sufficient to cause prosopagnosia.[20]

3. Visual object agnosia (see also Visual form imperception)

Clinical Indicators

a_1. Failure to recognize visually presented familiar objects; touching and listening to the sound of the object is prevented
a_2. Relatively preserved matching and discrimination of visually presented objects

a_3. Failure of all means of demonstrating visual object recognition (see Table 9–1)

Associated Features

a. Possibility that objects that cannot be recognized visually may be recognized by touch or by hearing a sound associated with the object
b. Preserved ability to draw objects that cannot be visually recognized
c. Recognition of pictures and line drawings of objects possibly worse than recognition of the actual objects
d. Naming or describing the use of visually presented objects possibly worse than pointing to objects named by the examiner
e. Impaired recognition of previously familiar faces (see Prosopagnosia)
f. Impaired recognition of previously familiar landmarks (see Topographical agnosia)
g. Impaired written language (see Chap. 13)
h. Impaired object color recognition (see Color agnosia)
i. Impaired color naming (see Stimulus-specific aphasia)
j. Impaired matching and discrimination of colors (see Color imperception)
k. Impaired learning and retention of new verbal information (see Verbal anterograde amnesia)
l. The presence of homonymous hemianopsia (loss of visual acuity in one visual half-field, usually the right) or quandrantanopsia (loss of acuity in one quadrant of the visual field of each eye, usually the right superior quadrant)

Factors to Rule Out

a. Impaired matching and discrimination of objects as a result of any of the following disorders:
   1) Loss of visual acuity so severe that it prevents objects from being seen regardless of where in the visual field they are presented
   2) Visual form imperception (see Chap. 5)
   3) Failure to detect portions of visual stimuli as a result of stimulus neglect (see Chap. 4)
b. Unfamiliarity with the objects before the onset of the brain lesion
c. Inability to demonstrate object recognition through language as a result of oral language impairment (see Chap. 12)
d. Inability to demonstrate object recognition through pantomime of the object's use as a result of any of the following disorders:
   1) Impaired execution of skilled movements on command (see Apraxia)
   2) Motor weakness
   3) Impaired initiation of movements (see Akinesia)
   4) Impaired maintenance of ongoing movements (see Motor impersistence)
   5) Impaired ability to stop ongoing movements (see Motor perseveration)

Lesion Locations

a. Combined temporal and occipital lobes, particularly the lingual, fusiform, and posterior-inferior temporal gyri, including interruption of the inferior longitudinal fasciculus, sometimes in combination with a corpus callosum (splenium) lesion[21–25]

b. Occipital lobe[26]

Lesion Lateralization

a. Bilateral lesions documented in virtually all reported cases

4. Finger agnosia (see also Finger mislocalization)

Clinical Indicators

a_1. Failure to visually recognize individual fingers of the hands

a_2. Relatively preserved matching and discrimination of visually presented fingers

a_3. Failure of all means of demonstrating finger recognition (see Table 9–1)

Associated Features

a. Impaired writing (see Agraphia)

b. Impaired calculation ability (see Acalculia)

c. Impaired discrimination of the right and left sides of the body, of space, or both (see Right-left disorientation)

NOTE: When finger agnosia occurs together with agraphia, acalculia, and right-left disorientation, the complex of disorders is referred to as Gerstmann's syndrome.

d. Deficits in verbal or global intellectual functioning (see Verbal and global intellectual decline)

e. Impaired oral language (see Chap. 12)

Factors to Rule Out

a. Impaired visual matching and discrimination of fingers as a result of any of the following disorders:

1) Loss of visual acuity so severe that it prevents fingers from being seen regardless of where in the visual field they are presented
2) Visual form imperception (see Chap. 5)
3) Failure to detect portions of visual stimuli as a result of stimulus neglect (see Chap. 4)

b. Unfamiliarity with the names of specific fingers prior to the onset of the brain lesion

c. Inability to demonstrate finger recognition as a result of oral language impairment (see Chap. 12)

d. Inability to demonstrate finger recognition through pantomime of the finger's use as a result of any of the following disorders:

1) Impaired execution of skilled movements on command (see Apraxia)
2) Motor weakness
3) Impaired initiation of movements (see Akinesia)
4) Impaired maintenance of ongoing movements (see Motor impersistence)
5) Impaired ability to stop ongoing movements (see Motor perseveration)

Lesion Locations

a. Parietal lobe, particularly the angular gyrus, supramarginal gyrus, and superior parietal lobule[27–30]

Lesion Lateralization

a. Language-dominant hemisphere, usually the left.

b. Agnosia typically extending to fingers of both hands even when the lesion is unilateral

5. Astereognosis (also called tactile object agnosia; see also Tactual form imperception)

Clinical Indicators

a_1. Failure to recognize tactually presented objects that were previously familiar; seeing and listening to the objects prevented

a_2. Relatively preserved matching and discrimination of tactually presented objects

a_3. Failure of all means of demonstrating tactual object recognition (see Table 9–1)

Associated Features

a. Deficit more likely to be present unilaterally than bilaterally

b. Left hand more likely to be impaired than the right

c. A recent history of decreased sensation in the astereognosic hand or hands

d. Impaired localization of stimuli on the astereognosic hand or hands (see Stimulus mislocalization)

e. Palpation of objects with the astereognosic hand or hands is hesitant (i.e., the object is only briefly palpated) or stereotyped (i.e., the patient manipulates all objects the same way, regardless of their shape)

f. Stimuli not recognized by touch possibly recognized when seen or when their characteristic sound is heard

g. Impaired perception of spatial information (see Spatial imperception)

h. Impaired judgment of direction when traveling a route (see Topographical disorientation)

Factors to Rule Out

a. Impaired tactual matching and discrimination of objects as a result of any of the following disorders:
   1) Loss of tactile sensitivity
   2) Tactual form imperception (see Chap. 5)
   3) Failure to detect portions of tactual stimuli as a result of stimulus neglect (see Chap. 4)

b. Unfamiliarity with the objects before the onset of the brain lesion

c. Inability to demonstrate tactual object recognition as a result of oral language impairment (see Chap. 12)

d. Inability to demonstrate tactual object recognition through pantomime of the object's use as a result of any of the following disorders:
   1) Impaired execution of skilled movements on command (see Apraxia)
   2) Motor weakness
   3) Impaired initiation of movements (see Akinesia)
   4) Impaired maintenance of ongoing movements (see Motor impersistence)
   5) Impaired ability to stop ongoing movements (see Motor perseveration)

Lesion Locations

a. Parietal lobe[31–33]
b. Posterior temporal lobe in combination with insular cortex[31]
c. Brainstem, causing interruption of the medial lemniscus[34,35]
d. Cervical spinal cord, specifically the nucleus cervicalis lateralis within the medial lemniscus[36–38]
e. Brachial plexus[39]

Lesion Lateralization

a. May follow right- or left-sided lesions
b. Impairment contralateral to the side of the lesion

6. Auditory agnosia (see also Auditory pattern imperception)

Clinical Indicators

a_1. Failure to recognize previously familiar sounds
a_2. Relatively preserved matching and discrimination of sounds
a_3. Failure of all means of demonstrating sound recognition (see Table 9–1)
b_1. Failure to recognize previously familiar works of music
b_2. Relatively preserved matching and discrimination of musical patterns
b_3. Failure of all means of demonstrating music recognition (see Table 9–1)

Associated Features

a. Some degree of impaired auditory pattern perception (see Auditory pattern imperception)
b. Extinction to bilateral simultaneous auditory stimulation (see Sensory extinction)
c. Impaired oral language, particularly pure word deafness (see Chap. 12)

Factors to Rule Out

a. Impaired matching and discrimination of object sounds or music as a result of any of the following disorders:
    1) Loss of auditory acuity
    2) Severe auditory pattern imperception (see Chap. 5)
b. Unfamiliarity with the object sounds or music before the onset of the brain lesion
c. Inability to demonstrate object sound or music recognition as a result of oral language impairment (see Chap. 12)
d. Inability to demonstrate object sound recognition through pantomime of the use of the object associated with the sound (music recognition cannot be assessed in this manner; see Table 9–1) as a result of any of the following disorders:
    1) Impaired execution of skilled movements on command (see Apraxia)
    2) Motor weakness
    3) Impaired initiation of movements (see Akinesia)
    4) Impaired maintenance of ongoing movements (see Motor impersistence)
    5) Impaired ability to stop ongoing movements (see Motor perseveration)

Lesion Locations

a. Temporal lobe (cortical or subcortical), particularly the middle and superior temporal gyri, with frequent involvement of the insular cortex and the frontal and parietal lobes[40–45]
b. Thalamus, in conjunction with internal capsule[46]
c. Ventricular enlargement without documented parenchymal damage[47]

Lesion Lateralization

a. Bilateral lesions in virtually all published cases

7. Topographical agnosia (see also Topographical disorientation)

Clinical Indicators

a_1. Failure to recognize previously familiar landmarks
a_2. Relatively preserved matching and discrimination of landmarks
a_3. Failure of all means of demonstrating landmark recognition (see Table 9–1)

Associated Features

a. Impaired perception of direction when traveling routes (see Topographical disorientation)
b. Impaired remembrance of previously familiar routes (topographical amnesia)
c. Impaired ability to learn and retain new routes (topographical amnesia)
d. Impaired recognition of previously familiar faces (see Prosopagnosia)
e. Impaired recognition of previously familiar objects (see Visual object agnosia)

Factors to Rule Out

a. Impaired matching and discrimination of landmarks as a result of any of the following disorders:
   1) Loss of visual acuity so severe that it prevents landmarks from being seen regardless of where in the visual field they are presented
   2) Visual form imperception (see Chap. 5)
   3) Failure to detect portions of visual stimuli as a result of stimulus neglect (see Chap. 4)
b. Unfamiliarity with the landmarks before the onset of the brain lesion when pictures of famous landmarks are used during testing; pictures of landmarks in the patient's home, job, or community should be substituted in these instances
c. The delusion that familiar landmarks have been transported to new locations (see Reduplication)
d. Inability to demonstrate landmark recognition through language as a result of oral language impairment (see Chap. 12)

Lesion Locations

a. Posterior cerebral hemisphere (without further localization)[48]
b. Combined temporal and occipital lobes[8,12,18]
c. Medial occipital lobe[18]
d. Medial parietal lobe[18]

Lesion Lateralization

a. Right-sided or bilateral lesions in most reported cases

ETIOLOGY

Cases of associative agnosia are rare, and the causes reported have primarily been cerebrovascular accident and, occasionally, traumatic brain injury. Often, the lesions that lead to the agnosias are bilateral. Thus, patients may present with a history of multiple strokes. Neoplasm is a less likely cause of agnosia, unless the tumor extends subcortically and medially so that it not only impairs unilateral hemisphere functioning but also interrupts callosal input from the preserved hemisphere.

DISABLING CONSEQUENCES

The disabling consequences of the associative agnosias vary from minor to severe. Finger agnosia is unlikely to produce significant disability, because use of the fingers is not impaired. People are rarely asked to name the fingers, and few negative consequences occur for failing to do so. Color agnosia produces little disability except in cases in which the patient is in a profession that requires judgments about color (e.g., fine arts, home decorating, fashion design). For individuals in these or similar occupations, color agnosia can cause the end of a career; however, for the average person, color agnosia is apt to be an annoyance rather than a disability.

Auditory agnosia, similarly, is disabling for individuals in specialized fields. Musicians, sound and recording engineers, and radio broadcasters, among others, are impacted to the greatest degree by this disorder. Physicians base some diagnostic decisions on sounds produced by body organs and also may suffer some disability from auditory agnosia. Nonverbal sounds play a less significant role in the livelihood of the average person. The only important nonverbal sounds regularly encountered by most people are ringing telephones, car horns, clock alarms, and doorbells. In these cases, perception of the sound volume and direction often is sufficient to allow the patient to compensate for any initial confusion regarding the nature of the sound.

Although the average person does not suffer occupational restrictions as a result of auditory agnosia, he or she may experience considerable restriction of leisure. Television programs, movies, and radio broadcasts make ample use of nonverbal sounds, and full appreciation of these programs is diminished by auditory agnosia. The greatest impact, however, is on the enjoyment and appreciation of music. What makes the music of each generation special are the memories, be they pleasant or bittersweet, that the music evokes. To lose those associations with the music of one's past is to lose a part of oneself.

For most individuals, visual interpretation of objects predominates over tactile interpretation. Thus, astereognosis may not be disabling, even for people in occupations that require the use of tools. One feature that accompanies astereognosis is a deficit in the ability to palpate objects. Patients handle objects reluctantly or in a stereotyped manner not appropriate for the specific object being grasped. No studies have been done on whether this palpation deficit leads to clumsy and inept handling of objects in realistic settings when vision is unobscured. If the palpation deficit does extend to these situations, astereognosis may be disabling for people in tool trades or other occupations requiring tool use. Blind persons rely on hearing and touch for object interpretation and are affected by auditory agnosia and astereognosis to a greater extent than sighted persons.

Prosopagnosia has great potential for both social embarrassment and occupational disability. After overcoming their initial distress, the patient's relatives are likely to accept his or her prosopagnosia. Social acquaintances who are not aware of the disorder and do not understand its nature are apt to be less forgiving of the patient's recognition failure. Prosopagnosia is a problem particularly when the patient attempts to establish new interpersonal relationships. Previous acquaintances may be recognizable from some familiar physical or personal characteristic, but no such memories are available to aid in recognizing new acquaintances. Occupational disability is prominent in business and consulting fields, in which advancement partially depends on social skills and the ability to form relationships.

Topographical and visual object agnosia have the greatest potential for disability. Individuals with topographical agnosia may continually become lost, even in their own neighborhoods, and these patients often require supervision when they travel. Jobs that require routine travel are impossible. Visual object agnosia can limit independent functioning almost as much as blindness. Without being in direct physical contact with objects, the visual agnosic may exist in an environment that seems to be full of bewildering and incomprehensible gadgets. Performance of virtually all jobs and domestic chores is restricted severely or rendered impossible.

Some agnosics function better in their natural environment than in the clinic. The patient's natural environment provides contextual information and an opportunity for using multiple senses to explore stimuli. These factors probably account for the patient's increase in level of functioning in familiar settings. Determination of the degree of disability suffered by an individual agnosic patient requires observation of the patient not only in the clinic but in the patient's daily environment as well.

ASSESSMENT INSTRUMENTS

Stimulus Recognition Procedures

Stimulus recognition tests are *not commercially available*.

Few stimulus recognition tests are commercially available; therefore, an examiner wishing to assess stimulus recognition is required to improvise materials and procedures. Tables 9–2 through 9–9 present procedures I employ for documenting agnosia. The materials are drawn either from commercially available tests or can be readily constructed. Responses are recorded on the answer sheets shown in Tables 9–2 through 9–9.

Object color is assessed by asking the patient the color of various common objects (Table 9–2). If the patient cannot name the color, he or she is given verbal or visual multiple-choice options. The color stimulus card from the Western Aphasia

Table 9–2. **COLOR STIMULUS RECOGNITION PROCEDURE**

OBJECT COLOR ("WHAT IS THE COLOR OF:")		
	Name*	**Multiple-Choice Options†**
1. Grass	+/−	Red Green Blue
2. Clouds	+/−	White Brown Red
3. Blood	+/−	Yellow Blue Red
4. Apples	+/−	Red Blue Black
5. Bananas	+/−	Blue Red Yellow
6. Charcoal	+/−	Green Black Brown
7. Tomatoes	+/−	Red White Blue
8. Corn	+/−	Blue Black Yellow

*A plus or minus is used to record a correct or incorrect response, respectively.
†Circle: Visual/verbal.

Battery (WAB)[49] is used for the visual multiple-choice trials in patients whose language deficits prevent verbal identification of color. When a visual multiple-choice response mode is selected, care must be taken to document that color perception is preserved; see Chapter 5 for assessment instruments.

Recognition of visual objects and forms (Tables 9–3 and 9–4) is assessed using drawings of objects and forms also from the WAB.[49] When patients are unable to demonstrate recognition through any response modality, deficits in visual form perception must be ruled out through additional testing; see Chapter 5 for assessment instruments.

The facial recognition procedure (Table 9–5) uses faces of United States presidents (Fig. 9–1). Response modalities include naming, description of the person, and verbal multiple choice. When assessing the ability to describe the presidents, the examiner looks not for a physical description but for a description of the person's life in such a manner that it is unmistakably clear that recognition has occurred. In cases of recognition failure, deficits in facial perception can be ruled out using the assessment procedures discussed in Chapter 5.

Table 9–3. **VISUAL OBJECT RECOGNITION PROCEDURE***

VISUAL OBJECTS ("WHAT OBJECT IS THIS?")			
	Name†	**Multiple-Choice Options**	**Use†‡**
1. Matches	+/–	Lighter Cigarette Matches	+/–
2. Cup	+/–	Cup Bowl Saucer	+/–
3. Comb	+/–	Brush Rake Comb	+/–
4. Screwdriver	+/–	Hammer Screwdriver Saw	+/–
5. Pencil	+/–	Knife Pencil Straw	+/–
6. Flower	+/–	Flower Funnel Pencil	+/–

*Stimuli are from the Western Aphasia Battery.[49]
†A plus or minus is used to record a correct or incorrect response, respectively.
‡Circle: Describe/demonstrate.

I use drawings of the hands from the Benton Finger Localization test[50] to assess finger agnosia (Table 9–6). Before testing, patients should be asked to remove all rings, which might cue them to the identity of a particular finger. Patients can be asked to describe or show an activity that involves the exclusive use of the thumb (hitchhiking), ring finger (wearing a wedding ring), and the index finger (pointing) if they fail otherwise to demonstrate recognition of these fingers. When asking for a description or demonstration, the examiner must be careful not to cue the patient to the target activity; the target activity must be generated spontaneously by the patient. Patients who fail to demonstrate visual recognition of the fingers should be assessed for possible deficits in visual form perception; see Chapter 5 for assessment instruments.

Landmark recognition is assessed in a manner analogous to that for facial recognition (Table 9–7) using pictures of landmarks (Fig. 9–2).

The Tactile Object Recognition Procedure uses stimuli from Forms I and II of the Fuld Object-Memory Evaluation.[51] Vision is occluded throughout the procedure. The objects are felt with either the left or right hand, as indicated in Table 9–8. Recognition is assessed through naming, through verbal multiple-choice options, or through describing or demonstrating object use. The multiple-choice items are also from the Fuld Object-Memory Evaluation, with the exception of the options listed for object 4 (card). In the Fuld Evaluation, a photograph is the first of the multiple-choice

Table 9–4. **VISUAL FORM RECOGNITION PROCEDURE***

VISUAL FORM ("WHAT IS THIS SHAPE CALLED?")		
	Name†	**Multiple-Choice Options**
1. Square	+/−	Triangle Cube Square
2. Triangle	+/−	Square Triangle Circle
3. Circle	+/−	Square Triangle Circle
4. Arrow	+/−	Triangle Arrow Rectangle
5. Cross	+/−	Cross Cube Pyramid
6. Cylinder	+/−	Rectangle Circle Cylinder

*Stimuli are from the Western Aphasia Battery.[49]
†A plus or minus is used to record a correct or incorrect response, respectively.

Table 9–5. **FACIAL RECOGNITION PROCEDURE**

FACES ("WHICH PRESIDENT IS THIS?")			
	Name*	**Describe***	**Multiple-Choice Options**
1. Nixon	+/−	+/−	Reagan Nixon Eisenhower
2. Kennedy	+/−	+/−	Kennedy Ford Roosevelt
3. Carter	+/−	+/−	Coolidge Carter Ford
4. Ford	+/−	+/−	Jackson Johnson Ford
5. Reagan	+/−	+/−	Carter Kennedy Reagan
6. Johnson	+/−	+/−	Johnson Nixon Bush

*A plus or minus is used to record a correct or incorrect response, respectively.

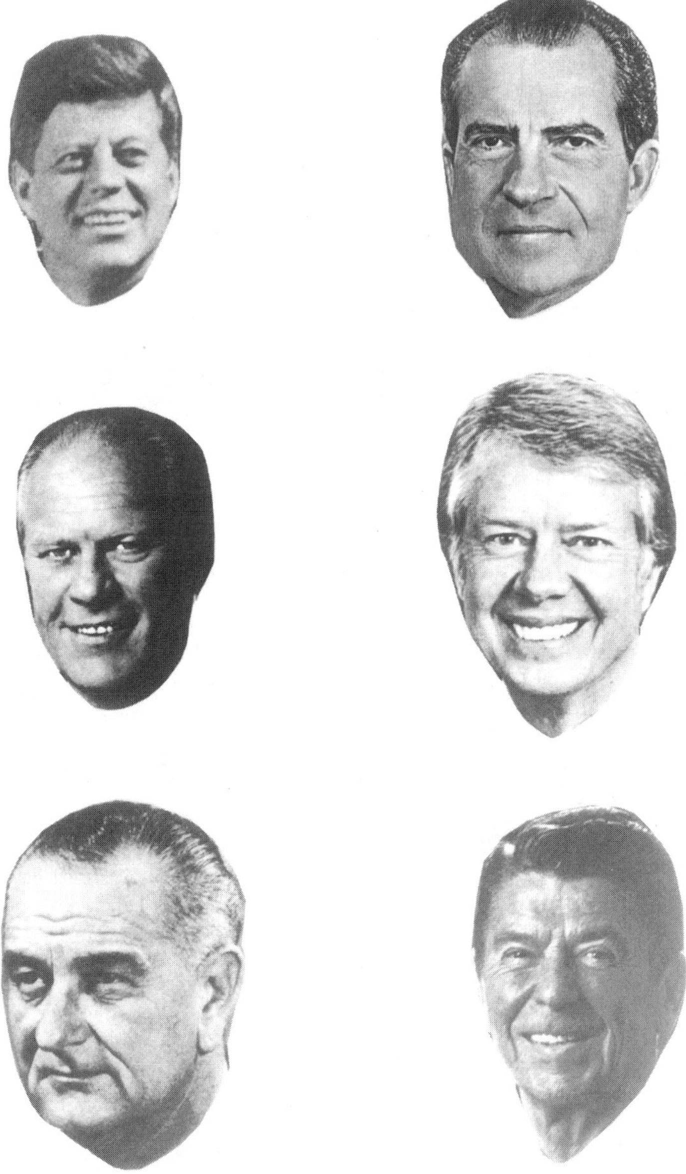

FIGURE 9–1. Facial recognition stimuli. (Adapted from *A Pictorial History of the Presidents of the United States*, LMG Crocker, Hong Kong, 1991, pp. 30–31; and Holland, B: *Hail to the Chiefs*, Ballantine Books, New York, 1990, pp. 241 and 249.)

Table 9–6. **FINGER RECOGNITION PROCEDURE**

FINGERS ("WHICH FINGER IS THIS?")			
	Name*	**Multiple-Choice Options**	**Use*†**
1. Thumb	+/−	Ring Thumb Little	+/−
2. Ring finger	+/−	Index Middle Ring	+/−
3. Index or pointer finger	+/−	Index Little Thumb	+/−
4. Little or baby finger	+/−	Thumb Little Middle	
5. Middle finger	+/−	Middle Index Ring	

*A plus or minus is used to indicate a correct or incorrect response, respectively.
†Circle: Describe/demonstrate.

Table 9–7. **LANDMARK RECOGNITION PROCEDURE**

LANDMARKS ("WHAT FAMOUS PLACE OR THING IS THIS?")			
	Name*	**Describe***	**Multiple-Choice Options**
1. Statue of Liberty	+/−	+/−	Colossus of Rhodes Statue of Athena Statue of Liberty
2. Eiffel Tower	+/−	+/−	Leaning Tower of Pisa Eiffel Tower Tower of London
3. White House	+/−	+/−	White House Buckingham Palace Taj Mahal
4. Sphinx	+/−	+/−	Sphinx King Tut's Tomb Great Pyramid
5. Washington Monument	+/−	+/−	Jefferson Memorial Lincoln Memorial Washington Monument

*A plus or minus is used to record a correct or incorrect response, respectively.

items. In Table 9–8, an envelope is substituted for the photograph because of the difficulty of distinguishing between a card and a photograph by touch alone. Tactile perception deficits can be ruled out using the procedures described in Chapter 5 when patients fail to demonstrate tactile object recognition.

Music recognition is assessed using an audiotape on which the specified bars

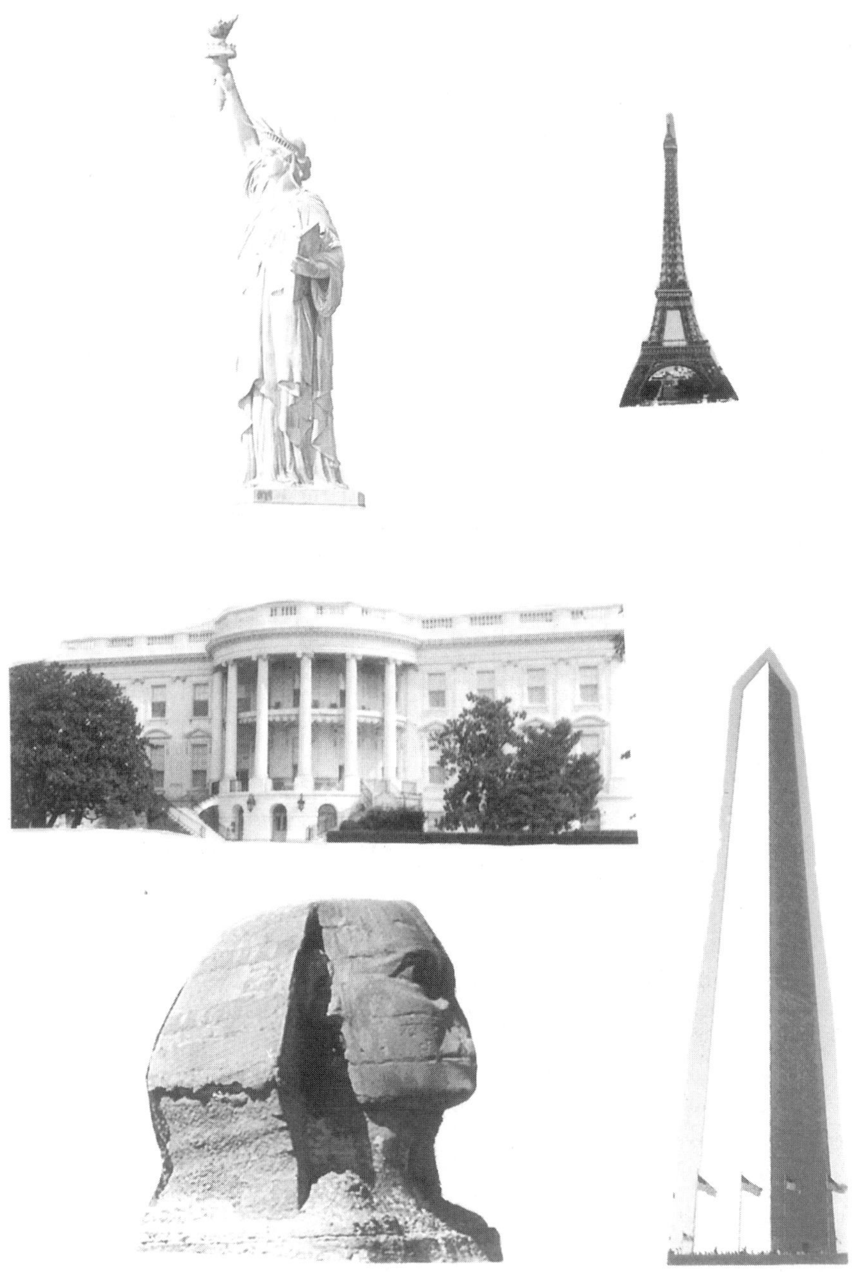

FIGURE 9–2. Landmark recognition stimuli. (Adapted from *Baedeker's New York*, Baedeker, Stuttgart, Germany, 1991, p. 8; Grossman, S: *Essential Paris*, Little, Brown and Company, Boston, 1990, p. 4; *Prince's Color Picture Guide Book of Washington*, Prince Lithograph Co., Fairfax, Virginia, p. 17; *Self-Guided Egypt*, Langenscheidt, New York, 1990, p. 55; and *Washington, DC Souvenier Book*, LB Prince, Fairfax, Virginia, 1992.)

Table 9–8. **TACTILE OBJECT RECOGNITION PROCEDURE***

TACTILE OBJECTS ("WHAT OBJECT DO YOU FEEL?")			
Hand/Object	**Name†**	**Multiple-Choice Options**	**Use†‡**
1. Left/ball	+/−	Stone Block Ball	+/−
2. Right/bottle	+/−	Lightbulb Bottle Box	+/−
3. Right/button	+/−	Coin Buckle Button	+/−
4. Left/card	+/−	Envelope Card Stamp	+/−
5. Left/cup	+/−	Spoon Saucer Cup	+/−
6. Right/key	+/−	Key Can opener Nail file	+/−
7. Right/matches	+/−	Lighter Toothpick Matches	+/−
8. Left/nail	+/−	Nail Screw Pencil	+/−
9. Left/ring	+/−	Bracelet Ring Thimble	+/−
10. Right/scissors	+/−	Scissors Knife Pliers	+/−

*Stimuli are from the Fuld Object-Memory Evaluation.[51]
†A plus or minus is used to record a correct or incorrect response, respectively.
‡Circle: Describe/demonstrate.

of the tunes listed in Table 9–9 are recorded. Recognition can be demonstrated by naming the tune, providing an unmistakable description, or by selecting the correct name from multiple-choice options. A successful description may consist of reciting lyrics from the tune, identifying the subject of the lyrics (e.g., "a Christmas song about riding in a sleigh" for "Jingle Bells"), or identifying a musician associated with the tune (e.g., Louis Armstrong for "When the Saints Come Marching In"). Simply identifying a context in which the tune is likely to be played is insufficient. For example, it is not enough to say that "Jingle Bells" is played at Christmas, or that "On Top of Old Smokey" may be sung around a campfire. Tests for assessing auditory perception deficits are discussed in Chapter 5 and should be employed if music recognition failure occurs.

Table 9–9. **MUSIC RECOGNITION PROCEDURE**

MUSIC ("WHAT TUNE IS THIS?")			
	Name*	**Describe***	**Multiple-Choice Options**
1. Yankee Doodle (bars 1–4)	+/−	+/−	Happy Birthday Yankee Doodle Pop Goes the Weasel
2. When the Saints Come Marching In (bars 5–8)	+/−	+/−	Saints Moonlight in Vermont Long, Long Ago
3. On Top of Old Smokey (bars 1–8)	+/−	+/−	Row, Row, Row Your Boat Little Brown Jug Smokey
4. Jingle Bells (bars 17–20)	+/−	+/−	Jingle Bells Joy to the World We Wish You a Merry Christmas
5. We Shall Overcome (bars 1–4)	+/−	+/−	Amazing Grace We Shall Overcome Rock of Ages
6. Auld Lang Syne (bars 1–5)	+/−	+/−	My Wild Irish Rose Silent Night Auld Lang Syne

*A plus or minus is used to record a correct or incorrect response, respectively.

Clinical experience must guide interpretation of the stimulus recognition procedures, because normative data are not available. Most healthy adults make no more than one error on any section of the procedure, with the exception of landmark identification. Identification of landmarks tends to be the most challenging task, because many of the items are known to people through pictures rather than personal experience. The Eiffel Tower, Washington Monument, and Sphinx are the items least likely to be recognized, and educational level may be a determinant of how well an individual performs on these items. Patients may fail to recognize the White House because many other buildings have similar architectural features, and the absence of context thwarts recognition of the particular building.

The stimulus recognition procedures are recommended for administration and interpretation only by experienced behavioral neurologists and neuropsychologists. The stimulus recognition procedures are most readily administered in office and laboratory settings, although some are not too cumbersome for bedside administration.

Sound Recognition Test

The Sound Recognition Test[52] can be obtained from *Neuropsychology Laboratory, University of Victoria, Victoria, British Columbia, V8W 3P5, Canada.*

This test consists of an audiotape of a variety of environmental sounds, which the patient is asked to identify. Recognition of the sounds may be demonstrated verbally, by naming or describing the object producing the sound, or by selecting multiple-choice options in the form of printed names or pictures. The Sound Recognition Test is available in two alternate forms, which correlate .68 to .79 across adult samples.[53] Norms are based on 79 non-brain-damaged adults. The validity of the test has been recently reviewed.[53]

The Sound Recognition Test is the only commercially available test of auditory object agnosia with known reliability and validity and a normative database. It provides a thorough assessment of auditory object agnosia and incorporates multiple formats for demonstrating recognition. It does not include a sound-matching component, and examiners must rule out auditory discrimination deficits in patients who perform poorly on the Sound Recognition Test. The test is most appropriate for office and laboratory administration because of the sound equipment required. The test can be administered and interpreted by experienced neurologists, neuropsychologists, and speech pathologists.

Halstead-Reitan Battery Sensory Perceptual Examination, Astereognosis Subtest

The Halstead-Reitan Battery (HRB) Sensory Perceptual Examination (SPE), Astereognosis Subtest, can be obtained from *Reitan Neuropsychological Laboratory, 1338 East Edison Street, Tucson, AZ 85719.*

The HRB-SPE Astereognosis Subtest requires patients to identify by touch a penny, a nickel, and a dime. Unilateral and simultaneous bilateral trials are included, and the patient is asked to give a verbal response.

The Astereognosis Subtest is omitted from some versions of the SPE (see Chaps. 4 and 5 for further discussion of the SPE subtests), and thorough investigation of its reliability and validity is lacking. The Astereognosis Subtest fails to provide an adequate assessment of tactile object recognition in that successful performance on the subtest is highly dependent on tactile sensory perception (even normal persons may have difficulty in distinguishing a penny and dime by touch), and all avenues for demonstrating recognition of the coins are not incorporated. In addition, limiting the stimuli to members of one class of objects may not fully capture the scope of a patient's recognition deficit.

The Astereognosis Subtest requires no special equipment or materials other than two sets of coins. It can be administered at bedside, in the office, or in the laboratory and can be interpreted by experienced neurologists and neuropsychologists. Specific training in administering the HRB is also advisable. Incorporation of other tests of tactile recognition, exploration of all avenues for demonstrating recognition of tactile objects, and assessment of tactile sensory loss are essential before attempting an interpretation of results of the Astereognosis Subtest.

Boston Spatial-Quantitative Battery, Finger Agnosia Subtest

See discussion of the Boston Spatial-Quantitative Battery (BSQB), Finger Agnosia Subtest, in Chapter 8.

NEUROPSYCHOLOGICAL TREATMENT

No systematic treatment approaches have been developed for the associative agnosias, perhaps because of their rarity. Some basis for treatment can be obtained from what is known about the relative strengths and weaknesses of agnosics. Because agnosia is often confined to one sensory modality, encouraging multisensory exploration of stimuli may facilitate recognition. The context in which stimuli appear also aids recognition. Thus, an object that is not initially recognized may be recognized after the patient considers the situation in which the object appears. For example, noting that an object is hanging over the bathroom sink next to several similar objects may cue the patient's realization that he or she is looking at a toothbrush.

Patients with prosopagnosia may recognize people based on specific physical details or mannerisms. Astereognosis patients may determine what an object is after noting the object's individual properties. Encouraging patients to mentally note the individual qualities of stimuli, whether they are faces or objects, may aid in their ability to identify the object.

Compensatory strategies may facilitate independent travel in patients with topographical agnosia. These strategies include providing a written set of directions with landmarks described rather than simply named or providing a map with detailed photographs that the patient can match to what he or she sees in the environment. The patient is most likely to be successful in learning short routes that are habitually traveled rather than long or highly varying routes.

It is hoped that in the future researchers will address not only the mechanisms underlying the associative agnosias, but also the efficacy of various treatment approaches. Although the scarcity of agnosic patients precludes large-scale treatment-outcome research, much can be gleaned from investigation of treatment effects in single subjects, provided that care is taken to establish pretreatment baseline values to which post-treatment stimulus recognition can be compared. The disability suffered by individual agnosics certainly justifies attention to treatment issues, even if the incidence of agnosia is low.

CASE ILLUSTRATIONS

CASE 9–1

R.A. was a 68-year-old man with a high-school education who worked as a cashier to earn money to supplement his Social Security retirement income. He suffered an embolic left-hemisphere cerebrovascular accident; his computed tomographic (CT) scans showed an infarction in the left posterior temporal-parietal area. Neurological and neuropsychological examinations revealed normal strength, speed, and coordination of movements in both upper extremities; no difficulty executing skilled movements of the hands; and a right visual-field cut.

R.A.'s speech consisted of fluent, neologistic jargon; he was unable to repeat phrases accurately; his comprehension of speech was severely impaired; but his comprehension of written language was preserved for individual words and phrases of moderate length. This pattern of language performance is consistent with pure word deafness (see Chap. 12). The patient's writing also consisted of jargon words. His written calculations were incorrect as a result of a failure to interpret arithmetic signs correctly (see Alexic acalculia). The patient's ability to distinguish right from left was assessed using written commands and revealed significant confusion of the right and left sides of his body and of the examiner's body.

R.A. correctly identified, by wiggling, fingers touched by the examiner while his vision was occluded. He was, however, unable to match fingers to their correct written names, making five errors in five trials. Similarly, when shown a finger and asked to indicate by head gestures whether it was, for example, a thumb or index finger (the patient was given two choices for each finger, with choices both spoken and written), he responded correctly on only 6 trials in 10. When he was asked in written format to show how the thumb and index fingers could be used, he failed to produce any response. When asked specifically to point and to pretend to hitchhike, R.A. had no difficulty. He was able to match without error fingers shown to him by the examiner with fingers drawn on a diagram.

Similar procedures were used to assess R.A.'s ability to point to body locations (excluding the fingers) corresponding to written words, to match pictures of objects with their written names, and to match the faces of United States presidents with their written names. The patient made no errors on any of these tasks, with the exception of misidentifying one object.

DISCUSSION

The patient in Case 9–1 presented with finger agnosia. Assessment was complicated by his language impairment, but the sparing of reading ability provided a means of assessing his recognition ability. The striking dissociation between the patient's recognition of fingers and other body parts lends further support to the diagnosis of finger agnosia. It is also notable that the patient has impaired writing, calculation, and right-left disorientation. Thus, the patient showed the complex of neuropsychological disorders that comprise Gerstmann's syndrome.

CASE 9–2

E.M. was a 74-year-old widow who had completed high school and worked as a homemaker. She suffered a left-hemisphere cerebrovascular accident; CT and magnetic resonance imaging (MRI) scans revealed left frontal and parietal infarctions and lacunar infarcts in the basal ganglia. Her history was positive for renal insufficiency, anemia, and a myocardial infarction 3 years ago. Her initial neurological examination revealed right hemiparesis, buccofacial apraxia (see Chap. 11), and global aphasia (see Chap. 12).

By the time of E.M.'s neuropsychological examination, her aphasia had recovered to the point that she was able to comprehend two-step commands and say some automatic phrases. Using a multiple-choice format, the patient identified via head gestures the names of objects, colors, and familiar faces. No errors were made on any trial, with the exception of her misidentifying one object. She also was able to trace with her finger the nonverbal items of Ishihara's plates (see Ishihara's Test for Color Blindness). A multiple-choice format, in which the patient indicated the correct color name through head gestures when spoken by the examiner, was also used to assess her ability to identify colors associated with objects. No correct responses were obtained in eight trials. Performance improved marginally (two correct responses in eight trials) when the task was repeated while the patient responded by pointing to the color associated with each object.

DISCUSSION

The patient in Case 9–2 showed color agnosia with other forms of stimulus recognition preserved. This is the only unambiguous case of color agnosia I have encountered.

CASE 9–3

C.C. was a 61-year-old man who had an 11th-grade education and worked as a decorator until he suffered a cardiac arrest with cerebral anoxia. Neurological examination revealed a severe global anterograde amnesia (see Chap. 16) but was otherwise normal. Neuropsychological examination was performed to assess subtle aspects of cognition. Testing revealed full visual fields and no significant deficits in any aspect of elementary or skilled movement, including strength, initiation, perseverance, and coordination, in either upper extremity. C.C. showed no evidence of aphasia (see Chap. 12) and was able to comprehend commands, repeat phrases, and express his ideas in fluent, grammatical sentences. There was also no evidence of stimulus neglect (see Chap. 4) in his line bisection or response to unilateral and bilateral simultaneous stimulation in the visual, auditory, and tactile modalities. Performance on the Benton Facial Recognition Test and Benton Visual Recognition Test was within normal limits.

C.C. accurately perceived colors and could identify the colors associated with common objects. Similarly, he had no difficulty in identifying environmental sounds or familiar melodies.

Nursing staff members noted that C.C. had mistaken the identity of family members during visits. The patient was shown a series of faces and asked to name them. He had no idea who the people were. He was then told that they were faces of United States presidents. He then proceeded to guess the names of each one, but made no correct responses (e.g., Kennedy was identified as Roosevelt, Nixon was identified as Carter). When asked to tell the examiner about each president, his responses were accurate for the person he thought each picture represented, but because he was wrong in his recognition of the faces, the information he provided was also inappropriate for the person. C.C. was then asked to point to the president named by the examiner, which resulted in two correct responses in six trials. He was then asked a series of questions about the presidents (e.g., "Which recent president was assassinated?") and correctly named each of the last six presidents in response to these questions.

Analogous assessment procedures were performed with drawings of famous landmarks. C.C.'s performance was as poor for landmarks as it was for faces. He could, however, recognize actual landmarks such as his room, the hospital cafeteria, and the nursing station.

C.C. identified real objects and furniture without error, but could not identify any drawings of objects or geometric forms from the Visual Object and Visual Form Recognition Procedures. These items were readministered, and the patient was required only to point to the pictures named by the examiner. Under this condition, he correctly identified only one of six objects and two of six forms. He was unable to describe or demonstrate the correct use of any of the objects that he misidentified. Matching of objects and forms was not impaired.

The Tactual Object Recognition Procedure was administered. C.C. correctly identified by touch only 3 of 10 objects. He named the other objects incorrectly and failed to describe or demonstrate their use. Providing multiple-choice options failed to improve his performance. Tactual matching was preserved. When shown the objects immediately after palpating them, the patient was still unable to identify them, and in one case misidentified an object he had just correctly named while holding it. When he was allowed to both see and hold the objects, he was able to demonstrate their use.

DISCUSSION

The patient in Case 9–3 showed the greatest range of recognition deficits. He met criteria for prosopagnosia, visual object agnosia, astereognosis, and topographical agnosia. This patient had greater difficulty in recognizing drawings of objects and landmarks than he did in recognizing actual landmarks. The cues provided by context probably greatly helped his performance. His recognition of actual objects deteriorated when he was required to palpate the objects before seeing them. It is possible that his visual recognition system could not cope with the erroneous associations triggered by palpating the objects. The patient's recognition was most accurate when he simultaneously held and viewed objects; the multisensory input apparently facilitated his recognition performance.

REFERENCES

1. American Psychiatric Association: Diagnostic and Statistical Manual of Mental Disorders, Fourth Edition. American Psychiatric Association, Washington, DC, 1994.
2. The International Classification of Diseases, Ninth Revision, Clinical Modification. Med-Index Publications, Salt Lake City, 1991.
3. DeVreese, LP: Two systems for colour-naming defects: Verbal disconnection vs colour imagery disorder. Neuropsychologia 29:1, 1991.
4. Dumont, I, et al: About a case of visual agnosia with prosopagnosia and colour agnosia. Acta Psychiatr Belg 81:25, 1981.
5. Sergent, J, and Signoret, JL: Functional and anatomical decomposition of face processing: Evidence

from prosopagnosia and PET study of normal subjects. Philosophical Transactions of the Royal Society of London, Series B: Biological Sciences 335:55, 1992.
6. DeHaan, EH, Young, AW, and Newcombe, F: Covert and overt recognition in prosopagnosia. Brain 114:2575, 1991.
7. Tyrrell, PJ, et al: Progressive degeneration of the right temporal lobe studied with positron emission tomography. J Neurol Neurosurg Psychiatry 53:1046, 1990.
8. Campbell, R, et al: Sensitivity to eye gaze in prosopagnosic patients and monkeys with superior temporal sulcus ablation. Neuropsychologia 28:1123, 1990.
9. Sergent, J, and Poncet, M: From covert to overt recognition of faces in a prosopagnosic patient. Brain 113:989, 1990.
10. Renault, B, et al: Brain potentials reveal covert facial recognition in prosopagnosia. Neuropsychologia 27:905, 1989.
11. Levine, DN, and Calvanio, R: Prosopagnosia: A defect in visual configural processing. Brain Cogn 10:149, 1989.
12. Landis, T, et al: Prosopagnosia and agnosia for noncanonical views. An autopsied case. Brain 111:1287, 1988.
13. Bauer, RM, and Verfaellie, M: Electrodermal discrimination of familiar but not unfamiliar faces in prosopagnosia. Brain Cogn 8:240, 1988.
14. DeRenzi, E, et al: Apperceptive and associative forms of prosopagnosia. Cortex 27:213, 1991.
15. Landis, T, et al: Are unilateral right posterior cerebral lesions sufficient to cause prosopagnosia? Clinical and radiological findings in six additional patients. Cortex 22:243, 1986.
16. Campbell, R, Landis, T, and Regard, M: Face recognition and lipreading. A neurological dissociation. Brain 109:509, 1986.
17. Trobe, JR, and Bauer, RM: Seeing but not recognizing. Surv Ophthalmol 30:328, 1986.
18. Landis, T, et al: Loss of topographic familiarity. An environmental agnosia. Arch Neurol 43:132, 1986.
19. Sparr, SA, et al: A historic case of visual agnosia revisited after 40 years. Brain 114:789, 1991.
20. Benton, A: Facial recognition 1990. Cortex 26:491, 1990.
21. Kawahata, N, and Nagata, K: A case of associative visual agnosia: Neuropsychological findings and theoretical considerations. J Clin Exp Neuropsychol 11:645, 1989.
22. Gomori, AJ, and Hawryluk, GA: Visual agnosia without alexia. Neurology 34:947, 1984.
23. Albert, ML, et al: The anatomic basis of visual agnosia. Neurology 29:876, 1979.
24. Mack, JL, and Boller, F: Associative visual agnosia and its related deficits: The role of the minor hemisphere in assigning meaning to visual perceptions. Neuropsychologia 15:345, 1977.
25. Benson, DF, Segarra, J, and Albert, M: Visual agnosia–prosopagnosia. Arch Neurol 30:307, 1974.
26. Hecaen, H, et al: A new case of object agnosia. A deficit in association or categorization specific for the visual modality. Neuropsychologia 12:447, 1974.
27. Cipolotti, L, Butterworth, B, and Denes, G: A specific deficit for numbers in a case of dense acalculia. Brain 114:2619, 1991.
28. Moore, MR, et al: Right parietal stroke with Gerstmann's syndrome. Appearance on computed tomography, magnetic resonance imaging, and single-photon emission computed tomography. Arch Neurol 48:432, 1991.
29. Matsuoka, H, et al: Impairment of parietal cortical functions associated with episodic prolonged spike-and-wave discharges. Epilepsia 27:432, 1986.
30. Roeltgen, DP, Sevush, S, and Heilman, KM: Pure Gerstmann's syndrome from a focal lesion. Arch Neurol 40:46, 1983.
31. Caselli, RJ: Rediscovering tactile agnosia. Mayo Clin Proc 66:129, 1991.
32. Mauguiere, F, Desmedt, JE, and Courjon, J: Astereognosis and dissociated loss of frontal or parietal components of somatosensory evoked potentials in hemispheric lesions. Detailed correlations with clinical signs and computerized tomographic scanning. Brain 106:271, 1983.
33. Bruyer, R, et al: Pure bilateral agraphia, right astereognosia and arithmetic defects associated with a left parietal tumor. Acta Neurol Belg 78:193, 1978.
34. Endtz, LJ, and Frenay, JJ: Studies on astereognosis and amyotrophy of the hand in brainstem syndromes. Relation to the symptomatology of tumours at the spinocranial junction. J Neurol Sci 44:241, 1980.
35. Feinsod, M, et al: Brainstem tumor presenting with unilateral astereognosis. Ann Neurol 8:191, 1980.
36. Weidenfeld, J, Finkelstein, Y, and Bental, E: Astereognosis as a presenting symptom in cervical meningioma. Acta Neurochir 90:67, 1988.
37. Lesoin, F, et al: Astereognosis and amyotrophy of the hand with neurinoma of the second cervical nerve root. J Neurol 233:57, 1986.

38. Frenay, JJ, Groen, JJ, and Endtz, LJ: Tumours at the spinocranial junction: Some clinical and electromyographic aspects in relation to the symptomatology. Clin Neurol Neurosurg 81:13, 1979.
39. Halpern, L: Astereognosis not of cortical origin. J Neurol Sci 7:245, 1968.
40. Kazui, S, et al: Subcortical auditory agnosia. Brain Lang 38:476, 1990.
41. Buchtel, HA, and Stewart, JD: Auditory agnosia: Apperceptive or associative disorder? Brain Lang 37:12, 1989.
42. Ho, KJ, et al: Neurologic, audiologic, and electrophysiologic sequelae of bilateral temporal lobe lesions. Arch Neurol 44:982, 1987.
43. Marshall, RC, Rappaport, BZ, and Garcia-Bunuel, L: Self-monitoring behavior in a case of severe auditory agnosia with aphasia. Brain Lang 24:297, 1985.
44. Rosati, G, et al: Clinical and audiological findings in a case of auditory agnosia. J Neurol 227:21, 1982.
45. Spreen, O, Benton, AL, and Fincham, RW: Auditory agnosia without aphasia. Arch Neurol 13:84, 1965.
46. Motomura, N, et al: Auditory agnosia. Analysis of a case with bilateral subcortical lesions. Brain 109:379, 1986.
47. Lambert, J, et al: Auditory agnosia with relative sparing of speech perception. Cortex 25:71, 1989.
48. Aimard, G, et al: Spatial disorientation. Report of 5 cases. Rev Neurol 137:97, 1981.
49. Kertesz, A: The Western Aphasia Battery Test Manual. Grune and Stratton, Orlando, FL, 1982.
50. Benton, AL, et al: Contributions to Neuropsychological Assessment. A Clinical Manual. Oxford University Press, New York, 1983.
51. Fuld, PA: Fuld Object-Memory Evaluation. Instruction Manual. Stoelting Company, Chicago, IL, 1977.
52. Spreen, O, and Benton, AL: A sound recognition test for clinical use, 1963. Cited in Spreen, O, and Strauss, E: A Compendium of Neuropsychological Tests. Administration, Norms, and Commentary. Oxford University Press, New York, 1991.
53. Spreen, O, and Strauss, E: A Compendium of Neuropsychological Tests. Administration, Norms, and Commentary. Oxford University Press, New York, 1991.

DISORDERS OF INTERHEMISPHERIC TRANSFER

10

The disorders of interhemispheric transfer involve a failure of information transfer from one cerebral hemisphere to the other as a result of damage to the pathways connecting the hemispheres. These pathways, collectively called the "cerebral commissures," consist of the massive corpus callosum, the anterior commissure, the hippocampal commissure, and the massa intermedia. The 10 subtypes of interhemispheric transfer disorders are listed under "Variety of Presentation" in the chapter outline. Many of these disorders consist of unilateral presentations of disorders discussed elsewhere in this book. For example, unilateral anomia is a unilateral presentation of anomic aphasia (see Chap. 12) that arises when the hemisphere that is nondominant for language loses access to contralateral language-processing areas.

Unilateral anomia is readily demonstrated in the visual and olfactory modalities; unilateral naming deficits are not expected in these sensory modalities in patients who lack callosal lesions. Unfortunately, this is not the case in the tactual modality. Tactual object recognition deficits (see Astereognosis) are often unilateral in presentation and arise in patients who do not have callosal lesions. The clinician may not always succeed in ruling out astereognosis in patients with callosal lesions who are suspected of having unilateral tactile anomia unless some means can be found for the patient to demonstrate recognition of the stimulus that he or she cannot name. Careful observation of the way in which a patient handles objects may aid in differentiating unilateral tactile anomia from astereognosis. Patients with the latter handle objects in an awkward, stereotyped manner that is not evident in those with unilateral tactile anomia.

In *pseudoneglect,* the deficit (i.e., failure to acknowledge stimuli present in a part of space) also occurs unilaterally, but the side of space that is ignored differs according to the type of response required. When verbal responses are required, stimuli ipsilateral to the language-dominant hemisphere appear to be neglected. When the right hand responds, the left side of space is ignored; the converse occurs somewhat less frequently when the left hand responds. Pseudoneglect has also been reported in normal persons during tasks such as tactile line bisection when performed using only one hand in the opposite side of space (e.g., when the right hand bisects a line in left hemispace, it tends to bisect slightly to the right of true center).[1] Consequently, this normal degree of perceptual inaccuracy must be ruled out when attempting to diagnose pseudoneglect in patients with callosal lesions.

In *diagonistic apraxia,* the patient's hands conflict with each other. For example, one hand may turn on a light while the other reaches to turn it off. In some cases, the two hands physically struggle with each other (e.g., one hand reaching to perform a task, while the other grasps it to restrain it). In milder cases, the patient simply verbalizes the feeling of having lost control over one hand. Diagonistic apraxia arises in patients with commissural lesions because the two hemispheres appear to form separate behavioral intentions that are not shared and integrated.

Finally, the disorder referred to in this text as *somesthetic disconnection* arises when patients with commissural lesions are unable to compare sensory information presented to the two sides of the body. Failure to locate stimuli to one side of the body with the contralateral hand and failure to replicate passively assumed hand postures with the contralateral hand are included under somesthetic disconnection.

In formulating the clinical indicators for the disorders of interhemispheric transfer, the left hemisphere was assumed to be dominant for language and for the ability to voluntarily perform skilled movement (praxis). Left-hemisphere dominance for language means that the left hemisphere is more adept at processing verbal information and is the primary location for storage of linguistic skills. Similarly, left-hemisphere dominance for praxis means that the left hemisphere is the primary location for storage of previously learned motor skills (i.e., "motor engrams" or "motor memories"). This is not meant to imply that the right hemisphere does not participate in language and praxis, but the right hemisphere is less adept at these activities in most people.

The pattern of right- and left-sided symptoms following callosal section is reversed for the few people who are right-hemisphere–dominant for language and praxis. The symptom pattern following commissural lesions is less predictable for the small percentage of people who have mixed dominance (e.g., left-hemisphere dominance for language and right-hemisphere dominance for praxis) or weak lateralization (e.g., both hemispheres appear approximately equal in their ability to mediate language, praxis, or both). Tests for determining handedness and degree of lateralization are in Chapter 11.

NOMENCLATURE

Only the nonspecific diagnoses "Cognitive Disorder Not Otherwise Specified" and "Mild Neurocognitive Disorder" are available in DSM-IV[2] for coding interhemispheric transfer disorders. In ICD-9-CM,[3] unilateral anomia can be coded with anomia under the label "Other Symbolic Dysfunction." Pseudoneglect can be coded as "Psychophysical Visual Disturbance" if the patient presents with primarily visual symptoms. Unilateral verbal dichotic suppression may be coded under the ICD-9-CM diagnosis "Abnormal Auditory Perception, Unspecified."

A variety of neuropsychological disorders are clustered in ICD-9-CM under the label "Other Symbolic Dysfunction"; these include alexia, agraphia, and apraxia. It is reasonable to use the same generic label to code the unilateral presentations of these disorders that result from callosal lesions. "Other Symbolic Dysfunction" can also be used for diagonistic apraxia. No specific code exists in ICD-9-CM for constructional disability. This disorder sometimes is referred to as "constructional apraxia" in the neurology literature. Although debate continues about whether constructional disability is an apraxia, no other coding is available in ICD-9-CM; therefore the label "Other Symbolic Dysfunction" must suffice.

Coding somesthetic disconnection presents a particular problem. In ICD-9-CM, the label "Disturbance of Skin Sensation" is used to code tactile discrimination and localization deficits, whereas the failure to recognize palpated objects (astereognosis) is listed under the highly generic label "Other General Symptoms," which includes such diverse conditions as retrograde amnesia, generalized pain, and chills. This label is far too generic for use in neuropsychological diagnostic coding. "Disturbance of Skin Sensation," although not an ideal label, comes closer to capturing the essence of somesthetic disconnection.

RULES FOR DIAGNOSIS

Clinical Indicators: Each is independent (only one must be observed for the disorder to be suspected) *except* when subscripting is used. Subscripted numbers (a_1, a_2) denote an indicator with multiple parts that must be considered together.
Associated Features: These are listed to give a more complete picture of the disorders. The presence or absence of these features does not affect the diagnosis.
Factors to Rule Out: All must be taken into account. Failure to rule out even one of these factors makes a firm diagnosis impossible.
Lesion Locations: Each location stands alone; damage in only one of the listed areas is sufficient to produce the disorder.

VARIETY OF PRESENTATION

1. Unilateral anomia* (see also Astereognosis)

Clinical Indicators

a_1. Inaccurate naming of object pictures exposed for a maximum of 200 msec in the left visual half-field (LVF) while the eyes are held at a central fixation point

a_2. Relatively accurate naming of object pictures similarly presented in the right visual half-field (RVF)

a_3. An object not named when presented in an LVF trial, selected from a set of foils by the left hand using pointing or some other nonverbal response; this nonverbal multiple-choice trial to immediately follow the LVF naming trial
NOTE: This phenomenon is termed unilateral visual anomia.

b_1. Inability to name colors presented in the LVF with the eyes held at central fixation

b_2. Relatively preserved naming of colors presented to the RVF
NOTE: This phenomenon is termed unilateral color anomia.

c_1. Inaccurate naming of odors presented to the right nostril with vision occluded†

c_2. Relatively accurate naming of odors presented to the left nostril
NOTE: This phenomenon is termed unilateral verbal anosmia or unilateral olfactory anomia.

---

*The left hemisphere is presumed to be dominant for language, and the patient is presumed to be right-handed. The pattern of left- and right-sided indicators is reversed in left-handed patients with right-hemisphere language dominance. Patients with other dominance patterns have less predictable clinical findings.

†The right nostril projects to the right hemisphere, and the left nostril projects to the left hemisphere.

d_1. Inaccurate naming of objects presented to the left hand with vision occluded

d_2. Relatively accurate naming of objects presented to the right hand
NOTE: This phenomenon is termed unilateral tactile anomia.

Associated Features

a. Possibility that vague verbal descriptions may be given for unnamed stimuli
b. Slowness in initiating and performing movements (see Akinesia) in patients with unilateral olfactory anomia
c. Relatively preserved palpation and manipulation of objects that cannot be named by patients showing unilateral tactile anomia
d. Recent history (following onset of brain damage) of absent speech or other attempts at vocal communication (see Mutism)
e. Presence of other interhemispheric transfer disorders

Factors to Rule Out

a. Loss of sensation in the sensory modality in which unilateral anomia is suspected.
b. Inability to recognize and assign meaning to tactual objects (see Astereognosis) presented to the left hand in cases of suspected unilateral tactile anomia. Preserved recognition may be demonstrated by obtaining a verbal description or manual demonstration of how the object would be used.

Lesion Locations

For unilateral visual anomia

a. Middle to posterior half of the body of the corpus callosum and often including a portion of the splenium[4–6]

For unilateral color anomia

a. Combined corpus callosum (splenium) and combined right occipital and right medial temporal lobes, including the hippocampal gyrus, with extension into the precuneus and cingulate gyrus[7]

For unilateral verbal anosmia

a. Combined corpus callosum and anterior commissure transection[8,9]

For unilateral tactile anomia

a. Middle to posterior half of the body of the corpus callosum with occasional involvement of the splenium[4–6,10–12]

2. Pseudoneglect*

Clinical Indicators

a_1. Failure to consistently signal the presence of left-sided stimuli when allowed to use only the right hand or a verbal response for signaling

a_2. Relatively preserved signaling of the presence of left-sided stimuli when allowed to use the left hand for signaling

*The left hemisphere is presumed to be dominant for language, and the patient is presumed to be right-handed. The pattern of left- and right-sided indicators is reversed in left-handed patients with right-hemisphere language dominance. Patients with other dominance patterns have less predictable clinical findings.

- a_3. Possibility that deficit may occur in only one sensory modality or in several sensory modalities simultaneously
- b_1. Failure to consistently signal the presence of right-sided stimuli when allowed to use only the left hand for signaling
- b_2. Relatively preserved signaling of the presence of right-sided stimuli when allowed to use the right hand or a verbal response for signaling
- b_3. Possibility that deficit may occur in only one sensory modality or in several sensory modalities simultaneously
- c_1. Failure to completely explore or draw the left sides of objects or other stimuli when using the right hand
- c_2. Relatively preserved exploration or drawing of the left sides of objects or other stimuli when using the left hand
- c_3. Deficit accentuated or may appear only when the right hand must perform in the left side of space
- d_1. Failure to completely explore or draw the right sides of objects or other stimuli when using the left hand
- d_2. Relatively preserved exploration or drawing of the right sides of objects or other stimuli when using the right hand
- d_3. Deficit accentuated or may appear only when the left hand must perform in the right side of space

Associated Features

a. Slowness in initiating and performing movements (see Akinesia)
b. Recent history (following onset of brain damage) of absent speech or other attempts at vocal communication (see Mutism)
c. Presence of other interhemispheric transfer disorders

Factors to Rule Out

a. Sensory loss sufficient to account for the deficit in any sensory modality in which pseudoneglect is suspected, ruled out by demonstrating that the deficit is no longer present when the response mode is changed
b. Loss of strength or coordination in the responding hand or arm, ruled out by demonstrating that the deficit occurs only when responding to stimuli on one side
c. In patients who show indicators c_1 and c_2, a normal degree of perceptual inaccuracy when performing visual or tactual tasks with the right hand in the left side of space
d. In patients who show indicators d_1 and d_2, a normal degree of perceptual inaccuracy when performing visual or tactual tasks with the left hand in the right side of space

Lesion Locations

a. Body of the corpus callosum, alone in a minority of cases but in conjunction with medial frontal, medial temporal and occipital, basal ganglia, thalamic, pontine, or more extensive callosal lesions in the majority of cases[13–18]

3. **Unilateral verbal dichotic extinction (see Sensory extinction)**

4. **Unilateral constructional disability***

Clinical Indicators

a_1. Inaccuracy in making a drawing of a model when using the right hand as indicated by any of the following signs:

1) The drawing is a simplified version of the model with individual parts or details omitted.
2) The individual parts of the drawing are misaligned or otherwise incorrectly placed relative to each other.
3) The proportionate sizes of the parts of the drawing do not match the corresponding parts of the model.
4) The three-dimensional perspective present in a model is lost in the drawing.
5) Part or all of the drawing is rotated so its orientation on the page no longer matches that of the model.

a_2. Relatively preserved ability to make a drawing of a model using the left hand

a_3. Preserved ability to detect and point out error or inaccuracy in the drawing done with the right hand

a_4. Inability to produce a substantially better drawing with the right hand despite awareness of the inaccuracy of the original attempted drawing

b_1. Inaccuracy in constructing a three-dimensional representation of a model with the right hand as evidenced by any of the following signs:

1) The construction is a simplified version of the model with individual parts omitted.
2) The individual parts of the construction are misaligned or otherwise incorrectly placed relative to each other.
3) The overall spatial configuration or design of the model is lost in the attempted construction so that it no longer resembles the model in its overall shape.
4) Part or all of the construction is rotated so that its orientation on the table top no longer matches that of the model.

b_2. Relatively preserved ability to make a construction of a two- or three-dimensional model using the left hand

b_3. Preserved ability to detect and point out error or inaccuracy in the construction done with the right hand

b_4. Inability to produce a substantially better construction with the right hand despite awareness of the inaccuracy of the original attempted construction

*The left hemisphere is presumed to be dominant for language, and the patient is presumed to be right-handed. The pattern of left- and right-sided indicators is reversed in left-handed patients with right-hemisphere language dominance. Patients with other dominance patterns have less predictable clinical findings.

Associated Features

a. Possibility that drawings and constructions done by the left hand may contain misaligned or incorrectly placed parts despite their relative preservation compared to right-hand drawings and constructions
b. Presence of other interhemispheric transfer disorders

Factors to Rule Out

a. Loss of visual acuity in both eyes sufficient to prevent a model from being seen
b. Visual stimulus imperception (see Chap. 5) so severe that it prevents accurate perception of the model, ruled out by demonstrating preserved ability to detect and point out errors in the attempted drawing or construction
c. Spatial imperception (see Chap. 6) so severe that it prevents accurate perception of the model, ruled out by demonstrating preserved ability to detect and point out errors in the attempted drawing or construction
d. Weakness of the muscles of the right arm or hand sufficient to prevent drawing or construction
e. Impaired coordination of the muscles of the right arm or hand sufficient to prevent drawing or construction
f. Impaired ability to initiate right arm or hand movements (see Akinesia)
g. Impaired ability to persist with ongoing right arm or hand movements (see Motor impersistence)
h. Impaired ability to perform skilled movements on demand (see Ideomotor apraxia)
i. Impaired ability to terminate ongoing movements (see Motor perseveration)

Lesion Locations

a. Middle to posterior trunk of the corpus callosum[4–6,10–12]

5. Unilateral alexia (also called hemialexia)*

Clinical Indicators

a_1. Inaccurate reading of words exposed for a maximum of 200 msec in the LVF
a_2. Relatively accurate reading of words similarly presented in the RVF
a_3. An object associated with a word not read in the LVF successfully retrieved or pointed to by the left hand

Associated Features

a. Performance in the LVF possibly better for words that have strong emotional connotations (e.g., "rape," "maim," "joy")
b. Presence of other interhemispheric transfer disorders

---

*The left hemisphere is presumed to be dominant for language, and the patient is presumed to be right-handed. The pattern of left- and right-sided indicators is reversed in left-handed patients with right-hemisphere language dominance. Patients with other dominance patterns have less predictable clinical findings.

Factors to Rule Out

a. Presence of homonymous hemianopsia: loss of acuity in one visual half-field
b. Failure to detect stimuli on one side of space (see Stimulus neglect)
c. Normal RVF superiority for reading briefly exposed words as a result of left-hemisphere language dominance, ruled out by demonstrating successful retrieval of objects associated with the words using the left hand

Lesion Locations

a. Splenium of the corpus callosum, sometimes in conjunction with posterior part of trunk[6,19]
b. Medial, inferior occipital lobe, including underlying white matter[20]

6. Unilateral agraphia (also called hemiagraphia)*

Clinical Indicators

a_1. A decline in the ability to write with the left hand in response to dictation or a stimulus (e.g., a picture that the patient is asked to describe in a sentence or paragraph) as evidenced by any of the following errors:
  1) Horizontal or vertical rotations of letters
  2) Poorly formed letters that may progress to the point of unrecognizable scrawling
  3) Omission of letters or words
  4) Incorrect selection of letters (misspelling) during writing

a_2. Relatively preserved writing with the right hand

Associated Features

a. Relatively preserved copying of letters with the left hand
b. Spelling with the use of cut-out letters (i.e., anagram letters) that improves left-hand performance in some but not all patients
c. Presence of other interhemispheric transfer disorders, particularly unilateral apraxia
d. Relatively preserved oral spelling
e. Relatively preserved reading when no limits are placed on the length of word exposure or location of words in the visual field

Factors to Rule Out

a. Weakness of the muscles of the left arm or hand sufficient to account for the writing deficit
b. Impaired coordination of the muscles of the left arm or hand sufficient to account for the writing deficit
c. Impaired ability to initiate left arm or hand movements (see Akinesia) sufficient to account for the writing deficit

*The left hemisphere is presumed to be dominant for language, and the patient is presumed to be right-handed. The pattern of left- and right-sided indicators is reversed in left-handed patients with right-hemisphere language dominance. Patients with other dominance patterns have less predictable clinical findings.

d. Impaired ability to persist with ongoing left arm or hand movements (see Motor impersistence) sufficient to account for the writing deficit
e. Impaired ability to perform skilled movements on demand (see Ideomotor apraxia and Unilateral ideomotor apraxia) sufficient to account for the writing deficit
f. Impaired ability to terminate ongoing left arm or hand movements (see Motor perseveration) sufficient to account for the writing deficit
g. Normal superiority of the right hand for writing as a result of left-hemisphere language dominance

Lesion Locations

a. Middle to posterior portion of the trunk of the corpus callosum, with occasional involvement of larger callosal areas[4–6,11,12,21–24]
b. Medial frontal-parietal cortex and white matter flanking the corpus callosum, interrupting the outflow of the middle portion of the trunk[25]

7. Unilateral ideomotor apraxia (also called hemiapraxia)*

Clinical Indicators

a_1. Inaccurate pantomime of skilled movements of the left arm and hand on verbal demand as evidenced by any of the following errors:
  1) Performance of an incorrect but recognizable movement (*parapraxia*)
  2) Performance of a partial movement that is an abridgement of the target movement
  3) Performance of a distorted and unrecognizable movement
  4) Use of a body part as if it were an object
  5) Incorrect orientation of the arm, hand, or fingers for the movement being attempted
  6) Substitution of a verbal response (e.g., a description) for the target movement

a_2. Inaccurate imitation of pantomimed skilled movements using the left arm and hand as a result of any of the errors listed previously

a_3. Inaccurate performance of skilled movements of the left arm and hand when using objects as evidenced by any of the following errors:
  1) Performance of a movement not appropriate for the object
  2) Performance of a partial movement that is an abridgement of the target movement
  3) Incorrect orientation of the arm, hand, or fingers with respect to the object
  4) Incorrect orientation of the object in space
  5) Use of a body part as if it were an object

---

*The left hemisphere is presumed to be dominant for language, and the patient is presumed to be right-handed, with memories of previously learned motor skills contained in the left hemisphere. The pattern of left- and right-sided indicators is reversed in left-handed patients with right-hemisphere language dominance and motor memories contained in the right hemisphere. Patients with other dominance patterns have less predictable clinical findings.

a_4. Relatively preserved pantomime of skilled movements of the right arm and hand
a_5. Relatively preserved imitation of skilled movements using the right arm and hand
a_6. Relatively preserved use of objects with the right arm and hand

Associated Features
a. Pantomime on demand possibly more impaired than imitation and object use
b. Imitation of pantomimed movements possibly more impaired than object use
c. Slowness in initiating and performing movements (see Akinesia)
d. Recent history (following onset of brain damage) of absent speech or other attempts at vocal communication (see Mutism)
e. Presence of other interhemispheric transfer disorders, particularly unilateral agraphia

Factors to Rule Out
a. Weakness of the muscles of the left arm or hand sufficient to account for the deficits in skilled movement
b. Impaired coordination of the muscles of the left arm or hand sufficient to account for the deficits in skilled movement
c. Impaired ability to initiate left arm or hand movements (see Akinesia) sufficient to account for the deficits in skilled movement
d. Impaired ability to persist with movements of the left arm or hand (see Motor impersistence) sufficient to account for the deficits in skilled movement
e. Impaired ability to terminate ongoing left arm or hand movements (see Motor perseveration) sufficient to account for the deficits in skilled movement
f. Failure to comprehend commands as a result of oral language disorder (see Chap. 12), ruled out by demonstrating preserved performance of skilled movements on verbal demand when using the right hand

Lesion Locations
a. Trunk (anterior more commonly than posterior) of the corpus callosum, with occasional extension to the genu and more common extension to the medial frontal lobe, including the cingulate gyrus, supplementary motor area, and subcortical white matter[5,11,12,23,26–29]
b. Subcortical (white matter) frontal lobe, interrupting the pathway from premotor cortex to corpus callosum[30]

Lesion Lateralization
a. Left hemisphere in right-handed patients having subcortical frontal white matter lesions[30]

8. **Unilateral disassociation apraxia***

Clinical Indicators

a_1. Inaccurate pantomime of skilled movements of the left arm and hand on verbal demand

a_2. Relatively preserved pantomime of skilled movements of the right arm and hand on verbal demand

a_3. Relatively preserved bilateral imitation of pantomimed skilled movements of the arms and hands

a_4. Relatively preserved bilateral performance of skilled movements of the arms and hands when an object is present to facilitate the target movements

NOTE: This pattern of unilaterally impaired pantomime on verbal demand with preserved imitation and object use is termed unilateral verbal-motor disassociation apraxia.

b_1. Inaccurate imitation of pantomimed skilled movements using the left arm and hand

b_2. Relatively preserved imitation of pantomimed skilled movements using the right arm and hand

b_3. Relatively preserved bilateral pantomime of skilled movements of arms and hands on verbal demand

b_4. Relatively preserved bilateral performance of skilled movements of the arms and hands when an object is present to facilitate the target movements

NOTE: This pattern of unilaterally impaired imitation with preserved pantomime on verbal demand and object use is termed unilateral visuomotor disassociation apraxia.

c_1. Inaccurate performance of skilled movements by the left arm and hand when using objects

c_2. Relatively preserved performance of skilled movements by the right arm and hand when using objects

c_3. Relatively preserved bilateral pantomime of skilled movements of the arms and hands on verbal demand

c_4. Relatively preserved bilateral imitation of pantomimed skilled movements of the arms and hands

NOTE: This pattern of unilaterally impaired object use with preserved pantomime on verbal demand and imitation is termed unilateral tactile-motor disassociation apraxia.

Associated Features

a. Preserved recognition of pantomimed movements
b. Presence of other interhemispheric transfer disorders
c. Relatively preserved bilateral performance of skilled movements of the

*The left hemisphere is presumed to be dominant for language, and the patient is presumed to be right-handed, with memories of previously learned motor skills contained in the left hemisphere. The pattern of left- and right-sided indicators is reversed in left-handed patients with right-hemisphere language dominance and motor memories contained in the right hemisphere. Patients with other dominance patterns have less predictable clinical findings.

arms and hands when an appropriate context (e.g., wanting to wave to someone through a window) is present to elicit target movements

Factors to Rule Out

a. Weakness of the muscles of the left arm or hand sufficient to account for the deficits in skilled movement, ruled out by demonstrating preserved pantomime, imitation, or object use
b. Impaired coordination of the muscles of the left arm or hand sufficient to account for the deficits in skilled movement, ruled out by demonstrating preserved pantomime, imitation, or object use
c. Impaired initiation of movements of the left arm or hand (see Akinesia) sufficient to account for the deficits in skilled movement, ruled out by demonstrating preserved pantomime, imitation, or object use
d. Impaired ability to persist with movements of the left arm or hand (see Motor impersistence) sufficient to account for the deficits in skilled movement, ruled out by demonstrating preserved pantomime, imitation, or object use
e. Impaired ability to terminate left arm or hand movements (see Motor perseveration) sufficient to account for the deficits in skilled movement, ruled out by demonstrating preserved pantomime, imitation, or object use

Lesion Locations

For visuomotor and verbal-motor disassociation apraxia

a. Middle to anterior two thirds of corpus callosum, with occasional extension to the medial frontal lobe[4,31]

For tactile-motor disassociation apraxia

Insufficient information available

9. Diagonistic apraxia (also called the alien hand)*

Clinical Indicators

a. Left and right hands acting at cross-purposes (e.g., the right hand turns on a light and immediately afterward, the left hand reaches to turn it off)
b. Left and right hands pushing, slapping, impeding, or otherwise openly conflicting with each other *(intermanual conflict)*

c_1. Left hand carrying out unintended but well-coordinated and sometimes complex actions (e.g., turning the pages of a book)

c_2. Left hand described by patient as acting outside of his or her control, as if it had purposes and intentions of its own

c_3. Inability to stop an unintended activity being performed by the left hand except by physically intervening with the right hand

*The left hemisphere is presumed to be dominant for language, and the patient is presumed to be right-handed. The pattern of left- and right-sided indicators is reversed in left-handed patients with right-hemisphere language dominance. Patients with other dominance patterns have less predictable clinical findings.

Associated Features

a. Critical or derogatory comments about the left hand accompanying the report of the left hand as being out of control *(autocriticism)*
b. Slowness in initiating and performing movements (see Akinesia)
c. Recent history (following onset of brain damage) of absent speech or other attempts at vocal communication (see Mutism)
d. Presence of other interhemispheric transfer disorders
e. A positive grasp reflex: involuntary grasping movement when the palm of the hand is stimulated
f. Inappropriate grasping and use of objects in the immediate vicinity that are unrelated to any ongoing activity *(utilization behavior)*

Factors to Rule Out

a. Intentional or unconscious avoidance of responsibility for socially unacceptable actions of the left hand; disorder not including or limited to socially unacceptable behavior

Lesion Locations

a. Trunk of the corpus callosum with occasional extension to the splenium and genu[4,6,11–14,26,27]
b. Medial frontal lobe, including the supplementary motor area and anterior cingulate, usually in association with an anterior callosal lesion and with occasional extension to the gyrus rectus, subcallosal area, basal ganglia, internal capsule, and thalamus[28,32–37]
c. Combined temporal and occipital lobes in combination with the splenium of the corpus callosum and thalamus[38]

Lesion Lateralization

a. Left hand affected (i.e., experienced as “alien”) in patients with left-hemisphere language dominance and lesions confined to the callosum
b. Contralateral hand affected in patients with medial frontal lobe lesions

10. Somesthetic disconnection

Clinical Indicators

a_1. Following palpation of an object with one hand, selection of an object from a larger set of objects that serve as foils inaccurate with the opposite hand (vision occluded throughout this procedure)
a_2. Relatively preserved selection of the object from a set of foils with the same hand that originally palpated it (vision occluded throughout this procedure)
a_3. Deficit occurring regardless of which hand initially palpates the object
b_1. Hand and finger postures impressed on one hand by the examiner inaccurately replicated by the opposite hand (vision occluded throughout this procedure)
b_2. Relatively preserved replication of hand and finger postures by the hand on which they were initially impressed (vision occluded throughout this procedure)

b_3. Deficit occurring regardless of which hand the postures are initially impressed on

c_1. Places on one side of the body that are touched by the examiner inaccurately pointed to using the hand opposite to the side of the body that was touched (vision occluded throughout this procedure)

c_2. Relatively preserved location of places touched on one side of the body using the ipsilateral hand (vision occluded throughout this procedure)

c_3. Deficit occurring regardless of which side of the body is touched

Associated Features

a. Slowness in initiating and performing movements (see Akinesia)
b. Recent history (following onset of brain damage) of absent speech or other attempts at vocal communication (see Mutism)
c. Presence of other interhemispheric transfer disorders

Factors to Rule Out

a. Impaired position sense so that hand and finger postures are not perceived, ruled out by demonstrating preserved same-hand replication of postures
b. Muscle weakness that prevents hand and finger posture replication, ruled out by demonstrating preserved same-hand replication of postures
c. Poor muscle coordination that prevents hand and finger posture replication, ruled out by demonstrating preserved same-hand replication of postures
d. Impaired ability to initiate movement (see Akinesia) that prevents hand and finger posture replication, ruled out by demonstrating preserved same-hand replication of postures
e. Impaired ability to persist with movements (see Motor impersistence) that prevents hand and finger posture replication, ruled out by demonstrating preserved same-hand replication of postures
f. Impaired ability to perform skilled movements on demand (see Apraxia) that prevents hand and finger posture replication, ruled out by demonstrating preserved same-hand replication of postures
g. Impaired ability to terminate ongoing movements (see Motor perseveration) that prevents hand and finger posture replication, ruled out by demonstrating preserved same-hand replication of postures

Lesion Locations

a. Trunk of corpus callosum, with occasional extension to the genu and splenium[11,12,39,40]

ETIOLOGY

Most naturally occurring adult cases of interhemispheric transfer disorder result from cerebrovascular disease involving pericallosal arteries. Hemorrhage from an anterior communicating artery aneurysm or vertebrobasilar artery infarction can produce various constellations of interhemispheric transfer disorder. Callosal damage can also result from traumatic brain injury or neoplasm. Additionally, the corpus callosum may degenerate when patients are exposed to toxic levels of substances such as ethanol, which produces Marchiafava-Bignami disease. Some of the best-studied cases of interhemispheric transfer disorder resulted from surgical ablation of the cerebral commissures in the treatment of severe epilepsy. Regardless of the cause, the nature and severity of the interhemispheric disorder depends on which portions of the cerebral hemispheres are disconnected from each other.

DISABLING CONSEQUENCES

Most of the disorders of interhemispheric transfer are not disabling and are not apparent in social situations. Unilateral anomia, for example, is rarely apparent except during clinical testing. Rather unusual circumstances would be required for this disorder to become manifest in the natural environment. Similarly, unilateral alexia, unilateral agraphia, and inflexible dichotic suppression do not pose problems for most patients.

Pseudoneglect, however, can be as disabling as the other stimulus neglect disorders. It prevents successful performance of occupations that require drawing (e.g., drafting, architecture). Depending on the severity of the disorder, the patient may be unable to drive, read, or perform any task requiring attention to visual or tactual details.

Patients who have somesthetic disconnection, unilateral apraxia, or diagonistic apraxia are impaired in performing any vocational or leisure task that requires coordinated, simultaneous use of the hands. This impairment is particularly evident in highly demanding situations with multiple distractors preventing the patient from constantly monitoring what his or her hands are doing. Additionally, diagonistic apraxia can be socially stigmatizing. An individual whose hands constantly reverse tasks done by each other is likely to be misunderstood and ostracized. Although unilateral constructional disability carries some disabling potential, most drawing tasks can be accomplished with one hand assuming the dominant role while the other aids by holding materials steady.

ASSESSMENT INSTRUMENTS

Because of infrequency of disorders of interhemispheric transfer in the average neuropsychological practice, little incentive has been created for the marketing of standardized commissural tests. The examiner wishing to test for interruption of interhemispheric transfer has several options. The examiner can use behavioral monitoring to detect intermittently occurring problems such as diagonistic apraxia. Tests used to detect disorders that normally affect both sides of the body can be adapted so that they also detect unilateral presentations of the disorder. Thus, standard tests of apraxia, agraphia, stimulus neglect, and constructional disability can be administered in a modified fashion to detect unilateral presentations of the disorders described previously.

Clinical laboratory procedures can be specifically designed to detect interhemispheric transfer disorders. Such procedures generally have not been subjected to large-scale normative study. This may not be a serious problem because most of these procedures are readily performed by virtually all normal individuals and depend on a comparison within the person rather than with a normative group. For example, the Visual Hemifield Reading Procedure compares how well stimuli are read from the LVF and RVF within the same person rather than comparing the individual with a normative group. Materials used in many of the procedures are not commercially available and must be constructed by the clinician.

Beery Development Test of Visual-Motor Integration

See discussion of this test in Chapter 7.

Halstead-Reitan Battery Aphasia Screening Test, Spatial Relations and Written Language Items

See discussion of this test in Chapter 12.

Boston Diagnostic Aphasia Examination, Written Language Subtests

See discussion of this test in Chapter 12.

Western Aphasia Battery, Written Language Subtests

See discussion of this test in Chapter 12.

Boston Spatial-Quantitative Battery, Apraxia Subtest

See discussion of this test in Chapter 11.

Western Aphasia Battery, Apraxia Subtest

See discussion of this test in Chapter 11.

Dichotic Listening Test

See discussion of this test in Chapter 4.

Visual Hemifield Reading Procedure

The Visual Hemifield Reading Procedure is *not commercially available.*

This procedure is administered via computer. A digit is presented at the center of the monitor along with a word 1/2 inch to the right or left of the digit. Stimuli are shown in Table 10–1. Words appear in capital letters and are white or amber on a black background screen. The patient sits in front of the monitor with the chin resting in a chin rest or in his or her cupped hands with the elbows bent and placed

Table 10–1. **HEMIFIELD READING STIMULI**

	Practice Stimuli	
1.	7	Stamp
2.	Knife	3
3.	Pencil	8
	Test Stimuli	
1.	Ball	6
2.	8	Bottle
3.	6	Button
4.	Card	2
5.	Cup	4
6.	9	Key
7.	4	Matches
8.	Nail	5
9.	Ring	9
10.	4	Scissors
11.	Button	2
12.	Bottle	3
13.	5	Ball
14.	Scissors	3
15.	Key	4
16.	8	Ring
17.	Matches	7
18.	1	Cup
19.	3	Nail
20.	1	Card

firmly on the table. The height of the monitor is adjusted so that the stimuli appear approximately at eye level. The monitor must also be positioned so that the center of the monitor, where the digit appears, is at the patient's midline.

Each trial begins with the word *READY* appearing for 5 seconds at the center of the screen, followed by the test stimulus, which is followed by a row of asterisks completely covering the area where the test stimulus previously appeared, to mask any afterimage. Test stimuli appear for 200 msec, and the mask stays on until a new trial begins. A new trial is not initiated until the space bar is pressed by the patient or examiner. Three practice and 20 test trials are presented (see Table 10–1). On each trial, patients are asked to keep their eyes at the center of the screen where the ready signal appears. Patients must first report the digit and then the word. No credit is given on a trial if the patient cannot report the digit because this response suggests that his or her eyes were not at central fixation. Each word appears once to the left and once to the right of the central digit, and digit-word combinations are random.

Stimuli are drawn from the Fuld Object-Memory Evaluation, Form I.[41] The Fuld objects are scattered randomly on the table adjacent to the computer. The patient is asked to select an object corresponding to the word that appeared on the monitor on any trial in which he or she fails to read the word. Selection of the object is permitted using only the hand ipsilateral to the target word. For example, if the target word appears to the left of central fixation, the left hand is used to select the corresponding object.

Reading words with greater accuracy to one or the other side of fixation (usually the right side) is expected and does not necessarily indicate pathology. Most individuals, however, should be able to read at least one half of the words presented in the nonpreferred visual field. Failure to read any words in the nonpreferred field may raise suspicion of a callosal lesion. Further support for this suspicion is provided if the patient additionally manages to manually locate objects corresponding to words he or she failed to read. This phenomenon must occur consistently in one visual field for the disorder to be interpreted as callosal in origin.

Reliability, validity, and normative data are not available for the Visual Hemifield Reading Procedure. Interpretation rests on the finding of a pathological pattern of performance rather than on a particular level of performance, although the two types of analysis are not mutually exclusive. Although the procedure is not commercially available, most computer programmers should be able to write a routine that administers stimuli in the manner described. Most nonprogrammers should be able to design a program to administer the stimuli via computer using the Micro Experimental Laboratory (MEL).[42] MEL requires some practice before it can be used, but it is learned fairly easily and brings "programming" within the reach of nonprogrammers.

Olfactory Recognition Procedure

The Olfactory Recognition Procedure is *not commercially available*.

In this procedure, 10 odors (Table 10–2) are presented, and patients attempt to name the odors. If they fail to name an odor, multiple-choice options are given. The correct odors are underlined in Table 10–2. Bottles of flavor extract, available in most grocery stores, are used to produce the odors. Labels must be removed from the bottles or the patient must be blindfolded during testing. If the labels are removed, the identical bottles can be coded numerically.

The odors can be administered simultaneously to both nostrils or to one nostril only by asking the patient to compress the other nostril with his or her finger. The test can be subsequently administered to the closed nostril. During odor presentation, the bottle cap is removed and the bottle held directly under the nostril or nostrils for 5 seconds while the patient smells the contents of the bottle. The cap is replaced immediately, and a minimum of 30 seconds is allowed to pass, during which a response can be obtained, before another odor is presented.

Reliability, validity, and normative data are not available for this procedure. My clinical experience suggests that normal individuals can accurately identify at least seven of the odors when given the multiple-choice options. The most useful comparison is between nostrils in the same patient. A large discrepancy between nostrils may suggest combined anterior callosum and anterior commissure lesions. Table 10–2 includes several preliminary questions about factors (e.g., nasal congestion) that could invalidate test results in a given patient.

Table 10–2. **OLFACTORY RECOGNITION PROCEDURE**

Do you presently have a cold or the flu?

Are you presently suffering from any type of sinus problem or nasal congestion?

Have you noticed any changes in your ability to smell?

Have you noticed anything unusual in the way food tastes?

Check: ______ Unilateral presentation (circle: R L nostril)

______ Bilateral presentation

Odor	Naming	Multiple-Choice Options*		
1.	+/−	Grape	Pineapple	Strawberry
2.	+/−	Banana	Rum	Almond
3.	+/−	Orange	Pineapple	Cherry
4.	+/−	Lemon	Rum	Maple
5.	+/−	Cherry	Mint	Strawberry
6.	+/−	Banana	Orange	Lemon
7.	+/−	Rum	Almond	Coconut
8.	+/−	Grape	Lemon	Mint†
9.	+/−	Orange	Lime	Peach
10.	+/−	Apricot	Rum	Maple

Total correct naming: ______/10

Total correct multiple choice: ______/10

*Underscoring indicates the correct answer.
†Accept peppermint or spearmint as correct alternatives.

The olfactory recognition procedure should be used only by experienced neurologists and neuropsychologists because of the absence of a normative database to guide interpretation. The procedure is most appropriate for office or laboratory administration, although bedside administration is feasible.

University of Florida Hand Posture Transfer Procedure

The University of Florida Hand Posture Transfer Procedure is *not commercially available.*

Figure 10–1 presents a series of hand postures that can be used to detect somesthetic disconnection. One of the patient's hands is moved into the target posture while his or her vision is occluded. The patient is then asked to replicate the posture using the same or the opposite hand. Trials are balanced so that the initial posture is introduced to the left and right hands an equal number of times. The posture is replicated with the same hand as often as it is replicated with the opposite hand. The posture must be transferred from the left to the right hand as often as from the right to the left hand.

Replication of postures with the same hand requires that the posture first be released, adding a memory component to the task. To preserve the equivalency of the trials, the posture should also be released before replication is attempted with the opposite hand. On any trial, the posture can be demonstrated again if it is forgotten

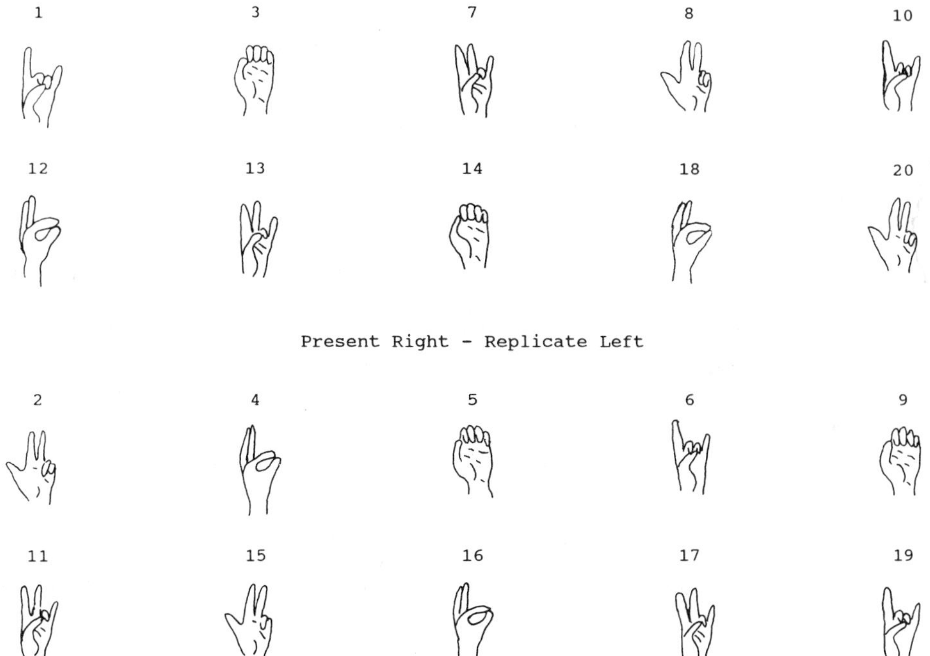

FIGURE 10–1. University of Florida Hand Posture Transfer Procedure.

before it can be replicated, but this should be noted in the margin on the answer sheet.

Reliability and validity data are not available for this procedure. My clinical experience suggests that the task is performed with few or no errors by patients who do not have callosal lesions. The most important comparison is within the individual rather than between individuals. Markedly poorer replication of postures with the opposite hand compared to same-hand replication suggests an interruption of callosal transmission. The deficit should be present regardless of which hand initially receives the target posture.

The Hand Posture Transfer Procedure can be administered at bedside, in the office, or in laboratory settings. The results of the procedure should be interpreted by a neuropsychologist, neurologist, neurosurgeon, or physiatrist.

Behavioral Monitoring Procedure

See discussion of this procedure in Chapter 3.

Diagonistic apraxia occurs intermittently and cannot always be elicited by asking the patient to perform certain tasks and activities. The Behavioral Monitoring Procedure can be used to document the intermittent occurrence of diagonistic apraxia, provided that the disorder is described in specific and objective terms that can be easily identified by all monitoring staff. Additionally, patients often can give rich descriptions of the disorder and in some instances can monitor its occurrence themselves. The Neuroemotional-Neuroideational-Neurobehavioral Symptom Survey discussed in Chapter 18 includes items that measure the patient's awareness and recollection of instances of diagonistic apraxia.

NEUROPSYCHOLOGICAL TREATMENT

No specific treatments exist for the disorders of interhemispheric transfer. This is partly the result of the lack of associated disability. Few patients seek treatment for disorders that are virtually unnoticeable. The more disabling of the interhemispheric transfer disorders do require treatment. Pseudoneglect, unilateral constructional disability, and the unilateral apraxias are approached in a manner similar to that for the analogous bilateral disorders. Treatment techniques are discussed in Chapters 4, 7, and 11.

When no treatment is rendered, patients with disorders of interhemispheric transfer nonetheless learn to compensate for their deficits to the degree that specialized clinical testing is needed to reveal the continued presence of impairment. In patients with only a partial disconnection of the hemispheres, information may begin to transfer from one hemisphere to the other via spared pathways. Alternatively, the hemispheres may learn to signal each other indirectly through gestures and characteristic physiological reactions. For example, the left hemisphere may attain some awareness of erotic stimuli tachistoscopically presented to the right hemisphere by noting the occurrence of physiological changes associated with sexual arousal.

It is possible that this naturally occurring compensation can be hastened or increased by providing therapeutic practice in the areas in which the patient is deficient. Thus, providing practice in comparing stimuli presented to the two sides of the body, in verbally identifying information targeted to the right hemisphere, or in coordinating the use of the two hands may lead to improved performance in patients with commissural deficits.

Practice-based treatments are more effective when the tasks challenge the patient, yet make success highly probable. One way of accomplishing this is to initially present material that is to be identified verbally to both cerebral hemispheres. Gradually reducing the amount of information sent to the left hemisphere while continuing to present full information to the right hemisphere may make it possible to maintain a desirable level of success. For example, a word can be tachistoscopically presented to both hemispheres, with letters systematically dropped from the end of the word presented to the left hemisphere while the full word continues to be presented to the right hemisphere.

Other commissural deficits can be addressed in a similar manner. However, treatment in this area remains a speculative endeavor, with no empirical guidelines available to guide the clinician's approach.

CASE ILLUSTRATION

CASE 10–1

P.H. was a right-handed, 37-year-old man who had completed 2 years of college and worked as a marketing consultant. He was taken to an emergency department after complaining to his wife of a severe headache and subsequently losing consciousness. The initial computed tomography (CT) scans revealed a large subarachnoid hemorrhage whose epicenter appeared to be in the territory of the anterior communicating artery. There was a large collection of blood in the interhemispheric fissure. A collection of blood between the frontal horns measured 1 cm. There was also an intraventricular hemorrhage, primarily in the right lateral ventricle, with hydrocephalus. The patient underwent a ventriculostomy to relieve the hydrocephalus. Subsequent CT scans showed a hematoma in the rostrum of the corpus callosum, and the development of an infarct in the left basal ganglia. The aneurysm appeared to seal itself; therefore, no additional surgery was necessary.

After a 2-week coma, P.H. became more alert, but was transiently mute and had a mild right hemiparesis. He received outpatient rehabilitation for several weeks before being admitted to a day rehabilitation program for continued intensive treatment. At the time of admission to this program, P.H. was able to converse normally and had only minimal right-sided weakness. A neuropsychological examination revealed that P.H. was functioning in the average range of intelligence. He had difficulty in dividing his concentration between two simultaneous tasks and was severely impaired in problem solving. He retained full visual fields, and visual acuity was 20/20 in each eye.

When the patient attempted to sort cards by various physical attributes, intermanual conflict was observed. He was sorting with his right hand when his left hand grabbed the right, yanked it back to prevent it from putting down the card in the pile just chosen, and tried to force the right hand to place the card elsewhere. When asked what was happening, P.H. responded that his left hand "had a mind of its own" and was "stubborn." He denied having any control over the left hand when it carried out these behaviors.

P.H.'s copies of the HRB Aphasia Screening Test, Spatial Relations Items, are shown in Figure 10–2. Considerable spatial distortion and omission of detail, particularly in the key, is present in the drawings done with the left hand. P.H. also failed to draw the right half of the cross. Although they are certainly not fully intact, P.H.'s drawings with the right hand are spatially accurate and are more complete, although details again are omitted from the key. The quality of P.H.'s drawings did not vary as a function of where the model was placed, whether to his right, to his left, or at his midline. P.H. expressed embarrassment at his poor left-hand performance, commenting that his key "wasn't shaped much like a key" and noting the absence of one side of his cross. He was also able to point out the poor quality of his square and triangle, particularly noting the absence of sharp angles. In contrast to what was seen on drawing tasks, no notable differences were present in writing samples obtained from each hand.

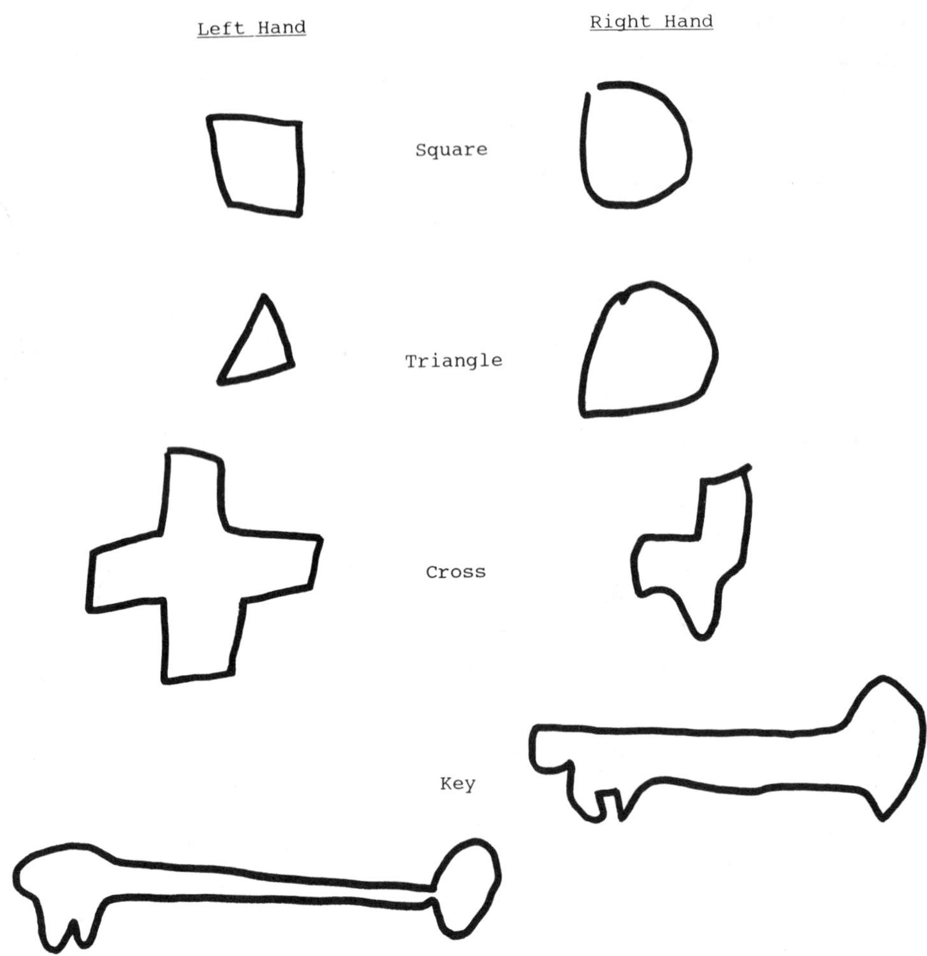

FIGURE 10–2. P.H.'s copies of the Aphasia Screening Test Spatial Relations items.

Table 10–3 presents the results of procedures used to assess P.H.'s capacity for interhemispheric transfer. The patient was equivalent in his pantomime of movements with each hand. He was also equally successful in naming odors regardless of the nostril to which they were presented. The patient succeeded in directing attention to the appropriate ear on demand under conditions of dichotic digit presentation. He was twice as proficient at reading words presented in the right visual half-field compared to words presented in the left visual half-field; however, he was unable to correct his errors by pointing or picking up objects corresponding to the words presented. On the Hand Posture Transfer Procedure, P.H. was twice as accurate when replicating positions with the same hand as when replicating positions with the contralateral hand.

Table 10–3. **PERFORMANCE ON TESTS OF INTERHEMISPHERIC TRANSFER**

Test or Procedure	Correct Responses	
	Right	**Left**
Western Aphasia Battery, Apraxia Subtest (upper limb and instrumental pantomime upon demand)	10/10	9/10
Olfactory Recognition Procedure	4/10	4/10
Dichotic Listening Test		
Attention directed to right ear	55	4
Attention directed to left ear	7	55
Visual Hemifield Reading Procedure		
Words read	9/10	4/10
Manual corrections	0	0
	Same Hand	**Opposite Hand**
University of Florida Hand Posture Transfer Procedure	8	4

DISCUSSION

P.H. presented with several interhemispheric transfer disorders. The intermanual conflict observed during the patient's test performance led to a diagnosis of diagonistic apraxia. Because the behavior did not occur in the context of avoidance of responsibility, there appear to be no competing explanations for the observed conflict. The patient's intact pantomime of movement with either hand ruled out the presence of a unilateral apraxia. Writing was equivalent in both hands, but at first glance, the data on visual half-field reading might appear to suggest the presence of unilateral alexia. P.H. was more proficient at reading words presented to the right visual half-field, but this can be explained by left-hemisphere language dominance without resorting to an assumption of callosal disconnection. If he had been able to point to objects with his left hand that represented words he failed to read in the left visual half-field, then the evidence for unilateral alexia would have been stronger.

Somesthetic disconnection was suggested by P.H.'s relative weakness at opposite-hand replication of postures. He was successful at indicating the appropriate ear during dichotic stimulation. He was poor at naming odors, but no difference between nostrils was apparent.

Unilateral constructional disability was suggested by P.H.'s drawings (see Fig. 10–2). This deficit cannot be accounted for by motor impairment, because his spared left hand performed worse than the mildly hemiparetic right hand. The quality of the left-hand performance was worse than would be expected simply because he was using his nondominant hand. It is surprising that performance was worse with the left hand because the opposite pattern is usually found. Although P.H.'s hemifield reading data suggest that he is left-hemisphere dominant for language, it is possible that other perceptual abilities are lateralized in an atypical manner. As noted previously, when callosal patients have mixed dominance, unusual patterns of performance can occur.

Inspection of P.H.'s left-hand drawing of a cross led to suspicion of right-sided hemispatial neglect (see Fig. 10–2). When P.H. drew the cross with his right hand, however, the right-sided neglect was no longer evident. A diagnosis of pseudoneglect is suggested by this finding. The presence of pseudoneglect does not, in this case, obviate the diagnosis of unilateral constructional disability because P.H.'s left-hand drawings were poor even when there was no evidence that a portion of the model was neglected.

Radiological data suggest that only the anterior portion of P.H.'s corpus callosum has sustained damage. This diagnosis fits well with the pattern of deficits seen in this patient. An anterior callosal lesion can account for P.H.'s diagonistic apraxia. Anterior lesions also are associated with pseudoneglect. Less is known about the precise part of the corpus callosum that must be damaged to produce unilateral constructional disability. Reading, writing, and dichotic listening should not be affected by anterior callosal lesions; these functions are spared in P.H. Unilateral olfactory anomia is associated with anterior lesions. Olfactory information can, however, cross from one hemisphere to another via the anterior commissure, which is spared in this patient.

Somesthetic information crosses the corpus callosum more posteriorly; thus, it is somewhat surprising to find somesthetic disconnection in a patient with an anterior lesion. However, it should be noted that the task used to assess somesthetic transfer involved hand movement. It is likely that the replication of hand postures required the participation of not only posterior somesthetic cortex but also anterior portions of the brain involved in motor control. Disconnection of motor areas in P.H.'s two hemispheres as a result of the anterior callosal lesion may be responsible for lowering his performance on the Hand Posture Transfer Procedure.

REFERENCES

1. Bowers, D, and Heilman, KM: Pseudoneglect: Effects of hemispace on a tactile line bisection task. Neuropsychologia 18:491, 1980.
2. American Psychiatric Association: Diagnostic and Statistical Manual of Mental Disorders, Fourth Edition. American Psychiatric Association, Washington, DC, 1994.
3. The International Classification of Diseases, Ninth Revision, Clinical Modification. Med-Index Publications, Salt Lake City, 1991.
4. Rosa, A, et al: Marchiafava-Bignami disease, syndrome of interhemispheric disconnection, and right-handed agraphia in a left hander. Arch Neurol 48:986, 1991.
5. Habib, M, Ceccaldi, M, and Poncet, M: Callosal disconnection syndrome caused by left hemisphere infarction. Rev Neurol 146:19, 1990.
6. Degos, JD, et al: Posterior callosal infarction. Clinicopathological correlations. Brain 110:1155, 1987.
7. Zihl, J, and von Cramon, D: Colour anomia restricted to the left visual hemifield after splenial disconnexion. J Neurol Neurosurg Psychiatry 43:719, 1980.
8. Gazzaniga, MS, et al: Psychologic and neurologic consequences of partial and complete commissurotomy. Neurology 25:10, 1975.
9. Gordon, HW, and Sperry, RW: Lateralization of olfactory perception in the surgically separated hemispheres of man. Neuropsychologia 7:111, 1969.
10. Boldrini, P, et al: Partial hemispheric disconnection syndrome of traumatic origin. Cortex 28:135, 1992.

11. Leiguarda, R, Starkstein, S, and Berthier, M: Anterior callosal haemorrhage. A partial interhemispheric disconnection syndrome. Brain 112:1019, 1989.
12. Starkstein, SE, Berthier, ML, and Leiguarda, R: Disconnection syndrome in a right-handed patient with right hemispheric speech dominance. Eur Neurol 28:187, 1988.
13. Watson, RT, Heilman, KM, and Bowers, D: Magnetic resonance imaging (MRI, NMR) scan in a case of callosal apraxia and pseudoneglect. Brain 108:535, 1985.
14. Heilman, KM, Bowers, D, and Watson, RT: Pseudoneglect in a patient with partial callosal disconnection. Brain 107:519, 1984.
15. Kashiwagi, A, et al: Hemispatial neglect in a patient with callosal infarction. Brain 113:1005, 1990.
16. Loring, DW, Meador, KJ, and Lee, GP: Differential-handed response to verbal and visual spatial stimuli: Evidence of specialized hemispheric processing following callosotomy. Neuropsychologia 27:811, 1989.
17. Goldenberg, G: Neglect in a patient with partial callosal disconnection. Neuropsychologia 24:397, 1986.
18. Dimond, SJ, et al: Functions of the centre section (trunk) of the corpus callosum in man. Brain 100:543, 1977.
19. Abe, T, et al: Partial disconnection syndrome following penetrating stab wound of the brain. Eur Neurol 25:233, 1986.
20. Castro-Caldas, A, and Salgado, V: Right hemifield alexia without hemianopia. Arch Neurol 41:84, 1984.
21. Kawamura, M, Hirayama, K, and Yamamoto, H: Different interhemispheric transfer of kanji and kana writing evidenced by a case with left unilateral agraphia without apraxia. Brain 112:1011, 1989.
22. Yamadori, A, Nagashima, T, and Tamaki, N: Ideogram writing in a disconnection syndrome. Brain Lang 19:346, 1983.
23. Watson, RT, and Heilman, KM: Callosal apraxia. Brain 106:391, 1983.
24. Sugishita, M, et al: Unilateral agraphia after section of the posterior half of the truncus of the corpus callosum. Brain Lang 9:215, 1980.
25. Gersh, F, and Damasio, AR: Praxis and writing of the left hand may be served by different callosal pathways. Arch Neurol 38:634, 1981.
26. Jason, GW, and Pajurkova, EM: Failure of metacontrol: Breakdown in behavioral unity after lesion of the corpus callosum and inferomedial frontal lobes. Cortex 28:241, 1992.
27. Graff-Radford, NR, Welsh, K, and Godersky, J: Callosal apraxia. Neurology 37:100, 1987.
28. Goldenberg, G, et al: Apraxia of the left limbs in a case of callosal disconnection: The contribution of medial frontal lobe damage. Cortex 21:135, 1985.
29. Satomi, K, Kinoshita, Y, and Hirakawa, S: Disturbances of cross-localization of fingertips in a callosal patient. Cortex 27:327, 1991.
30. Ferro, JM, et al: Crossed optic ataxia: Possible role of the dorsal splenium. J Neurol Neurosurg Psychiatry 46:533, 1983.
31. Tanaka, Y, Iwasa, H, and Obayashi, T: Right hand agraphia and left hand apraxia following callosal damage in a right-hander. Cortex 26:665, 1990.
32. Feinberg, TE, et al: Two alien hand syndromes. Neurology 42:19, 1992.
33. Della-Sala, S, Marchetti, C, and Spinnler, H: Right-sided anarchic (alien) hand: A longitudinal study. Neuropsychologia 29:1113, 1991.
34. Hanakita, J, and Nishi, S: Left alien hand sign and mirror writing after left anterior cerebral artery infarction. Surg Neurol 35:290, 1991.
35. Tanaka, Y, Iwasa, H, and Yoshida, M: Diagonistic dyspraxia: Case report and movement-related potentials. Neurology 40:657, 1990.
36. Banks, G, et al: The alien hand syndrome. Clinical and postmortem findings. Arch Neurol 46:456, 1989.
37. Goldberg, G, Mayer, NH, and Toglia, JU: Medial frontal cortex infarction and the alien hand sign. Arch Neurol 38:683, 1981.
38. Levine, DN, and Rinn, WE: Opticosensory ataxia and alien hand syndrome after posterior cerebral artery territory infarction. Neurology 36:1094, 1986.
39. Risse, GL, et al: Interhemispheric transfer in patients with incomplete section of the corpus callosum. Anatomic verification with magnetic resonance imaging. Arch Neurol 46:437, 1989.
40. Bentin, S, Sahar, A, and Moscovitch, M: Intermanual information transfer in patients with lesions in the trunk of the corpus callosum. Neuropsychologia 22:601, 1984.
41. Fuld, PA: Fuld Object-Memory Evaluation Instruction Manual. Stoelting Company, Chicago, 1977.
42. Schneider, W: Micro Experimental Laboratory: An integrated system for IBM PC compatibles. Behavior Research Methods, Instruments, and Computers 20:206, 1988.

DISORDERS OF VOLUNTARY COGNITIVE CONTROL OF MOVEMENT

11

Elementary disorders of movement such as paresis (weakness), ataxia (incoordination), and chorea are generally not the focus of attention in neuropsychological examinations, except as factors that can impede valid testing of other aspects of behavior. The notable exception to this is the inclusion of tests of strength, speed, and coordination in assessment batteries that are designed to localize lesions or predict performance in vocational settings. More generally, neuropsychologists become interested in movement at the point at which it intersects with cognition. In addition, it is primarily movements of the face and hands that are of concern. Deficits in the ability to initiate, sustain, alternate, terminate, inhibit, access, and sequence skilled movements of the face and hands are the focus of this chapter. All disorders in these areas involve a fault in the cognitive component of movement.

Unilateral verbal-motor disassociation apraxia, unilateral ideomotor apraxia, and diagonistic apraxia are discussed in Chapter 10 with other disorders of interhemispheric transfer. Constructional apraxia, a disorder of visual-motor integration, is discussed in Chapter 7 (see Constructional disability). Dressing apraxia, a failure to dress one half of the body, is an aspect of hemispatial neglect and is discussed in Chapter 4. Apraxic agraphia is discussed in Chapter 13 with other disorders of written language. Psychogenic motor dysfunction is not the result of a brain lesion, but is included in this chapter because it may accompany and exaggerate the presentation of other movement disorders. When a psychogenic problem is suspected, neuropsychological examination is often done to confirm or refute the suspicion.

Melokinetic apraxia, also called "limb kinetic apraxia," is an inability to perform precise movements of the fingers, such as picking up small objects or rapidly tapping a finger. The lesion responsible for this disorder is unclear, and it is difficult to distinguish this disorder conceptually from a simple lack of fine motor coordination. Consequently, melokinetic apraxia is not included in this text.

Elementary movement disorders are included in this chapter only as factors to rule out when diagnosing the disorders of voluntary cognitive control of movement. Tests and procedures for detecting elementary movement disorders are listed.

NOMENCLATURE

The terms used to label the disorders included in this chapter are in fairly common use in the neurology and neuropsychology literature. It should be noted that the term *adiadochokinesia* is used more broadly in this book than is customary. *Adiadochokinesia* refers to a deficit in the ability to perform rapid alternating movements. Very basic movements are used in neurological examinations to assess rapid alternation; patients may be asked to pat their hands on the table top or to alternate between pronation and supination of the hands. Such tests are sensitive to cerebellar dysfunction. Luria[1] introduced a number of more complex alternation tasks that are sensitive to cerebellar and frontal lobe dysfunction. These tasks are variously referred to as "dynamic motor activities" or "Luria's motor programs," among other terms. Because these more complex tasks still tap the patient's capacity to rapidly alternate between two or more successive movements, dysfunction in this area is treated as a complex form of adiadochokinesia in this text.

Limited coding options for disorders of voluntary cognitive control of movement are available in DSM-IV.[2] Akinesia can be coded as "Catatonic Disorder Due to a General Medical Condition." Psychogenic motor dysfunction can be coded as a conversion disorder if the symptoms are unconsciously produced, as somatization disorder if the symptoms occur as part of a long series of questionable somatic complaints, as factitious disorder if the symptoms are consciously produced with the goal being the assumption of the role of patient, or as malingering if the symptoms are consciously produced in order to obtain tangible compensation. Apraxia is listed in DSM-IV as a symptom of dementia. The nonspecific diagnoses "Cognitive Disorder Not Otherwise Specified" and "Mild Neurocognitive Disorder" can be used if a more specific code is not appropriate for a given patient.

ICD-9-CM[3] includes many additional options for coding movement disorders. No code exists for akinesia, but dyskinesia can be coded as "Lack of Coordination." Dyskinesia, however, typically refers to aberrant movement (e.g., tardive dyskinesia) rather than to decreased initiation. Dysdiadochokinesia is also coded as lack of coordination in ICD-9-CM. Perseveration and apraxia are included under the "Other" subcategory of "Other Symbolic Dysfunction."

ICD-9-CM includes an additional option for coding psychogenic motor dysfunction. It may be coded as "Psychogenic Dyskinesia" under "Other and Unspecified Special Symptoms or Syndromes, Not Elsewhere Classified." This rather vague term includes such disparate behaviors as hair pulling and masturbation and offers no advantages over the codes for psychogenic motor dysfunction available in DSM-IV. No codes exist in ICD-9-CM for echopraxia or motor impersistence.

RULES FOR DIAGNOSIS

Clinical Indicators: Each is independent (only one must be observed for the disorder to be suspected) *except* when subscripting is used. Subscripted numbers (a_1, a_2) denote an indicator with multiple parts that must be considered together.
Associated Features: These are listed to give a more complete picture of the disorders. The presence or absence of these features does not affect the diagnosis.
Factors to Rule Out: All must be taken into account. Failure to rule out even one of these factors makes a firm diagnosis impossible.
Lesion Locations: Each location stands alone; damage in only one of the listed areas is sufficient to produce the disorder.

VARIETY OF PRESENTATION

1. Akinesia (includes hypokinesia, bradykinesia, and hemiakinesia)

Clinical Indicators

a_1. Failure to initiate (spontaneously or on demand) movements of the face, trunk, and limbs

a_2. Absence of meaningful interaction with the environment

a_3. Preserved random and stimulus-tracking movements of the eyes

a_4. Preserved eye blink

b_1. The presence of either of the following signs:

1) Failure to initiate movement in, or otherwise use, a limb on one side of the body *(hemiakinesia)*
2) Failure to initiate movement in, or otherwise use, both limbs when positioned in the left or right but not both sides of space

b_2. The presence of either of the following signs:

1) Increased use of an affected limb when attention is directed specifically to the limb
2) Increased use of affected limbs when they are moved to the opposite side of space

c. Decreased speed of movements on one or both sides of the body (*hypokinesia* or *bradykinesia*)

d_1. Spontaneous deviation of the head or eyes to the left or right of midline

d_2. Infrequent spontaneous movement of the head or eyes away from the side of deviation (e.g., if the head or eyes are deviated to the right, they will travel to the left of midline infrequently)

d_3. Relatively preserved ability to move the head or eyes to either side of midline on demand or when following a stimulus

Associated Features

a. Absence of speech (see Mutism)
   NOTE: When complete akinesia (absence of all trunk and limb movements with preserved tracking) occurs with mutism, the complex of disorders is variously referred to as akinetic mutism, coma-vigil, apallic state, or persistent vegetative state.
b. Weakness on one or both sides of the body
c. Presence of a tremor when limbs are at rest *(resting tremor)*
d. Failure to notice or detect stimuli on one or both sides of space, the body, or both (see Stimulus neglect)
e. A decrease in intrinsic motivation and interest (see Abulia)
f. Failure to sustain ongoing movements (see Motor impersistence)
g. Reflexive sucking movements in response to stimulation around the mouth *(positive suck reflex)* in patients who have akinetic mutism
h. Raising and pulling back of the upper lip in response to stimulation above the lips *(positive snout reflex)* in patients who have akinetic mutism
i. Grasping in response to a stroke across the palm *(positive grasp reflex)* in patients who have akinetic mutism

j. Preserved chewing and swallowing when food is placed in the mouth in patients who have akinetic mutism
k. Preserved walking when placed in a standing position in some cases of akinetic mutism
l. Transient return of motor and verbal behavior in response to sudden or intense stimulation in patients who have akinetic mutism
m. Transient improvement of motor performance when movements require close visual guidance (e.g., when climbing stairs or stepping over an object)
n. Markedly decreased size of writing *(micrographia)*
o. Rigidity of the limbs when they are moved by the examiner

Factors to Rule Out

a. Weakness sufficient to account for the failure to move
b. The locked-in syndrome: inability to move, speak, or interact with the environment except through purposeful blinking (e.g., once for "yes," twice for "no") or directional movements of the eyes (e.g., right for "yes," left for "no"), ruled out by documenting the inability to learn a communication code involving eye movements or blinks
c. Catatonic behavior: absence of movement or assumption of inflexible postures in patients who have schizophrenia, assessment procedures for detecting schizophrenia discussed in Chapter 18
d. Intentional or unconscious failure to respond to the environment (see Psychogenic unresponsiveness and Psychogenic motor dysfunction)
e. Recent use of antipsychotic drugs known to produce transient akinesia

Lesion Locations

a. Basal ganglia, often with additional involvement of the substantia nigra, locus coeruleus, subthalamic nuclei, centrum medianum of the thalamus, superior colliculis, Meynert's nucleus, of diagonal band of Broca, septal nuclei, frontal cortex, and pons[4–9]
b. Thalamus, particularly the medial thalamic nuclei[10,11]
c. Hypothalamus[12,13]
d. Reticular activating system in the brainstem (pons) and mesencephalon[14,15]
e. Medial frontal lobe, particularly the cingulate gyrus and supplementary motor area[16–20]
f. Combined temporal, parietal, and occipital lobes[21]
g. Diffuse cortical and subcortical involvement, particularly of the white matter[22–25]

Lesion Lateralization

a. May follow unilateral (right or left) or bilateral lesions
b. In unilateral cases, deficit is greatest contralateral to the lesion

2. Motor impersistence (includes motor extinction)

Clinical Indicators

a. Inability to sustain an ongoing movement
b_1. Inability to sustain or marked slowing of movement in one limb when the contralateral limb is moving *(motor extinction)*

b_2. Relatively preserved ability to sustain movement in the affected limb when the contralateral limb is still

c. Inability to maintain a specified posture or position

Associated Features

a. Weakness on one or both sides of the body

b. Failure to notice or detect stimuli on one or both sides of the body (see Stimulus neglect)

c. Absent or slow spontaneous and responsive movement (see Akinesia)

Factors to Rule Out

a. Weakness in the impersistent limb sufficient to account for the failure to sustain movements or postures, ruled out in patients with motor extinction by documenting that movement is sustained in the affected limb when the other is still

b. Automatic slowing of movement in a strong limb to keep pace with the rate of movement possible in a weak (hemiparetic) limb during bilateral simultaneous rapid motor activity, ruled out by demonstrating that the strong limb moves even more slowly than the weak limb during bilateral simultaneous movement

Lesion Locations

a. Cerebral hemisphere, particularly the parietal lobe or combined frontal, temporal, and parietal lobes[26–32]

b. Precentral gyrus, paracentral lobule[33]

c. Anterior limb of internal capsule[34]

d. Caudate nucleus of basal ganglia[35]

e. Ventral lateral thalamic nucleus[36]

Lesion Lateralization

a. More frequent following right-sided lesions

3. Adiadochokinesia and dysdiadochokinesia

Clinical Indicators

a_1. Inaccurate rapid alternation or sequencing of elementary movements as evidenced by any of the following errors:

1) Failure to learn the sequence of movements
2) Performance of movements out of sequence
3) Repetitive performance of portions of the sequence
4) Hesitant, slow, and effortful performance of the movements

a_2. Relatively preserved production or imitation of individual movements in the sequence when rapid alternation or sequencing is not required

Associated Features

a. Performance of the movement sequence improving when each movement is labeled and named as it is attempted

b. Failure to terminate movements at the required time (see Motor perseveration)

c. Inability to inhibit imitation of observed movements (see Echopraxia)

d. Weakness on one or both sides of the body
e. Impaired coordination on one or both sides of the body
f. Global decline in intellectual functioning (see Global intellectual decline)

Factors to Rule Out

a. Weakness severe enough to prevent performance of the desired movements, ruled out by documenting adequate performance of individual movements within the sequence when rapid alternation or sequencing is not required
b. A coordination deficit severe enough to prevent performance of the desired movements, ruled out by documenting adequate performance of individual movements in the sequence when rapid alternation or sequencing is not required
c. Inability to learn movement sequences as a result of severe memory impairment (see Global anterograde amnesia)

Lesion Locations

a. Cerebellum, sometimes with extension to the pons and inferior olive[37]
b. Medial frontal lobe, supplementary motor area[16]

Lesion Lateralization

Insufficient information available

4. Motor perseveration (see also Behavioral perseveration)

Clinical Indicator

a. Failure to terminate movements at the required or specified time

Associated Features

a. Perseveration most evident on motor tasks that require a set number of repetitions
b. Inaccurate rapid alternation or sequencing of movements (see Adiadochokinesia)
c. Inability to inhibit imitation of observed movements (see Echopraxia)
d. Involuntary grasping in response to stimulation of the palm *(positive grasp reflex)*
e. Impaired speech production with relatively preserved oral language comprehension and speech repetition (see Transcortical motor aphasia)
f. Failure of transfer of information from one cerebral hemisphere to the other (see Chap. 10)
g. Global decline in intellectual functioning (see Global intellectual decline)

Factor to Rule Out

a. Failure to comprehend the specified point at which a movement should be terminated

Lesion Locations

a. Frontal lobe, particularly medial lesions including the supplementary motor area, with occasional extension to the temporal lobe[17,38–41]
b. Occipital lobe in conjunction with posterior corpus callosum[42]
c. Diffuse cerebral hemisphere[43,44]
d. Basal ganglia[45]

Lesion Lateralization

a. May follow left- or right-sided lesions

5. Echopraxia

Clinical Indicators

a_1. Spontaneous imitation of observed movements

a_2. Inability to inhibit the tendency to imitate

Associated Features

a. Most evident on tasks that require a movement from the patient opposite to or at variance with observed movements

b. Inaccurate rapid alternation or sequencing of movements (see Adiadochokinesia)

c. Failure to terminate movements at the required time (see Motor perseveration)

d. Global decline in intellectual functioning (see Global intellectual decline)

Factor to Rule Out

a. Failure to comprehend the movement expected on tasks requiring a movement from the patient that is opposite to or at variance with observed movements

Lesion Locations

a. White matter beneath the angular gyrus in conjunction with thalamus[46]

Further lesion specification is not possible because of the limited data available from studies including radiologic or postmortem lesion verification.

Lesion Lateralization

Insufficient information available

6. Oculomotor apraxia (also called gaze apraxia and psychic paralysis of gaze)

Clinical Indicators

a_1. Impaired movement of the eyes on demand, as indicated by any of the following signs:

1) Failure to shift the eyes in several specified directions or toward several specified targets
2) Inability to break fixation on a point without occluding the eyes (i.e., by blinking or covering)
3) Inability to move the eyes without also moving the head in the same direction

a_2. Preserved movement of the eyes when following a target or when vision is occluded (e.g., moving the eyes beneath closed lids)

Associated Features

a. Inaccurate visual guidance of the hands when reaching (see Optic ataxia)

b. Inability to perceive more than one stimulus at a time (see Simultanagnosia)

NOTE: When optic ataxia and simultanagnosia occur with oculomotor apraxia, the entire complex is referred to as Balint's syndrome.

Factors to Rule Out

a. Weakness of the eye muscles sufficient to account for the deficit in eye movement on demand, ruled out by documenting preserved ability to follow targets or move the eyes with vision occluded

b. Decreased speed of eye movements or absence of spontaneous eye movements in a particular direction (see Akinesia) sufficient to account for the deficit in eye movement on demand, ruled out by documenting that the deficit occurs in multiple directions

Lesion Locations

a. Frontal lobe, often with extension to the parietal lobe[47–49]

For oculomotor apraxia limited to vertical gaze

a. Dorsal lateral thalamic nucleus[50]

Lesion Lateralization

a. Usually follows a bilateral lesion, although unilateral lesion cases have been reported[48]

7. Buccofacial apraxia (also called buccolingual apraxia and oral apraxia)

Clinical Indicators

a_1. Inaccurate pantomime of skilled movements of the lower face, lips, tongue, pharynx, or larynx on demand, as evidenced by either of the following errors:

1) Performance of an incorrect movement
2) Substitution of a verbal response (e.g., a description) for the target movement

a_2. Inaccurate imitation of pantomimed skilled movements of the lower face, lips, tongue, pharynx, or larynx

a_3. Deficits in pantomime and imitation on demand occur on both sides of the face

a_4. Relatively preserved performance of skilled movements of the lower face, lips, tongue, larynx, and pharynx, when an object (e.g., a straw or cigarette) is present to facilitate target movements

a_5. Relatively preserved performance of skilled movements of the lower face, lips, tongue, larynx, and pharynx when an appropriate context (e.g., needing to whistle for a taxi) present to elicit target movements

Associated Features

a. Relatively preserved performance of movements involving the upper face on demand

b. Unilateral weakness of the muscles of the face

c. Oral language disorders, particularly Broca's aphasia, conduction aphasia, and mutism (see Chap. 12)

d. Impaired performance of skilled movements of the arms and hands on demand (see Ideomotor and ideational apraxia)

e. Relatively preserved facial expression of emotion both on demand and in situations that elicit emotional reactions

Factors to Rule Out

a. Weakness of the muscles of the face sufficient to account for the deficit in pantomime and imitation of skilled movements, ruled out by documenting preserved elicitation of facial movements by objects
b. Poor coordination of the muscles of the face sufficient to account for the deficit in pantomime and imitation of skilled movements, ruled out by documenting preserved elicitation of facial movements by objects
c. Impaired initiation of facial movements (see Akinesia), ruled out by documenting preserved elicitation of facial movements by objects
d. Impaired ability to sustain movements of the face (see Motor impersistence), ruled out by documenting preserved elicitation of facial movements by objects
e. Failure to terminate facial movements at the required time (see Motor perseveration), ruled out by documenting preserved performance when objects are present to facilitate facial movements
f. Failure to comprehend commands as a result of oral language disorders (see Chap. 12 for assessment procedures)

Lesion Locations

a. Cerebral hemisphere without further localization[51]
b. Perisylvian, predominantly the frontal operculum, but often also including central operculum, anterior insula, and the first temporal convolution, with occasional extension to the parietal lobe, lenticular nucleus of the basal ganglia, and paraventricular white matter[52–56]
c. Combined basal ganglia, anterior limb of internal capsule, and anterior paraventricular white matter[56]

Lesion Lateralization

a. Language-dominant hemisphere or bilateral lesions, although cases of "crossed" buccofacial apraxia following lesions in the hemisphere nondominant for language have been reported[51]

8. Disassociation apraxia (see also Unilateral disassociation apraxia)*

Clinical Indicators

a_1. Inaccurate pantomime of skilled movements of the arms and hands on both sides of the body on verbal demand
a_2. Relatively preserved bilateral imitation of pantomimed skilled movements of the arms and hands
a_3. Relatively preserved bilateral performance of skilled movements of the arms and hands when an object (e.g., a comb or key) present to facilitate the target movements
NOTE: This pattern of impaired pantomime on verbal demand with preserved imitation and object use is termed verbal-motor disassociation apraxia.

*This disorder must be considered putative because there are relatively few published cases.

b_1. Inaccurate imitation of pantomimed skilled movements of the arms and hands on both sides of the body

b_2. Relatively preserved bilateral pantomime of skilled movements of arms and hands on verbal demand

b_3. Relatively preserved bilateral performance of skilled movements of the arms and hands when an object (e.g., a comb or key) is present to facilitate the target movements

NOTE: This pattern of impaired imitation with preserved pantomime on verbal demand and with object use is termed visuomotor disassociation apraxia.

c_1. Inaccurate performance of skilled movements of the arms and hands on both sides of the body when using objects

c_2. Relatively preserved bilateral pantomime of skilled movements of the arms and hands on verbal demand

c_3. Relatively preserved bilateral imitation of pantomimed skilled movements of the arms and hands

NOTE: This pattern of impaired object use with preserved pantomime on verbal demand and imitation is termed tactile-motor disassociation apraxia.

Associated Features

a. Preserved recognition of pantomimed movements in patients who have verbal-motor disassociation apraxia
b. Relatively preserved bilateral performance of skilled movements of the arms and hands when an appropriate context (e.g., wanting to wave to someone through a window) present to elicit target movements in patients who have verbal-motor or visuomotor disassociation apraxia
c. A recent history of ideomotor apraxia in patients who have verbal-motor disassociation apraxia

Factors to Rule Out

a. Weakness of the muscles of the arms or hands sufficient to account for the deficits in performance of skilled movements, ruled out by demonstrating preserved use of the arms and hands during pantomime, imitation, or object use
b. Unilateral verbal-motor disassociation apraxia (see Chap. 10), can be ruled out only when assessment is possible on both sides of the body
c. Impaired coordination of the muscles of the arms or hands sufficient to account for the deficits in performance of skilled movements, ruled out by documenting preserved use of the arms and hands during pantomime, imitation, or object use
d. Impaired initiation of movements of the arms or hands (see Akinesia) sufficient to account for the deficits in performance of skilled movements, ruled out by documenting preserved use of the arms and hands during pantomime, imitation, or object use
e. Impaired ability to sustain movements of the arms or hands (see Motor im-

persistence) sufficient to account for the deficits in performance of skilled movements, ruled out by documenting preserved use of the arms and hands during pantomime, imitation, or object use

f. Failure to terminate movements at the required time (see Motor perseveration), ruled out by documenting preserved use of the arms and hands during pantomime, imitation, or object use

g. Failure to comprehend commands as a result of oral language disorder sufficient to account for a deficit in pantomime on verbal demand (see Chap. 12 for assessment procedures)

Lesion Locations

Insufficient data available

Lesion Lateralization

Insufficient data available

9. Unilateral verbal-motor disassociation apraxia (see Chap. 10)

10. Ideomotor apraxia (see also Unilateral ideomotor apraxia)

Clinical Indicators

a_1. Inaccurate pantomime of skilled movements of the arms and hands on both sides of the body on verbal demand as evidenced by any of the following errors:

1) Performance of an incorrect but recognizable movement *(parapraxia)*
2) Performance of a partial movement that is an abridgement of the target movement
3) Performance of a distorted and unrecognizable movement
4) Use of a body part as if it were an object
5) Incorrect orientation of the arm, hand, or fingers for the movement being attempted
6) Substitution of a verbal response (e.g., a description) for the target movement

a_2. Inaccurate imitation of pantomimed skilled movements of the arms and hands on both sides of the body as a result of any of the errors listed previously

a_3. Inaccurate performance of skilled movements of the arms and hands when using objects as a result of any of the following errors:

1) Performance of a movement not appropriate for the object
2) Performance of a partial movement that is an abridgement of the target movement
3) Incorrect orientation of the arm, hand, or fingers with respect to the object
4) Incorrect orientation of the object in space
5) Use of a body part as if it were an object

Associated Features

a. Pantomime on demand possibly impaired more than imitation and object use

b. Imitation of pantomimed movements possibly impaired more than object use
c. Axial movements (i.e., movements involving the head and trunk) possibly preserved
d. Object use and imitation of pantomimed movements recovering first, leaving a verbal-motor disassociation apraxia
e. Weakness of the muscles on one side of the body (hemiparesis)
f. Impaired oral language (see Chap. 12)
g. Recognition of pantomimed movements may be impaired
h. Difficulty learning new motor skills
i. Impaired sequencing of a series of movements (see Ideational apraxia)

Factors to Rule Out

a. Unilaterally impaired pantomime of skilled movements on demand (see Unilateral ideomotor apraxia), can be ruled out only when assessment is possible on both sides of the body
b. Weakness of the muscles of the arms or hands sufficient to account for the deficits in performance of skilled movements
c. Impaired coordination of the muscles of the arms or hands sufficient to account for the deficits in performance of skilled movements
d. Impaired initiation of movements of the arms or hands (see Akinesia) sufficient to account for the deficits in performance of skilled movements
e. Impaired ability to sustain movements of the arms or hands (see Motor impersistence) sufficient to account for the deficits in performance of skilled movements
f. Failure to terminate arm or hand movements at the required time (see Motor perseveration) sufficient to account for the deficits in skilled movements
g. Failure to comprehend commands as a result of oral language disorder sufficient to account for the deficits in performance of skilled movements (see Chap. 12 for assessment techniques)

Lesion Locations

a. Parietal lobe, particularly the parietal operculum, supramarginal and angular gyri, and subjacent white matter,* with occasional extension to the frontal lobe[57–62]
b. Supplementary motor area of the medial frontal lobe, with occasional extension to the corpus callosum[17,62]
c. Insular cortex and adjacent white matter, with extension to medial surface of the combined frontal, temporal, and parietal operculum[63]
d. Basal ganglia, particularly the caudate nucleus and lenticular nuclei, with occasional extension to the anterior limb of the internal capsule or thalamus[64,65]

*Patients with lesions in these areas are likely to be impaired in their recognition of movements pantomimed by the examiner, but if the lesion is confined to subjacent white matter, recognition may be spared.

Lesion Lateralization

a. More common following left-sided lesions[66]

11. Unilateral ideomotor apraxia (see Chap. 10)

12. Ideational apraxia

Clinical Indicators

a_1. Inaccurate sequencing of the individual steps within a goal-directed series of actions, as evidenced by any of the following errors:
   1) Confusion of the sequential order of the series
   2) Omission of one or more steps within the series
   3) Substitution of incorrect actions for one or more of the actions in the series
   4) Inability to use a tool to act on another object

a_2. Relatively preserved performance of individual actions within the series on verbal demand

a_3. Relatively preserved imitation of individual actions within the series

Associated Features

a. High variability in the occurrence of sequencing errors
b. Sequencing errors occurring regardless of which hand is used
c. Inaccurate pantomime of skilled movements on demand (see Ideomotor apraxia)
d. Oral language disorders (see Chap. 12)
e. Inaccurate drawing of models or construction of two- or three-dimensional puzzles (see Constructional disability)
f. Decreased global intellectual functioning (see Global intellectual decline)
g. Confused ideation (see Ideational disorientation and confusion)
h. Impaired recognition of the fingers of the hands (see Finger agnosia)
i. Failure to terminate movements at the required time (see Motor perseveration)

Factors to Rule Out

a. Impaired pantomime of skilled movements on demand (see Ideomotor and disassociation apraxia) sufficient to account for the sequencing deficit, ruled out by documenting the preservation of individual actions within the series
b. Weakness of the muscles of the arms or hands sufficient to account for the sequencing deficit, ruled out by documenting preserved imitation of individual actions within the series
c. Impaired coordination of the muscles of the arms or hands sufficient to account for the sequencing deficit, ruled out by documenting preserved imitation of individual actions within the series
d. Impaired initiation of movements of the arms or hands (see Akinesia) sufficient to account for the sequencing deficit, ruled out by documenting preserved imitation of individual actions within the series
e. Impaired ability to persist with movements of the arms or hands (see Motor impersistence)

f. Failure to terminate movements at the required time (see Motor perseveration)
g. Failure to comprehend commands as a result of oral language disorder sufficient to account for the sequencing deficit (see Chap. 12 for assessment procedures)
h. Failure to recall the steps required to accomplish the goal

Lesion Locations

a. Frontal lobe, particularly the anterior insula, precentral gyrus, foot of the inferior and middle frontal gyri, and supplementary motor area, alone or with extension to the temporal and parietal lobes[67,68]
b. Temporal lobe, particularly the lateral surface, alone or with extension to the frontal and parietal lobes[67,68]
c. Parietal lobe, particularly the inferior-posterior aspect, alone or with extension to the frontal and temporal lobes[67–69]

13. Constructional apraxia (see Constructional disability)

14. Dressing apraxia (see Hemispatial neglect)

15. Diagonistic apraxia (see Chap. 10)

16. Apraxic agraphia (see Chap. 13)

17. Psychogenic motor dysfunction

Clinical Indicators

a_1. Severity of motor impairment exceeds the known extent of the illness or brain lesion

a_2. Atypical course or presentation of the motor impairment, as evidenced by any of the following signs:
1) Absence of a clear precipitating illness or brain lesion
2) An unaccountable lag between the onset of the illness or lesion and the onset of the motor impairment
3) Inconsistent motor performance across equivalent examinations
4) Inconsistent motor performance across equivalent situations (e.g., situations that place equal demands on motor performance and that are equally likely to elicit or facilitate motor performance)

a_3. Motivational factors contribute to the presence of the motor impairment, as evidenced by any of the following signs:
1) Failure to exert the effort required to perform motor tasks
2) Motor impairment permitting avoidance of unpleasant consequences or responsibilities
3) Motor impairment leading to, or expected to soon produce, emotional benefits or material compensation

Associated Features

a. Some degree of impaired motor performance as a result of neurological illness or a brain lesion
b. Depressed mood or major depressive disorder

c. Fear or anxiety
d. Hysterical conversion disorder: a mental disorder characterized by the unconscious expression of mental and emotional conflicts and stress via physical symptoms
e. Pain when performing movements
f. Post-traumatic stress disorder: a mental disorder arising after the experience of intense emotional or physical trauma and stress, characterized by panic, a tendency to re-experience the source of trauma in dreams or waking flashbacks, and re-enactment of behavior shown at the time of the original trauma
g. Malingering: deliberate feigning of symptoms to obtain a goal
h. Factitious disorder: a mental disorder characterized by intentional feigning of symptoms as a result of a need to assume a sick role
i. Somatization disorder: a mental disorder characterized by a history of multiple physical complaints of uncertain cause

Factor to Rule Out

a. Neurological illness or a brain lesion of sufficient extent to account for the motor impairment, ruled out by documenting the excessiveness of the motor impairment and an atypical pattern or course of impairment

Lesion Location

Not associated with structural brain damage

ETIOLOGY

The most common cause of disorders of voluntary cognitive control of movement is cerebrovascular disease. The apraxias are often the result of an embolic or thrombotic infarction in the distribution of the middle cerebral artery. Adiadochokinesia may be seen in patients who have cerebrovascular disease involving the vertebrobasilar arteries. Traumatic brain injury, particularly involving direct or contrecoup damage to the frontal portions of the brain, may produce motor impersistence, adiadochokinesia, motor perseveration, or echopraxia. Parkinson's disease includes akinesia as one of its core symptoms. Akinesia may also be seen in cases of progressive supernuclear palsy, Shy-Drager syndrome, and diffuse Lewy body formation, as well as in a rare form of Huntington's disease.[7]

Neoplasm in the areas associated with the various movement disorders is another etiologic factor. Degenerative diseases (e.g., Alzheimer's disease) are closely associated with ideational and ideomotor apraxia but can also lead to any of the other disorders discussed in this chapter.

As its name implies, psychogenic motor dysfunction has a psychological or motivational etiology. The patient consciously or unconsciously chooses not to perform motor tasks that are within his or her physical capacity. When this choice is conscious, it serves to abet the avoidance of undesirable situations or to increase the likelihood of emotional or material compensation. Patients who experience pain during certain motor activities and who have a limited pain tolerance may also develop psychogenic motor dysfunction as a means of avoiding pain. Even when the cause of the pain has been successfully treated or the patient has been given analgesics, he or she may continue to avoid certain motor activities because of the anticipation of pain.

When the motor dysfunction is produced unconsciously, an underlying mental disorder usually is found. The most extreme presentations of the disorder occur in patients who have hysterical conversion reactions, factitious disorder, or somatization disorder, and in some patients with post-traumatic stress disorder. Less severe manifestations of psychogenic motor dysfunction can occur in depressed patients who lack the motivation to perform. Similarly, psychogenic motor dysfunction can occur in highly anxious patients who cannot perform certain motor tasks (often tasks that involve a risk of falling) because of fearfulness or a lack of confidence in their own ability.

Although psychogenic motor dysfunction does not have a direct physiological cause, it often accompanies physical illness, including neurological disease. This association must not be overlooked when diagnosing and treating patients with this disorder.

DISABLING CONSEQUENCES

The ability to drive is compromised by all the movement disorders except buccofacial apraxia. Disassociation apraxia, depending on the specific manner in which movement is interrupted, may or may not impede driving. When the apraxia is limited to pantomime and does not impact actual object use, the ability to drive may be preserved. Even in these cases, careful evaluation of driving safety in realistic road conditions is essential.

Work that requires fine or gross movements, ambulation, or rapid performance is impossible for patients who have moderate or severe degrees of akinesia, echopraxia, impersistence, motor perseveration, or apraxia. Even mild presentations of these disorders can restrict work performance. Adiadochokinesia primarily impedes work that requires speed and finely coordinated movements of the hands. Performance of domestic chores is also likely to be impeded by these movement disorders, and if the deficits are sufficiently severe, patients may not be safe when left alone for extended periods of time.

Ordinarily, buccofacial apraxia disables only people in highly specialized occupations such as acting. However, when buccofacial apraxia and oral language disorder occur together, the potential for disability rises. Not only is communication restricted, but the likelihood that therapy will improve speech greatly diminishes. In general, when deficits in movement and oral language combine, patients are apt to be disabled severely for extended periods of time, if not permanently. Treatment of these patients is difficult and often produces less than optimal results.

Psychogenic motor dysfunction is temporarily disabling, but once it is diagnosed and treated, no permanent disability should occur. When psychogenic motor dysfunction accompanies physical illness, the disability attributable to the physical illness remains after treatment of the former condition.

ASSESSMENT INSTRUMENTS

Benton Motor Impersistence Test

The Benton Motor Impersistence Test (MIT)[70] can be obtained from *Oxford University Press, Incorporated, 200 Madison Avenue, New York, NY, 10016.*

The MIT consists of eight subtests requiring the maintenance of movements or postures for specified periods. Movements involve the eyes, tongue, mouth, and head. Adult normative data are based on 106 patients without brain damage, ranging in age from 16 to 66 years. The MIT appears to be sensitive to motor impersistence deficits in both brain-damaged and schizophrenic samples.[70] Tests requiring the patient to maintain eyelid closure are particularly sensitive measures of motor impersistence,[27] and such procedures are incorporated in the MIT.

Reliability studies, many of which were conducted in children, are summarized in the test manual. Inter-judge agreement is described as "satisfactory," whereas test-retest reliability results vary among studies, with some investigators reporting stability over time and others finding changes of two or more total points.[70]

The MIT can be used to document not only motor impersistence but also akinesia. I extend the examination to the upper extremities by having patients pat their hands palm side down on the table as rapidly as possible for 20 seconds. Each hand is tested separately; then both hands are tested together. Performance is rated qualitatively as adequate or impaired based on three factors:

1. The capacity to tap rapidly (at least 10 taps in 5 seconds)
2. The capacity to sustain a steady rate of tapping for the full 20 seconds
3. The capacity to maintain the same rate of tapping in each hand regardless of whether the opposite hand is also tapping

The MIT can be quickly administered, even with my additions. It is appropriate for bedside, office, or laboratory administration. Interpretation should be attempted only by neurologists, neurosurgeons, physiatrists, neuropsychologists, and occupational therapists because of the multiple cognitive and motor factors that can impact MIT results.

Rapid Alternating and Sequential Movements

The Rapid Alternating and Sequential Movements test is *not commercially available.*

Three rapid alternating movement sequences are described. The first is drawn from the standard neurological examination; the second and third are based on procedures used in Luria's Neuropsychological Investigation.[71]

1. Rapid pronation-supination: The patient places his or her open hands on a flat surface and is instructed to rapidly alternate the hands between pronation and supination. Each hand is tested separately, then both hands are tested simultaneously. I request that 15 alternations be performed in 10 seconds; one pronation plus one supination is counted as one alternation. A 5-second practice trial is allowed with each hand before the test trials begin. The total number of alternations within

10 seconds is recorded. A notation is made if the patient is unable to alternate between pronation and supination (e.g., begins to repetitively pat the table with the palm), is clumsy in alternating, or is markedly slow in his or her performance.

2. Alternating hand positions: The right hand is placed palm down on a flat surface with fingers clenched, while the left hand lies next to it with fingers open. The patient is asked to shift rapidly between clenching and unclenching the fingers of each hand so that one hand is flat while the other is clenched. I request that 20 shifts be performed in 10 seconds. A 5-second practice trial is allowed before the test trial begins. The number of shifts accomplished within the period is recorded. A notation is made if the patient is slow, clumsy, or begins simultaneously clenching and unclenching the fingers of both hands instead of alternating hands.

3. Fist-edge-palm sequence: The examiner demonstrates the sequence of hand positions (fist flat on the table, edge of hand on the table, palm on the table) and asks the patient to imitate the movements. After the patient successfully imitates the sequence, he or she is asked to continue without the examiner's modeling the movements. If the patient loses the sequence, he or she is instructed to imitate again and then to try the sequence alone. If the patient fails, each hand position is labeled ("fist," "edge," and "palm"), and the patient is asked to attempt the sequence with the examiner's verbal guidance. The patient should then attempt the sequence alone, intoning the label for each position as it is performed. If the patient still fails to perform the sequence independently, the task is discontinued.

After the patient can complete three independent runs through the entire sequence, with or without verbal labels, the examiner requests 10 more rapid executions of the entire sequence. No time limit is specified, but the patient is encouraged to execute the sequence as rapidly as possible. Testing is discontinued after 30 seconds. The number of correctly completed sequences and the time elapsed are recorded for the initial hand used by the patient.

The opposite hand is then tested without benefit of further instruction in the sequence. The patient does not have to reach a criterion of three correctly completed sequences and can proceed directly to attempting 10 rapid alternations with the other hand. The number of correct sequences and the elapsed time are recorded. Notations should be made whenever the patient confuses the order or leaves out steps in the sequence with either hand. Clumsiness and slowness should also be noted.

Empirically derived reliability and validity data are not available for these rapid alternating and sequential movement procedures. Most healthy individuals can perform the movements with ease within the established time limits. My experience suggests that normal elderly individuals, however, may have difficulty maintaining the order of the fist-edge-palm sequence and may show slowing of performance in all three procedures.

Besides cognitive dysfunction, performance of these three procedures can be affected by pain in the upper extremities, poor coordination, or weakness. The multiple factors that must be considered when attempting to interpret the results of these procedures requires the examiner be experienced with patients with neurological problems. The procedures are recommended for use only by neurologists, neurosurgeons, physiatrists, neuropsychologists, and occupational therapists. Bedside, office, and laboratory administration are all feasible.

Tandem Reciprocal Movements

The Tandem Reciprocal Movements procedure, also called Contrasting Motor Programs, is *not commercially available.*

This procedure is drawn from Luria's Neuropsychological Investigation.[71] The patient is asked to hold up two fingers when the examiner holds up one finger and one finger when the examiner holds up two fingers. The instructions are given without initially stating the number of fingers that are to be held up. Instead, the examiner states, "When I do this," while holding up one finger, "you do this," while holding up two fingers. If the patient cannot demonstrate what is required in response to the examiner's one- and two-finger signals, the number of fingers each person is to hold up may be explicitly stated. If the patient still fails to respond correctly, testing should be discontinued.

After it is clear that the patient comprehends the procedure, the examiner proceeds with testing. The examiner attempts to establish a response set by holding up the same number of fingers for several trials and then suddenly shifting to a different number of fingers to see if the patient shifts his or her response accordingly. The number of trials can vary from patient to patient, but to standardize the procedure, I prefer to administer 11 trials, shifting after every second response (e.g., one finger, one finger, two fingers, two fingers, one finger). A second block of 16 trials is then administered, with the shift occurring after every third response. Trial 11 from the first block is the first trial in the second block, so that no interruption occurs between blocks. In this manner, each trial block contains an opportunity for five shifts.

When the patient responds incorrectly during the procedure, he or she should be quickly corrected (e.g., "No, you should have held up two fingers") and the test continued. One or both hands may be tested. No repetition of instructions is required after completing testing with one hand unless performance is grossly impaired. The number of correct responses in 27 trials is recorded separately for each hand. Incorrect responses that the patient rapidly (within 3 seconds) self-corrects are counted as correct. Two types of error are noted: slavish imitation of the examiner's movement (e.g., holding up one finger when the examiner holds up one finger) and failing to shift to a new response when the examiner shifts to a different number of fingers.

Reliability and validity data are unavailable. My experience has been that reciprocal movements are easily performed by healthy individuals with no more than one or two errors expected. The procedure is appropriate for bedside, office, or laboratory administration. Interpretation is relatively straightforward, and the procedure is appropriate for use by neuropsychologists, neurologists, neurosurgeons, physiatrists, and occupational therapists.

Repetitive Graphomotor Sequences

The Repetitive Graphomotor Sequences (triple loops and alternating "m" and "n") are *not commercially available.*

These procedures are derived from Luria's Neuropsychological Investigation.[71] Patients are shown a drawing of a triple loop (Fig. 11–1) and are asked to copy it exactly as shown. The number of requested reproductions varies from setting to setting. To standardize the procedure, I request 10 reproductions. More reproductions can be requested if subtle motor perseveration is suspected. Performance of the opposite hand can also be assessed. The graphic quality of the reproduction is less important than producing the correct number of loops. The number of extra loops in each reproduction is counted and summed separately for each hand. Patients who make fewer than three loops per reproduction are reinstructed in the procedure.

An alternative procedure involves showing the patient a series of alternating "m"s and "n"s written in connected cursive script. Usually, six letters (three "m"s and three "n"s in alternating sequence) are sufficient to demonstrate the task. The patient is asked to continue the alternating pattern for another three to five lines. One or both hands can be tested, and the number of letter perseverations (failure to alternate) are summed separately for each hand.

Reliability and validity data are not available for these procedures. My experience suggests that healthy individuals perform these tasks with no difficulty. The examiner should expect at most one or two errors on these tasks in normal populations, but even this number of errors raises suspicion of impairment and is justification for extending the number of trials. These procedures may be administered at bedside, in the office, or in the laboratory and are appropriate for use by physicians, psychologists, speech pathologists, and occupational therapists.

Oculomotor Apraxia Procedure

The Oculomotor Apraxia Procedure is *not commercially available.*

In random order, patients are told to look up, down, right, and left. Each direction is tested twice, and each trial is scored as passed or failed. Patients who cannot distinguish left from right can be requested to look at specific objects in each direction. Head turning is not permitted; in some instances, it may be necessary to hold the patient's head stationary during testing.

If his or her performance is defective, the patient is asked to follow the examiner's finger with his or her eyes. The examiner's finger is moved in each direction, and performance in each direction is scored as passed or failed. The latter trials help to distinguish weakness of the eye muscles from oculomotor apraxia. I have found it helpful with some patients to hold the eyelids shut while the patient moves his or her eyes in each direction. The movement of the eyes can usually be detected through the closed lids. Spared eye movements with the eyes closed helps to rule out motor weakness as a cause of the deficit when the eyes are open.

Oculomotor apraxia should be diagnosed only when the deficit in shifting gaze occurs in at least three directions. Elderly individuals may exhibit upgaze deficiencies alone, and hemiakinetic patients may show a deficit in moving their eyes or in tracking objects in one lateral direction. These findings should not be considered diagnostic of oculomotor apraxia. The Oculomotor Apraxia Procedure can be administered at bedside, in the office, or in the laboratory. It is recommended that interpretation be attempted only by neurologists, ophthalmologists, physiatrists, neuropsychologists, and neuro-optometrists because of the unavailability of empirically derived reliability and validity data.

Boston Spatial-Quantitative Battery, Apraxia Subtest

The Boston Spatial-Quantitative Battery (BSQB), Apraxia Subtest,[72] is *not commercially available.*

This test can be constructed from information provided by Goodglass and Kaplan.[72] The patient is asked to perform buccofacial, limb (ideomotor), whole-body, and serial (ideational) movements specified by the examiner. In the standard administration, performance is assessed in one hand under three conditions: pantomime to command, imitated pantomime, and using real objects. Imitation and use of real objects are assessed only when the patient fails to pantomime on command in the standard administration. I recommend, however, that the standard administration not be followed. Performance should be assessed separately in each hand. In addition, imitation and object use should be assessed in all patients regardless of whether they fail to pantomime on command. Failure to do so can lead to a failure to detect some apraxia subtypes. Notation of the specific type of errors exhibited by the patient is also important.

Reliability coefficients are not reported for the BSQB, and normative data are unavailable. Consequently, interpretation of the results should be attempted only by neurologists, neurosurgeons, physiatrists, neuropsychologists, speech pathologists, and occupational therapists with extensive experience in the diagnosis of apraxia. The test is appropriate for bedside, office, or laboratory administration.

Western Aphasia Battery, Apraxia Subtest

The Western Aphasia Battery (WAB), Apraxia Subtest,[73] can be obtained from *Grune & Stratton, Incorporated, Orlando, FL 32809.*

In this test, patients are asked to perform facial, upper limb, instrumental (ideomotor), and complex (ideational) pantomime movements. If patients fail to perform the movements on demand, their ability to imitate movements of the examiner is assessed. If this method fails, the patient's ability to perform movements using actual objects is assessed. Performance is assessed in one hand only. A previous version of the WAB Apraxia Subtest was normed on 215 aphasic patients and 63 normal and nonaphasic brain-damaged controls.[74] The prior version of the WAB had high intra-judge (.983 to .989) and inter-judge (.996) reliability, but lower test-retest reliability (.581).[75] The current version of the apraxia subtest correlates .97 with the previous version.[73] The validity studies conducted on the WAB have centered on the diagnosis of aphasia rather than apraxia. It should be noted, however, that the Apraxia Subtest appears to be capable of differentiating skilled movement deficits from language comprehension deficits in aphasic patients using the imitation and object-use trials.[74]

Once again, I recommend that the standard administration be expanded to permit more precise detection and diagnosis. Testing should be conducted separately in each hand for all commands involving the arms and hands, and imitation and object use should be assessed in all patients, regardless of whether they fail to pantomime on command. Notation of the specific types of errors exhibited by the patient is also important to incorporate in the examination. Interpretation of Apraxia Subtest results should be attempted only by neuropsychologists, neurologists, neurosurgeons, physiatrists, speech pathologists, and occupational therapists who have extensive experience in the diagnosis of apraxia. The subtest is appropriate for bedside, office, or laboratory administration.

Hand Dynamometer

The Hand Dynamometer can be obtained from *The Stoelting Company, Oakwood Center, 620 Wheat Lane, Wood Dale, IL 60191*.

The Hand Dynamometer is composed of a stirrup that moves a dial when it is gripped in the hand and squeezed. The dial records the strength of the patient's grip in kilograms. One practice trial and two test trials are performed with each hand; the score for each hand is the average of the test trials. Additional trials can be administered until two trials with results within 5 kg of each other are obtained.

Grip strength varies with age (elderly individuals tend to have weaker grips than young adults), gender (females tend to have weaker grips than males), and hand tested (the nondominant hand tends to be weaker than the dominant hand). Normative data for each hand are available for adults aged 20 to 80 years, with corrections for gender, age, and education.[76] Test-retest reliability coefficients vary from .52 to .96 among studies employing the Hand Dynamometer.[77–80] Grip strength has been reported to discriminate healthy from brain-damaged individuals and to differentiate between patients with left- and right-sided lesions.[81–83]

The Hand Dynamometer provides a quick means of detecting decreases in motor strength that could affect performance on tests of cognitive regulation of movement. Performance on the Hand Dynamometer is affected by motivation, and low grip-strength scores can sometimes be the result of emotional rather than neurological factors. The Hand Dynamometer can be administered in the office, laboratory, or at bedside, although the patient must either stand or sit on the side of the bed. The test can be used by physicians, psychologists, nurses, and occupational and physical therapists. If low motivation is suspected, results should be evaluated and interpreted by a neurologist, physiatrist, orthopedist, or psychologist.

Halstead-Reitan Battery, Finger-Tapping Test

The Halstead Reitan Battery (HRB), Finger-Tapping Test,[84] can be obtained from *Reitan Neuropsychological Laboratory, 1338 East Edison Street, Tucson, AZ 85719.*

In this test, patients tap a key with their index fingers as rapidly as possible for 10 seconds while a counter records the number of taps. Five trials are typically obtained using each hand, but some examiners administer as many trials as needed up to a maximum of 10 to obtain 5 trials for each hand that are within five taps of each other. The score is the average of all 5 trials or the average of the 5 trials that are within five points of each other, and separate scores are calculated for each hand. Normative data with demographic corrections are available for individuals aged 20 to 80 years.[76]

The Finger-Tapping Test has high internal consistency (.99).[85] Test-retest reliability coefficients reported in the literature vary from .24 to .81 among normal and patient samples.[86,87] The Finger-Tapping Test has been reported to discriminate normal control[88] and blind[89] persons from brain-damaged patients at statistically significant levels. It does not, however, appear to be sensitive to mild degrees of brain dysfunction.[90] Lateralized lesions typically produce a contralateral lowering of finger-tapping performance, but in my experience, it is not uncommon for lateralized lesions to lower performance in both hands. Even in these instances, the deficit typically is still more severe in the contralateral hand.

In addition to the contribution the Finger-Tapping Test makes to the HRB, on its own it provides a useful measure of motor speed and coordination. The test requires minimal visual guidance, as evidenced by the fact that blind individuals can perform the test at a level above that achieved by brain-damaged patients.[89] The Finger-Tapping Test can be administered in office and laboratory settings, or at bedside if a flat surface is available. Neuropsychologists trained and experienced in administering and interpreting the HRB are most qualified to interpret Finger-Tapping Test results.

Grooved Pegboard

The Grooved Pegboard can be obtained from *Psychological Assessment Resources, Incorporated, P.O. Box 998, Odessa, FL 33556.*

In this test, patients rotate ridged pegs to fit them into variously angled slots. Twenty-five slots, arranged in equal rows of five, must be filled as rapidly as possible while the examiner records the time to completion and the number of pegs dropped. Each hand is tested separately. Normative data are available for adults aged 20 to 80 years, with corrections for age, gender, and education.[76] Unilateral brain damage lowers the performance of the contralateral hand on Grooved Pegboard, but may also lower the performance of the ipsilateral hand.[91,92]

The Grooved Pegboard provides a quick measure of hand coordination. Empirical investigation of the reliability of the test is needed. The test is best administered in office and laboratory settings, but can be administered at bedside if a flat surface is available and the patient can assume a sitting position. It is recommended for use by psychologists, occupational therapists, and vocational evaluators.

Pin Test

The Pin Test[93] can be obtained from *Psychological Assessment Resources, P.O. Box 998, Odessa, FL 33556.*

The Pin Test measures fine motor coordination, visual guidance of movement, and hand dominance by requiring patients to punch holes through a response sheet as indicated by a printed pattern of dots. Holes are punched using a straight pin. Two 30-second trials are administered for each hand, and the score consists of a tally of the holes punched by each hand. An "advantage index" can be calculated by dividing the total number of holes punched with the dominant hand by the total number of holes punched with the nondominant hand. The advantage index provides a measure of handedness in patients who do not have unilateral motor deficits.

Normative data are based on 598 healthy volunteers ranging in age from 16 to 69 years. A significant age effect was found in the normative sample, with Pin Test scores peaking in the 30- to 39-year-old age range and decreasing for individuals older than 40 years of age.[93] Age-stratified normative tables are included in the manual. A significant decline in test performance with increasing age and the absence of norms for individuals aged 70 years or older make the Pin Test unsuitable for neurological patients of very advanced age. Pin Test performance increases slightly with practice but not enough that this poses an interpretive problem across the two trials administered to each hand.[93] Test-retest reliability coefficients of .83 for the dominant hand and .74 for the nondominant hand are reported over a test-retest interval of 5 to 20 days.[93] The Pin Test is reported in the manual to classify virtually all normals correctly in terms of their self-reported handedness and to be sensitive to the motor effects of traumatic brain injury.

The Pin Test can be administered at bedside if a flat surface is available, in the office, and in the laboratory. Interpretation is relatively straightforward and can be attempted by physicians, psychologists, and occupational therapists.

Behavioral Monitoring Procedure

The Behavioral Monitoring Procedure is *not commercially available.*

Intermittent motor regulation disorders (e.g., motor perseveration, echopraxia) are not always elicited by direct testing. In these instances, diagnosis may depend on sustained observation of the patient and assessment when the disorder happens to manifest itself. A Behavioral Monitoring Procedure is presented in Chapter 3 for use in detecting concentration deficits. The same procedure and forms can be adapted for use with intermittent motor regulation disorders.

Modified Annett Handedness Inventory

The Modified Annett Handedness Inventory is *not commercially available*, but can be constructed from published accounts.[94] The original Annett Handedness Inventory consisted of 12 questions about which hand the patient uses to perform functions such as write, throw, play racquet games, cut with scissors, thread a needle, deal cards, use a hammer, and use a toothbrush. The original inventory has been modified by adding questions that request information on the handedness of parents and siblings and information on eye dominance.[94] A strength-of-preference scale has also been added, permitting patients to respond "always left," "usually left," "no preference," "usually right," or "always right" to each hand preference question. Responses are scored using a point system that assigns positive values to right-hand answers and negative values to left-hand answers, with "no preference" scored as a zero. The addition of the strength-of-preference scale permits more accurate determination of ambidexterity.[94]

The original Annett Inventory was reported to have a test-retest reliability (kappa) coefficient of .80 in a normal sample, using a retest interval of 14 weeks.[95] Kendall's coefficient of concordance was high ($W = .92, p < .001$) for the 12 items of the inventory scored using the strength-of-preference scale in a sample of 1599 college students. The high concordance coefficient suggests good agreement among the 12 items of the inventory dealing with patient handedness. Studies examining the correlation of inventory responses and observed hand preferences during performance of actual tasks are necessary to evaluate the Annett Inventory's validity. The Annett Inventory provides a simple and quick method for determining hand preferences that can be administered at bedside, in the office, or in the laboratory by most health care professionals.

NEUROPSYCHOLOGICAL TREATMENT

Treatment of the disorders of voluntary cognitive control of movement is not a part of the practice of most neuropsychologists. Buccofacial apraxia is usually addressed by speech therapists. Occupational therapists address the other disorders when they manifest themselves in the upper extremities or in general self-care or vocational activities. Speech therapists may work with patients having upper extremity apraxia, perseveration, impersistence, and akinesia, because these disorders affect written communication. Recreation therapists, through the use of crafts, board games, social activities, and community outings, are also able to provide appropriate and challenging situations for patients with impaired movement.

The neuropsychologist's contribution to the treatment of these disorders usually takes the form of recommendations for optimizing treatment success. Neuropsychological examination may reveal that an apraxic patient's performance greatly improves when he or she is allowed to imitate a model. A patient with adiadochokinesia may be observed to improve when allowed to perform alternating movements at a slower speed. A patient with impaired sequencing as a result of ideational apraxia may show improvement when instructed to talk his or her way through the sequence, stating what should come first, second, and so on. When communicated to speech, occupational, and recreation therapists, these observations can have an important impact on the treatment of movement-impaired patients.

Psychotherapy is central to the treatment of psychogenic motor dysfunction. Treatment focuses on any underlying mental disorders (e.g., anxiety, post-traumatic stress disorder), as well as on the motor dysfunction itself. As with other psychological disorders that mimic neurological illness, successful treatment includes a combination of emotional support, insight-oriented interpretation, confrontation, and behavior-management techniques. Emotional support is necessary to create an environment in which the patient can trust the therapist enough to relinquish the motor symptoms. These symptoms serve an important psychological function for the patient, and will not be abandoned unless the therapist establishes a trusting alliance.

Within the context of this trusting alliance, the patient's dysfunctional behaviors can be pointed out and their relationship to psychological and motivational factors explored. Patients gain insight gradually, often as a result of observing the variability of and inconsistencies in their disorder. Case 11–2 describes a patient with psychogenic motor dysfunction; this patient became aware of the emotional basis for her deficits only when a vacation away from her husband led to a temporary remission of her disorder. When she returned to her home, the disorder also returned. Even with such a clear pattern, the patient would have been likely to reject the psychologist's interpretation if a trusting alliance had not already been established.

Physiologically based motor disorders usually cannot be treated without effort and cooperation from the patient. The patient who has psychogenic motor dysfunction in addition to a physiological disorder often cannot exert the effort required for physical and occupational therapy. Confronting the patient about his or her psychogenic deficits can be attempted in hopes of bringing about an early remission so that treatment of the physiologically based deficits can proceed. Often it is best to assign responsibility for confrontation to the physician member of the treatment team so that the psychologist can continue to work with the patient in a more supportive and insight-oriented manner.

Behavioral management techniques should be instituted concurrently with confrontation. This includes specifying desirable behaviors, providing concrete rewards when these behaviors occur, specifying negative consequences that will occur when the patient fails to meet expectations, monitoring progress, and providing clear feedback to the patient about his or her progress. As with any behavioral program, emphasis should be placed on reinforcing desirable behaviors rather than on punishing undesirable ones. Positive reinforcement should be given in response to even slight increases in desirable behaviors.

When psychogenic motor dysfunction is the result of conscious malingering, psychotherapy is not indicated and is not likely to be successful. The most appropriate intervention is to let the patient know that the deception has been detected and that no success in manipulating the health care team can be expected.

CASE ILLUSTRATIONS

CASE 4–5

R.M. was a 50-year-old man with a high-school education. Following triple coronary artery bypass grafting, he developed atrial fibrillation and an anoxic encephalopathy. Magnetic resonance imaging (MRI) scans revealed bilateral watershed area infarctions (C-shaped infarctions extending from the frontal to the occipital poles), with greater damage evident in the right hemisphere.

Details of the patient's neuropsychological examination are presented in Chapters 4, 7, 8, and 13. The patient tolerated extensive examination despite having numerous cognitive deficits. His motivation remained high throughout the examination, and his effort to perform was always evident. There was no history of psychiatric disorder, and no psychiatric symptoms were present during the examination.

When R.M. was initially approached, his eyes were deviated to the right of center. He was unable to move his eyes in any direction commanded by the examiner and instead turned his head in the specified direction. When his head was held stationary, he struggled unsuccessfully to follow the command. He followed the examiner's finger with his eyes as far as the midline, but failed to track the finger any farther to the right. When his eyelids were held shut, R.M. was able to move his eyes in all directions; the movement was observed through the closed lids.

R.M. had reduced strength in both arms; the left deficit was worse than that in the right. He was unable to perform any movements with his left hand or arm. His right arm was capable of coordinated movement despite its mild weakness. He was impaired in his pantomime of movements on demand with his right hand, showing confusion and the absence of any response, but correctly imitated movements and had no difficulty using objects, with one exception. He tended to confuse the order of complex, multistep movements.

Confusion of the sequence of movements was evident both in the complex movements of the WAB Apraxia Subtest and in everyday movements involving objects. For example, when asked to pick up a pencil and place it in a pencil holder, R.M. repeatedly picked up the pencil holder instead of the pencil. Each time he made this mistake, he looked perplexed and mumbled "no" to himself, but on trying again, he still picked up the pencil holder instead of the pencil. He was unable to perform the task until the pencil was placed directly in his hand, preventing him from making his previous mistake. No other deficits were evident in his motor performance.

DISCUSSION

Oculomotor apraxia was evident in this patient. However, this diagnosis is complicated by the patient's rightward gaze deviation, a finding that could indicate weakness of the eye muscles or could reflect akinesia for eye movements to the left of midline. Muscle weakness was ruled out by the observation that the eyes could travel in all directions when the patient's vision was occluded. The patient was akinetic for eye movements to the left, but this alone cannot account for his inability to shift his gaze in any direction on demand. Thus, an additional diagnosis of oculomotor apraxia is justified.

The patient in Case 4–5 also presented with ideational apraxia. He was unable to sequence individual steps in complex goal-directed actions. The fact that he could carry out the individual steps of the sequence when his errors were prevented rules out the possible confounding influence of other movement disorders. The test items were from the WAB Apraxia Subtest, which uses movement sequences containing logically related steps that are familiar to most adults. Consequently, the memory demands of the test items were minimal, and forgetting the steps in the sequence is an unlikely explanation of the patient's deficient performance.

CASE 11–1

S.S. was a 48-year-old man with a business degree who had worked as an aircraft mechanic until suffering a right combined parietal and occipital cerebrovascular accident involving both cortical and subcortical tissue. Carotid angiography revealed right middle cerebral artery occlusion. Following medical stabilization, S.S. underwent a comprehensive rehabilitation program. The patient was right-hand dominant and had left hemiparesis. Strength (assessed using the Hand Dynamometer), speed (assessed using the HRB Finger-Tapping Test), and coordination (assessed using the Grooved Pegboard) were within normal limits in the right hand. The patient was normal in oculomotor, oral, limb, and ideational praxis; the latter two were assessed only in the right hand.

Figure 11–1 shows the patient's attempts to copy triple loops. Although he succeeded at his first attempt, subsequent attempts were notably perseverative. On the final attempt, S.S. stopped making loops only when the examiner told him to do so.

S.S. was able to alternate rapidly between palm-up and palm-down positions. He was able to learn the fist-edge-palm movement sequence and performed it correctly with his right hand through three repetitions before he began confusing the sequence. He completed two more correct repetitions of the sequence, then performed the incorrect sequence fist-edge-fist. This was followed by fist-edge-fist-palm and palm-edge-fist-palm before the patient again succeeded in performing the

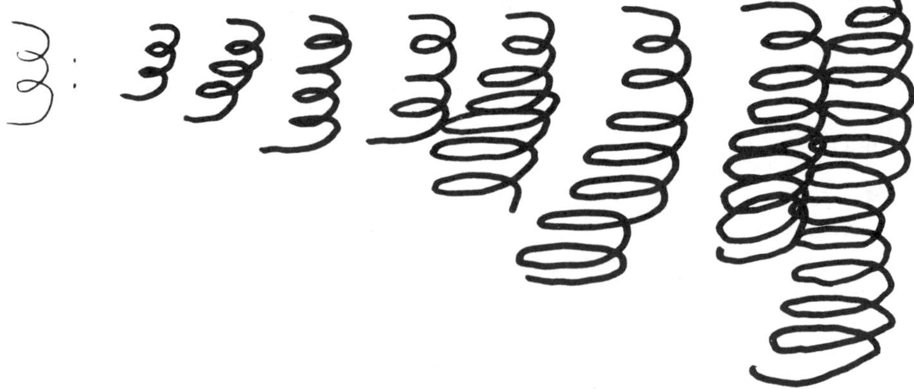

FIGURE 11–1. Triple loops copied by patient S.S.

correct sequence. On a subsequent set of trials, the patient was given a verbal label for each movement and instructed to name the movements as he made them. Under this condition, the patient made no errors. He had no difficulty with the goal-directed movement sequences from the WAB Apraxia Subtest or with any other motor task presented to him.

DISCUSSION

A diagnosis of motor perseveration was made in Case 11–1. This patient also showed an inability to rapidly perform the fist-edge-palm sequence, although he succeeded once he was given verbal labels for the movements. He did not have difficulty with simpler rapid alternating movements. Adiadochokinesia was diagnosed, with the notation that the deficit appeared only with more complex series. Notably, the patient had no difficulty with goal-directed movement sequences, distinguishing him from patients who have ideational apraxia.

CASE 11–2

H.M. was a right-handed, 54-year-old woman with a bachelor's degree. The patient presented with complaints of decreased coordination, impaired memory, difficulty performing calculations, and difficulty finding words to express her ideas. During the past 17 months, she had undergone numerous medical examinations because she feared that she had Alzheimer's disease. With the exception of documenting considerable anxiety and depression, all examinations, including computed tomography (CT) and MRI scans, were negative. The patient was placed on an antidepressant and began a course of psychotherapy.

H.M. did not accept the negative findings and came to the current examiner for another opinion. This was her third neuropsychological examination. Only results relevant to her motor functioning are discussed here; additional test results are presented in Chapter 16. The patient was unable to pantomime on demand oral movements that involved the pretended use of objects. For example, when asked to pantomime sucking through a straw, she stuck her finger in her mouth and exhaled. Errors involving use of a body part as an object also occurred bilaterally when she pantomimed movements involving the arms and hands. Her performance remained impaired even when imitating oral and limb movements, although it was slightly better than her performance of pantomime on demand. When she was using actual objects, her performance was correct on all but one trial. She performed goal-directed sequences of movement without error.

H.M. was unable to learn the fist-edge-palm movement sequence and could not perform the sequence with either hand even when guided by verbal labels for the movements. She was unable to place a single peg in the holes with either hand on the Grooved Pegboard and was in the severely impaired range on the HRB Finger-Tapping Test, both hands being equally impaired.

In an interview, H.M. reported great difficulty with motor tasks in her home environment, particularly around her husband. She spoke of her husband as being perfectionistic and controlling. She could identify no accident, illness, or other event that preceded and might have accounted for her decline in motor performance. She stated that her motor deficits had worsened during the past 17 months, with the exception of a 2-week period during which she had taken a vacation without her husband. During this period, she was not bothered by her usual clumsiness and other motor problems. The problems returned, however, once she was back home.

A Minnesota Multiphasic Personality Inventory (MMPI) was administered, with a valid clinical profile resulting. The profile was consistent with the presence of anxiety, agitation, tension, and depression. Patients obtaining similar profiles usually present with multiple unsubstantiated somatic complaints. They are also likely to be lacking in assertiveness and frequently do not express uncomfortable feelings directly. Feelings of despair and worthlessness are also correlates of H.M.'s personality profile.

DISCUSSION

Case 11–2 is a classic presentation of psychogenic motor dysfunction. The patient presented with an apparently severe apraxia that had no clear precipitating event and did not fit with the absence of any documented neurological disease. The course of the disorder was atypical in that it remitted during a vacation away from her husband. Although this patient did not initially discuss her marriage in detail, her description of her husband made it clear that she did not view him positively. Her MMPI suggested she was agitated and depressed and was unlikely to express feelings in a direct and assertive manner. It is possible that her motor problems gave vent to her feelings, and they probably provided her with a means of escaping from what she perceived as her husband's perfectionistic control.

CASE 11–3

L.K. was a right-handed, 59-year-old woman who worked as a grade-school teacher. She underwent right carotid endarterectomy because of 100% stenosis of the right carotid artery. The patient developed an embolic right temporal-parietal infarction subsequent to surgery, which resulted in left hemiparesis and left-sided stimulus neglect (see Chap. 4). Strength, speed, coordination, and praxis were intact in the right hand. No language deficits were present. The patient showed notable motor perseveration when copying triple loops with her right hand. During the tandem reciprocal movement procedure, she made 17 errors. Her errors consisted of inadvertent imitation of the examiner's movements rather than performance of the movement she had been instructed to perform. Although the task was repeatedly explained to her, and although she was able to demonstrate the desired movements immediately after instruction, she continued to make imitative errors during testing.

DISCUSSION

A diagnosis of motor perseveration was made in the patient in Case 11–3. This patient also showed echopraxia during the tandem reciprocal movement procedure, despite frequent reinstruction in the rules of the task.

REFERENCES

1. Christensen, AL: Luria's Neuropsychological Investigation Text. Spectrum Publications, New York, 1975.
2. American Psychiatric Association: Diagnostic and Statistical Manual of Mental Disorders, Fourth Edition. American Psychiatric Association, Washington, DC, 1994.
3. The International Classification of Diseases, Ninth Revision, Clinical Modification. Med-Index Publications, Salt Lake City, 1991.
4. Taniwaki, T, et al: Positron emission tomography (PET) in "pure akinesia." J Neurol Sci 107:34, 1992.
5. Matsuo, H, et al: Pure akinesia: An atypical manifestation of progressive supranuclear palsy. J Neurol Neurosurg Psychiatry 54:397, 1991.
6. Riley, DE, et al: Cortical-basal ganglionic degeneration. Neurology 40:1203, 1990.
7. Albin, RL, et al: Striatal and nigral neuron subpopulations in rigid Huntington's disease: Implications for the functional anatomy of chorea and rigidity-akinesia. Ann Neurol 27:357, 1990.
8. Quinn, NP, et al: Pure akinesia due to Lewy body Parkinson's disease: A case with pathology. Mov Disord 4:85, 1989.
9. Takahashi, K, et al: Pallido-nigro-luysial atrophy associated with degeneration of the centrum medianum. A clinicopathologic and electron microscopic study. Acta Neuropathol (Berl) 37:81, 1977.
10. Szirmai, I, Guseo, A, and Molnar, M: Bilateral symmetrical softening of the thalamus. J Neurol 217:57, 1977.
11. Freemon, FR: Akinetic mutism and bilateral anterior cerebral artery occlusion. J Neurol Neurosurg Psychiatry 34:693, 1971.
12. Cairns, H, et al: Akinetic mutism with an epidermoid cyst of the 3rd ventricle (with a report of the associated disturbance of brain potentials). Brain 64:273, 1941.
13. Ross, ED, and Stewart, RM: Akinetic mutism from hypothalamic damage: Successful treatment with dopamine agonists. Neurology 31:1435, 1981.
14. Cravioto, H, Silberman, J, and Feigin, I: A clinical and pathological study of akinetic mutism. Neurology 10:10, 1960.
15. Daly, DD, and Love, JG: Akinetic mutism. Neurology 8:238, 1958.
16. Laplane, D, et al: Clinical consequences of corticectomies involving the supplementary motor area in man. J Neurol Sci 34:301, 1977.
17. Watson, RT, et al: Apraxia and the supplementary motor area. Arch Neurol 43:787, 1986.
18. Nemeth, G, Hegedus, K, and Molnar, L: Akinetic mutism associated with bicingular lesions: Clinicopathological and functional anatomical correlates. Eur Arch Psychiatry Neurol Sci 237:218, 1988.
19. Skultely, FM: Clinical and experimental aspects of akinetic mutism. Arch Neurol 19:1, 1968.
20. Barris, RW, and Schuman, HR: Bilateral anterior cingulate gyrus lesions. Syndrome of the anterior cingulate gyri. Neurology 3:44, 1953.
21. Rosselli, M, et al: Topography of the hemi-inattention syndrome. Int J Neurosci 27:165, 1985.
22. Perry, RH, et al: Senile dementia of Lewy body type. A clinically and neuropathologically distinct form of Lewy body dementia in the elderly. J Neurol Sci 95:119, 1990.
23. Gutling, E, Landis, T, and Kleihues, P: Akinetic mutism in bilateral necrotizing leukoencephalopathy after radiation and chemotherapy: Electrophysiological and autopsy findings. J Neurol 239:125, 1992.
24. Devinsky, O, et al: Akinetic mutism in a bone marrow transplant recipient following total-body irradiation and amphotericin B chemoprophylaxis. A positron emission tomographic and neuropathologic study. Arch Neurol 44:414, 1987.
25. Aoki, N: Reversible leukoencephalopathy caused by 5-fluorouracil derivatives, presenting as akinetic mutism. Surg Neurol 25:279, 1986.

26. Bogousslavsky, J, and Regli, F: Response-to-next-patient-stimulation: A right hemisphere syndrome. Neurology 38:1225, 1988.
27. DeRenzi, E, Gentilini, M, and Bazolli, C: Eyelid movement disorders and motor impersistence in acute hemisphere disease. Neurology 36:414, 1986.
28. Kertesz, A, et al: Motor impersistence: A right hemisphere syndrome. Neurology 35:662, 1985.
29. Hier, DB, Mondlock, J, and Caplan, LR: Behavioral abnormalities after right hemisphere stroke. Neurology 33:337, 1983.
30. Levin, HS: Motor impersistence and proprioceptive feedback in patients with unilateral cerebral disease. Neurology 23:833, 1973.
31. Carmon, A: Impaired utilization of kinesthetic feedback in right hemispheric lesions. Possible implications for the pathophysiology of "motor impersistence." Neurology 20:1033, 1970.
32. Heilman, KM, and Valenstein, E: Mechanisms underlying hemispatial neglect. Ann Neurol 5:166, 1979.
33. Nishimura, M, et al: Chronic progressive spinobulbar spasticity with disturbance of voluntary eyelid closure. Report of a case with special reference to MRI and electrophysiological findings. J Neurol Sci 96:183, 1990.
34. Viader, F, Cambier, J, and Pariser, P: Left motor extinction due to an ischemic lesion of the anterior limb of the internal capsule. Rev Neurol 138:213, 1982.
35. Valenstein, E, and Heilman, KM: Unilateral hypokinesia and motor extinction. Neurology 31:445, 1981.
36. Velasco, F, and Velasco, M: A reticulothalamic system mediating proprioceptive attention and tremor in man. Neurosurgery 4:30, 1979.
37. Orozco-Diaz, G, et al: Autosomal dominant cerebellar ataxia: Clinical analysis of 263 patients from a homogeneous population in Holguin, Cuba. Neurology 40:1369, 1990.
38. Gelmers, HJ: Non-paralytic motor disturbances and speech disorders: The role of the supplementary motor area. J Neurol Neurosurg Psychiatry 46:1052, 1983.
39. Goldberg, G, Mayer, NH, and Toglia, JU: Medial frontal cortex infarction and the alien hand sign. Arch Neurol 38:683, 1981.
40. Shahani, B, Burrows, PT, and Whitty, CW: The grasp reflex and perseveration. Brain 93:181, 1970.
41. Luria, AR: Two kinds of motor perseveration in massive injury of the frontal lobes. Brain 88:1, 1965.
42. Denes, G, et al: An unusual case of perseveration sparing body-related tasks. Cortex 26:269, 1990.
43. Sandson, J, and Albert, ML: Perseveration in behavioral neurology. Neurology 37:1736, 1987.
44. Goldberg, E: Varieties of perseveration: A comparison of two taxonomies. J Clin Exp Neuropsychol 8:710, 1986.
45. Sandson, J, and Albert, ML: Varieties of perseveration. Neuropsychologia 22:715, 1984.
46. Pirozzolo, FJ, et al: Neurolinguistic analysis of the language abilities of a patient with a "double disconnection syndrome": A case of subangular alexia in the presence of mixed transcortical aphasia. J Neurol Neurosurg Psychiatry 44:152, 1981.
47. Monaco, F, et al: Acquired ocular-motor apraxia and right-sided cortical angioma. Cortex 16:159, 1980.
48. Waltz, AG: Dyspraxias of gaze. Arch Neurol 5:638, 1961.
49. Cogan, DG, and Adams, RD: A type of paralysis of conjugate gaze (ocular motor apraxia). Arch Ophthalmol 50:434, 1953.
50. Mills, RP, and Swanson, PD: Vertical oculomotor apraxia and memory loss. Ann Neurol 4:149, 1978.
51. Mani, RB and Levine, DN: Crossed buccofacial apraxia. Arch Neurol 45:581, 1988.
52. Groswasser, Z, Groswasser-Reider, I, and Korn, C: Biopercular lesions and acquired mutism in a young patient. Brain Inj 5:331, 1991.
53. Graswasser, Z, et al: Mutism associated with buccofacial apraxia and bihemispheric lesions. Brain Lang 34:157, 1988.
54. Kramer, JH, Delis, DC, and Nakada, T: Buccofacial apraxia without aphasia due to a right parietal lesion. Ann Neurol 18:512, 1985.
55. Tognolo, G, and Vignolo, LA: Brain lesions associated with oral apraxia in stroke patients: A clinico-neuroradiological investigation with the CT scan. Neuropsychologia 18:257, 1980.
56. Alexander, MP, et al: Neuropsychological and neuroanatomical dimensions of ideomotor apraxia. Brain 115:87, 1992.
57. Basso, A, and Capitani, E: Spared musical abilities in a conductor with global aphasia and ideomotor apraxia. J Neurol Neurosurg Psychiatry 48:407, 1985.

58. Rothi, LJ, Heilman, KM, and Watson, RT: Pantomime comprehension and ideomotor apraxia. J Neurol Neurosurg Psychiatry 48:207, 1985.
59. Heilman, KM, Rothi, LJ, and Valenstein, E: Two forms of ideomotor apraxia. Neurology 32:342, 1982.
60. Benson, DF, et al: Conduction aphasia: A clinico-pathologic study. Arch Neurol 28:339, 1973.
61. Poncent, M, Habib, M, and Robillard, A: Deep left parietal lobe syndrome: Conduction aphasia and other neurobehavioural disorders due to a small subcortical lesion. J Neurol Neurosurg Psychiatry 50:709, 1987.
62. Kertesz, A, and Ferro, JM: Lesion size and location in ideomotor apraxia. Brain 107:921, 1984.
63. Berthier, M, Starkstein, S, and Leiguarda, R: Behavioral effects of damage to the right insula and surrounding regions. Cortex 23:673, 1987.
64. Basso, A, and Della-Sala, S: Ideomotor apraxia arising from a purely deep lesion. J Neurol Neurosurg Psychiatry 49:458, 1986.
65. Agostoni, E, et al: Apraxia in deep cerebral lesions. J Neurol Neurosurg Psychiatry 46:804, 1983.
66. DeRenzi, E, Motti, F, and Nichelli, P: Imitating gestures. A quantitative approach to ideomotor apraxia. Arch Neurol 37:6, 1980.
67. DeRenzi, E, and Lucchelli, F: Ideational apraxia. Brain 111:1173, 1988.
68. Ochipa, C, Rothi, LJ, and Heilman, KM: Ideational apraxia: A deficit in tool selection and use. Ann Neurol 25:190, 1989.
69. Matsuoka, H, et al: Impairment of parietal cortical functions associated with episodic prolonged spike-and-wave discharges. Epilepsia 27:432, 1986.
70. Benton, AL, et al: Contributions to Neuropsychological Assessment. A Clinical Manual. Oxford University Press, New York, 1983.
71. Christensen, AL: Luria's Neuropsychological Investigation Manual. Spectrum Publications, New York, 1975.
72. Goodglass, H, and Kaplan, E: The Assessment of Aphasia and Related Disorders, Second Edition. Lea & Febiger, Philadelphia, 1983.
73. Kertesz, A: The Western Aphasia Battery Test Manual. Grune & Stratton, Orlando, FL, 1982.
74. Kertesz, A: Aphasia and Associated Disorders: Taxonomy, Localization, and Recovery. Grune & Stratton, New York, 1979.
75. Shewan, CM, and Kertesz, A: Reliability and validity characteristics of the Western Aphasia Battery (WAB). Journal of Speech and Hearing Disorders 45:308, 1980.
76. Heaton, RK, Grant, I, and Matthews, CG: Comprehensive Norms for an Expanded Halstead-Reitan Battery. Psychological Assessment Resources, Odessa, FL, 1991.
77. Raddon, JR, et al: Hand dynamometer: Effects of trials and sessions. Percept Mot Skills 61:1195, 1985.
78. Dunn, JM: Reliability of selected psychomotor measures with mentally retarded adult males. Percept Mot Skills 46:295, 1978.
79. Matarazzo, JD, et al: Psychometric and clinical test-retest reliability of the Halstead Impairment Index in a sample of healthy, young, normal men. J Nerv Ment Dis 158:37, 1974.
80. Provins, KA, and Cunliffe, P: The reliability of some motor performance tests of handedness. Neuropsychologia 10:199, 1972.
81. York Haaland, K, and Delaney, HD: Motor deficits after left or right hemisphere damage due to stroke or tumor. Neuropsychologia 19:17, 1981.
82. Finlayson, MA, and Reitan, RM: Effect of lateralized lesions on ipsilateral and contralateral motor functioning. J Clin Neuropsychol 2:237, 1980.
83. Hom, J, and Reitan, RM: Effect of lateralized cerebral damage upon contralateral and ipsilateral sensorimotor performances. J Clin Neuropsychol 4:249, 1982.
84. Reitan, RM, and Davison, LA: Clinical Neuropsychology: Current Status and Applications. H.V. Winston, New York, 1974.
85. Charter, RA, et al: Reliability of the WAIS, WMS, and Reitan Battery: Raw scores and standardization scores corrected for age and education. International Journal of Clinical Neuropsychology 9:28, 1987.
86. Matarrazzo, JD, et al: Psychometric and clinical test-retest reliability of the Halstead Impairment index in a sample of healthy, young, normal men. J Nerv Ment Dis 158:37, 1974.
87. Goldstein, G, and Watson, JR: Test-retest reliability of the Halstead-Reitan battery and the WAIS in a neuropsychiatric population. The Clinical Neuropsychologist 3:265, 1989.
88. O'Donnell, JP, et al: Neuropsychological test findings for normal, learning disabled and brain damaged young adults. J Consult Clin Psychol 51:726, 1983.

89. Bigler, ED, and Tucker, DM: Comparison of verbal IQ, Tactual Performance, Seashore Rhythm and Finger Oscillation Tests in the blind and brain-damaged. J Clin Psychol 37:849, 1981.
90. Prigatona, GP, et al: Neuropsychological test performance in mildly hypoxic patients with chronic obstructive pulmonary disease. J Consult Clin Psychol 51:108, 1983.
91. Haaland, KY, Cleeland, CS, and Carr, D: Motor performance after unilateral hemispheric damage in patients with tumor. Arch Neurol 34:556, 1977.
92. Haaland, KY, and Delaney, HD: Motor deficits after left or right hemisphere damage due to stroke or tumor. Neuropsychologia 19:17, 1981.
93. Satz, P, and D'Elia, L: The Pin Test Professional Manual. Psychological Assessment Resources, Odessa, FL, 1989.
94. Briggs, GG, and Nebes, RD: Patterns of hand preference in a student population. Cortex 11:230, 1975.
95. McMeekan, ERL, and Lishman, WA: Retest reliabilities of the Annett Hand Preference Questionnaire and the Edinburgh Handedness Inventory. J Psychol 66:53, 1975.

DISORDERS OF ORAL LANGUAGE

12

In the disorders of oral language, one or more aspects of oral communication are compromised. For example, verbal expression may be compromised as a result of an inability to generate the words necessary to express an idea, a failure to arrange words into sentences according to syntactic rules, or a frequent production of incorrect speech sounds. Comprehension of oral language may be compromised because of an inability to recognize and interpret speech sounds, an inability to interpret the meaning of words, or an inability to appreciate and comprehend syntax.

The oral language disorders include the subtypes listed under "Variety of Presentation" in the chapter outline. In the first 12 subtypes, multiple aspects of oral communication are impaired simultaneously. In addition, written communication is almost always impaired (see also Aphasic alexia-agraphia). In contrast, the deficit is restricted to a single aspect of oral communication in stimulus-specific aphasia, mutism, and pathological reiteration. Two types of pathological reiteration are included in this text: a tendency to repeat one's own verbalizations, termed *palilalia,* and a tendency to repeat someone else's verbalizations, termed *echolalia.*

Oral language impairment typically follows cortical lesions in the language-dominant hemisphere. Subcortical lesions can also produce oral language impairment, and many texts include subcortical aphasia as a distinct subtype.[1,2] Full characterization of a syndrome or syndromes of subcortical aphasia is still under way. The clinical profiles of most cases of subcortical aphasia resemble the profiles of patients diagnosed with one of the traditional oral language disorders, although the full pattern of deficits usually is not present. For example, some patients with thalamic aphasia perform similarly to transcortical sensory aphasics on speech production and repetition tests, but unlike transcortical sensory aphasics, they may be intact or minimally impaired in their comprehension.

Rather than attempting to define a specific set of behaviors characteristic of subcortical aphasia, this text contains a notation in the lesion location sections of the traditional oral language disorders when a subcortical lesion is known to be associated with a partial presentation of the disorder. Further clarification of the language deficits produced by subcortical lesions may lead to a more precise delineation of differences between subcortical aphasia and the traditional aphasic disorders.

NOMENCLATURE

Aphasia can be coded in DSM-IV[3] as "Expressive Language Disorder," "Mixed Receptive-Expressive Language Disorder," or "Communication Disorder Not Otherwise Specified." As discussed later, the expressive-receptive dichotomy is misleading, and in most instances a diagnosis of "Expressive Language Disorder" does not capture an aphasic patient's presentation. ICD-9-CM[4] includes a single diagnostic code for aphasia and all other subtypes of oral language disorder, with the exception of anomia (anomic aphasia) and pathologic reiteration (echolalia and palilalia), which are listed under "Other Symbolic Dysfunction."

The neurology literature is replete with schemes for subtyping the disorders of oral language, beginning with such early classification systems as that of Lichtheim[5] and continuing to the present era with classification systems proposed by Luria,[6] the aphasiologists of the Boston Veterans Administration Hospital,[1] and Hecaen and Albert.[7] This proliferation of classification systems has long created confusion among aphasiologists. Benson[1] has argued, however, that beyond surface differences in terminology, considerable agreement can be found in the way the classification systems cluster symptoms and in the neuropathology believed to underlie the clusters.

The terminology employed in the Boston Veterans Administration Hospital aphasia classification system,[1] with some additions and modifications, is used in this text. Corresponding terms in Luria's[6] and Hecaen and Albert's[7] systems are listed. Readers interested in the correspondence between these contemporary systems and earlier aphasia classifications are referred to Benson.[1]

The additions to the Boston classification system include optic, tactile, and stimulus-specific aphasia. Optic and tactile aphasia are rarely reported disorders that have not been included in the major classification systems. *Stimulus-specific aphasia* is the term I use for the syndromes of color anomia, color aphasia, and aphasia for body parts, which also are rarely reported. These putative disorders are included because their presence implies a lesion location that is somewhat distinct from that of the other aphasias. In addition, these disorders deserve greater clinical attention and empirical study if for no other reason than the possibility that they may eventually provide information about the organization of language in the brain.

Brief mention is made of the unfortunate dichotomy that is made in some clinical settings between "receptive" and "expressive" aphasia. By *receptive aphasia*, the clinician usually means Wernicke's or transcortical sensory aphasia, in which reception (comprehension) of oral language is impaired. *Expressive aphasia* corresponds to Broca's or transcortical motor aphasia, characterized by striking deficits in the expression of speech. The expressive-receptive dichotomy obscures the fact that there are receptive and expressive deficits in all of the previously mentioned aphasias. Consequently, this dichotomy provides an inaccurate picture of the aphasias. The only real advantage of the expressive-receptive distinction is its simplicity, and this probably accounts for its continued use in some clinical settings. This terminology is not used in this book.

Finally, the term *mixed nonfluent aphasia* is sometimes used for patients who would be classified as Broca's aphasics were it not for their having greater comprehension impairment than is typical in Broca's aphasia. The term can also be applied to global aphasics who have recovered to the point where they are producing some

RULES FOR DIAGNOSIS

Clinical Indicators: Each is independent (only one must be observed for the disorder to be suspected) *except* when subscripting is used. Subscripted numbers (a_1, a_2) denote an indicator with multiple parts that must be considered together.
Associated Features: These are listed to give a more complete picture of the disorder. The presence or absence of these features does not affect the diagnosis.
Factors to Rule Out: All must be taken into account. Failure to rule out even one of these factors makes a firm diagnosis impossible.
Lesion Locations: Each location stands alone; damage in only one of the listed areas is sufficient to produce the disorder.

intelligible speech. It is likely that these patients represent points along the continuum of recovery rather than a distinct subtype of aphasia. According to the following clinical indicators, these patients are classified as global aphasics.

Patients within a diagnostic category can vary considerably from each other, particularly when observed at different points in their recovery. Although they serve many useful functions, diagnostic labels alone cannot communicate everything of value about a given patient's clinical presentation. This is particularly true in aphasia, in which many variables go into establishing membership within a diagnostic subtype. Determining a patient's oral language diagnosis is not sufficient; careful delineation of the specific strengths and weaknesses of each patient is vital to ensure accurate communication in settings in which aphasic patients are examined and treated.

VARIETY OF PRESENTATION

1. Broca's aphasia (also called motor and efferent motor aphasia; see also Aphasic alexia-agraphia)

Clinical Indicators

a_1. Dysfluent spontaneous and responsive speech and writing as evidenced by any of the following signs:

1) Speech and writing limited to simple, repetitively produced word fragments
2) Speech and writing limited to isolated concrete words
3) Speech and writing terse and telegraphic, consisting of simple phrases (e.g., verb and object combinations)
4) Slow, laborious, and effortful speech and writing

a_2. Agrammatic speech and writing as evidenced by any of the following signs:

1) Absence of articles (e.g., "a," "an," "the")
2) Absence of prepositions (e.g., "with," "to")
3) Absence of conjunctions (e.g., "and," "or")
4) Absence of auxiliary verbs (e.g., "would," "should," "could," "may," "can," "do")
5) Absence of inflectional changes in verbs to indicate the correct tense (e.g., "We run yesterday" rather than "We ran yesterday"), number (e.g., "Jan and Michael agrees" rather than "Jan and Michael agree"), or person (e.g., "He go" rather than "He goes")
6) Absence of words indicating the relationship between objects (e.g., "in," "on")

a_3. Dysfluent and agrammatic immediate repetition of oral phrases and oral reading (see signs of agrammatism)

a_4. Impaired comprehension of the syntactic elements of spoken and written sentences as evidenced by any of the following signs:

1) Incorrect performance of commands or incorrect responses to questions that hinge on the prepositions "with" or "to" (e.g., "Point to the pencil with the paper.")

2) Incorrect performance of commands or incorrect responses to questions that hinge on prepositions that specify location (e.g., "on," "under," "behind," "in front")
3) Confusion of actor with object acted upon in sentences spoken or written in the passive voice
4) Failure to comprehend possessive relationships when both the possessor and the object possessed belong to the same semantic category (e.g., "Is my wife's brother a man or a woman?")
5) Difficulty in determining differences in the subjects referred to by verbs in syntactically similar verb complement phrases (e.g., "John asked his father to mail the letter, and he did. Who mailed the letter?" versus "Susan promised her mother to bake some brownies, and she did. Who baked the brownies?")[8]

a_5. Relatively preserved comprehension of the vocabulary (i.e., the lexical elements as distinct from grammar and syntax) of spoken or written sentences

Associated Features

a. Impaired naming of objects (see also Anomic aphasia), improving slightly when contextual cues (e.g., describing the object's use) or phonetic cues (e.g., presenting the initial speech sounds of the object's name) are provided
b. Unilateral (usually right-sided) motor weakness (hemiparesis)
c. Impaired ability to perform skilled movements on demand (see Apraxia)
d. In some multilingual patients, a dissociation in the severity of the deficit seen across languages so that communication in one language appears less impaired or even spared
e. Relatively preserved ability to utter obscenities when frustrated or otherwise emotionally aroused
f. Relatively preserved ability to utter overlearned sequences of speech (e.g., the days of the week, months of the year)
g. Less impaired or even spared ability to sing previously learned songs
h. Impaired ability to express verbal prosody: a deficit in the ability to vary tone of voice, pitch, rate of speech, and word stress to coincide with the intended meaning or purpose of an utterance (e.g., the patient cannot turn the statement "Cathy is driving" into a question by raising the pitch of his or her voice at the end and stressing the last word)
i. In some patients, presence of phonemic (literal) paraphasias in oral expression, including spontaneous speech, responsive speech, and speech repetition (phonemic paraphasias are incorrect speech sounds substituted for the target sounds in words)
j. A recent history of global aphasia (see later text)

Factors to Rule Out

a. Impaired articulation as a result of weakness of the speech muscles (*anarthria* or *dysarthria*) sufficient to account for the deficits in oral language, ruled out by documenting the agrammatic qualities of the speech and the extension of the deficit to written language

b. Impaired ability to carry out skilled movements of the speech muscles on demand (see Buccofacial apraxia) sufficient to account for the deficits in oral language, ruled out by documenting the extension of the deficit to written language

Lesion Locations

a. Broca's area in the frontal operculum (posterior portion of inferior frontal gyrus), with the lesion typically extending to subjacent white matter, the anterior parietal lobe, the insula, and both banks of the Rolandic fissure[9,10]

Lesion Lateralization

a. Language-dominant (usually left) hemisphere

2. Wernicke's aphasia (also called sensory aphasia; see also Aphasic alexia-agraphia)

Clinical Indicators

a_1. Impaired comprehension of the vocabulary (i.e., lexical elements, distinct from grammar and syntax) of spoken or written sentences

a_2. Fluent but impaired immediate repetition of oral phrases and oral reading as a result of the presence of any of the following errors:

1) Addition of extra words or phrases to the target phrases being repeated or read
2) Substitution of incorrect speech sounds for the target sounds in words (*phonemic* or *literal paraphasia*)
3) Word substitution errors semantically related to the target words that should have been repeated *(semantic paraphasia)* or read *(semantic paralexia)*
4) Random word substitution errors that have no meaningful relation to the target words that should have been repeated *(random paraphasia)* or read *(random paralexia)*
5) Substitution of nonsense words that have no linguistic meaning (*neologisms* or *jargon words*) for the target words that should have been repeated or read

   NOTE: Semantic paraphasias, random paraphasias, and neologisms are collectively referred to as verbal paraphasias; *the term* verbal paralexia *is used when the errors occur during reading.*

a_3. Impaired or indecipherable spontaneous and responsive speech and writing as a result of the occurrence of any of the following errors:

1) Addition of extra words or phrases to the target phrases being spoken or written
2) Phonemic paraphasias
3) Verbal paraphasias, including semantic and random paraphasias and neologisms (the term *paragraphia* is used when the errors occur during writing)

4) Substitution of nonspecific words (e.g., "it," "thing") for concrete words (i.e., "empty speech")
5) Substitution of one grammatical function word for another (e.g., "to" substituted for "with")
6) Tangled juxtaposition of phrases that have no meaningful relationship to each other
NOTE: The term paragrammatism *is used to describe the incorrect grammar of these patients as a result of substitution errors involving function words, verbal paraphasias, and the meaningless juxtaposition of phrases.*

a_4. Speech and writing fluent and unrestricted and in some cases occurring at a greater than normal rate and in a greater than normal amount

Associated Features

a. Unawareness of the speech deficit as a result of a failure to monitor own speech
b. Frustration at the seemingly inexplicable failure of others to comprehend own utterances
c. Impaired naming of objects (see also Anomic aphasia) that does not improve when contextual cues (e.g., describing the object's use) or phonetic cues (e.g., presenting the initial speech sounds of the object's name) are provided
d. The presence of homonymous hemianopsia: loss of acuity in one visual half-field
e. Impaired ability to perform skilled movements on demand (see Apraxia)
f. In some multilingual patients, a dissociation in the severity of the deficit seen across languages such that communication in one language appears less impaired or even spared
g. Impaired ability to perceive verbal prosody: a deficit in the ability to appreciate variations in another speaker's tone of voice, pitch, rate of speech, and word stress that coincide with the speaker's intended meaning or purpose (e.g., the patient may fail to interpret the phrase "Cathy is driving" as a question because he or she does not perceive that the last word is stressed and spoken in a higher pitch)
h. Impaired ability to identify the fingers of the hand (see Finger agnosia)
i. Impaired discrimination of the right and left sides of the body, of space, or both (see Right-left disorientation)

Factors to Rule Out

a. Hearing loss sufficient to account for the failure to comprehend oral language, ruled out by audiologic assessment or by documenting the presence of additional deficits in oral expression and written language
b. Schizophrenia and related psychiatric disorders in which speech is idiosyncratic and neologistic, and comprehension is compromised by confusion and disorganization (see Chap. 18 for assessment techniques)

Lesion Locations

a. Wernicke's area (posterior portion of the superior temporal gyrus)[10,11]
b. Combined basal ganglia (head of caudate nucleus, rostral portion of lenticular nucleus) and internal capsule[12,13]

Lesion Lateralization

a. Language-dominant (usually left) hemisphere

3. **Pure word deafness (also called auditory speech agnosia and auditory verbal agnosia)**

Clinical Indicators

a_1. Impaired comprehension of the meaning of spoken sentences; deficit possibly so severe that the speech of others sounds muffled, foreign, or like meaningless noise

a_2. Fluent but impaired immediate repetition of oral phrases as a result of either of the following errors:

1) Omission of target words or word fragments
2) Rare or transient phonemic (also called literal) paraphasias: incorrect speech sounds substituted for the target sounds in words

a_3. Impaired writing to dictation as a result of omission of many target letters or words

a_4. Fluent and relatively preserved spontaneous speech and writing

a_5. Fluent and relatively preserved speech and writing in response to written questions or pictures

a_6. Relatively preserved oral reading

a_7. Relatively preserved reading comprehension

Associated Features

a. Context cues (e.g., embedding words in sentences, presenting new information that is closely related to information already presented and understood) possibly improving oral comprehension
b. Reducing the rate at which oral information is presented may improve oral comprehension
c. Impaired discrimination of elementary speech sounds *(phonemes)*
d. Extinction to auditory bilateral simultaneous stimulation (see Sensory extinction)
e. Impaired ability to find words to express ideas (see also Anomic aphasia)
f. Presence of auditory hallucinations (see Auditory hallucinosis)
g. Suspicious thoughts and feelings related to what people are saying
h. Transiently euphoric mood
i. A recent history of Wernicke's aphasia

Factors to Rule Out

a. Hearing loss sufficient to account for the deficit in comprehension of oral language, ruled out by audiologic examination or by demonstrating intact perception of nonverbal sounds
b. Schizophrenia and related psychiatric disorders in which speech compre-

hension is compromised by confusion and disorganization, auditory hallucinations are common, and suspiciousness may be present (see Chap. 18 for assessment techniques)

c. Lithium carbonate toxicity in patients taking this medication,[14] ruled out by laboratory determination of lithium blood level

Lesion Locations

a. Temporal lobe, particularly the middle and posterior part of superior temporal gyrus and often including part of Wernicke's area and Heschl's gyrus, with frequent extension to the subcortical white matter, including internal capsule and geniculate-temporal auditory radiation; parietal lobe, particularly the supramarginal and angular gyri; thalamus; and basal ganglia[15–23]

Lesion Lateralization

a. Although most reported cases have bilateral lesions, a few have lesions confined to the language-dominant (usually the left) hemisphere.[16,17,20,23]

4. Conduction aphasia (also called afferent motor aphasia; see also Aphasic alexia-agraphia)

Clinical Indicators

a_1. Impaired immediate repetition of oral phrases as a result of any of the following errors:
   1) Omission of target words or word fragments
   2) Phonemic (also called literal) paraphasias: incorrect speech sounds substituted for the target sounds in words
   3) Substitution of nonsense words that have no linguistic meaning (*neologisms* or *jargon words*) for the target words that should have been repeated

a_2. Impaired oral reading as a result of the presence of phonemic paraphasias

a_3. Fluent but impaired spontaneous and responsive speech as a result of phonemic paraphasias and neologisms

a_4. Fluent but impaired writing as a result of incorrect selection of letters (misspelling)

a_5. Relatively preserved comprehension of the meaning of oral and written words, phrases, and sentences

Associated Features

a. Relatively preserved immediate repetition of numbers
b. Particular difficulty with immediate repetition of polysyllabic words or phrases that contain an abundance of pronouns and grammatical function words
c. Awareness of deficits in speech and repetition with efforts to self-correct errors
d. Impaired naming of objects as a result of phonemic paraphasias and neologisms
e. Impaired ability to perform skilled movements on demand (see Apraxia)
f. Extinction to auditory bilateral simultaneous stimulation (see Sensory extinction)
g. A recent history of Wernicke's aphasia

Factors to Rule Out

a. Impaired speech articulation sufficient to account for the deficit in immediate oral repetition, ruled out by documenting, during attempts at repetition, the presence of well-articulated speech sounds that nonetheless fail to match the target sounds presented
b. Schizophrenia and related psychiatric disorders in which speech is neologistic (see Chap. 18 for assessment techniques)

Lesion Locations

a. Arcuate fasciculus, anywhere along its course[10,11,13,24–29]
b. Combined temporal and parietal lobes, particularly Wernicke's area, with sparing of the arcuate fasciculus[29,30]

Lesion Lateralization

a. Language-dominant (usually left) hemisphere

5. Global aphasia (see also Aphasic alexia-agraphia)

Clinical Indicators

a_1. Dysfluent spontaneous and responsive speech and writing as evidenced by any of the following signs:
   1) Speech and writing limited to simple, repetitively produced word fragments
   2) Speech and writing limited to isolated, concrete words
   3) Speech and writing terse and telegraphic, consisting of simple phrases (e.g., verb and object combinations)
   4) Slow, laborious, and effortful speech and writing

a_2. Agrammatic speech and writing as evidenced by any of the following signs:
   1) Absence of articles (e.g., "a," "an," "the")
   2) Absence of prepositions (e.g., "with," "to")
   3) Absence of conjunctions (e.g., "and," "or")
   4) Absence of auxiliary verbs (e.g., "would," "should," "could," "may," "can," "do")
   5) Absence of inflectional changes in verbs to indicate the correct tense (e.g., "We run yesterday" rather than "We ran yesterday"), number (e.g., "Jan and Michael agrees" rather than "Jan and Michael agree"), or person (e.g., "He go" rather than "He goes")
   6) Absence of words indicating the relation between objects (e.g., "in," "on")

a_3. Dysfluent and agrammatic immediate repetition of oral phrases and oral reading (see signs of agrammatism)

a_4. Impaired comprehension of the meaning of spoken and written words, phrases, and sentences

Associated Features

a. Impaired naming of objects (see also Anomic aphasia)
b. Unilateral (usually right-sided) motor weakness (hemiparesis)

c. Impaired ability to perform skilled movements on demand (see Apraxia)
d. The presence of homonymous hemianopsia: Loss of acuity in one visual half-field
e. Impaired ability to express verbal prosody: a deficit in the ability to vary tone of voice, pitch, rate of speech, and word stress to coincide with the intended meaning or purpose of an utterance (e.g., the patient cannot turn the statement "Cathy is driving" into a question by raising the pitch of his or her voice at the end and stressing the last word)
f. Impaired ability to perceive verbal prosody: a deficit in the ability to appreciate variations in another speaker's tone of voice, pitch, rate of speech, and word stress that coincide with the speaker's intended meaning or purpose
g. Impaired ability to identify the fingers of the hand (see Finger agnosia)
h. Impaired discrimination of the right and left sides of the body, space, or both (see Right-left disorientation)

Factors to Rule Out

a. Impaired articulation as a result of weakness of the speech muscles (*anarthria* or *dysarthria*) sufficient to account for the deficits in oral language, ruled out by documenting the agrammatic qualities of the speech or the extension of the deficit to written language
b. Impaired ability to carry out skilled movements of the speech muscles on demand (see Buccofacial apraxia) sufficient to account for the deficits in oral language, ruled out by documenting the extension of the deficit to written language
c. Hearing loss sufficient to account for the failure to comprehend oral language, ruled out by audiologic assessment or by documenting the presence of deficits in oral expression and written language

Lesion Locations

a. Entire perisylvian area, including portions of the insula and frontal lobe (particularly Broca's area), temporal lobe (particularly Wernicke's area or medial geniculate-temporal auditory radiation), and parietal lobe (particularly the supramarginal gyrus, angular gyrus, inferior parietal lobule, or superior parietal lobule), with frequent extension to the basal ganglia and internal capsule[10,11,31–37]
b. Combined basal ganglia and internal capsule (anterior or posterior limbs), sometimes with extension to thalamus, paraventricular white matter, or perisylvian area[33,34,38,39]

Lesion Lateralization

a. Language-dominant (usually left) hemisphere

6. Transcortical motor aphasia (also called dynamic aphasia; see also Aphasic alexia-agraphia)

Clinical Indicators

a_1. Dysfluent spontaneous and responsive speech and writing as evidenced by any of the following signs:

1) Speech and writing limited to simple, repetitively produced word fragments
2) Speech and writing limited to isolated concrete words
3) Speech and writing terse and telegraphic, consisting of simple phrases (e.g., verb and object combinations)
4) Speech and writing slow, laborious, and effortful

a_2. Relatively preserved repetition of recently heard oral phrases

a_3. Relatively preserved comprehension of the meaning of spoken and written words, phrases, and sentences

Associated Features

a. A tendency to repeat recently heard phrases, which the patient is unable to inhibit (see Echolalia)
b. In some patients, the presence of impaired naming of objects, impaired word finding during conversation, or both (see also Anomic aphasia); naming and word finding improving slightly when phonetic cues (e.g., presenting the initial speech sounds of the word) are provided
c. Unilateral (usually right-sided) motor weakness (hemiparesis)
d. Impaired ability to perform skilled movements on demand (see Apraxia)
e. Speech fluency possibly improving slightly during the course of an ongoing conversation but declining rapidly following termination of the conversation
f. Occasional production of fluent and grammatical sentences
g. Relatively preserved oral reading in some cases
h. Relatively preserved ability to respond to questions that can be answered with one word
i. A recent history of mixed transcortical aphasia (see later text) or Broca's aphasia (see earlier text)

Factors to Rule Out

a. Impaired articulation as a result of weakness of the speech muscles (*anarthria* or *dysarthria*) sufficient to account for the deficits in oral language, ruled out by documenting the extension of the deficit to written language or by documenting the preserved repetition of recently heard phrases
b. Impaired ability to carry out skilled movements of the speech muscles on demand (see Buccofacial apraxia) sufficient to account for the deficits in oral language, ruled out by documenting the extension of the deficit to written language or by documenting the preserved repetition of recently heard phrases

Lesion Locations

a. Medial frontal lobe, particularly the supplementary motor area and white matter anterior and lateral to the frontal horn of lateral ventricle[40–42]
b. Basal ganglia (lenticular nucleus)[12]

Lesion Lateralization

a. Language-dominant (usually left) hemisphere

7. Transcortical sensory aphasia (also called acoustic amnestic aphasia; see also Aphasic alexia-agraphia)

Clinical Indicators

a_1. Impaired comprehension of the vocabulary (i.e., the lexical elements distinct from grammar and syntax) of spoken or written sentences

a_2. Relatively preserved repetition of recently heard oral phrases

a_3. Impaired or indecipherable spontaneous and responsive speech and writing as a result of the occurrence of any of the following errors:

1) Addition of extra words or phrases to the target phrases being spoken or written
2) Substitution of incorrect speech sounds for the target sounds in words (*phonemic* or *literal paraphasia*)
3) Word substitution errors that are semantically related to the target words that should have been spoken *(semantic paraphasia)* or written *(semantic paragraphia)*
4) Random word substitution errors that have no meaningful relation to the target words that should have been spoken *(random paraphasia)* or written *(random paragraphia)*
5) Substitution of nonsense words that have no linguistic meaning (*neologisms* or *jargon words*) for the target words that should have been spoken or written

   NOTE: Semantic paraphasias, random paraphasias, and neologisms are collectively referred to as verbal paraphasias; *the term* paragraphia *is used when the errors occur during writing.*
6) Substitution of nonspecific words (e.g., "it," "thing") for concrete words (i.e., "empty speech")
7) Substitution of one grammatical function word for another (e.g., "to" substituted for "with")
8) Tangled juxtaposition of phrases that have no meaningful relationship to each other

   NOTE: The term paragrammatism *is used to describe the incorrect grammar of these patients as a result of substitution errors involving function words, verbal paraphasias, and the meaningless juxtaposition of phrases.*

a_4. Speech and writing fluent and unrestricted, in some cases occurring at a greater than normal rate and in a greater than normal amount

Associated Features

a. A tendency to repeat recently heard phrases, which the patient is unable to inhibit (see Echolalia)
b. Failure to monitor speech so that the patient is unaware that it is meaningless or impaired
c. Frustration at the seemingly inexplicable failure of others to comprehend own utterances
d. Impaired naming of objects (see also Anomic aphasia) that does not im-

prove when contextual cues (e.g., describing the object's use) or phonetic cues (e.g., presenting the initial speech sounds of the object's name) are provided

e. The presence of homonymous hemianopsia: loss of acuity in one visual half-field
f. Impaired ability to perform skilled movements on demand (see Apraxia)
g. Relatively preserved ability to sing the lyrics of songs learned before the onset of brain damage
h. Relatively preserved ability to recite passages (e.g., poems, prayers) learned before the onset of brain damage

Factors to Rule Out

a. Hearing loss sufficient to account for the failure to comprehend oral language, ruled out by documenting preserved repetition of recently heard phrases
b. Schizophrenia and related psychiatric disorders in which speech is idiosyncratic and neologistic, and comprehension is compromised by confusion and disorganization (see Chap. 18 for assessment techniques)

Lesion Locations

a. Medial or lateral parietal lobe, particularly the angular gyrus, with occasional extension to the occipital lobe[43,44]
b. Thalamus, particularly the pulvinar nucleus[45–50]*

Lesion Lateralization

a. Language-dominant (usually left) hemisphere

8. Mixed transcortical aphasia

Clinical Indicators

a_1. Total or near-total absence of spontaneous speech and writing

a_2. Dysfluent responsive speech and writing as evidenced by any of the following signs:
   1) Repetition of examiner's statements or questions with no additional speech
   2) Speech and writing are limited to simple, repetitively produced word fragments
   3) Speech and writing limited to isolated, concrete words
   4) Speech and writing terse and telegraphic, consisting of simple phrases (e.g., verb and object combinations)
   5) Speech and writing slow, laborious, and effortful

a_3. Relatively preserved repetition of recently heard oral phrases

a_4. Impaired comprehension of the meaning of spoken and written words, phrases, and sentences

---

*The aphasic disorder seen in some cases of thalamic hemorrhage or infarction can be characterized as a partial transcortical sensory aphasia. Speech production may be paraphasic and neologistic, whereas repetition is spared or minimally impaired. Comprehension is impaired in most cases, but to a lesser degree than in cases of transcortical sensory aphasia following cortical lesions.

Associated Features

a. A tendency to repeat recently heard phrases, which the patient is unable to inhibit (see Echolalia)
b. Impaired naming of objects (see also Anomic aphasia), which does not improve when contextual cues (e.g., showing the object being used) or phonetic cues (e.g., presenting the initial speech sounds of the object's name) are provided
c. Relatively preserved ability to complete overlearned phrases (e.g., a line from a poem or proverb), the initial part of which is provided by the examiner
d. Relatively preserved ability to sing familiar songs

Factors to Rule Out

a. Impaired articulation as a result of weakness of the speech muscles (*anarthria* or *dysarthria*) sufficient to account for the deficits in oral language, ruled out by documenting the preserved repetition of recently heard oral phrases
b. Impaired ability to carry out skilled movements of the speech muscles on demand (see Buccofacial apraxia) sufficient to account for the deficits in oral language, ruled out by documenting the extension of the deficit to written language or by documenting the preserved repetition of recently heard oral phrases
c. Hearing loss sufficient to account for the failure to comprehend oral language, ruled out by documenting the preserved repetition of recently heard oral phrases

Lesion Locations

a. Perisylvian area (cortical or subcortical white matter, or both), including portions of the frontal, temporal, and parietal lobes[51,52]
b. Combined medial frontal lobe, particularly the supplementary motor area, and medial parietal lobe, particularly the supplementary sensory area, with frequent extension to the temporal lobe but sparing the perisylvian area[41,53]
c. Frontal lobe, particularly Broca's area, premotor cortex, and prefrontal cortex[54]
d. Combined parietal and occipital lobes[55]
e. White matter subjacent to the angular gyrus and thalamus[56]

Lesion Lateralization

a. Language-dominant (usually left) hemisphere

9. Anomic aphasia (also called anomia, amnestic aphasia, and semantic aphasia)

Clinical Indicators

a_1. Diminished ability to name visually and tactually presented familiar objects or object parts
a_2. Diminished ability to find substantive words to express ideas
a_3. Speech fluent and unrestricted, but contains many pauses as a result of an inability to find the words the patient wishes to say

a_4. Relatively preserved ability to describe the use of objects that cannot be named

a_5. Relatively preserved repetition of recently heard oral phrases

a_6. Relatively preserved comprehension of the meaning of oral words, phrases, and sentences

a_7. No current preponderance of clinical indicators of another disorder of oral communication

Associated Features

a. Presence of semantic paraphasias in some patients: word substitution errors that are semantically related to the target words that should have been spoken
b. Substitution of descriptions of target words when the word itself cannot be found *(circumlocution)*
c. Speech appearing empty of meaning as a result of the lack of substantive words
d. Impaired ability to identify the fingers of the hand (see Finger agnosia)
e. Impaired discrimination of the right and left sides of the body, space, or both (see Right-left disorientation)
f. Impaired ability to write (see Agraphia)
g. Impaired calculation ability (see Acalculia)
NOTE: When finger agnosia, right-left disorientation, agraphia, and acalculia occur together in the same patient, the entire complex is referred to as Gerstmann's syndrome.
h. Impaired ability to read (see Alexia)
i. A recent history of another disorder of oral communication

Factors to Rule Out

a. Normal decline in naming ability with advancing age
b. Current presence of another subtype of aphasia in which naming and word finding are characteristically impaired
c. A premorbidly poor vocabulary as a result of limited education or learning disability
d. Lithium carbonate toxicity in patients prescribed this medication,[14] ruled out by laboratory determination of lithium blood level

Lesion Locations

a. Frontal lobe[11,57]
b. Temporal lobe[11,57,58]
c. Parietal lobe, particularly the angular gyrus, usually with additional involvement of temporal lobe[11,57,59]

Lesion Lateralization

a. Language-dominant (usually left) hemisphere

10. Unilateral anomia (see Chap. 10)

11. Optic aphasia (see also Visual object agnosia)

Clinical Indicators

a_1. Inaccurate oral naming of visually presented familiar objects, regardless of where in the visual field they are presented, as evidenced by any of the following signs:

1) Failure to respond
2) An incorrect but semantically related name
3) Naming a visually similar but incorrect object
4) Repeating a response that was correct on a previous trial but is not correct on the current trial (see Ideational perseveration)
5) A response unrelated to the object
6) Extended delay in responding

a_2. Relatively preserved recognition of visually presented familiar objects, as evidenced by either of the following signs:
1) Relatively preserved ability to demonstrate the use of objects that cannot be named
2) Relatively preserved ability to point to objects that previously could not be named when they are named by the examiner

a_3. Relatively preserved ability to name tactually presented familiar objects

Associated Features

a. Relatively preserved ability, in some cases, to write the names of objects that cannot be named orally
b. A recent history of impaired recognition of visually presented familiar objects (see Visual object agnosia)
c. Presence of (usually right-sided) homonymous hemianopsia: loss of acuity in one visual half-field
d. Impaired reading with relatively preserved ability to write (see Pure alexia)

Factors to Rule Out

a. Impaired perception of visually presented objects as a result of any of the following disorders:
   1. Loss of visual acuity so severe that it prevents objects from being seen regardless of where in the visual field they are presented
   2. Visual form imperception (see Chap. 5)
   3. Failure to detect portions of visual stimuli as a result of stimulus neglect (see Chap. 4)
b. Unfamiliarity with the objects before the onset of the brain lesion
c. Inability to make intelligible oral responses as a result of the presence of another oral language disorder

Lesion Locations

a. Occipital lobe alone, but usually in conjunction with posterior and inferior temporal lobes, with extension to the posterior forceps[60–65]

Lesion Lateralization

a. Language-dominant (usually left) hemisphere

12. Tactile Aphasia* (see also Astereognosis)

Clinical Indicators

a_1. Inaccurate oral naming of tactually presented familiar objects while vision is occluded, regardless of which hand explores the object

*This disorder must be considered putative because there are few clinical reports available.

a_2. Relatively preserved ability to demonstrate the use of objects that cannot be named

a_3. Relatively preserved oral naming of visually presented objects

Associated Features

a. Impaired verbal description of the use of tactually presented familiar objects while vision is occluded

Factors to Rule Out

a. Impaired perception of tactually presented objects as a result of any of the following disorders:
   1. Loss of tactile sensation so severe that it prevents objects from being perceived by touch
   2. Tactual form imperception (see Chap. 5)
   3. Failure to detect portions of tactual stimuli as a result of stimulus neglect (see Chap. 4)

b. Unfamiliarity with the objects before the onset of the brain lesion

c. Inability to make intelligible oral responses as a result of the presence of another oral language disorder

Lesion Locations

a. Combined temporal lobe, posterior part of second temporal convolution; parietal lobe, angular gyrus; and subcortical white matter, including the inferior longitudinal fasciculus, occipital vertical fasciculus, arcuate fasciculus, occipital-frontal fasciculus, and the thalamic radiations[66]

Lesion Lateralization

a. Language-dominant (usually left) hemisphere

13. Stimulus-specific aphasia (includes color aphasia and color anomia)*

Clinical Indicators

a_1. Diminished ability to orally communicate about colors, as evidenced by any of the following signs:
   1) Inability to name the characteristic colors of familiar objects
   2) Reduced color fluency: the patient able to generate only a few colors when asked to name all the colors that he or she knows
   3) Inability to name objects that share a common color
   4) Inability to name colors that are visually presented
   5) Inability to point to colors that are named

a_2. Deficit in communication about color disproportionate to any other oral language impairment that may be present

NOTE: The terms color anomia *and* color aphasia *have been used to describe patients with various combinations of these signs.*

b_1. Diminished ability to communicate orally about body parts, as evidenced by either of the following signs:

---

*This disorder must be considered putative because there are few clinical reports available.

1) Inability to name body parts
2) Inability to indicate body parts named by the examiner

b_2. Deficit in communication about body parts disproportionate to any other oral language impairment that may be present

b_3. Relatively preserved ability to visually recognize body parts, as indicated by either of the following signs:
1) Relatively accurate oral or written description of how body parts are used
2) Relatively accurate indication of how body parts are used by pointing to pictures of activities that can be done with particular body parts

Associated Features

a. The presence of (usually right-sided) homonymous hemianopsia: loss of acuity in one visual half-field
b. Muscle weakness that is usually mild and on one side of the body, usually the right
c. The presence of other disorders of oral language
d. Some degree of impairment in the recognition of the colors associated with common objects (see Color agnosia) when assessed with nonverbal tasks; the impairment is exacerbated when the patient attempts to verbalize answers while performing manually
e. Impaired reading with relatively preserved ability to write (see Pure alexia)
f. Severely impaired memory (see Amnesia)

Factors to Rule Out

a. The presence of impaired matching and discrimination of colors in patients who are unable to name visually presented colors or point to colors named; matching and discrimination deficits possibly the result of any of the following disorders:
   1. Loss of visual acuity so severe that it prevents colored stimuli from being seen regardless of where in the visual field they are presented
   2. Color imperception (see Chap. 5)
   3. Failure to detect portions of visual stimuli as a result of stimulus neglect (see Chap. 4)
b. The presence of impaired recognition of object colors (see Color agnosia) sufficient to account for the deficit in patients who are unable to name colors of objects or objects having a common color
c. The presence of impaired visual recognition of body parts (see Finger agnosia) in patients who are unable to name body parts or who are unable to point to body parts named by the examiner, ruled out by documenting preserved ability to describe or indicate nonverbally the use of the body part
d. The presence of impaired body part localization in response to nonverbal stimuli (see Finger mislocalization and Autotopagnosia) in patients who are unable to indicate body parts named by the examiner; if this factor cannot be ruled out, diagnosis based on assessment of patient's ability to name body parts

Lesion Locations

a. Combined lesions of the occipital lobe, involving the cuneus and the fusiform and lingual gyri; medial temporal lobe, particularly the parahippocampal gyrus and the hippocampus; and corpus callosum, involving the splenium, posterior forceps, or both,* with frequent extension to the precuneus and occasional extension to the thalamus (geniculate bodies), optic radiations, fornix, and cingulate gyrus[67–71]

Lesion Lateralization

a. Language-dominant (usually left) hemisphere

14. Pathological reiteration (palilalia and echolalia)

Clinical Indicators

a_1. Spontaneous multiple repetitions of own syllables, words, or phrases *(palilalia)*
a_2. Inability to inhibit the tendency to repeat
b_1. Spontaneous repetition of someone else's words or phrases *(echolalia)*
b_2. Inability to inhibit the tendency to repeat

Associated Features

a. Speed of utterance increasing with each repetition in patients with palilalia
b. Voice volume decreasing with each repetition of an utterance in patients with palilalia
c. Terminal sounds, words, phrases, or sentences in an utterance tending to be repeated by patients with palilalia
d. Presence of other oral language disorders, particularly transcortical sensory, transcortical motor, and mixed transcortical aphasia
e. Global decline in intellectual functioning (see Global intellectual decline)

Factors to Rule Out

a. Use of repetition of phrases and commands as a strategy to facilitate comprehension, performance, or memory, ruled out by documenting that the patient cannot inhibit the repetition
b. Schizophrenia and related psychiatric disorders in which speech is idiosyncratic and may include spontaneous reiterations (see Chap. 18 for assessment techniques)
c. Verbal tics that can be distinguished from pathologic reiteration by their content (e.g., barks, grunts, obscenities) and onset (typically in childhood without a clear precipitant)
d. Stuttering that can be distinguished from pathologic reiteration by the great effort required to utter words by stutterers and by the tendency of stutterers to repeat only the initial sounds in words

Lesion Locations

Palilalia

a. Combined medial thalamus, subthalamic nucleus, and midbrain[72]

---

*If right homonymous hemianopsia is present, the lesion need not include the corpus callosum.

b. Basal ganglia with extension to subthalamic nucleus, substantia nigra, or cerebral cortex[73,74]
c. Cerebral hemisphere, particularly the combined frontal and parietal lobes[75,76]

Echolalia

a. Thalamus with extension to posterior limb of internal capsule, paraventricular white matter, or rostral midbrain[39,77,78]
b. Basal ganglia with extension to cerebral cortex[79]
c. Cerebral hemisphere, particularly the combined frontal, parietal, and temporal lobes[52,80]

Lesion Lateralization

a. Palilalia most commonly reported following bilateral lesions[73]
b. Echolalia most commonly reported following left-sided lesions

15. Mutism (including aphemia*)

Clinical Indicator

a. Absence of all speech sounds, whether spontaneous, imitative, or in response to questions

Associated Features

a. With recovery, low-volume (hypophonic), effortful, slow speech becoming possible
b. When assessable, writing in response to a command or stimulus relatively preserved
c. When assessable, comprehension of written and spoken sentences relatively preserved
d. When assessable, writing relatively free of syntactic and grammatical errors (when speech becomes possible, it is also relatively free of syntactic and grammatical errors)
e. When assessable, naming and ability to find words to express ideas relatively preserved.
f. May precede the occurrence of another oral language disorder, particularly in patients with subcortical lesions
g. Impaired ability to perform skilled movements of the mouth, face, and speech muscles on demand (see Buccofacial apraxia)
h. Impaired ability to express verbal prosody after speech becomes possible: a deficit in the ability to vary tone of voice, pitch, rate of speech, and word stress to coincide with the intended meaning or purpose of an utterance (e.g., the patient cannot turn the statement "Cathy is driving" into a question by raising the pitch of his or her voice at the end of the phase and stressing the last word)
i. Impaired or absent initiation of all movements (see Akinesia)
NOTE: When akinesia and mutism occur together in a patient, the entire complex is referred to as akinetic mutism.

---

*Aphemia is also called *pure word dumbness* and *subcortical motor aphasia*.

Factors to Rule Out

a. Loss of ability to make all vocal sounds *(aphonia)* as a result of damage of the vocal organs. When even nonlinguistic verbalizations are absent, medical consultation for examination of the vocal organs and air passages is required.
b. Deliberate or unconscious avoidance of speech as a result of recent emotional trauma or to avoid unpleasant consequences or situations.

Lesion Locations

a. Frontal lobe, particularly the operculum, cingulate gyrus, and supplementary motor area[81–86]
b. Basal ganglia, particularly the lenticular nucleus and head of caudate, with frequent extension to the anterior or posterior limbs of the internal capsule[86–89]
c. Thalamus[86,90,91]
d. Reticular activating system in the brainstem (pons) and mesencephalon[92–94]
e. Pericollicular area[95]
f. Hypothalamus, with occasional extension to the medial forebrain bundle[96,97]
g. Diffuse white matter[98–100]

ETIOLOGY

Cerebrovascular accident involving the middle cerebral artery is the most common cause of the oral language disorders. Transcortical motor aphasia may follow infarction in the territory of the anterior cerebral or anterior choroidal arteries, or it may follow anterior watershed infarctions in the border zone between areas supplied by the anterior cerebral and middle cerebral arteries.[101] Transcortical sensory aphasia may follow posterior cerebral artery infarctions or posterior watershed infarctions in the border zone between areas supplied by the posterior cerebral artery and the middle cerebral artery.[43] Optic aphasia is associated with posterior communicating artery infarctions, whereas color aphasia tends to follow posterior cerebral artery infarctions.

Traumatic brain injury, particularly when secondary hemorrhages occur, can also lead to oral language impairment. Oral language can also be compromised in demyelinating disease and the advanced stages of degenerative diseases such as Alzheimer's. Neoplasm is a less common cause of oral language impairment. Pathologic reiteration may be seen in diseases of the basal ganglia, such as Parkinson's disease, and in idiopathic cerebral calcinosis. Leukoencephalopathy following chemotherapy and radiotherapy for cancer is a rarely reported cause of mutism. Finally, cerebral anoxia may compromise the ability to produce oral language.

DISABLING CONSEQUENCES

Patients with persistent disorders of oral language must, in most cases, be considered totally disabled. Communication is essential in virtually all occupational settings. This is as true for the attorney who must argue cases before juries as it is for the janitor who must follow the verbal directions of a supervisor. Even jobs involving unskilled manual labor require the individual to follow verbal directions and to communicate meaningfully with supervisors and coworkers. Patients with minimal to mild deficits in verbal communication may fare better in modified and heavily structured work settings, but even in these cases, competitive employability might not be achieved.

Disability in these patients usually extends to domestic and community settings. Preparing grocery lists, following recipes, reading and responding to business correspondence, placing orders in restaurants, and other everyday tasks may be beyond the patient. Even the communication of basic needs for food or access to lavatory facilities may be a problem. The patient's inability to communicate may make it impossible for him or her to obtain aid independently in an emergency.

The patient who has compromised oral language skills is apt to experience considerable social isolation and restriction of leisure activity. Movies, television, radio, and books are of little use to a person who cannot comprehend the language contained in these media. An individual who enjoyed church attendance, taking classes, or going to dinner parties may avoid these activities now that he or she cannot communicate adequately.

Virtually all aspects of the ability to function independently are diminished in patients who have severe oral language disorders. Extensive, long-term support from society, the patient's immediate family, and other caretakers is often required.

ASSESSMENT INSTRUMENTS

Boston Diagnostic Aphasia Examination

The Boston Diagnostic Aphasia Examination (BDAE)[8] can be obtained from *Williams & Wilkins, Rose Tree Corporate Center, Building II, Suite 5025, 1400 North Providence Road, Media, PA 19063-2043.*

The BDAE assumes that various components of language can be selectively impaired and that these components can be assessed with relative independence, provided that the patient can shift flexibly between input channels and response modes. Both of these assumptions are compatible with the approach taken in this text.

The BDAE provides a thorough and comprehensive assessment of oral and written language. Oral language subtests measure fluency (speech articulation, phrase length, and intonation), auditory comprehension, naming, speech repetition, the presence of paraphasic errors in speech, and the ability to produce overlearned automatic phrases. The written language subtests measure oral reading, reading comprehension, and written and oral spelling. Supplementary language tests allow for a more refined assessment of comprehension, repetition, and expression. For example, the supplementary tests contrast repetition of indicative, interrogative, and conditional phrases. The BDAE results lead directly to a classification of oral and written language disorder consistent with the one used in this book and a rating of the severity of the language disorder.

Internal consistency reliability coefficients computed using the Kuder-Richardson formula and reported in the test manual vary from .68 to .98 among the BDAE oral and written language subtests. In addition to the severity rating scale, the BDAE includes rating scales for speech intonation, phrase length, speech articulation, grammatical form, paraphasia, repetition, word finding, and auditory comprehension, based on mean percentiles of four subtests. Inter-rater reliability coefficients varied from .68 to .96, with both the lowest and highest correlations occurring on subtests included in the auditory comprehension rating.

Normative data are reported in the manual on 242 patients with aphasia and 147 neurologically normal English-speaking men. In most cases, normal controls obtained the maximum possible scores on the BDAE subtest measures computed for them. The few low scorers were normal persons older than 60 years of age who had fewer than 9 years of education. Some caution in interpreting BDAE performance in the elderly or in patients who have had limited education appears to be warranted.

Factor analysis of the BDAE results in the aphasic sample reported in the manual produced eight language-related factors and two factors with loadings primarily from supplementary nonverbal tests. The eight language-related factors were identified as fluency, repetition-recitation, auditory comprehension, writing, verbal paraphasia, nonverbal oral agility (see Buccofacial apraxia), naming, and freedom from paraphasia factors. Additional factor analyses are discussed in the test manual, but overall, similar factors tended to emerge in analyses that included all or most of the BDAE subtests.

A discriminant function analysis is also reported in the manual. The results suggested that five BDAE scores are most effective in classifying prototypical Broca's, Wernicke's, conduction, and anomic aphasics:

1. Body-part identification
2. Repetition of high-probability sentences
3. Verbal paraphasia
4. Articulatory agility rating
5. Automatized sequences

Cross-validation of these results was not attempted.

The BDAE incorporates state-of-the-art diagnostic procedures and is one of the best available oral and written language batteries. It does not, however, incorporate procedures based on the newer cognitive subtypes of written language disorder (see Chap. 13). The BDAE is most readily administered in office and laboratory settings, although bedside testing is feasible. Interpretation depends not only on the BDAE normative data, but also on the experience of the clinician. Consequently, the test is recommended for use only by speech pathologists, neurologists, and neuropsychologists who have considerable experience in the diagnosis of language disorder.

Western Aphasia Battery

The Western Aphasia Battery (WAB)[102] can be obtained from *Grune & Stratton, Incorporated, Orlando, FL 32809.*

The WAB consists of subtests measuring oral language (spontaneous speech, comprehension, naming, and repetition), written language (reading and writing), calculation ability, and associated nonverbal functions. The WAB leads to a diagnostic classification compatible with the system used in this text. Classification is achieved based on the range of the patient's scores on fluency, comprehension, repetition, and naming subtests. Disorders not included in the classification system can nonetheless be diagnosed using data from the WAB and the criteria specified in this book.

The current version of the WAB is a revision of a previously published version that was standardized on 215 patients with aphasia and 63 normal and nonaphasic brain-damaged controls,[103] with high reliability and demonstrated ability to differentiate aphasic from nonaphasic groups.[104] The correlations between the revised and original WAB oral language subtests range between .85 and .99.[102] The written language subtests show more variable correlations, ranging from .54 to .99. The test manual reports that comparison of revised and previous WAB subtests yielded no statistically significant differences. Direct investigation of the reliability and validity of the revised WAB is necessary to fully substantiate clinical use of the WAB.

The WAB is most appropriate for office or laboratory administration, but bedside administration is also feasible. The test is recommended for use by neurologists, speech pathologists, and neuropsychologists with extensive experience in the diagnosis of oral and written language disorder because of the uncertainty regarding the psychometric properties of the revised WAB. The WAB is similar to the BDAE, which is also reviewed in this chapter. The WAB provides a quicker but less comprehensive assessment of a patient's language abilities. When comprehensiveness and rigorous standardization are vital, the BDAE is the instrument of choice. When brevity and practicality are vital, the WAB may be the better option.

Boston Naming Test

The Boston Naming Test[105] can be obtained from *Williams & Wilkins, Rose Tree Corporate Center, Building II, Suite 5025, 1400 North Providence Road, Media, PA 19063-2043.*

In this test, patients attempt to name drawings of objects. Object names range from high-frequency to low-frequency words. The examiner gives phonemic (first sound in the word) or semantic cues if the patient's initial response is incorrect or if the patient is unable to give an answer. The use of two types of cues helps to distinguish patients with naming deficits who may benefit from phonemic but not semantic cues from patients who fail to recognize or do not know the name of a target stimulus.

The normative data accompanying the test are based on 84 normal adults ranging in age from 18 to 59 years.[105] Age and education effects are not apparent in these data but have been documented in other normative samples.[106] The latter investigators provide cut-off scores by 5-year age cohorts for individuals aged 60 to 85 years.

The reliability of the current version of the Boston Naming Test has not been well investigated. The test appears to have good concurrent validity; it correlates at .81 with the BDAE Visual Confrontation Naming subtest and at .71 with the BDAE Responsive Naming subtest.[8] The Boston Naming Test is intended to be sensitive to subtle naming deficits that may be missed by the naming subtests of the BDAE and WAB, which employ more common objects. Empirical investigation has supported the sensitivity of the Boston Naming Test and of several shortened versions (e.g., tests using odd or even items only) to naming deficits in various patient populations.[107,108]

The Boston Naming Test can be administered at bedside, in the office, or in the laboratory. Interpretation should be attempted only by neuropsychologists, behavioral neurologists, and speech pathologists. Care must be taken to avoid confusing the effects of age and education and the effects of brain damage. Reliance on age and education norms is critical for the proper interpretation of Boston Naming Test results.

Halstead-Reitan Battery Aphasia Screening Test

The Halstead-Reitan Battery (HRB) Aphasia Screening Test (AST)[109] can be obtained from *Reitan Neuropsychological Laboratory, 1338 East Edison Street, Tucson, AZ 85719.*

The HRB-AST is a brief screening device designed to detect language disorder and its associated features. Language items assess comprehension of speech, oral expression, speech repetition, naming, oral reading, reading comprehension, and writing. Additional items require the patient to solve simple oral and written calculations, to distinguish right from left, and to draw a square, triangle, cross, and key from a model. The drawing tasks are sometimes referred to as "spatial relations" items. Test results are usually presented descriptively, but a simple scoring system for the test is available that leads to separate scores reflecting the language and constructional components of the AST.[110] Age, education, and gender corrections are also available.[111]

Because the HRB-AST is typically not scored, little research has been done on its psychometric properties. The HRB-AST has been reported to discriminate cerebral dysfunction from psychiatric patient samples at the .01 level of statistical significance before scores were corrected for age and intelligence quotient (IQ) and at the .001 level of significance after age and IQ correction.[112]

The HRB-AST can be administered at bedside, in the office, or in laboratory settings. It is recommended for use only by neuropsychologists experienced in the diagnosis of oral and written language disorders and in the use of the HRB. The HRB-AST was not designed to provide a comprehensive and thorough assessment of language, nor does it lead directly to a classification of oral and written language disorder subtypes. Whenever possible, the AST should be supplemented with additional language tests.

NEUROPSYCHOLOGICAL TREATMENT

Treatment of oral language disorders is the province of speech therapists. They alone have the necessary training and expertise to address this group of disorders.

Neuropsychologists have only a limited, adjunctive role, and typically they are not consulted unless a patient who seems to have good potential for improvement fails to participate in and respond to speech therapy.

Patients may not respond to speech therapy because they lack motivation for treatment and doubt that they can make progress. Several steps can be taken to alleviate this problem. First, the neuropsychologist must identify what stimuli are uniquely rewarding to the patient. Potential rewards can range from a simple approving handshake to an opportunity to listen to favorite music. These activities can then be made contingent on the patient's active participation in speech therapy. In patients who have sufficiently intact language comprehension, the relation between therapy participation and the rewards can be explained verbally. Other patients may require the contingency to be demonstrated (i.e., immediately after they show any amount of effort, the reward should be given).

The length of time for which active participation can be maintained before a reward is given must be determined, often by trial and error. After the patient begins to respond to rewards, the length of time he or she must work before another reward is given should be lengthened gradually. For patients who have drastically limited motivation, rewards should be given initially just for coming to speech therapy and agreeing to sit attentively for a moment. As they begin to respond, they can be shaped in the direction of better participation.

Providing feedback about progress is also an effective motivational technique. Such feedback is more convincing when it comes not only from the speech therapist but also from relatives and friends. Audiotaping and videotaping the patient at successive points in time is another way of convincingly demonstrating progress to the patient. Progress can be graphically diagrammed each week on a wall chart hung in a prominent place. In my clinic, a "wall of fame" has been designated where graphs of all patients' progress are displayed and updated in a weekly meeting. Patients who are making progress are congratulated by the staff and given a round of applause by the other patients. Even patients who simply maintain the same consistent level of effort are rewarded with a handshake from the therapist and a pat on the back from other patients.

Aphasic patients may fail to benefit from speech therapy if other emotional and neuropsychological disorders that interfere with progress are present. Depression is often encountered in aphasic patients and can manifest itself subtly as a lack of enthusiasm and effort or more overtly as near-constant tearfulness during therapy sessions. Impaired ability to concentrate, reduced capacity to learn and retain new information, declines in intellectual functioning, and perceptual disorders, among other factors, can interfere with efforts to remediate language. Behavioral problems such as aggression or sexually disinhibited acts can halt progress and sabotage the working relationship between the patient and speech therapist.

Neuropsychological examination of patients with oral language disorders can help reveal other disorders that may be present. Once identified, these disorders can be addressed either directly by the speech therapist (e.g., when a memory disorder is present) or by intervention from the neuropsychologist or other rehabilitation professional. The neuropsychologist should at least be able to suggest ways of modifying speech therapy to accommodate the full range of deficits present in a patient.

Even simple changes, such as giving a tearfully depressed patient 5 minutes at the end of each session to vent his or her feelings, can enhance the effectiveness of speech therapy with difficult patients. Specific treatment approaches are listed under each category of neuropsychological disorder in this book.

CASE ILLUSTRATIONS

CASE 12–1

H.S. was a 64-year-old man with a 12th-grade education. He suffered an embolic left middle cerebral artery cerebrovascular accident secondary to atrial fibrillation. His medical history was positive for a previous myocardial infarction. There was no history of psychiatric disorder, nor were there any indications of hallucinations. Neurological examination revealed right hemiparesis and a right homonymous hemianopsia. His hearing appeared to be normal. The patient's speech was dysarthric. The content of his speech consisted of unintelligible jargon expressed in a highly melodic voice; he often appeared to be singing when he spoke. When he was frustrated, the volume of his voice increased, and his tone became unmistakably angry. The patient was unable to follow even simple commands, and extensive neuropsychological testing was not possible.

Results of the oral language subtests of the WAB are presented in Table 12–1. The Aphasia Quotient is consistent with the presence of a severe oral language disorder. H.S.'s subtest scores indicated that he was severely impaired in comprehension, repetition, and naming at the time of testing. His speech was fluent and rhythmic, but consisted of jargon words that conveyed no information. Written language, including all aspects of reading and writing, was as impaired as oral language in this patient. For illustrations of written language disorder, see Chapter 13.

DISCUSSION

Because this patient completed the WAB, the classification criteria from this test can be used to aid in making a diagnosis. H.S.'s fluent speech in the context of severely impaired comprehension, repetition, and naming met criteria established for a diagnosis of Wernicke's aphasia. The WAB does not provide criteria for pure word deafness, which could also fit H.S.'s pattern of test scores. However, the fact that all aspects of written language were as impaired as oral language rules out pure word deafness. No difficulty in hearing was noted in the examination, and there was no history of psychiatric disorder. Although an extensive interview was not possible with this patient, at no point did his behavior suggest the possibility of psychiatric disorder.

CASE 12–2

H.L. was a 27-year-old man with a master's degree in business administration. He was in good health until he was found unconscious outside his apartment after

Table 12–1. **PERFORMANCE OF H.S. AND H.L. ON THE WESTERN APHASIA BATTERY (WAB)**

WAB Subtest	Maximum Possible Score	Patient H.S.	Patient H.L.
Spontaneous speech			
Information	10	0	7
Fluency	10	7	4
Total	20	7	11
Comprehension			
Yes/no	60	5	54
Word recognition	60	10	59
Commands	80	0	34
Total/20	10	0.75	7.4
Repetition			
Total/10	10	0	7.2
Naming			
Object naming	60	0	48
Word fluency	20	0	4
Sentence completion	10	0	8
Responsive speech	10	0	8
Total/10	10	0	6.8
Aphasia quotient	93.8 (cut-off)	15.5	64.8

returning from jogging. A computed tomography (CT) scan revealed a large infarction in the distribution of the middle cerebral artery, affecting both the temporal and parietal lobes.

The patient was admitted to a rehabilitation hospital approximately 1 month after his infarction. Neurological and neuropsychological examinations revealed a right hemiparesis that was worse in the upper extremity, decreased right-sided tactile sensation, and right-sided extinction to double simultaneous stimulation in the visual and auditory modalities (see Sensory extinction). Perceptual skills, nonverbal problem solving, and memory for visuospatial information were intact.

The WAB was administered; results are listed in Table 12–1. H.L.'s aphasia quotient is fairly high, suggesting that he had only moderate language deficits when tested. The information content of his speech was relatively high, but this content was communicated in a halting, telegraphic manner. For example, when asked to describe what was depicted in test picture 1 of the WAB (a picnic scene), H.L. replied:

> *"Well that's the flag [pause] that's all right. [Pause] Over there's the sailboat [pause] and on the other hand, [pause] it's the sail, [pause] on the other hand, [pause] looking like reading [pause] you see, that's it, you see. [Pause] Well it's, I don't know. [Pause] The table and chair [pause] all right."*

Besides being telegraphic, H.L.'s speech was filled with automatic phrases (e.g., "you see," "all right," "on the other hand") that acted as filler material but added little substantive content. Except for the table and chair, all items mentioned were actually in the picture. Writing samples obtained from H.L. were entirely consistent with his pattern of speech. Spontaneous writing was telegraphic, with omission of grammatical words and frequent misspellings.

The data in Table 12–1 also suggest that H.L.'s comprehension of speech was good, with the exception of his ability to carry out sequential commands. Inspection of the individual items of the WAB Sequential Commands Subtest suggested that the patient's difficulty was with syntactic comprehension. For example, he accurately carried out the command "Point to the pen and the book." However, he failed to correctly carry out the commands "Point with the pen to the book," and "Point to the pen with the book." These three commands involve the same number of steps, but the latter two require a greater appreciation of syntax than does the first. H.L.'s repetition was only slightly impaired. He performed at an 80 percent correct level on most naming tasks, with the exception of the Word Fluency Subtest, on which he showed greater impairment.

DISCUSSION

Using criteria provided by the WAB, the patient in Case 12–2 would be classified as having Broca's aphasia. Dysarthria could not account for the agrammatic, halting quality of his speech, nor could buccofacial apraxia account for the extension of his deficits in writing. It is notable that H.L.'s speech repetition is relatively preserved compared with his other deficits. He scored only 0.8 points below the cut-off for transcortical motor aphasia. It appears likely that the patient's aphasia is evolving. Although the current diagnosis is Broca's aphasia, reassessment in as little as 1 month will probably lead to a revision of the diagnosis.

CASE 12–3

I.L. was a 72-year-old woman with a high-school education who had worked as a legal secretary until her retirement. She was taken to the emergency department following a syncopal episode. A CT scan revealed a right intracerebral hematoma. The patient subsequently developed hydrocephalus and underwent ventriculostomy. Neuropsychological testing revealed impaired concentration, perceptual deficits, bilateral motor ataxia, intellectual functioning in the average range, intact problem solving, and intact memory for verbal information.

The HRB-AST was administered as part of the neuropsychological evaluation. The patient made poor copies of the figures included in this test, but made no errors in comprehension, reading, writing, repetition, or speech. She accurately named all pictured objects except for a fork, which she named on her third try after calling it a brush and a comb. She was aware of her incorrect naming of the fork and attempted to correct herself without prompting from the examiner.

Difficulty in word finding was also evident during conversations. I.L. paused frequently during conversations and voiced frustration over not being able to express herself. At such times, she would say that she could not think of the right word, and indicated that the word was on the "tip of [her] tongue." She typically was able to describe the concept she wanted to communicate even if the correct word never came to her. To further document this deficit, the Boston Naming Test was administered. I.L. was correct on only 42 of 60 trials and did not benefit from phonemic or semantic cues.

DISCUSSION

The patient in Case 12–3 presented with anomic aphasia. Limited education could not explain her inability to name common household objects such as forks. Additionally, the patient performed at a level below that of individuals of her approximate age on the Boston Naming Test; therefore, age-related decline in naming is not a likely alternative explanation. No other evidence of language impairment was present in this patient. Interestingly, her deficit arose after a right-hemisphere lesion.

CASE 10–1

P.H. was a 37-year-old man who had completed 2 years of college and worked as a marketing consultant. A rupture of a probable berry aneurysm originating from the anterior communicating artery resulted in subarachnoid, interhemispheric fissure and intraventricular hemorrhages. A hematoma was subsequently detected in the rostrum of the corpus callosum, and an infarct was found in the left basal ganglia.

P.H. was comatose for 2 weeks. After awakening, he made no verbalizations spontaneously or in response to questions. He failed to repeat words spoken to him, but would comply with other requests not involving speech. After several days, spontaneous verbalizations returned, but his volume was limited to a whisper.

Formal neuropsychological assessment was done approximately 4 months after the initial onset of bleeding. At that time, P.H. showed impaired problem solving and a number of deficits suggesting a partial disconnection of his cerebral hemispheres. For further discussion of the test results in this patient, see Chapter 10.

The HRB-AST was administered; the patient made errors only when he was required to perform calculations. His speech was completely intact except for a notable reduction in volume. Both the patient and his wife remarked about the change in his voice compared to before his hemorrhages. He had sung part-time with a band and had been known for his strong voice. He reported being unable to sing above the volume that he currently used for conversations.

DISCUSSION

The patient in Case 10–1 presented a history consistent with mutism. At the time of assessment, he had substantially recovered; the only residual sign was a reduction in voice volume. There was no evidence in his original medical examination of damage to his vocal organs, and his deficit did not occur in the context of an emotional trauma or an attempt to avoid an unpleasant situation. His basal ganglia lesion was also consistent with the diagnosis of mutism.

REFERENCES

1. Benson, DF: Aphasia. In Heilman, KM, and Valenstein, E (eds): Clinical Neuropsychology, Second Edition. Oxford University Press, New York, 1985.
2. Benson, DF, and Geschwind, N: Aphasia and Related Disorders: A Clinical Approach. In Mesulam, M-M (ed): Principles of Behavioral Neurology. F.A. Davis, Philadelphia, 1985
3. American Psychiatric Association: Diagnostic and Statistical Manual of Mental Disorders, Fourth Edition. American Psychiatric Association, Washington, DC, 1994.
4. The International Classification of Diseases, Ninth Revision, Clinical Modification. Med-Index Publications, Salt Lake City, 1991.
5. Lichtheim, L: On aphasia. Brain 7:433, 1885.
6. Luria, AR: Higher Cortical Functions in Man, Second Edition. Basic Books, New York, 1966.
7. Hecaen, H, and Albert, ML: Human Neuropsychology. John Wiley & Sons, New York, 1978.
8. Goodglass, H, and Kaplan, E: The Assessment of Aphasia and Related Disorders. Lea & Febiger, Philadelphia, 1983.
9. Mohr, JP: Broca's area and Broca's aphasia. Stroke 6:228, 1975.
10. Hayward, RW, Naeser, MA, and Zatz, LM: Cranial computed tomography in aphasia: Correlation of anatomical lesions with functional deficits. Radiology 123:653, 1977.
11. Naeser, MA, and Hayward, RW: Lesion localization in aphasia with cranial computed tomography and the Boston Diagnostic Aphasia Exam. Neurology 28:545, 1978.
12. Wallesch, CW: Two syndromes of aphasia occurring with ischemic lesions involving the left basal ganglia. Brain Lang 25:357, 1985.
13. Naeser, MA, and Hayward, RW: The resolving stroke and aphasia. A case study with computerized tomography. Arch Neurol 36:233, 1979.
14. Donaldson, JO, Hale, MS, and Klau, M: A case of reversible pure-word deafness during lithium toxicity. Am J Psychiatry 138:242, 1981.
15. Yaqub, BA, et al: Pure word deafness (acquired verbal auditory agnosia) in an Arabic speaking patient. Brain 111:457, 1988.
16. Roberts, M, Sadercock, P, and Ghadiali, E: Pure word deafness and unilateral right temporoparietal lesions: A case report. J Neurol Neurosurg Psychiatry 50:1708, 1987.
17. Takahashi, N, et al: Pure word deafness due to left hemisphere damage. Cortex 28:295, 1992.
18. Tanaka, Y, Yamadori, A, and Mori, E: Pure word deafness following bilateral lesions. A psychophysical analysis. Brain 110:381, 1987.
19. Buchman, AS, et al: Word deafness: One hundred years later. J Neurol Neurosurg Psychiatry 49:489, 1986.
20. Metz-Lutz, MN, and Dahl, E: Analysis of word comprehension in a case of pure word deafness. Brain Lang 23:13, 1984.
21. Coslett, HB, Brashear, HR, and Heilman, KM: Pure word deafness after bilateral primary auditory cortex infarcts. Neurology 34:347, 1984.
22. Auerbach, SH, et al: Pure word deafness. Analysis of a case with bilateral lesions and a defect at the prephonemic level. Brain 105:271, 1982.
23. Kirshner, HS, Webb, WG, and Duncan, GW: Word deafness in Wernicke's aphasia. J Neurol Neurosurg Psychiatry 44:197, 1981.
24. Demeurisse, G, and Capon, A: Brain activation during a linguistic task in conduction aphasia. Cortex 27:285, 1991.
25. Hyman, BT, and Tranel, D: Hemianesthesia and aphasia. An anatomical and behavioral study. Arch Neurol 46:816, 1989.
26. Poncet, M, Habib, M, and Robillard, A: Deep left parietal lobe syndrome: Conduction aphasia and other neurobehavioral disorders due to a small subcortical lesion. J Neurol Neurosurg Psychiatry 50:709, 1987.
27. Sheremata, W, Andrews, R, and Pandya, DN: Conduction aphasia from a frontal lobe lesion. Trans Am Neurol Assoc 99:249, 1974.
28. Damasio, H, and Damasio, AR: The anatomical basis of conduction aphasia. Brain 103:337, 1980.
29. Benson, DF, et al: Conduction aphasia: A clinicopathological study. Arch Neurol 28:339, 1973.

30. Mendez, MF, and Benson, DF: Atypical conduction aphasia. A disconnection syndrome. Arch Neurol 42:886, 1985.
31. Naeser, MA, et al: Late recovery of auditory comprehension in global aphasia. Improved recovery observed with subcortical temporal isthmus lesion vs. Wernicke's cortical area lesion. Arch Neurol 47:425, 1990.
32. Deleval, J, et al: Global aphasia without hemiparesis following prerolandic infarction. Neurology 39:1532, 1989.
33. Tranel, D, et al: Global aphasia without hemiparesis. Arch Neurol 44:304, 1987.
34. Vignolo, LA, Boccardi, E, and Caverni, L: Unexpected CT-scan findings in global aphasia. Cortex 22:55, 1986.
35. Ferro, JM: Global aphasia without hemiparesis. Neurology 33:1106, 1983.
36. Van Horn, G, and Hawes, A: Global aphasia without hemiparesis: A sign of embolic encephalopathy. Neurology 32:403, 1982.
37. Bogousslavsky, J: Global aphasia without other lateralizing signs. Arch Neurol 45:143, 1988.
38. DeRenzi, E, Colombo, A, and Scarpa, M: The aphasic isolate. A clinical-CT scan study of a particularly severe subgroup of global aphasics. Brain 114:1719, 1991.
39. Yang, BJ, et al: Three variant forms of subcortical aphasia in Chinese stroke patients. Brain Lang 37:145, 1989.
40. Freedman, M, Alexander, MP, and Naeser, MA: Anatomic basis of transcortical motor aphasia. Neurology 34:409, 1984.
41. Ross, ED: Left medial parietal lobe and receptive language functions: Mixed transcortical aphasia after left anterior cerebral artery infarction. Neurology 30:144, 1980.
42. Bogousslavsky, J, Assal, G, and Regli, F: Infarct in the area of the left anterior cerebral artery. II. Language disorders. Rev Neurol 143:121, 1987.
43. Kertesz, A, Sheppard, A, and MacKenzie, R: Localization in transcortical sensory aphasia. Arch Neurol 39:475, 1982.
44. Heilman, KM, et al: Transcortical sensory aphasia with relatively spared spontaneous speech and naming. Arch Neurol 38:236, 1981.
45. Graff-Radford, NR, et al: Nonhemorrhagic infarction of the thalamus: Behavioral, anatomic, and physiologic correlates. Neurology 34:14, 1984.
46. Kirshner, HS, and Kistler, KH: Aphasia after right thalamic hemorrhage. Arch Neurol 39:667, 1982.
47. Jenkyn, LR, Alberti, AR, and Peters, JD: Language dysfunction, somasthetic inattention, and thalamic hemorrhage in the dominant hemisphere. Neurology 31:1202, 1981.
48. Archer, CR, et al: Aphasia in thalamic stroke: CT stereotactic localization. J Comput Assist Tomogr 5:427, 1981.
49. Alexander, MP, and LoVerme, SR: Aphasia after left hemispheric intracerebral hemorrhage. Neurology 30:1193, 1980.
50. Cappa, SF, and Vignolo, LA: "Transcortical" features of aphasia following left thalamic hemorrhage. Cortex 15:121, 1979.
51. Grossi, D, et al: Mixed transcortical aphasia: Clinical features and neuroanatomical correlates. A possible role of the right hemisphere. Eur Neurol 31:204, 1991.
52. Trojano, L, et al: Mixed transcortical aphasia. On relative sparing of phonological short-term store in a case. Neuropsychologia 26:633, 1988.
53. Bogousslavsky, J, Regli, F, and Assal, G: Isolation of speech area from focal brain ischemia. Stroke 16:441, 1985.
54. Rapcsak, SZ, et al: Mixed transcortical aphasia without anatomic isolation of the speech area. Stroke 21:953, 1990.
55. Speedie, LJ, Coslett, HB, and Heilman, KM: Repetition of affective prosody in mixed transcortical aphasia. Arch Neurol 41:268, 1984.
56. Pirozzolo, FJ, et al: Neurolinguistic analysis of the language abilities of a patient with a double disconnection syndrome: A case of subangular alexia in the presence of mixed transcortical aphasia. J Neurol Neurosurg Psychiatry 44:152, 1981.
57. Kohn, SE, and Goodglass, H: Picture-naming in aphasia. Brain Lang 24:266, 1985.
58. Hadar, U, Jones, C, and Mate-Kole, C: The disconnection in anomic aphasia between semantic and phonological lexicons. Cortex 23:505, 1987.
59. Hadar, U, Ticehurst, S, and Wade, JP: Crossed anomic aphasia: Mild naming deficits following right brain damage in a dextral patient. Cortex 27:459, 1991.
60. Coslett, HB, and Saffran, EM: Optic aphasia and the right hemisphere: A replication and extension. Brain Lang 43:148, 1992.

61. Manning, L, and Campbell, R: Optic aphasia with spared action naming: A description and possible loci of impairment. Neuropsychologia 30:587, 1992.
62. Iorio, L, et al: Visual associative agnosia and optic aphasia. A single case study and a review of the syndromes. Cortex 28:23, 1992.
63. Coslett, HB, and Saffran, EM: Preserved object recognition and reading comprehension in optic aphasia. Brain 112:1091, 1989.
64. Pena-Casanova, J, et al: Optic aphasia, optic apraxia, and loss of dreaming. Brain Lang 26:63, 1985.
65. Gil, R, et al: Visuoverbal disconnection (optical aphasia) for objects, pictures, colors and faces with abstractive alexia. Neuropsychologia 23:333, 1985.
66. Beauvois, MF, et al: Bilateral tactile aphasia: A tacto-verbal dysfunction. Brain 101:381, 1978.
67. DeRenzi, E, Zambolin, A, and Crisi, G: The pattern of neuropsychological impairment associated with left posterior cerebral artery infarcts. Brain 110:1099, 1987.
68. Damasio, AR, and Damasio, H: The anatomic basis of pure alexia. Neurology 33:1573, 1983.
69. Damasio, AR, McKee, J, and Damasio, H: Determinants of performance in color anomia. Brain Lang 7:74, 1979.
70. Mohr, JP, et al: Right hemianopia with memory and color deficits in circumscribed left posterior cerebral artery territory infarction. Neurology 21:1104, 1971.
71. Geschwind, N, and Fusillo, M: Color-naming defects in association with alexia. Arch Neurol 15:137, 1966.
72. Yasuda, Y, et al: Paramedian thalamic and midbrain infarcts associated with palilalia. J Neurol Neurosurg Psychiatry 53:797, 1990.
73. Boller, F, Albert, M, and Denes, F: Palilalia. Br J Disord Commun 10:92, 1975.
74. Contamin, F, et al: Atrophy of the globus pallidus, substantia nigra, and nucleus subthalamicus. Akinetic syndrome with palilalia, oppositional rigidity and catatonia. Rev Neurol 124:107, 1971.
75. Horner, J, and Massey, EW: Progressive dysfluency associated with right hemisphere disease. Brain Lang 18:71, 1983.
76. Dierckx, RA, et al: Evolution of technetium-99m-HMPAO SPECT and brain mapping in a patient presenting with echolalia and palilalia. J Nucl Med 32:1619, 1991.
77. Papagno, C, and Guidotti, M: A case of aphasia following left thalamic hemorrhage. Eur Neurol 22:93, 1983.
78. Fenmore, C, et al: Language and memory disturbances from mesencephalothalamic infarcts. A clinical and computed tomography study. Eur Neurol 28:51, 1988.
79. Brunner, RJ, et al: Basal ganglia participation in language pathology. Brain Lang 16:281, 1982.
80. Bogousslavsky, J, Regli, F, and Assal, G: Acute transcortical mixed aphasia. A carotid occlusion syndrome with pial and watershed infarcts. Brain 111:631, 1988.
81. Groswasser, Z, Groswasser-Reider, I, and Korn, C: Biopercular lesions and acquired mutism in a young patient. Brain Inj 5:331, 1991.
82. Nemeth, G, Hegedus, K, and Molnar, L: Akinetic mutism associated with bicingular lesions: Clinicopathological and functional anatomical correlates. Eur Arch Psychiatry Neurol Sci 237:218, 1988.
83. Groswasser, Z, et al: Mutism associated with buccofacial apraxia and bihemispheric lesions. Brain Lang 34:157, 1988.
84. Skultely, FM: Clinical and experimental aspects of akinetic mutism. Arch Neurol 19:1, 1968.
85. Barris, RW, and Schuman, HR: Bilateral anterior cingulate gyrus lesions. Syndrome of the anterior cingulate gyri. Neurology 3:44, 1953.
86. Freemon, FR: Akinetic mutism and bilateral anterior cerebral artery occlusion. J Neurol Neurosurg Psychiatry 34:693, 1971.
87. Murdoch, BE, Chenery, HJ, and Kennedy, M: Aphemia associated with bilateral striato-capsular lesions subsequent to cerebral anoxia. Brain Inj 3:41, 1989.
88. Helgason, C, et al: Acute pseudobulbar mutism due to discrete bilateral capsular infarction in the territory of the anterior choroidal artery. Brain 111:507, 1988.
89. Levin, HS, et al: Mutism after closed head injury. Arch Neurol 40:601, 1983.
90. Szirmai, I, Guseo, A, and Molnar, M: Bilateral symmetrical softening of the thalamus. J Neurol 217:57, 1977.
91. Segarra, JM: Cerebral vascular disease and behavior. Arch Neurol 22:408, 1970.
92. Markand, ON, and Dyken, ML: Sleep abnormalities in patients with brain stem lesions. Neurology 26:769, 1976.
93. Cravioto, H, Silberman, J, and Feigin, I: A clinical and pathological study of akinetic mutism. Neurology 10:10, 1960.

94. Daly, DD, and Love, JG: Akinetic mutism. Neurology 8:238, 1958.
95. Chambers, AA, and McLennan, JE: Pericollicular syndromes. Neuroradiology 16:547, 1978.
96. Cairns, H, et al: Akinetic mutism with an epidermoid cyst of the 3rd ventricle (with a report of the associated disturbance of brain potentials). Brain 64:273, 1941.
97. Ross, ED, and Stewart, RM: Akinetic mutism from hypothalamic damage: Successful treatment with dopamine agonists. Neurology 31:1435, 1981.
98. Gutling, E, Landis, T, and Kleihues, P: Akinetic mutism in bilateral necrotizing leucoencephalopathy after radiation and chemotherapy: Electrophysiological and autopsy findings. J Neurol 239:125, 1992.
99. Devinsky, O, et al: Akinetic mutism in a bone marrow transplant recipient following total-body irradiation and amphotericin B chemoprophylaxis. A positron emission tomographic and neuropathologic study. Arch Neurol 44:414, 1987.
100. Aoki, N: Reversible leukoencephalopathy caused by 5-fluorouracil derivatives, presenting as akinetic mutism. Surg Neurol 25:279, 1986.
101. Evrard, S, et al: Watershed cerebral infarcts: Retrospective study of 24 cases. Neurol Res 14 (Suppl 2):97, 1992.
102. Kertesz, A: The Western Aphasia Battery Test Manual. Grune & Stratton, Orlando, FL, 1982.
103. Kertesz, A: Aphasia and Associated Disorders: Taxonomy, Localization, and Recovery. Grune & Stratton, New York, 1979.
104. Shewan, CM, and Kertesz, A: Reliability and validity characteristics of the Western Aphasia Battery (WAB). J Speech Hearing Dis 45:308, 1980.
105. Kaplan, EF, Goodglass, H, and Weintraub, S: The Boston Naming Test, Second Edition. Lea & Febiger, Philadelphia, 1983.
106. Van Gorp, WG, et al: Normative data on the Boston Naming Test for a group of normal older adults. J Clin Exper Neuropsychol 8:702, 1986.
107. Knopman, DS, et al: Recovery of naming in aphasia: Relationship of fluency, comprehension, and CT findings. Neurology 34:1461, 1984.
108. Williams, BW, Mack, W, and Henderson, VW: Boston Naming Test in Alzheimer's disease. Neuropsychologia 27:1073, 1989.
109. Reitan, RM, and Davison, LA: Clinical Neuropsychology: Current Status and Applications. H.V. Winston, New York, 1974.
110. Russell, EW, Neuringer, C, and Goldstein, G: Assessment of Brain Damage. A Neuropsychological Key Approach. Wiley-Interscience, New York, 1970.
111. Heaton, RK, Grant, I, and Matthews, CG: Comprehensive Norms for an Expanded Halstead-Reitan Battery. Demographic Corrections, Research Findings, and Clinical Applications. Psychological Assessment Resources, Odessa, FL, 1991.
112. Barnes, GW, and Lucas, GJ: Cerebral dysfunction vs. psychogenesis in Halstead-Reitan tests. J Nerv Ment Dis 158:50, 1974.

DISORDERS OF WRITTEN LANGUAGE (ALEXIA AND AGRAPHIA)

13

The desirability of a classification system based on an analysis of underlying pathological mechanisms is discussed in the introduction to this book. In most areas of neuropsychology, such an analysis remains a desire rather than a reality, but the study of written language has taken major strides in recent decades. By recording and analyzing reading and writing errors made by patients, cognitive neuropsychologists are constructing novel typologies of written language disorder based on the cognitive mechanisms that appear to be impaired.[1,2]

The new cognitive typology of written language disorder is subdivided into the following cognitive error patterns:

1. Phonological alexia (with visual paralexias)
2. Phonological agraphia (with visual paragraphias)
3. Deep alexia (with visual and semantic paralexias)
4. Deep agraphia (with visual and semantic paragraphias)
5. Surface alexia
6. Lexical agraphia (phonological spelling)
7. Letter-by-letter reading (spelling dyslexia)

A neurological typology of written language disorders predates the cognitive typology. The neurological typology divides written language disorder into the 10 subtypes listed under "Variety of Presentation" in the chapter outline.

The nascent cognitive typology is not ready to supplant the traditional neurological typology, which has the advantages of a long and reliable clinical diagnostic history and well-known lesion locations. In contrast, the cognitive typology has been explored in only a few patients, and the lesion locations of many of the subtypes are incompletely established. Rather than pitting the two typologies against each other, some authors have chosen to view them as complementary systems and have sought links between them based on clinical association or similarity in clinical presentation.[3] The latter approach is taken in this text.

The cognitive typology is integrated into the neurological system by listing the cognitive disorders as error patterns that may be observed in a given patient. For example, patients with pure alexia, a disorder from the neurological typology, may exhibit letter-by-letter reading, a disorder from the cognitive typology. Consequently, letter-by-letter reading is listed as one clinical indicator of pure alexia. In a similar manner, the other cognitive subtypes are merged with the traditional neurological subtypes.

The task of merging the two classification systems is difficult because of the sparse literature linking them. Letter-by-letter reading and phonological alexia have been observed in patients who meet the criteria for the diagnosis of pure alexia. In contrast, deep alexic error patterns have not been reported in patients having pure alexia. Before it can be concluded that deep alexic errors do not occur in patients with pure alexia, it must be considered that too few cases of deep alexia may have been reported to draw a final conclusion. At most, the only safe conclusion is that no relationship between deep alexic error patterns and pure alexia has been demonstrated thus far. Future cases may establish such a relationship, but until that time, deep alexic errors cannot be included in the clinical indicators of pure alexia. The cognitive error patterns listed in the following section for each of the neurological subtypes are based on relationships established in the current literature.

COGNITIVE ERROR PATTERNS

To simplify the later presentation of clinical indicators, the cognitive error patterns are listed and described in this section. Later, these patterns are referred to by label alone. Note that the term *paralexia* refers to reading errors and *paragraphia* refers to written spelling errors.

Phonological Paralexic Pattern (Phonological Alexia) with Visual Paralexias (Visual Alexia)

1. Inaccurate reading of uncommon (low-frequency) words
2. Inaccurate reading of pronounceable pseudowords (nonsense syllables)
3. Relatively preserved reading of common (high-frequency) words
4. Visual paralexias (also called visual alexia) occurring during reading, consisting of reading errors that are visually (i.e., orthographically) similar to the target words because they share many of the same letters

Phonological Paragraphic Pattern (Phonological Agraphia) with Visual Paragraphias

1. Inaccurate written or oral spelling of uncommon words
2. Inaccurate written or oral spelling of pronounceable pseudowords
3. Relatively preserved ability to spell common words
4. Visual paragraphias occurring during written or oral spelling, consisting of spelling errors that are visually (i.e., orthographically) similar to the target words because they share many of the same letters

Deep Paralexic Pattern (Deep Alexia) with Visual and Semantic Paralexias

1. Inaccurate reading of uncommon words.
2. Inaccurate reading of pronounceable pseudowords.
3. Inaccurate reading of function words, including conjunctions, prepositions, and adverbs, with the patient often substituting one function word for another.
4. Greater difficulty in reading verbs than adjectives.
5. Greater difficulty in reading adjectives than nouns.
6. Greater difficulty in reading low-imagery words than high-imagery words (e.g., "automobile" may be read more easily than "ability").
7. Visual paralexias occurring during reading.
8. Semantic paralexias occur during reading. These consist of oral reading errors that are semantically related to the target words (i.e., the error may be a synonym, antonym, subordinate, or meaningful associate of the target). For example, if the target word is "happiness," the patient may read "joy" (a

synonym) or "sadness" (an antonym); if the target word is "airplane," the patient may read "helicopter" (a meaningful associate).

9. The occurrence of derivational errors during reading (e.g., the word "take" may be read as "taken," "fix" may be read as "fixed").

Deep Paragraphic Pattern (Deep Agraphia) with Visual and Semantic Paragraphias

1. Inaccurate written or oral spelling of uncommon words.
2. Inaccurate written or oral spelling of pronounceable pseudowords.
3. Inaccurate written or oral spelling of function words.
4. Greater difficulty spelling verbs than adjectives.
5. Greater difficulty spelling adjectives than nouns.
6. Greater difficulty spelling low-imagery words than high-imagery words.
7. Visual paragraphias occur during written or oral spelling.
8. Semantic paragraphias occur during written or oral spelling. These consist of spelling errors that are semantically related to the target words (i.e., the error may be a synonym, antonym, subordinate, or meaningful associate of the target). If the target word has a homophone, the patient may mistakenly spell the homophone instead of the target. For example, if instructed to spell the word "male" as in "The opposite of female is male," the patient may produce "mail."
9. The occurrence of derivational errors during written or oral spelling.

Surface Paralexic Pattern (Surface Alexia)

1. Inaccurate oral reading of words whose pronunciation does not conform to English phonological rules (i.e., irregular words), with the patient attempting to pronounce the words as if they did conform to English phonology
2. Relatively preserved oral reading of words and pseudowords that conform to English phonological rules
3. Failure to comprehend or misinterpretation of the meaning of words that are read incorrectly

Lexical Paragraphic Pattern (Lexical Agraphia or Phonological Spelling)

1. Inaccurate written or oral spelling of irregular words.
2. Inaccurate written or oral spelling of words with ambiguous orthographies. Words with ambiguous orthographies have letters whose constituent sounds could be represented by different letters (e.g., "phony" could be spelled "fhony", "cow" could be spelled "kow").
3. Relatively preserved written and oral spelling of words and pseudowords that conform to English phonology.

4. Spelling errors are phonologically accurate (e.g., "bomb" spelled as "bom").

Letter-by-Letter Reading Pattern (Spelling Dyslexia)

1. Patients read words by first reading the individual letters silently or aloud.
2. When prevented from reading the individual letters, the patient may be unable to read the word.
3. Reading accuracy decreases as word length increases.

NOMENCLATURE

Written language disorders can be coded in DSM-IV[4] as "Reading Disorder" or "Disorder of Written Expression," depending on which aspect of written language is impaired. The residual diagnosis "Learning Disorder Not Otherwise Specified" is also available in the rare instance when one of the other diagnoses will not suffice. ICD-9-CM[5] includes adult-onset alexia and agraphia under the diagnostic label "Other Symbolic Dysfunction." The traditional neurological subtypes of alexia and agraphia are not included in ICD-9-CM or DSM-IV, and the cognitive subtypes are too recent to have affected the official nomenclature.

The cognitive subtypes of alexia and agraphia are in common use in the cognitive neuropsychology literature and are gradually being introduced in the clinical neurology literature. The classical neurological subtypes are well known in the clinical literature.

Two additional terms are used to describe reading error patterns. The term *literal alexia* refers to patients with impaired letter identification but preserved reading of words. *Verbal alexia* is the opposite pattern: preserved letter identification but impaired reading of words. The validity of these subtypes has been questioned, because most patients with literal alexia are impaired when they attempt to read words, and most verbal alexics are deficient in letter identification.[6] The terms *literal alexia* and *verbal alexia* fail to describe discrete syndromes and consequently are not used in this text.

VARIETY OF PRESENTATION

1. Pure alexia (also called alexia without agraphia, pure word blindness, subcortical alexia, agnosic alexia, and visual alexia)

Clinical Indicators

a_1. A decline in reading ability as indicated by any of the following signs:
   1) Inaccurate oral identification of individual letters
   2) Letter-by-letter reading pattern
   3) Phonological paralexic pattern with visual paralexias
   4) Inaccurate matching of words or sentences to pictures

5) Failure to carry out written commands accurately
6) Failure to answer questions about a written passage accurately when questions and answers are oral

a_2. Reading deficit occurring in both the left and right visual fields

a_3. Relatively preserved writing to dictation, to command, and in response to a stimulus

a_4. Relatively preserved written and oral spelling of words

Associated Features

a. Inability to read own writing
b. Relatively preserved ability to assign words to categories despite an inability to read or match the word to a picture
c. Impaired calculation ability (see Acalculia)
d. Impaired visual recognition of objects (see Visual object agnosia)
e. Impaired identification of the characteristic colors of objects (see Color agnosia)
f. Diminished ability to communicate orally about colors (see Stimulus-specific aphasia)
g. Loss of visual acuity in one (usually the right) visual field (i.e., homonymous hemianopsia)
h. Mild weakness on one (usually the right) side of the body

Factors to Rule Out

a. Decline in visual acuity sufficient to prevent seeing letters and words regardless of where they are presented in the visual field
b. Failure to notice all or a portion of visual test stimuli as a result of stimulus neglect (see Chap. 4)

RULES FOR DIAGNOSIS

Clinical Indicators: Each is independent (only one must be observed for the disorder to be suspected) *except* when subscripting is used. Subscripted numbers (a_1, a_2) denote an indicator with multiple parts that must be considered together.

Associated Features: These are listed to give a more complete picture of the disorder. The presence or absence of these features does not affect the diagnosis.

Factors to Rule Out: All must be taken into account. Failure to rule out even one of these factors makes a firm diagnosis impossible.

Lesion Locations: Each location stands alone; damage in only one of the listed areas is sufficient to produce the disorder.

c. Impaired speech articulation sufficient to prevent intelligible oral reading
d. The presence of oral language impairment sufficient to prevent intelligible reading (see Aphasic alexia-agraphia) or oral response to questions
e. Impaired visual recognition of objects (see Visual object agnosia) when pictures are used in the assessment of reading comprehension
f. A premorbid history of poor reading as a result of limited education or learning disability

Lesion Locations

a. Medial or lateral occipital lobe,* particularly the cuneus and fusiform, lingual, inferior, and superior calcarine gyri; the inferior longitudinal fasciculus; and the vertical occipital fasciculus, with frequent extension to the corpus callosum (splenium), parietal lobe (with rare involvement of angular gyrus), inferior or posterior medial temporal lobe, hippocampal gyrus, thalamus, optic radiation,† forceps major, and the posterior limb of the internal capsule[7–31]
b. White matter subjacent to the angular gyrus (*subangular alexia*‡)[32–35]
c. Combined temporal and parietal lobes[18,36]
d. Thalamus (lateral geniculate), with frequent extension to the splenium of the corpus callosum, optic radiation, anterior limb of the internal capsule, and forceps major[11,37,38]

Lesion Lateralization

a. Left hemisphere in most reported cases, but may follow right-sided lesions in patients with right-hemisphere written language dominance,[16,21,26] regardless of handedness and oral language dominance
b. Bilateral lesions in a few cases[9]

2. Pure agraphia (see also Apraxic agraphia)

Clinical Indicators

a_1. A decline in the ability to write in response to a command, to dictation, or to a stimulus (e.g., a picture the patient is asked to describe in a sentence or paragraph), as evidenced by any of the following signs:
   1) Horizontal or vertical rotation of letters
   2) Poorly formed letters, which may progress to the point of unrecognizable scrawling
   3) Omission of letters or words
   4) Incorrect selection of letters (misspelling)
   5) Phonological paragraphic pattern with visual paragraphias
   6) Lexical paragraphic pattern

a_2. Deficit in writing occurring in both hands

a_3. Use of anagram letters (i.e., cut-out letter models) failing to produce significant improvement of written spelling

---

*Lateral occipital lesions are likely to produce a transient disorder, whereas medial lesions produce chronic alexia.

†The presence of homonymous hemianopsia indicates extension of the lesion to the optic radiation.

‡Visual fields are typically full in patients who have subangular alexia.

a_4. Relatively preserved oral reading of individual letters, words, and sentences

a_5. Relatively preserved comprehension of written words and sentences

Associated Features

a. Written and oral spelling possibly not equally impaired; in some cases, oral spelling relatively preserved
b. Impaired calculation ability (see Acalculia)
c. Impaired recognition of the fingers of the hand (see Finger agnosia)
d. Impaired ability to distinguish right from left (see Right-left disorientation)
NOTE: When agraphia, acalculia, finger agnosia, and right-left disorientation occur together in the same patient, the entire complex is referred to as Gerstmann's syndrome.
e. Confused ideation (see Ideational disorientation and confusion)

Factors to Rule Out

a. Weakness of the muscles of the arm or hand sufficient to account for the writing deficit
b. Impaired coordination of the muscles of the arm or hand sufficient to account for the writing deficit
c. Impaired ability to initiate arm or hand movements (see Akinesia) sufficient to account for the writing deficit
d. Impaired ability to persist with ongoing arm or hand movements (see Motor impersistence) sufficient to account for the writing deficit
e. Impaired ability to terminate ongoing arm or hand movements (see Motor perseveration) sufficient to account for the writing deficit
f. Impaired ability to perform the movements involved in writing on demand (see Apraxic agraphia) sufficient to account for the writing deficit, ruled out by documenting impaired spelling even when anagram letters are used
g. Impaired ability to guide the hand perceptually during writing (see Constructional agraphia) sufficient to account for the writing deficit, ruled out by documenting impaired spelling even when anagram letters are used
h. The presence of oral language impairment sufficient to account for writing and anagram spelling deficits (see Aphasic alexia-agraphia)
i. Impaired visual recognition of objects (see Visual object agnosia) if pictures are used as a stimulus for writing words or sentences
j. A premorbid history of poor writing as a result of limited education or learning disability

Lesion Locations

a. Posterior or inferior temporal lobe, or both, particularly white matter[39–41]
b. Combined superior and posterior parietal lobes, including the precuneus, angular gyrus, white matter subjacent to the angular gyrus, supramarginal gyrus, and superior parietal lobule, with occasional extension to the occipital lobe, temporal lobe, insula, and forceps major[42–51]
c. Foot of the second frontal gyrus[52]

d. Dorsal precentral gyrus[53]
e. Basal ganglia (caudate nucleus) and internal capsule[54]

Lesion Lateralization

a. Left hemisphere in most reported cases, but may follow right-sided lesions in patients with right-hemisphere written language dominance,[49,51] regardless of handedness and oral language dominance

3. Alexia with agraphia (also called alexic agraphia, agraphic alexia, agraphia with alexia, parietal alexia, and parietal agraphia)

Clinical Indicators

a_1. A decline in reading ability, as indicated by any of the following signs:
  1) Inaccurate oral identification of individual letters
  2) Phonological paralexic pattern with visual paralexias
  3) Surface paralexic pattern
  4) Inaccurate matching of words or sentences to pictures
  5) Failure to carry out written commands accurately
  6) Failure to answer questions about a written passage accurately when questions and answers are oral

a_2. A decline in the ability to write in response to a command, to dictation, or to a stimulus (e.g., a picture the patient is asked to describe in a sentence or paragraph), as evidenced by any of the following signs:
  1) Horizontal or vertical rotation of letters
  2) Poorly formed letters, which may progress to the point of unrecognizable scrawling
  3) Omission of letters or words
  4) Incorrect selection of letters (misspelling)
  5) Phonological paragraphic pattern with visual paragraphias

a_3. The reading deficit occurs in both the left and right visual fields

a_4. The deficit in writing occurs in both hands

a_5. Use of anagram letters (i.e., cut-out letter models) fails to produce significant improvement of written spelling

Associated Features

a. Relatively preserved ability to assign words to categories despite an inability to read or match the word to a picture
b. Impaired ability to name objects (see Anomic aphasia)
c. Impaired calculation ability
d. Impaired recognition of the fingers of the hand (see Finger agnosia)
e. Impaired ability to distinguish right from left (see Right-left disorientation)
   NOTE: When agraphia, acalculia, finger agnosia, and right-left disorientation occur together in the same patient, the entire complex is referred to as Gerstmann's syndrome.
f. Confused ideation (see Ideational disorientation and confusion)
g. Impaired ability to perform skilled movements on demand (see Apraxia)

Factors to Rule Out

a. A decline in visual acuity sufficient to prevent seeing letters and words regardless of where they are presented in the visual field

b. Failure to notice all or a portion of visual test stimuli as a result of stimulus neglect (see Chap. 4)
c. Impaired speech articulation sufficient to prevent intelligible oral reading
d. Presence of oral language impairment sufficient to account for the deficits in reading, writing (see Aphasic alexia-agraphia), or oral responding to questions
e. Impaired visual recognition of objects (see Visual object agnosia) when pictures are used in the assessment of reading or writing
f. Weakness of the muscles of the arm or hand sufficient to account for the writing deficit
g. Impaired coordination of the muscles of the arm or hand sufficient to account for the writing deficit
h. Impaired ability to initiate arm or hand movements (see Akinesia) sufficient to account for the writing deficit
i. Impaired ability to persist with ongoing arm or hand movements (see Motor impersistence) sufficient to account for the writing deficit
j. Impaired ability to terminate ongoing arm or hand movements (see Motor perseveration) sufficient to account for the writing deficit
k. A premorbid history of poor reading and writing as a result of limited education or learning disability

NOTE: The primary means of distinguishing pure agraphia from apraxic and constructional agraphia is through assessment of anagram spelling, which is impaired in the first but not in the latter two disorders. Unfortunately for the diagnostician, anagram spelling may be impaired in some cases of alexia with agraphia not because of the agraphic component, but because the alexic component impedes reading of the anagram letters. Consequently, the agraphia in alexia with agraphia cannot always be distinguished from apraxic or constructional agraphia.

Lesion Locations

a. Medial and posterior-inferior temporal lobe, sometimes including the temporal isthmus and portions of Wernicke's area, with occasional extension to the parietal lobe[55–60]
b. Combined occipital and parietal lobes, particularly the angular gyrus, the superior parietal lobule, and the supramarginal gyrus, with occasional extension to the temporal lobe and the optic radiation[61–64]
c. Superior premotor cortex (Exner's area)[65]

Lesion Lateralization

a. Left hemisphere in virtually all reported cases

4. Aphasic alexia-agraphia

Clinical Indicators

a_1. Presence of an oral language disorder (see Chap. 12) that parallels the written language disorder in severity and pattern of errors

a_2. A decline in reading ability as indicated by any of the following signs:
   1) Inaccurate oral identification of individual letters
   2) Phonological paralexic pattern with visual paralexias

3) Surface paralexic pattern
4) Deep paralexic pattern with semantic paralexias
5) The presence of random paralexias: word substitution errors that are not meaningfully related to the target words presented for reading
6) The presence of neologisms (nonsense words that have no linguistic meaning that are added to or substituted for target words presented for reading)

NOTE: Semantic paralexias, random paralexias, and neologisms that occur during reading are collectively called verbal paralexias *and are analogous to the verbal paraphasias seen in some oral language disorders (see Chap. 12).*

7) Inaccurate matching of words or sentences to pictures
8) Failure to carry out written commands accurately

a_3. A decline in the ability to write in response to a command, to dictation, or to a stimulus (e.g., a picture the patient is asked to describe in a sentence or paragraph) as evidenced by any of the following signs:
1) Horizontal or vertical rotation of letters
2) Poorly formed letters that may progress to the point of unrecognizable scrawling
3) Omission of letters or words
4) Incorrect selection of letters (misspelling)
5) Phonological paragraphic pattern with visual paragraphias
6) Deep paragraphic pattern with semantic paragraphias

a_4. Reading deficit occurring in both the left and right visual fields

a_5. Deficit in writing occurring in both hands

a_6. Use of anagram letters failing to produce significant improvement of written spelling

Associated Features

a. Unilateral (usually right-sided) muscle weakness
b. Impaired ability to perform skilled movements on demand (see Apraxia)
c. Loss of visual acuity in one (usually the right) visual half-field (i.e., homonymous hemianopsia)
d. Impaired calculation ability
e. Impaired recognition of the fingers of the hand (see Finger agnosia)
f. Impaired ability to distinguish right from left (see Right-left disorientation)
NOTE: When agraphia, acalculia, finger agnosia, and right-left disorientation occur together in the same patient, the entire complex is referred to as Gerstmann's syndrome.
g. Confused ideation (see Ideational disorientation and confusion)

Factors to Rule Out

a. A decline in visual acuity sufficient to prevent seeing letters and words regardless of where they are presented in the visual field
b. Failure to notice all or a portion of visual test stimuli as a result of stimulus neglect (see Chap. 4)
c. Impaired speech articulation that prevents intelligible oral reading
d. Impaired visual recognition of objects when pictures are used in the assessment of reading or writing

e. Weakness of the muscles of the arm or hand sufficient to account for the writing deficit
f. Impaired coordination of the muscles of the arm or hand sufficient to account for the writing deficit
g. Impaired ability to initiate arm or hand movements (see Akinesia) sufficient to account for the writing deficit
h. Impaired ability to persist with ongoing arm or hand movements (see Motor impersistence) sufficient to account for the writing deficit
i. Impaired ability to terminate ongoing arm or hand movements (see Motor perseveration) sufficient to account for the writing deficit
j. A premorbid history of poor reading, writing, or both as a result of limited education or learning disability

NOTE: The primary means of distinguishing pure agraphia from apraxic and constructional agraphia is through assessment of anagram spelling, which is impaired in the first disorder but not in the latter two disorders. Unfortunately for the diagnostician, anagram spelling may be impaired in some cases of aphasic alexia-agraphia, not because of the agraphic component, but because the aphasic or alexic components impede reading of the anagram letters. Consequently, the agraphia in aphasic alexia-agraphia cannot always be distinguished from apraxic or constructional agraphia.

Lesion Locations*

a. Cerebral hemisphere, without further localization[66,67]
b. Combined anterior and inferior supramarginal gyri, in the context of a larger hemispheric lesion[68]
c. Combined frontal lobe (middle frontal and precentral gyri and the operculum of the inferior frontal gyrus), temporal lobe (superior temporal gyrus and temporal operculum), and parietal lobe (postcentral, supramarginal, and angular gyri)[69]

Lesion Lateralization†

a. Language-dominant (usually the left) hemisphere

5. Apraxic agraphia‡

Clinical Indicators

a_1. The production of poorly formed letters, which may progress to the point of unrecognizable scrawling when writing in response to a command, to dictation, or to a stimulus
a_2. Deficit present in both hands
a_3. Relatively preserved spelling with anagram letters

Associated Features

a. Relatively preserved oral spelling in some but not all cases
b. Copying letters and words may be less impaired than writing in response to a command, to dictation, or to a stimulus

---

*Also see lesion locations of the associated oral language disorder.
†See lesion lateralization of the associated oral language disorder.
‡The term *pure apraxic agraphia* can be used when alexia is absent.

c. Impaired ability to perform skilled movements on demand, including movements unrelated to writing (see Apraxia)

Factors to Rule Out

a. Weakness of the muscles of the arm or hand sufficient to account for the writing deficit
b. Impaired coordination of the muscles of the arm or hand sufficient to account for the writing deficit
c. Impaired ability to initiate arm or hand movements (see Akinesia) sufficient to account for the writing deficit
d. Impaired ability to persist with ongoing arm or hand movements (see Motor impersistence) sufficient to account for the writing deficit
e. Impaired ability to terminate ongoing arm or hand movements (see Motor perseveration) sufficient to account for the writing deficit
f. Impaired ability to perceptually guide the hand during writing (see Constructional agraphia) sufficient to account for the writing deficit
g. The presence of oral language impairment sufficient to account for the writing deficit (see Aphasic alexia-agraphia), ruled out by documenting preserved anagram spelling
h. Impaired visual recognition of objects (see Visual object agnosia) if pictures are used as a stimulus for writing words or sentences
i. A premorbid history of poor writing as a result of limited education or learning disability

Lesion Locations

a. Parietal lobe, including the angular gyrus, with occasional extension to the temporal lobe, the occipital lobe, or the internal capsule[70–75]
b. Superior frontal lobe[76]
c. Medial centrum semiovale[77]

Lesion Lateralization

a. Left hemisphere in most reported cases, but may follow right-sided lesions in patients with right-hemisphere written language dominance[72]

6. Constructional agraphia (also called spatial and visuospatial agraphia)

Clinical Indicators

a_1. Inaccurate writing of individual letters in response to a command, to dictation, or to a stimulus or when copying, as evidenced by any of the following signs:
   1) Reiteration of letter strokes
   2) Inability to write in a straight horizontal line
   3) Insertion of excessive blank space between the letters within a word

a_2. Deficit present in both hands
a_3. Relatively preserved oral spelling
a_4. Relatively preserved spelling with anagram letters

Associated Features

a. Failure to notice all or a portion of visual stimuli (see Stimulus neglect); during writing, may manifest itself as writing on only one half of the page

Factors to Rule Out

a. Weakness of the muscles of the arm or hand sufficient to account for the writing deficit
b. Impaired coordination of the muscles of the arm or hand sufficient to account for the writing deficit
c. Impaired ability to terminate ongoing arm or hand movements (see Motor perseveration) sufficient to account for the writing deficit, particularly if the writing deficit is confined to a reiteration of strokes
d. Impaired visual recognition of objects (see Visual object agnosia) if pictures are used as a stimulus for writing words or sentences
e. A premorbid history of poor writing as a result of limited education or learning disability

Lesion Locations

a. Parietal lobe[78]
b. Premotor cortex[79]

Lesion Lateralization

a. Can follow left- or right-sided lesions

7. **Unilateral alexia (see Chap. 10)**
8. **Unilateral agraphia (see Chap. 10)**
9. **Alexic acalculia (see Chap. 15)**
10. **Agraphic acalculia (see Chap. 15)**

ETIOLOGY

The major causes of written language disorder parallel the causes of oral language disorder discussed in Chapter 12. Cerebrovascular disease, particularly involving the posterior cerebral artery; brain trauma; demyelinating disease; degenerative disease; and, less commonly, neoplasm can lead to written language impairment. In addition, written language is often impaired in patients who have compromised brain metabolism or electrolyte imbalance secondary to organ failure or nutritional deficiencies. Migraine has been reported to produce a transient pure alexia with hemianopsia.[80]

DISABLING CONSEQUENCES

Although literacy was not always a prerequisite for success in some segments of society, it has become a necessity in the modern world. There are virtually no jobs that do not require reading and writing, whether in the application stage, during the workday itself, or when the paycheck is received. When facility in reading and writing is lost, the patient at best requires the aid of others to perform most jobs, and at worst is in jeopardy of losing his or her job. One resourceful executive, who became alexic and agraphic following a stroke, resorted to dictating all written reports. Once typed, the reports had to be read into a tape recorder by his secretary for him to play back and correct—a process that greatly lengthened the time needed to complete even a single written project. The more circumscribed deficits seen in apraxic agraphia and constructional agraphia are more readily compensated for and may be less disabling.

The limitations imposed by alexia and agraphia are not confined to the workplace. Driving can be compromised if the patient is unable to read road signs and street names. The patient may require someone else to read personal mail, to respond to correspondence, and to write checks. Sales and service contracts, insurance policies, labels on grocery items, and product descriptions in catalogs may be inaccessible. To the extent that reading and writing are pursued by a given patient for personal enjoyment, leisure time may be less rewarding. Added to these factors is the social stigma faced by illiterate people, even when that illiteracy is acquired and the result of circumstances beyond their control. Depending on the importance of literacy in a patient's occupation and leisure time, he or she may experience significant disability as a result of alexia and agraphia.

ASSESSMENT INSTRUMENTS

Boston Diagnostic Aphasia Examination, Written Language Sections

See discussion of this test in Chapter 12.

Western Aphasia Battery, Written Language Section

See discussion of this test in Chapter 12.

Halstead-Reitan Battery Aphasia Screening Test, Written Language Items

See discussion of this test in Chapter 12.

Luria's Neuropsychological Investigation, Section K

See discussion of this test in Chapter 19.

Battery of Adult Reading Function

The Battery of Adult Reading Function (BARF)[81] can be obtained from *Audiology and Speech Pathology Service (126), Veterans Administration Medical Center, Gainesville, FL 32602.*

The BARF is designed to identify neuropsychological mechanisms underlying written language disorders in adult neurological patients. It consists of six basic subtests and two appendices that contain supplementary tests. Subtests 1 through 4 contain pronounceable pseudowords, regular words, rule-governed words, and irregular words, respectively. Patients are asked to read these words aloud while the examiner records responses and notes the types of errors (i.e., semantic, phonologic, visual, visual/phonologic, derivational, or other) made by the patient. Subtests 2 through 4 are equivalent in their average word frequency. All four subtests are balanced in the average number of graphemes (the graphic representation of the sounds of spoken words) per word.

Subtests 5 and 6 are used in patients whose oral language impairment prevents them from taking subtests 1 through 4. Subtest 5 consists of pairs of nonhomographic homophones, one of which matches a picture. The patient must select which of the homophones matches the picture (i.e., discriminate target homophones from foils). The average target homophone word frequency matches the average word frequency of the foils. Target homophones and foils are also closely matched in average number of graphemes. Adequate performance on this subtest requires use of the orthographic, whole-word approach to reading, because the word pairs are identical in their phonology.

Subtest 6 items are pseudowords that match one of three pictures. The matching picture depicts the meaning of a real word that is homophonic with (i.e., shares the phonology of) the pseudoword. For example, Item 1 of Subtest 6 is the pseudoword *coam*; the patient must match this word to a picture of a comb (correct choice), a cone, or a coat. The foil pictures (cone and coat in this example) depict the meaning of words that begin with the same phoneme or grapheme as the pseudoword. Adequate performance on this subtest requires use of the phonological approach to reading, because pseudowords cannot be read orthographically.

Appendix A of the BARF contains 60 words, 30 of which are contentives (i.e., nouns, adjectives, and verbs) and 30 of which are functors. The contentives and functors are equivalent in their average word frequency and number of graphemes per word. Appendix B uses the same word pairs as Subtest 5; however, they are dictated to the patient.

Four different administrations of the BARF are possible. The oral reading administration uses Subtests 1 through 4 and Appendix A. The silent-reading administration, for oral-language–impaired patients who cannot take Subtests 1 through 4, uses Subtests 5 and 6. A written administration of the BARF for assessment of agraphia employs Subtests 1 through 4 and Appendices A and B. A written or oral screening version of the BARF employs Items 1 through 10 of Subtests 1 through 4 and Items 1 through 20 of Appendix A. The screening items in Subtests 1 through 4 and Appendix A are balanced in average word frequency and word length.

The BARF is one of the few reading batteries designed to aid in the identification of cognitive subtypes of written language disorder. It is a well-designed and potentially valuable addition to the neuropsychological examination. The test has not yet been published, and reliability and validity data are not available. It is hoped that the necessary validation of the test will be completed and that the test will be marketed, because its composition is virtually unparalleled by any other available written language battery. At present, the BARF should be used in conjunction with other reading tests having known psychometric properties and an established normative database. Interpretation of the BARF should be attempted only by experienced speech pathologists, neuropsychologists, and behavioral neurologists. The BARF can be administered at bedside, in the office, or in laboratory settings.

NEUROPSYCHOLOGICAL TREATMENT

Neuropsychologists have little involvement in the treatment of alexia and agraphia; these disorders fall within the domain typically handled by the speech therapist. As with oral communication disorders, the neuropsychologist is consulted only when treatment of a written communication disorder fails to proceed as expected. The neuropsychologist then becomes a resource for the speech therapist to draw on in tackling a patient's motivational problems and in assessing and alleviating the impact of other emotional and neuropsychological disorders on treatment. Specific techniques the neuropsychologist can use in aiding the speech therapist are discussed in Chapter 12.

CASE ILLUSTRATIONS

The following cases illustrate both the difficulty of diagnosing written language disorders and the great frustration that can be engendered by taking extensive written language tests.

CASE 4–5

R.M. was a 50-year-old man with a high-school education. Following triple coronary artery bypass grafting, he developed atrial fibrillation and an anoxic encephalopathy. Magnetic resonance imaging (MRI) scans revealed bilateral watershed area infarctions (C-shaped infarctions extending from the frontal to the occipital poles), with greater damage evident in the right hemisphere.

Results of R.M.'s neuropsychological assessment were presented in Chapters 4, 7, 8, and 11, and are summarized briefly here. The patient presented with multiple neuropsychological disorders, including left-sided stimulus neglect, simultanagnosia, stimulus mislocalization, possible optic ataxia, and oculomotor apraxia. He also had bilateral weakness and reduced coordination in his arms, but the right arm and hand had sufficient strength and coordination for him to attempt writing.

The patient was able to learn and correctly sequence series of movements with his right hand but showed confusion of the order of some goal-directed movements (see Ideational apraxia). He did not show perseveration or impersistence in his motor performance. Constructional skills were severely impaired to the point at which he could not copy even simple line drawings, and his perceptual deficits prevented him from identifying the errors he made in drawings.

Figure 13–1 shows R.M.'s attempts to write the alphabet (he gave up after the letter H) and the numbers 0 through 20 (he gave up after reaching 9). His production consists of an illegible scrawl; only the merest portions of some letters

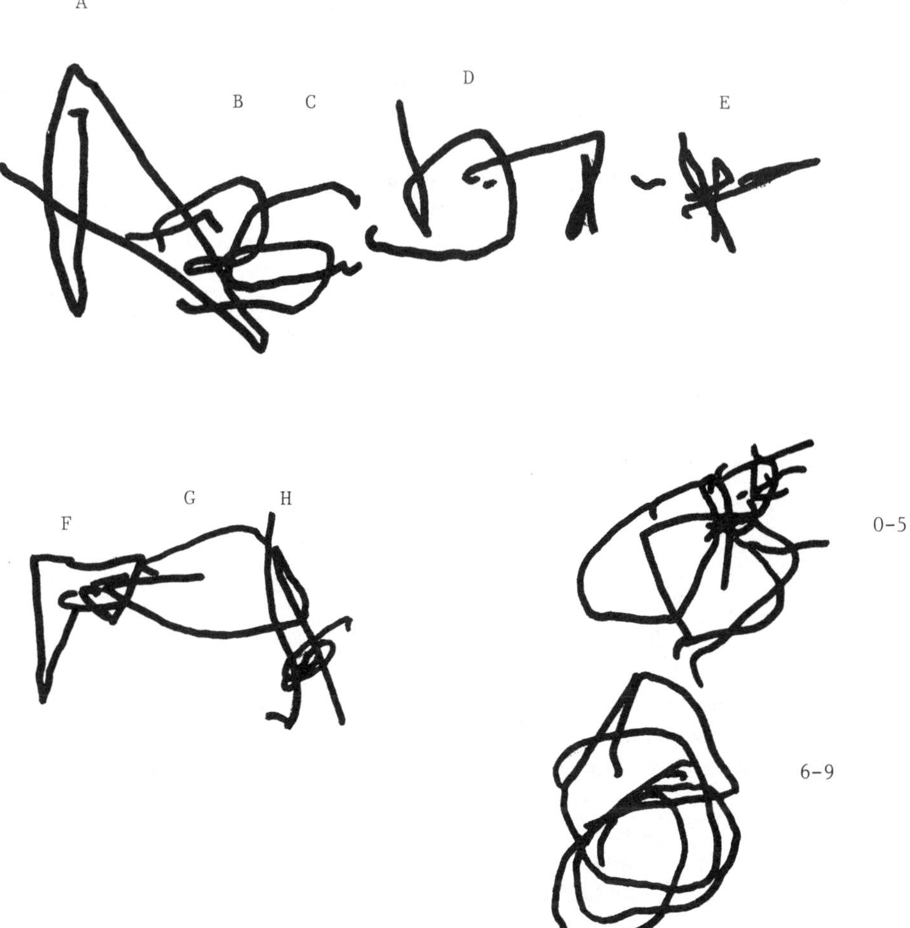

FIGURE 13–1. Patient R.M.'s attempt to write the alphabet and the numbers 0 through 20. The patient discontinued writing after the letter H and the number 9.

and numbers are recognizable. Performance could not be assessed with the left hand because of its greater weakness. The patient's oral spelling, contrastingly, was preserved. He had minimal difficulty with oral spelling items from the WAB. An attempt was made to assess his use of anagram letters. He could spell successfully under this condition, but because of his visual perceptual deficits, he required maximum assistance in finding the letters he wanted and in aligning them to make a word. Although he usually was able to tell the examiner what anagram letter should come next, so much assistance was required that the validity of the procedure was questionable.

DISCUSSION

The patient in Case 4–5 presented with possible apraxic agraphia. However, constructional agraphia could not be ruled out in this patient. Nor could the examiner entirely rule out the possibility that reduced strength in the right arm and hand contribute substantially to the deficient graphic production. In addition, it was not possible to assess writing in the left hand because of its severe weakness. Definitive diagnosis is impossible in this case.

The effort of attempting to narrow the diagnosis to one or two possibilities in Case 4–5 was worthwhile, however, because it led to treatment recommendations that were implemented by the speech therapist. Specifically, it was recommended that the patient be approached as a probable apraxic agraphic. It was advised to have the patient practice the mechanics of writing (e.g., tracing letters) and to train him to use compensatory devices (e.g., press-on anagram letters, typewriter) to facilitate written communication. The compensatory approach led to some success, because the patient was already familiar with the typewriter keyboard and could target his fingers to the right keys based on tactile feedback.

CASE 12–2

H.L. was a 27-year-old man with a master's degree in business administration. He was in good health until he was found unconscious outside his apartment after returning from jogging. A computed tomography (CT) scan revealed a large infarction in the distribution of the middle cerebral artery, affecting both the temporal and parietal lobes.

The patient was admitted to a rehabilitation hospital approximately 1 month after his infarction. Neurological and neuropsychological examinations revealed right hemiparesis that was worse in the upper extremity, decreased right-sided tactile sensation, and right-sided extinction to double simultaneous stimulation in the visual and auditory modalities (see Stimulus neglect). Perceptual skills, nonverbal problem solving, and memory for visuospatial information were intact. Results of this patient's oral language assessment are presented in Chapter 12. H.L. evidenced a moderately severe Broca's aphasia that was thought to be evolving toward transcortical motor aphasia.

Written language was assessed with the BARF. The patient failed to read any pseudowords correctly, but read correctly 80 percent of regular words, 50 percent of rule-governed words, and 80 percent of irregular words. He correctly matched all of the homophones with pictures on Subtest 5 of the BARF, but was correct on only 40 percent of the trials of Subtest 6, which required him to match pseudowords to pictures based on their phonologic similarity to real words. Functors (BARF Appendix A) were read with only 10 percent accuracy. When the written version of the BARF was taken with the patient using his nondominant hand, a different pattern of results was obtained. The patient failed to score above 60 percent on any subtest, and was as poor at writing irregular words as he was at writing pseudowords. It is notable that all individual letters were well formed. The patient was unable to write any functors correctly and refused further testing after attempting the written version of Appendix A.

DISCUSSION

The patient in Case 12–2 presented with aphasic alexia-agraphia. Striking effects of word class on his reading performance are evident. He showed features of the deep paralexic pattern, although the deep paragraphic pattern was not seen when his writing was considered. Writing could not be assessed in both hands because of weakness on the right side, but because of the nature of his lesion, it is unlikely that the agraphia was unilateral.

CASE 13–1

J.S. was a 51-year-old man with a 9th-grade education. He reported having failed several grades, but denied difficulty in learning to read or write. The patient suffered a traumatic brain injury with a subsequent intracranial hemorrhage. CT scans showed a large area of hemorrhage in the left parietal lobe and compression of the left lateral ventricle. His history was positive for substance abuse (primarily alcohol) and renal insufficiency. At the time of neuropsychological examination, the patient was ambulating and performing all self-care activities independently. He had no clinically significant weakness or other movement disorders, although he showed a general reduction in endurance. He had anomic aphasia (see Chap. 12), but otherwise his oral language was preserved.

The Written Language Section of the WAB were administered and yielded the following significant results. The patient failed all items assessing comprehension of written sentences and comprehension of written commands. No errors were made when he attempted to point to written words read by the examiner, but he was correct on only three of six trials involving matching actual objects to written words. Even on trials in which he correctly matched pictures and words, he was not always able to read the word orally. For example, he could not read the word "screwdriver," but was aware that the word referred to some type of tool, and this allowed him to match it with the correct object.

J.S. was poor at spelling words (one correct response in six trials) and at identifying words spelled to him (two correct responses in six trials). Use of anagram letters failed to improve his spelling performance. He was able to write his name but could write only a portion of his address. He was notably telegraphic when attempting to write a description of a picture; he simply listed isolated items in the picture. This was in marked contrast to his fluent (with the exception of word-finding difficulty) and grammatical speech. Spelling errors were notable throughout his spontaneous writing (e.g., he wrote "woaman" for "woman"). J.S. accurately wrote dictated numbers and letters, but when asked to write the entire alphabet on his own, he omitted the "D," continued as far as the letter "F," then indicated he could not do more. Similarly, when attempting to write up to the number 20, he got to number "3," wrote "F," and became confused to the point where he could not continue. His ability to copy a sentence was also poor as a result of letter substitutions, and the patient again discontinued out of frustration before he reached the end of the sentence. No differences in writing ability were apparent when the two hands were compared.

DISCUSSION

Case 13–1 presented a fairly straightforward profile. The patient showed both reading and writing errors, although his reading appeared somewhat more impaired than his writing. The primary differential is between aphasic alexia-agraphia and alexia with agraphia. Because the patient's anomic aphasia results only in word-finding difficulty, the oral language deficits do not parallel the written language deficits in any way. Alexia with agraphia is the most likely diagnosis. An interesting associated feature was the patient's occasional success in "categorizing" words that he was unable to read orally. Thus, it was possible for him to match a screwdriver with the corresponding written word, which he could not read but knew was a tool. The only major confounding factor was the patient's premorbid history of educational failure. Because he denied having trouble learning to read and write and because of the considerable consternation his current performance caused him, it is unlikely that these deficits were a part of his life before his illness.

CASE 13–2

C.M. was a 59-year-old man with degrees in law and meteorology. He suffered a left-hemisphere cerebrovascular accident with involvement of the left posterior temporal lobe, corona radiata, and the anterior and posterior limbs of the internal capsule, documented by CT scans. His history was positive for excessive alcohol use, left carotid stenosis documented by angiography, and carotid endarterectomy 5 months before his stroke. Neuropsychological and neurological examination revealed right-sided motor weakness; preserved ability to initiate, sustain, sequence, and discontinue movements at specified times; full visual fields with no evidence of stimulus neglect (see Chap. 4); preserved stimulus recognition (see Chap. 9); and aphasia (see Chap. 12) of moderate severity. The patient's oral language was characterized by fluent but paraphasic speech, impaired comprehension, and impaired repetition.

Written language was assessed with the HRB-AST and the BARF. Reading comprehension was severely impaired, but the patient was more successful at orally reading the stimuli from the HRB-AST, making only occasional paraphasic errors (e.g., "pog" for "dog," and "plendly" for "friendly"). C.M. was unable to spell orally any of the items from this test. The patient's great frustration when required to read forced the examiner to limit testing with the BARF to two subtests. C.M. succeeded in reading irregular words with 80 percent accuracy but dropped to 40 percent accuracy when reading pseudowords. He would not attempt to read functors and declined to take the written version of the BARF.

DISCUSSION

The patient in Case 13–2 presented with aphasic alexia-agraphia. His reading errors paralleled his fluent but paraphasic speech. The patient's oral language disorder appeared to be consistent with Wernicke's aphasia (see Chap. 12). Unfortunately, testing was truncated by the patient's increasing level of frustration. It appears that his reading errors are consistent with a phonological paralexic pattern with visual paralexias, although further assessment would likely have revealed additional effects of word class on his reading, which would alter interpretation of his error pattern. Writing could not be examined thoroughly in this case, but the prominent oral spelling errors suggest that a writing deficit confined to one hand would be an unlikely finding.

CASE 19–1

P.P. was a 68-year-old man who had completed 1 year of college and was retired from a lumber business. He suffered a left intracerebral and intraventricular hematoma at age 61 years and a second left-hemisphere stroke at age 64 years. He is reported to have made a good recovery in the months following both of these incidents. At age 67 years, the patient's family noted increased irritability, emotional lability, and the development of unfounded jealous suspicions concerning his wife, which led to violent threats when other family members tried to defend her. Neuropsychological testing was requested. Results of the assessment are discussed in detail in Chapter 19; only selected findings are presented here.

P.P. had a right homonymous hemianopsia but was otherwise free of perceptual deficits, including stimulus neglect (see Chap. 4) and constructional disability (see Chap. 7). He had no difficulty in recognizing object pictures or colors, although he was anomic (see Anomic aphasia). His naming improved when he was given a phonemic cue, and he was consistently able to describe any stimulus or concept that he failed to name. The patient showed no indications of reduced strength or coordination, perseveration, decreased motor speed and initiation, apraxia, or any other movement disorder (see Chap. 11).

Reading and writing were assessed using Section K of Luria's Neuropsychological Investigation and the BARF. P.P. read letters with only occasional errors (e.g., "W" read as "U"). Ideograms (acronyms) and syllables of up to four letters in length could be read without error. Words could be read, but only by the patient spelling them, aloud or silently, one letter at a time. Consequently, reading was a slow and laborious process. Word class did not affect the patient's reading performance, but word length was a major factor in how well he did. Reading by spelling was not successful for longer words. When confronted with a word such as "astrocytoma," the patient would spell the initial few syllables, then guess the identity of the word, in this instance guessing "astrodome."

P.P. was able to copy block letters and write in cursive script using his right or left hand with minimal difficulty. Occasional letter substitutions were noted in his production, however. Copying was better than writing to dictation, in that letter substitutions were more frequent in the latter. At no point did his writing problems even marginally approach the severity of impairment seen in his reading. Copying words failed to improve P.P.'s subsequent ability to read them.

DISCUSSION

The patient in Case 19–1 presented with pure alexia. Although he made some spelling errors, his writing deficit was minimal in comparison to his reading deficit. This patient's reading was not facilitated by writing the words first. His performance illustrates the letter-by-letter reading pattern. The deficit arose in this patient in the context of possible verbal intellectual decline (see Chap. 19) brought on by multiple cerebrovascular accidents occurring since his 61st birthday.

REFERENCES

1. Roeltgen, D: Agraphia. In Heilman, KM, and Valenstein, E (eds): Clinical Neuropsychology, Second Edition. Oxford University Press, New York, 1985, p 75.
2. Coltheart, M, Patterson, K, and Marshall, JC (eds): Deep Dyslexia. Routledge and Kegan Paul, London, 1980.
3. Friedman, RB, and Albert, ML: Alexia. In Heilman, KM, and Valenstein, E (eds): Clinical Neuropsychology, Second Edition. Oxford University Press, New York, 1985, p 49.
4. American Psychiatric Association: Diagnostic and Statistical Manual of Mental Disorders, Fourth Edition. American Psychiatric Association, Washington, DC, 1994.
5. The International Classification of Diseases, Ninth Revision, Clinical Modification. Med-Index Publications, Salt Lake City, 1991.
6. Benson, DF, Brown, J, and Tomlinson, EB: Varieties of alexia. Neurology 21:951, 1971.
7. Coslett, HB, et al: Reading in pure alexia. The effect of strategy. Brain 116:21, 1993.
8. Quint, DJ, and Gilmore, JL: Alexia without agraphia. Neuroradiology 34:210, 1992.
9. DeVreese, LP: Two systems for colour-naming defects: Verbal disconnection vs. colour imagery disorder. Neuropsychologia 29:1, 1991.
10. Naranjo, IC, et al: Alexia without agraphia: A new case studied by CT-scan. Neuroradiology 31:199, 1989.
11. Coslett, HB, and Saffran, EM: Evidence for preserved reading in "pure alexia." Brain 112:327, 1989.
12. Leegaard, OF, Riis, JO, and Andersen, G: "Pure alexia" without hemianopia or colour anomia. Acta Neurol Scand 78:501, 1988.
13. Mochizuki, H, and Ohtomo, R: Pure alexia in Japanese and agraphia without alexia in kanji. The ability dissociation between reading and writing kanji vs. kana. Arch Neurol 45:1157, 1988.
14. Fukuzawa, K, et al: Internal representations and the conceptual operation of color in pure alexia with color naming defects. Brain Lang 34:98, 1988.
15. DeRenzi, E, Zambolin, A, and Crisi, G: The pattern of neuropsychological impairment associated with left posterior cerebral artery infarcts. Brain 110:1099, 1987.
16. Pillon, B, Bakchine, S, and Lhermitte, F: Alexia without agraphia in a left-handed patient with a right occipital lesion. Arch Neurol 44:1257, 1987.
17. Caffarra, P: Alexia without agraphia or hemianopia. Eur Neurol 27:65, 1987.
18. Weisberg, LA, and Wall, M: Alexia without agraphia: Clinical-computed tomographic correlations. Neuroradiology 29:283, 1987.
19. Henderson, VW, et al: Left hemisphere pathways in reading: Inferences from pure alexia without hemianopia. Neurology 35:962, 1985.
20. Grossi, D, et al: Residual reading capability in a patient with alexia without agraphia. Brain Lang 23:337, 1984.
21. Winkelman, MD, and Glasson, CC: Unilateral right cerebral representation of reading in a familial left-hander. Neuropsychologia 22:621, 1984.

22. Damasio, AR, and Damasio, H: The anatomic basis of pure alexia. Neurology 33:1573, 1983.
23. Nicole, S, Nardi, P, and Fortuna, A: Alexia without agraphia. A case studied by means of computed axial tomography. Eur Neurol 21:361, 1982.
24. Mani, SS, Fine, EJ, and Mayberry, Z: Alexia without agraphia: Localization of the lesion by computerized tomography. Comput Tomogr 5:95, 1981.
25. Johansson, T, and Fahlgren, H: Alexia without agraphia: Lateral and medial infarction of left occipital lobe. Neurology 29:390, 1979.
26. Erkulvrawatr, S: Alexia and left homonymous hemianopia in a non-right-hander. Ann Neurol 3:549, 1978.
27. Hirose, G, Kin, T, and Murakami, E: Alexia without agraphia associated with right occipital lesion. J Neurol Neurosurg Psychiatry 40:225, 1977.
28. Binder, JR, and Mohr, JP: The topography of callosal reading pathways. A case-control analysis. Brain 115:1807, 1992.
29. Prior, M, and McCorriston, M: Acquired and developmental spelling dyslexia. Brain Lang 20:263, 1983.
30. Speedie, LJ, Rothi, LJ, and Heilman, KM: Spelling dyslexia: A form of cross-cuing. Brain Lang 15:340, 1982.
31. Beauvois, MF, and Derouesne, J: Phonological alexia: Three dissociations. J Neurol Neurosurg Psychiatry 42:1115, 1979.
32. Iragui, VJ, and Kritchevsky, M: Alexia without agraphia or hemianopia in parietal infarction. J Neurol Neurosurg Psychiatry 54:841, 1991.
33. Pirozzolo, FJ, et al: Neurolinguistic analysis of the language abilities of a patient with a "double disconnection syndrome": A case of subangular alexia in the presence of mixed transcortical aphasia. J Neurol Neurosurg Psychiatry 44:152, 1981.
34. Greenblatt, SH: Subangular alexia without agraphia or hemianopsia. Brain Lang 3:229, 1976.
35. Ducarne, B, Bergego, C, and Gardeur, D: "Sub-angular" alexis and associated neuropsychologic signs: Clinical and tomodensitometric study. Cortex 19:115, 1983.
36. Staller, J, et al: Alexia without agraphia: An experimental case study. Brain Lang 5:378, 1978.
37. Stommel, EW, Friedman, RJ, and Reeves, AG: Alexia without agraphia associated with spleniogeniculate infarction. Neurology 41:587, 1991.
38. Silver, FL, et al: Resolving metabolic abnormalities in a case of pure alexia. Neurology 38:730, 1988.
39. Yokota, T, et al: Pure agraphia of kanji due to thrombosis of the Labbe vein. J Neurol Neurosurg Psychiatry 53:335, 1990.
40. Soma, Y, et al: Lexical agraphia in the Japanese language. Pure agraphia for kanji due to left posteroinferior temporal lesions. Brain 112:1549, 1989.
41. Rosati, G, and DeBastiani, P: Pure agraphia: A discrete form of aphasia. J Neurol Neurosurg Psychiatry 42:266, 1979.
42. Trillet, M, Croisile, B, and Laurent, B: Pure agraphia. Apropos of 2 cases. Rev Neurol 145:720, 1989.
43. Levine, DN, Mani, RB, and Calvanio, R: Pure agraphia and Gerstmann's syndrome as a visuospatial-language dissociation: An experimental case study. Brain Lang 35:172, 1988.
44. Auerbach, SH, and Alexander, MP: Pure agraphia and unilateral optic ataxia associated with a left superior parietal lobule lesion. J Neurol Neurosurg Psychiatry 44:430, 1981.
45. Roeltgen, DP, and Heilman, KM: Lexical agraphia: Further support for the two-system hypothesis of linguistic agraphia. Brain 107:811, 1984.
46. Miceli, G, Silveri, C, and Caramazza, A: Cognitive analysis of a case of pure dysgraphia. Brain Lang 25:187, 1985.
47. Basso, A, Taborelli, A, and Vignolo, LA: Dissociated disorders of speaking and writing in aphasia. J Neurol Neurosurg Psychiatry 41:556, 1978.
48. Mazzocchi, E, and Vignolo, LA: Localization of lesions in aphasia: Clinical CT scan correlations in stroke patients. Cortex 15:627, 1979.
49. Kirk, A, et al: Phonolexical agraphia. Superimposition of acquired lexical agraphia on developmental phonological dysgraphia. Brain 114:1977, 1991.
50. Croisile, B, et al: Lexical agraphia caused by left temporoparietal hematoma. Rev Neurol 145:287, 1989.
51. Gonzalez-Rothi, LJ, Roeltgen, DP, and Kooistra, CA: Isolated lexical agraphia in a right-handed patient with a posterior lesion of the right cerebral hemisphere. Brain Lang 30:181, 1987.
52. Aimard, G, et al: Agraphie pure (dynamique?) d'origine frontale. A propos d'une observation. Rev Neurol 131:505, 1975.

53. Rapcsak, SZ, Arthur, SA, and Rubens, AB: Lexical agraphia from focal lesion of the left precentral gyrus. Neurology 38:1119, 1988.
54. Laine, T, and Marttila, RJ: Pure agraphia: A case study. Neuropsychologia 19:311, 1981.
55. Kawahata, N, Nagata, K, and Shishido, F: Alexia with agraphia due to the left posterior inferior temporal lobe lesion—neuropsychological analysis and its pathogenetic mechanisms. Brain Lang 33:296, 1988.
56. Kawamura, M, et al: Alexia with agraphia of kanji (Japanese morphograms). J Neurol Neurosurg Psychiatry 50:1125, 1987.
57. Day, JT, Fisher, AG, and Mastaglia, FL: Alexia with agraphia in multiple sclerosis. J Neurol Sci 78:343, 1987.
58. Lüders, H, et al: Basal temporal language area demonstrated by electrical stimulation. Neurology 36:505, 1986.
59. Friedman, RB, and Kohn, SE: Impaired activation of the phonological lexicon: Effects upon oral reading. Brain Lang 38:278, 1990.
60. Rapcsak, SZ, Gonzalez-Rothi, LJ, and Heilman, KM: Phonological alexia with optic and tactile anomia: A neuropsychological and anatomical study. Brain Lang 31:109, 1987.
61. Freedman, L, et al: Posterior cortical dementia with alexia: Neurobehavioural, MRI, and PET findings. J Neurol Neurosurg Psychiatry 54:443, 1991.
62. Benson, DF, Davis, RJ, and Snyder, BD: Posterior cortical atrophy. Arch Neurol 45:789, 1988.
63. Sevush, S, and Heilman, KM: A case of literal alexia: Evidence for a disconnection syndrome. Brain Lang 22:92, 1984.
64. Alexander, MP, et al: Lesion localization of phonological agraphia. Brain Lang 43:83, 1992.
65. Anderson, SW, Damasio, AR, and Damasio, H: Troubled letters but not numbers. Domain specific cognitive impairments following focal damage in frontal cortex. Brain 113:749, 1990.
66. Rapcsak, SZ, Beeson, PM, and Rubens, AB: Writing with the right hemisphere. Brain Lang 41:510, 1991.
67. Glosser, G, and Friedman, RB: The continuum of deep/phonological alexia. Cortex 26:343, 1990.
68. Roeltgen, DP, Sevush, S, and Heilman, KM: Phonological agraphia: Writing by the lexical-semantic route. Neurology 33:755, 1983.
69. Bub, D, and Kertesz, A: Deep agraphia. Brain Lang 17:146, 1982.
70. Crary, MA, and Heilman, KM: Letter imagery deficits in a case of pure apraxic agraphia. Brain Lang 34:147, 1988.
71. Coslett, HB, et al: Dissociations of writing and praxis: Two cases in point. Brain Lang 28:357, 1986.
72. Valenstein, E, and Heilman, KM: Apraxic agraphia with neglect-induced paragraphia. Arch Neurol 36:506, 1979.
73. Roeltgen, DP, and Heilman, KM: Apractic agraphia in a patient with normal praxis. Brain Lang 18:35, 1983.
74. Baxter, DM, and Warrington, EK: Ideational agraphia: A single case study. J Neurol Neurosurg Psychiatry 49:369, 1986.
75. Kinsbourne, M, and Rosenfield, D: Agraphia selective for written spelling, an experimental case study. Brain Lang 1:215, 1974.
76. Hodges, JR: Pure apraxic agraphia with recovery after drainage of a left frontal cyst. Cortex 27:469, 1991.
77. Croisile, B, et al: Pure agraphia after deep left hemisphere haematoma. J Neurol Neurosurg Psychiatry 53:263, 1990.
78. Imai, S, Kawashima, Y, and Ohye, C: Constructional agraphia in left parietal glioma—a case report. Rinsho Shinkeigaku 21:567, 1981.
79. Demeurisse, G, Coekaerts, MJ, and Hublet, C: Agraphia, cortical anarthria and planning disorders as a result of a lesion of the right hemisphere in a right-handed patient. Acta Neurol Belg 84:119, 1984.
80. Bigley, GK, and Sharp, FR: Reversible alexia without agraphia due to migraine. Arch Neurol 40:114, 1983.
81. Gonzalez Rothi, LJ, Coslett, HB, and Heilman, KM: Battery of Adult Reading Function, Experimental Edition. Unpublished manuscript, 1984.

DISORDERS OF EMOTIONAL COMMUNICATION

14

In addition to the semantic and grammatical components of communication, Monrad-Krohn[1] identified a third component, which he termed "prosody," having to do with changes in the rhythm, pitch, and stress with which words are spoken. This third component of communication can be as important as the previous two in determining the social meaning of an utterance. For example, the declarative sentence "Cathy is driving" can be changed to the interrogative "Cathy is driving?" simply by altering word stress and tone of voice. Prosody also functions as a means of communicating emotion. For example, the simple phrase "Thanks a lot" can indicate appreciation or sarcastic displeasure, depending on the speaker's use of prosody.

The ability to use nonemotional prosody to shape the social meaning of an utterance declines following left- or right-hemisphere brain damage.[2–6] Disturbances in emotional prosody, however, are more likely to arise after right-hemisphere brain damage,[7] whereas even left-hemisphere–damaged patients with Broca's aphasia (see Chap. 12) typically are able to communicate emotion through tone of voice.

Ross[8] introduced the term *aprosodia* to describe the syndrome of impaired emotional communication via prosody and facial gesture that typically follows right-hemisphere brain damage. Ross noted that aprosodia could be subtyped in a manner similar to the aphasias and theorized that the lesions in the right hemisphere that produce the aprosodia subtypes parallel the left-hemisphere lesions that produce the analogous aphasia subtypes. More than 30 cases of aprosodia have appeared in the literature, and the lesions have generally been located where Ross predicted.[7–15]

The subtypes of aprosodia are listed under "Variety of Presentation" in the chapter outline. Most of these subtypes involve deficits in both affective prosody and facial gesture. Although both prosody and facial gesture are impaired in a given case of aprosodia, the severity of the deficits seen in prosody and gesture often differs.[8,13]

The cases in the literature are not evenly divided among the subtypes of aprosodia. Most reported cases exemplify motor, sensory, and global aprosodia. The existence, clinical description, and lesion locations of the other aprosodia subtypes must be considered putative.

NOMENCLATURE

The terms *aprosody* and *aprosodia* are sometimes used interchangeably in the literature, although Ross and his colleagues restrict the use of "aprosodia" to disorders of emotional prosody and emotional facial gesture. This convention is followed in this text. The term *auditory affective agnosia* has also been used to describe deficits in perceiving affect. This term is not used in this text, although deficits in affect perception are present in several of the aprosodia subtypes. DSM-IV[16] and ICD-9-CM[17] do not contain specific diagnostic codes for the aprosodias. ICD-9-CM does contain codes for voice disturbance. The aprosodias can be coded as "Unspecified Voice Disturbance" or "Other Voice Disturbance," although more than voice is impaired in aprosodia.

VARIETY OF PRESENTATION

1. Motor aprosodia

Clinical Indicators

a_1. Impaired expression of emotional tones of voice on demand
a_2. Impaired expression of emotional facial gestures on demand
a_3. Impaired imitation of emotional tones of voice
a_4. Relatively preserved perception of emotional tones of voice
a_5. Relatively preserved perception of emotional facial expressions

Associated Features

a. Preserved ability to vary the volume of the voice
b. Transitory improvement in the expression of emotion via prosody and facial gesture during periods of high emotional arousal

Clinical Indicators: Each is independent (only one must be observed for the disorder to be suspected) *except* when subscripting is used. Subscripted numbers (a_1, a_2) denote an indicator with multiple parts that must be considered together.
Associated Features: These are listed to give a more complete picture of the disorder. The presence or absence of these features does not affect the diagnosis.
Factors to Rule Out: All must be taken into account. Failure to rule out even one of these factors makes a firm diagnosis impossible.
Lesion Locations: Each location stands alone; damage in only one of the listed areas is sufficient to produce the disorder.

c. Difference between severity of deficits in prosody and severity of deficits in facial expression
d. Clumsy groping or making unrelated and incorrect movements when attempting to express emotion via facial gestures
e. Recent history of global aprosodia
f. Unilateral (usually left-sided) muscle weakness (hemiparesis)
g. Lack of awareness of emotional communication deficits (see Anosognosia)

Factors to Rule Out

a. Depressed mood sufficient to account for the deficits in emotional expression
b. Impaired speech articulation sufficient to account for the deficits in emotional prosody
c. Reduced ability to make vocal sounds as a result of damage of the vocal organs (hypophonia) sufficient to account for the deficits in emotional prosody; medical consultation for examination of the vocal organs and air passages possibly required
d. Weakness or poor coordination of facial muscles sufficient to account for the deficits in emotional facial expression
e. Impaired initiation of movements of the face (see Akinesia) sufficient to account for the deficits in emotional facial expression

Lesion Locations

a. Combined frontal and anterior parietal opercula[8,10,18]
b. Basal ganglia[18]
c. Internal capsule[12]

Lesion Lateralization

a. Right hemisphere in most published cases

2. **Sensory aprosodia (also called "auditory affective agnosia")**

Clinical Indicators

a_1. Impaired perception of emotional tones of voice
a_2. Impaired perception of emotional facial expressions
a_3. Impaired imitation of emotional tones of voice
a_4. Relatively preserved expression of emotional tones of voice on demand
a_5. Relatively preserved expression of emotional facial gestures on demand

Associated Features

a. Overly happy or euphoric mood (see Moria)
b. Possible difference between severity of deficits in prosody and severity of deficits in facial expression
c. Loss of acuity in one (usually the left) visual half-field (homonymous hemianopsia)
d. Loss of somesthetic (touch, vibratory, and position) sensation on one (usually the left) side of the body
e. Impaired recognition of objects palpated in the hand (see Astereognosis)

Factors to Rule Out

a. Depressed mood sufficient to account for the deficits in the imitation of emotional tones of voice, ruled out by documenting preserved expression of emotional tones of voice on demand because a mood disorder does not selectively impair imitation
b. Impaired speech articulation sufficient to account for the deficits in the imitation of emotional tones of voice, ruled out by documenting preserved expression of emotional tones of voice on demand because an articulation deficit does not selectively impair imitation
c. Reduced ability to make vocal sounds as a result of damage of the vocal organs (hypophonia) sufficient to account for the deficits in imitation of emotional tones of voice, ruled out by documenting preserved expression of emotional tones of voice on demand because hypophonia does not selectively impair imitation
d. A bias toward or against the perception of some emotions as a result of the presence of a mood disorder or other intense emotional state

Lesion Locations

a. Combined posterior temporal and parietal opercula[8,10]
b. Combined thalamus and posterior limb of the internal capsule[15]
c. Combined basal ganglia and posterior limb of the internal capsule[18]

Lesion Lateralization

a. Right hemisphere

3. **Pure affective deafness (also called "pure prosodic deafness")***

Clinical Indicators

a_1. Impaired perception of emotional tones of voice

---

*This disorder must be considered putative because there are relatively few published cases.

a_2. Impaired imitation of emotional tones of voice
a_3. Relatively preserved perception of emotional facial expressions
a_4. Relatively preserved expression of emotional tones of voice on demand
a_5. Relatively preserved expression of emotional facial gestures on demand

Associated Features

No information available

Factors to Rule Out

a. Depressed mood sufficient to account for the deficits in imitation of emotional tones of voice, ruled out by documenting preserved expression of emotional tones of voice on demand because a mood disorder does not selectively impair imitation
b. Impaired speech articulation sufficient to account for the deficits in imitation of emotional tones of voice, ruled out by documenting preserved expression of emotional tones of voice on demand because an articulation deficit does not selectively impair imitation
c. Reduced ability to make vocal sounds as a result of damage of the vocal organs (hypophonia) sufficient to account for the deficits in imitation of emotional tones of voice, ruled out by documenting preserved expression of emotional tones of voice on demand because hypophonia does not selectively impair imitation
d. A bias toward or against the perception of some emotions as a result of the presence of a mood disorder or other intense emotional state

Lesion Locations

a. Anterior temporal lobe,* with damage to the ipsilateral primary auditory cortex and interruption of contralateral auditory fibers traveling across the corpus callosum[8–10]

Lesion Lateralization

a. Right hemisphere in most reported cases

4. Conduction aprosodia†

Clinical Indicators

a_1. Impaired imitation of emotional tones of voice
a_2. Relatively preserved perception of emotional tones of voice
a_3. Relatively preserved perception of emotional facial expressions
a_4. Relatively preserved expression of emotional tones of voice on demand
a_5. Relatively preserved expression of emotional facial gestures on demand

Associated Features

a. Difference between severity of deficits in prosody and severity of deficits in facial expression

---

*The lesion should spare the posterior-superior temporal lobe but isolate it from tonal input. Visual input continues to be received because occipital-temporal fibers are spared. All cases reported, however, have had more widespread lesions, preventing precise determination of the lesion responsible for pure affective deafness.

†This disorder must be considered putative because there are relatively few published cases.

Factors to Rule Out

a. Depressed mood sufficient to account for the deficits in imitating emotional tones of voice, ruled out by documenting preserved expression of emotional tones of voice on demand because a mood disorder does not selectively impair imitation
b. Impaired speech articulation sufficient to account for the deficits in imitating emotional tones of voice, ruled out by documenting preserved expression of emotional tones of voice on demand because an articulation deficit does not selectively impair imitation
c. Reduced ability to make vocal sounds as a result of damage of the vocal organs (hypophonia) sufficient to account for the deficits in imitating emotional tones of voice, ruled out by documenting preserved expression of emotional tones of voice on demand because hypophonia does not selectively impair imitation

Lesion Locations

a. Combined temporal and parietal lobes[18]
b. Superior frontal lobe[18]

Lesion Lateralization

a. Right hemisphere

5. Global aprosodia

Clinical Indicators

a_1. Impaired expression of emotional tones of voice on demand
a_2. Impaired expression of emotional facial gestures on demand
a_3. Impaired imitation of emotional tones of voice
a_4. Impaired perception of emotional tones of voice
a_5. Impaired perception of emotional facial expressions

Associated Features

a. Preserved ability to vary volume of voice
b. Transitory improvement in expression of emotion via prosody and facial gesture during periods of high emotional arousal
c. Possible difference between severity of deficits in prosody and severity of deficits in facial expression
d. Clumsy groping or making unrelated and incorrect movements when attempting to express emotion via facial gestures
e. Unilateral (usually left-sided) muscle weakness (hemiparesis)
f. Loss of acuity in one (usually the left) visual half-field (homonymous hemianopsia)
g. Loss of somesthetic (touch, vibratory, and position) sensation on one (usually the left) side of the body
h. Impaired recognition of objects palpated in the hand (see Astereognosis)

Factors to Rule Out

a. Depressed mood sufficient to account for deficits in expression of emotion

b. Impaired speech articulation sufficient to account for deficits in emotional prosody
c. Reduced ability to make vocal sounds as a result of damage of the vocal organs (hypophonia) sufficient to account for the deficits in emotional prosody, possibly requiring medical consultation for examination of the vocal organs and air passages
d. Weakness or poor coordination of the facial muscles sufficient to account for deficits in emotional facial expression
e. Inability to initiate movements of the face (see Akinesia) sufficient to account for the deficits in emotional facial expression
f. A bias toward or against the perception of some emotions as a result of the presence of a mood disorder or other intense emotional state

Lesion Locations

a. Perisylvian area, involving the frontal, parietal, and temporal lobes[8,10,18]

Lesion Lateralization

a. Right hemisphere in most reported cases

6. Transcortical motor aprosodia*

Clinical Indicators

a_1. Impaired expression of emotional tones of voice on demand
a_2. Impaired expression of emotional facial gestures on demand
a_3. Relatively preserved imitation of emotional tones of voice
a_4. Relatively preserved perception of emotional tones of voice
a_5. Relatively preserved perception of emotional facial expressions

Associated Features

a. Preserved ability to vary volume of voice
b. Transitory improvement in the expression of emotion via prosody and facial gesture during periods of high emotional arousal
c. Possible difference between severity of deficits in prosody and severity of deficits in facial expression
d. Clumsy groping or making unrelated and incorrect movements when attempting to express emotion via facial gestures
e. Recent history of mixed transcortical aprosodia
f. Unilateral (usually left-sided) muscle weakness (hemiparesis)

Factors to Rule Out

a. Depressed mood sufficient to account for the deficits in emotional expression†
b. Impaired speech articulation sufficient to account for the deficits in emotional prosody†

---

*This disorder must be considered putative because there are relatively few published cases.

†Demonstrating relatively preserved imitation of emotional tones of voice is insufficient to rule out this factor because imitation is often superior to production on demand in depressed, dysarthric, and hypophonic patients.

c. Reduced ability to make vocal sounds as a result of damage of the vocal organs (hypophonia) sufficient to account for the deficits in emotional prosody,* possibly requiring medical consultation for examination of the vocal organs and air passages
d. Weakness or poor coordination of the facial muscles sufficient to account for deficits in emotional facial expression
e. Inability to initiate movements of the face (see Akinesia) sufficient to account for deficits in emotional facial expression

Lesion Locations

a. Medial or anterior-superior frontal lobe[8,13]
b. Basal ganglia[8,10†]

Lesion Lateralization

a. Right hemisphere

7. Transcortical sensory aprosodia‡ (also called "auditory affective agnosia")

Clinical Indicators

a_1. Impaired perception of emotional tones of voice
a_2. Impaired perception of emotional facial expressions
a_3. Relatively preserved imitation of emotional tones of voice
a_4. Relatively preserved expression of emotional tones of voice on demand
a_5. Relatively preserved expression of emotional facial gestures on demand

Associated Features

a. Overly happy or euphoric mood (see Moria)
b. Possible difference between severity of deficits in prosody and severity of deficits in facial expression

Factors to Rule Out

a. Bias toward or against the perception of some emotions as a result of the presence of a mood disorder or other intense emotional state

Lesion Locations

a. Anterior-inferior temporal lobe[8,10]

Lesion Lateralization

a. Right hemisphere

8. Mixed transcortical aprosodia‡

Clinical Indicators

a_1. Impaired expression of emotional tones of voice on demand
a_2. Impaired expression of emotional facial gestures on demand
a_3. Relatively preserved imitation of emotional tones of voice

---

*Demonstrating relatively preserved imitation of emotional tones of voice is insufficient to rule out this factor, because imitation is often superior to production on demand in depressed, dysarthric, and hypophonic patients.

†This disorder may be transient when it follows a basal ganglial lesion.

‡This disorder must be considered putative because there are relatively few published cases.

a_4. Impaired perception of emotional tones of voice
a_5. Impaired perception of emotional facial expressions

Associated Features

a. Preserved ability to vary volume of voice
b. Transitory improvement in the expression of emotion via prosody and facial gesture during periods of high emotional arousal
c. Difference between severity of deficits in prosody and severity of deficits in facial expression.
d. Clumsy groping or making unrelated and incorrect movements when attempting to express emotion via facial gestures
e. Unilateral (usually left-sided) muscle weakness (hemiparesis)
f. Loss of acuity in one (usually the left) visual half-field (homonymous hemianopsia)
g. Loss of somesthetic (touch, vibratory, and position) sensation on one (usually the left) side of the body
h. Impaired recognition of objects palpated in the hand (see Astereognosis)

Factors to Rule Out

a. Depressed mood sufficient to account for the deficits in expression of emotion*
b. Impaired speech articulation sufficient to account for the deficits in emotional prosody*
c. Reduced ability to make vocal sounds as a result of damage of the vocal organs (hypophonia) sufficient to account for the deficits in emotional prosody,* possibly requiring medical consultation for examination of the vocal organs and air passages
d. Weakness or poor coordination of the facial muscles sufficient to account for the deficits in emotional facial expression
e. Inability to initiate movements of the face (see Akinesia) sufficient to account for the deficits in emotional facial expression
f. Bias toward or against the perception of some emotions as a result of the presence of a mood disorder or other intense emotional state

Lesion Locations

a. Frontal and parietal opercula with extension into the superior temporal lobe[8]

Lesion Lateralization

a. Right hemisphere

ETIOLOGY

Most cases of aprosodia reported in the literature and encountered in my clinical practice have resulted from cerebrovascular disease. A few patients diagnosed

*Demonstrating relatively preserved imitation of emotional tones of voice is insufficient to rule out this factor, because imitation is often superior to production on demand in depressed, dysarthric, and hypophonic patients.

with aprosodia have had right-hemisphere neoplasms.[13,18] As more cases of aprosodia are encountered and reported, other causes are likely to be identified.

DISABLING CONSEQUENCES

Patients in occupations that involve public speaking (e.g., teaching, law, ministry) or persuasion (e.g., sales) or that require skill in interpersonal interaction (e.g., counseling, medicine, secretarial fields) are likely to suffer the greatest disability from aprosodia. Although they do not become totally unable to work as a result of this disorder, these patients are likely to experience a considerable drop in their work performance and satisfaction.

Intact verbal ability is usually not sufficient to compensate for the absence of emotional expression. When a speaker's prosody and facial expression do not match the speaker's verbal content, he or she is likely to be perceived as insincere. For example, an elementary school teacher with aprosodia may have difficulty getting his or her pupils to stop misbehaving if they fail to detect sincere displeasure in the teacher's tone of voice, despite the verbal content of the communication.

Close interpersonal relationships may suffer as well because the patient's partner fails to detect warmth, caring, and sincerity in the patient's communications. Although it may be easier for a partner in an already established relationship to adjust to the change in the patient's emotional expression, the deficit can severely restrict the establishment and maintenance of new relationships.

ASSESSMENT INSTRUMENTS

Profile of Nonverbal Sensitivity

The Profile of Nonverbal Sensitivity (PONS)[19] can be obtained from *Johns Hopkins University Press, 2715 North Charles Street, Baltimore, MD 21218.*

The PONS measures comprehension of nonverbal emotional communications. It consists of a film of 220 2-second emotional scenes portrayed by a young woman. In each scene, only portions of the total communication are present. For example, in one set of scenes, only the woman's face is shown; another set of scenes shows only her body; in a third set, the words have been randomly scrambled to eliminate coherent meaning; in a fourth set, electronic filtering of high-frequency sounds is used to eliminate distinguishable words while preserving prosody. The remaining sets of scenes are combinations of these four elements. Patients view each scene, then select which of two printed statements correctly describes the scene.

The PONS has the advantage of being widely used; it has been given to more than 3000 subjects from 20 nations. It also provides a highly thorough and standardized assessment of comprehension of nonverbal emotional communications. Research has shown that the internal consistency reliability of the PONS ranges from .86 to .92, and its median test-retest reliability is .69.[20] The PONS has been shown to discriminate brain-damaged patients from normal controls, and left- from right-hemisphere damaged patients (the latter score lower).[20,21] The test should be administered for clinical purposes only by individuals trained in psychological or neuropsychological assessment. It is appropriate for office or laboratory use.

Perception of Emotions Test

The Perception of Emotions Test (POET)[22] can be obtained from *the author of the test.*

The POET consists of 128 6-second, videotaped emotional scenes portrayed by two men and two women. Separate sets of scenes present verbal content only, prosody only, facial expressions only, or a combination of the three. Following each scene, patients indicate what emotion was depicted by pointing to a sheet containing a drawing of a face showing anger, happiness, sadness, or neutrality. Each emotion is also written below the corresponding drawing. Normative data are based on 100 healthy college students. Test-retest reliability was .72 in a sample of 17 college students.[22] Left-cortical stroke patients performed significantly worse than right-cortical stroke patients on scenes containing verbal content only, whereas right-sided stroke patients aged 49 years or older performed significantly worse than left-sided stroke patients of the age group on the prosody-only scenes. The POET appears to be a promising measure, but further validation research is necessary before it can be used alone. The test should be administered for clinical purposes only by individuals trained in psychological or neuropsychological assessment. It is appropriate for office or laboratory use.

Affective Communication Test

The Affective Communication Test (ACT)[13] can be obtained from *the author of the test.* Separate sections of the ACT assess imitation and production of affective prosody, imitation of facial affect, production of facial affect, comprehension of affective prosody, and comprehension of affective facial expressions. The test also includes phonation, articulation, and motor screening sections, with items that assist the examiner in ruling out deficits in these areas that might alter the interpretation of the patient's affective performance.

The ACT has several disadvantages. It relies on the examiner's subjective judgment in rating patient responses. Additionally, it requires the examiner to act as a model of emotional expression. Reliability and validity data are based on a small subject population and thus must be viewed skeptically.[13] Inter-rater reliability was reported to be .71 for ratings of imitation of affective prosody and .99 for ratings of its production. Inter-rater reliability was .70 for imitation of affective facial expressions and .83 for ratings of their production. My experience with the ACT suggests that it does discriminate between normal controls and brain-damaged patients, but this has not been systematically studied in a large sample. At present, the instrument can be used only as a procedural guide for the examiner's bedside clinical examination of affective communication, but with further reliability and validity research, it may become a more useful instrument.

The principal reasons for recommending use of the ACT are that it is an improvement over the unstructured clinical examination procedures that are reported in the literature, and it does include an assessment of imitation and production of affect, which is omitted from the available standardized instruments. The ACT is appropriate for use by neurologists, neuropsychologists, and speech pathologists and is easily administered at bedside, in the office, or in the laboratory.

NEUROPSYCHOLOGICAL TREATMENT

There are no neuropsychological approaches to the treatment of the aprosodias. Speech therapists treat deficits in production and imitation of affective prosody but generally do not address impaired affective facial expression and identification of affect in others. Treatment of affective prosody deficits consists primarily of providing the patient with feedback about the affective quality of his or her communications, modeling affective prosody, and providing an opportunity for the patient to practice vocalization. The use of recording devices may provide particularly effective feedback to the patient about his or her affective communication skills.

Computer-based pitch analyzers are being used with increasing frequency to aid in the assessment and treatment of prosodic deficits.[23,24] These devices can provide feedback to the patient on the variability of his or her voice and keep a record over time of increases in variability with training. However, pitch analyzers are not capable of distinguishing one affect from another and thus can give feedback only about the variability in prosody and not about whether the patient's voice is approaching a more qualitative goal (e.g., being able to sound angry when anger is felt).

Neuropsychologists play a role in treating the aprosodias, particularly those subtypes that involve a deficit in affect perception. Psychological principles can be used to design effective remediation programs. One approach might involve pairing pictures of people showing different emotions with one-word verbal labels describing the emotion. As the patient learns to associate the facial expression with the label, the latter can be reduced one letter at a time until the patient can identify the expression without the label. For example, an angry expression would be paired with the word "ANGRY," a surprised expression with the word "SURPRISE," and so forth for several different emotional expressions. After several trials, the angry expression would appear with the label "ANGR_" and the surprised expression with the label "SURPRIS_." This should be enough to cue the patient that angry and surprised expressions are being shown. Additional letters are removed over time from each picture. If the patient's rate of correct responding drops, letters can be added to the labels until performance is again at an acceptable level. Over many trials, the patient should progress to the point where he or she can identify the facial expressions without verbal cues. Deficits in emotional prosody could similarly be approached by pairing emotional vocal statements with verbal labels and gradually fading the labels.

An alternative approach might involve teaching the patient to pay attention to discrete facial movements that are reliably associated with different emotional expressions. Several facial movement coding systems that relate facial movements to emotional expressions are available.[25,26] Simplified portions of these systems could be taught to patients, who could use them as compensatory aids when attempting to identify an emotional expression.

Approaches such as the ones described previously are not currently in use. This is clearly an area that needs exploration by and attention from rehabilitation neuropsychologists. Such programs may prove useful in dealing with aprosodic patients in occupations that place an emphasis on social and emotional communication.

CASE ILLUSTRATION

CASE 14–1

J.G. was a 30-year-old man who worked as a trial attorney.[13] Following the onset of seizures, he was diagnosed with a right frontal anaplastic astrocytoma in 1981. The tumor was removed in 1986 when the seizures were no longer controllable with medication. A magnetic resonance imaging scan obtained before surgery revealed that the tumor lay in the posterior and superior right frontal lobe. The bulk of the tumor was removed in two sections, which measured 3 by 2.5 by 1 cm and 3 by 1.5 by 0.4 cm. Tissue was also removed from the margins of the tumor in three aggregates, ranging from 3.5 by 2.5 by 1 cm to 1 by 0.5 by 0.2 cm. Following surgery, the patient was admitted to a rehabilitation facility.

In the initial examination, J.G. had a left hemiparesis that was worse in the upper extremity, mild lower left facial weakness, and a normal sensory examination. Neuropsychological examination revealed a 35-point discrepancy in his Verbal (113) and Performance (78) Intelligence Quotients from the Wechsler Adult Intelligence Scale–Revised; Full Scale IQ was 96. He was able to make spatially accurate copies of line drawings and was normal in his ability to make fine visual discriminations. The patient showed deficits in recall of verbal information. He scored within normal limits on tests of word fluency, problem-solving, and cognitive regulation of movement. Motor coordination and speed ranged from normal to mildly impaired in the right hand, whereas the left hand was too impaired for testing as a result of hemiparesis. The Minnesota Multiphasic Personality Inventory revealed little significant emotional pathology. The only elevation occurred on a scale sensitive to somatic complaints. The somatic complaints reported by J.G. included muscle twitching, poor balance, and poor general physical health, all of which were attributable to his neurologic status.

J.G.'s spontaneous speech was a monotone, and he showed little variability in facial expression, even when discussing his illness. Both J.G. and his relatives detected the change in his emotional expression, and it was of concern to him because he made his living as a litigator and depended on his ability to evoke emotional responses in juries during opening and summation speeches. To illustrate the change in his affective communication, J.G. obtained a videotape depicting him at a party 1 month prior to his surgery. In the videotape, J.G. had a full range of

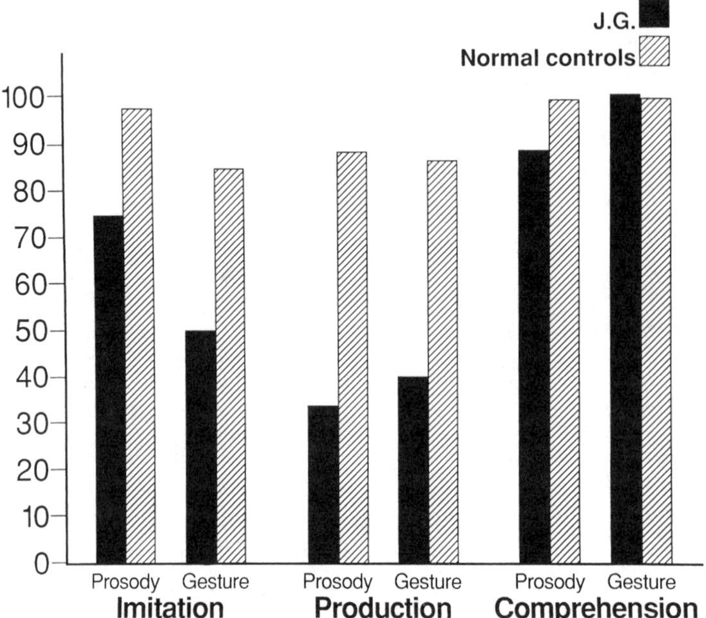

FIGURE 14–1. Affective Communication Test results for patient J.G. and a normal comparison group. (From Stringer and Hodnett,[13] p. 95, with permission.)

emotional expression, in stark contrast to his current wooden-appearing facial expressions and mechanical-sounding voice.

The ACT was administered to J.G. 7 months postsurgery. He obtained a perfect score on the phonation and articulation screening portion of the test and performed normally on items requiring him to make simple facial movements (e.g., pursing the lips, opening and closing the mouth, protruding and retracting the tongue, biting, blowing, and sniffing). However, he was markedly clumsy when asked to attempt complex facial movements (e.g., simultaneously knitting the brow, wrinkling the nose, and showing the teeth).

The results of the affective portion of the ACT are shown in Figure 14–1 for J.G. and a comparison group of men without brain damage ranging in age from 21 to 40 years (average, 33.1 years). These data represent the average of separate ratings made by two examiners. The results suggest that J.G.'s comprehension of affective prosody and facial gestures was comparable to that of the normal subjects. He had mild difficulty in imitating affective prosody but performed far below the normal subjects in his ability to produce affective prosody on demand. Both imitation and production of affective facial gestures were poor, although he performed slightly better when imitating a model.

DISCUSSION

J.G. showed a reduction in affective prosody and gesture done spontaneously and on demand, whereas imitation and perception of prosody and gesture were preserved. He showed no signs of depression, and his phonation and articulation were intact. His facial movements were not akinetic. The patient did show lower left facial weakness, but he was able to perform basic facial movements, showing difficulty only with complex, multistep movements. The clinical data suggest a diagnosis of transcortical motor aprosodia secondary to surgical removal of an astrocytoma in the posterior-superior right frontal lobe. A notable difference was found in the severity of the patient's deficits in prosody and gesture, along with a slight divergence in the pattern of deficits (e.g., both imitation and production of gesture were impaired, whereas only production of prosody was impaired). As discussed previously, a dissociation in the severity of prosodic and gestural deficits is common in aprosodic patients.

REFERENCES

1. Monrad-Krohn, GH: Dysprosody or altered "melody of language." Brain 70:405, 1947.
2. Blumstein, S, and Goodglass, H: The perception of stress as a semantic cue in aphasia. J Speech Hear Res 15:800, 1972.
3. Danly, M, Cooper, WE, and Shapiro, B: Fundamental frequency, language processing, and linguistic structure in Wernicke's aphasia. Brain Lang 19:1, 1983.
4. Danly, M, and Shapiro, B: Speech prosody in Broca's aphasia. Brain Lang 16:171, 1982.
5. Heilman, KM, et al: The comprehension of emotional and nonemotional prosody. Neurology (Suppl 2) 33:241, 1983.
6. Weintraub, S, Mesulam, MM, and Kramer, L: Disturbances in prosody. Arch Neurol 38:742, 1981.
7. Ross, ED, and Mesulam, MM: Dominant language functions of the right hemisphere? Prosody and emotional gesturing. Arch Neurol 36:144, 1979.
8. Ross, ED: The aprosodias. Functional-anatomic organization of the affective components of language in the right hemisphere. Arch Neurol 38:561, 1981.
9. Ross, ED, Anderson, B, and Morgan-Fisher, A: Crossed aprosodia in strongly dextral patients. Arch Neurol 46:206, 1989.
10. Ross, ED: Modulation of affect and nonverbal communication by the right hemisphere. In Mesulam, MM (ed): Principles of Behavioral Neurology. FA Davis, Philadelphia, 1985, p 239.
11. Ross, ED: Prosody and brain lateralization: Fact vs. fancy or is it all just semantics? Arch Neurol 45:338, 1988.
12. Ross, ED, et al: How the brain integrates affective and propositional language into a unified behavioral function. Hypothesis based on clinico-anatomic evidence. Arch Neurol 38:745, 1981.
13. Stringer, AY, and Hodnett, C: Transcortical motor aprosodia: Functional and anatomical correlates. Arch Clin Neuropsychol 6:89, 1991.
14. Weintraub, S, Mesulam, MM, and Kramer, L: Disturbances in prosody. A right-hemisphere contribution to language. Arch Neurol 38:742, 1981.
15. Wolfe, GI, and Ross, ED: Sensory aprosodia with left hemiparesis from subcortical infarction: Right hemisphere analogue of sensory-type aphasia with right hemiparesis? Arch Neurol 44:668, 1987.
16. American Psychiatric Association: Diagnostic and Statistical Manual of Mental Disorders, Fourth Edition. American Psychiatric Association, Washington, DC, 1994.
17. The International Classification of Diseases, Ninth Revision, Clinical Modification. Med-Index Publications, Salt Lake City, 1991.
18. Gorelick, PB, and Ross, ED: The aprosodias: Further functional-anatomic evidence for the organization of affective language in the right hemisphere. J Neurol Neurosurg Psychiatry 50:553, 1987.
19. Rosenthal, R, et al: Sensitivity to Nonverbal Communication: The PONS Test. Johns Hopkins University Press, Baltimore, 1979.
20. Rosenthal, R, and Benowitz, LI: Sensitivity to nonverbal communication in normal, psychiatric, and brain-damaged samples. In Blanck, PD, Buch, R, and Rosenthal, R (eds): Nonverbal Communication in the Clinical Context. Pennsylvania State University Press, University Park, PA, 1986.
21. Benowitz, LI, et al: Hemispheric specialization in nonverbal communication. Cortex 19:5, 1983.
22. Egan, G, et al: Assessment of emotional perception in right and left hemisphere stroke patients: A validation study. J Clin Exp Neuropsychol 12:51, 1990.

23. Ross, ED, et al: Acoustic analysis of affective prosody during right-sided Wada test: A within-subjects verification of the right hemisphere's role in language. Brain Lang 33:128, 1988.
24. Shapiro, B, and Danly, M: The role of the right hemisphere in the control of speech prosody in propositional and affective contexts. Brain Lang 25:19, 1985.
25. Ekman, P, and Friesen, WV: Unmasking the Face. Prentice-Hall, Englewood Cliffs, NJ, 1975.
26. Izard, CE: The Maximally Discriminative Facial Movement Coding System (Max). Instructional Resources Center, University of Delaware, Newark, DE, 1979.

CALCULATION DISORDERS (ACALCULIA)

15

The calculation disorders involve an impairment in the ability to perform operations using numbers. The modern subtyping of acalculia is based on the work of Hécaen and his colleagues in France.[1] Hécaen divides acalculia into four subtypes:

1. Number alexia (called *alexic acalculia* in this text)
2. Number agraphia (called *agraphic acalculia* in this text)
3. Spatial acalculia
4. Anarithmetria

The first three subtypes of acalculia involve noncomputational deficits that nonetheless impair the ability to calculate. Only the final subtype, anarithmetria, involves a deficit in performing arithmetic operations.

Whether alexic, agraphic, and spatial acalculia are disorders specific to numbers is debatable. Alexic acalculia may result from a general reading deficit that includes numbers (see Alexia). Similarly, agraphic acalculia may be a subtype of agraphia (see Chap. 13), and spatial acalculia may be a subtype of constructional disability (see Chap. 7).

The clinical association between acalculia and disorders of reading, writing, and visual-motor integration is undeniable. Yet the association is never 100 percent in large clinical series.[2] Thus, it is possible to be alexic or agraphic for numbers but not for letters and words and to have spatial acalculia without having constructional disability. For this reason, it seems justifiable to classify alexic, agraphic, and spatial acalculia as disorders specific to numbers, yet recognizing that in practice, related reading, writing, and constructional disorders are present and may contribute to the calculation deficit.

NOMENCLATURE

The term *acalculia* is common in the neurology and neuropsychology literature. DSM-IV[3] includes the diagnosis "Mathematics Disorder," which may be used to code acalculia. ICD-9-CM[4] includes acquired acalculia under the diagnosis "Other Symbolic Dysfunction." This diagnostic code can be used for the disorders discussed in this chapter, although the DSM-IV code is preferable because of its specificity.

VARIETY OF PRESENTATION

1. Alexic acalculia (also called "number alexia")

Clinical Indicators

a. Inaccurate reading of numbers or arithmetic signs as indicated by any of the following errors:
   1) Individual digits are incorrectly read aloud (e.g., "3" read as "five")
   2) Misinterpretation of the position of individual digits in multidigit numbers when reading aloud (e.g., "1003" read as "one hundred and three")
   3) Arithmetic signs incorrectly read aloud (e.g., "+" read as "multiplication sign")

RULES FOR DIAGNOSIS

Clinical Indicators: Each is independent (only one must be observed for the disorder to be suspected) *except* when subscripting is used. Subscripted numbers (a_1, a_2) denote an indicator with multiple parts that must be considered together.
Associated Features: These are listed to give a more complete picture of the disorder. The presence or absence of these features does not affect the diagnosis.
Factors to Rule Out: All must be taken into account. Failure to rule out even one of these factors makes a firm diagnosis impossible.
Lesion Locations: Each location stands alone; damage in only one of the listed areas is sufficient to produce the disorder.

4) No response or "I don't know" when asked to read numbers or arithmetic signs
5) Incorrect matching of spoken and written numbers
6) Incorrect matching of spoken and written arithmetic signs

b. Inability to comprehend the meaning of numbers or arithmetic signs as indicated by any of the following errors:
1) Inaccurate matching of written numbers and actual physical quantities
2) Errors on written calculation problems that would be correct responses if the arithmetic signs were different (e.g., when asked to calculate the answer to the written problem "$3 \times 4 =$," the patient responds "seven")

Associated Features

a. Impaired oral language (see Chap. 12)
b. Impaired written language (see Chap. 13)
c. Impaired ability to write numbers (see Agraphic acalculia)
d. Impaired ability to perform skilled movements on demand (see Apraxia)
e. Loss of acuity in one (usually the right) visual half-field (homonymous hemianopsia)
f. Decreased tactile sensation on one (usually the right) side of the body
g. Impaired ability to draw or to construct puzzles (see Constructional disability)
h. Confusion of the right and left sides of the body, of space, or both (see Right-left disorientation)
i. Impaired recognition of the fingers (see Finger agnosia)
NOTE: When acalculia, impaired written language (agraphia), right-left disorientation, and finger agnosia occur together in the same patient, the entire complex is referred to as Gerstmann's syndrome.

Factors to Rule Out

a. Oral language impairment sufficient to account for the deficit in reading numbers and arithmetic signs
b. Loss of visual acuity so severe that numbers and arithmetic signs cannot be perceived regardless of where they are presented in the visual field
c. Failure to detect portions of visual stimuli as a result of stimulus neglect (see Chap. 4)
d. Impaired speech articulation as a result of weakness or poor coordination of the speech muscles (dysarthria or anarthria) sufficient to preclude intelligible oral reading of numbers and arithmetic signs
e. Impaired ability to perform skilled movements of the mouth and speech muscles on demand (see Buccofacial apraxia) sufficient to preclude intelligible oral reading of numbers and arithmetic signs
f. A premorbid history of impaired ability to read numbers and arithmetic signs as a result of limited education or learning disability

Lesion Locations

a. Parietal lobe, alone or with extension to the frontal, temporal, and occipital lobes[5–7]
b. Junction of the temporal and occipital lobes[7]

Lesion Lateralization

a. May follow left- or right-hemisphere lesions, but more frequent and severe following left-sided lesions[8]

2. **Agraphic acalculia (also called "number agraphia")**

Clinical Indicators

a. Complete absence of graphic output when attempting to write numbers on demand or to dictation
b. No recognizable digits produced when attempting to write numbers on demand or to dictation
c. Production of recognizable but graphically distorted digits when attempting to write numbers on demand or to dictation
d. Production of recognizable but incorrect digits when attempting to write numbers on demand or to dictation (e.g., writes digits out of sequence or writes digits different from the ones requested or dictated)

Associated Features

a. Relatively preserved copying of digits
b. Impaired oral language (see Chap. 12)
c. Impaired written language (see Chap. 13)
d. Impaired ability to read numbers or arithmetic signs (see Alexic acalculia)
e. Impaired ability to perform skilled movements on demand (see Apraxia)
f. Loss of acuity in one (usually the right) visual half-field (homonymous hemianopsia)
g. Decreased tactile sensation on one (usually the right) side of the body
h. Impaired ability to draw or construct two- and three-dimensional puzzles (see Constructional disability)
i. Confusion of the right and left sides of the body, of space, or both (see Right-left disorientation)
j. Impaired recognition of the fingers (see Finger agnosia)
NOTE: When acalculia, impaired written language (agraphia), right-left disorientation, and finger agnosia occur together in the same patient, the entire complex is referred to as Gerstmann's syndrome.

Factors to Rule Out

a. Weakness of the muscles of the arm or hand sufficient to account for the writing deficit
b. Impaired coordination of the muscles of the arm or hand sufficient to account for the writing deficit
c. Impaired ability to initiate arm or hand movements (see Akinesia) sufficient to account for the writing deficit
d. Impaired ability to persist with ongoing arm or hand movements (see Motor impersistence) sufficient to account for the writing deficit
e. Impaired ability to terminate ongoing arm or hand movements (see Motor perseveration) sufficient to account for the writing deficit

f. Impaired ability to perform the movements involved in writing on demand (see Apraxic agraphia) sufficient to account for the writing deficit
g. Impaired ability to guide the hand perceptually during writing (see Constructional agraphia) sufficient to account for the writing deficit
h. The presence of oral language impairment (see Aphasic alexia-agraphia) sufficient to account for the writing deficit
i. A premorbid history of poor number writing as a result of limited education or learning disability

Lesion Locations

a. Parietal lobe, alone or with extension to the frontal, temporal, and occipital lobes[5,6]
b. Combined basal ganglia (caudate and putamen), anterior limb of internal capsule, and periventricular white matter[9]

Lesion Lateralization

a. May follow left- or right-hemisphere lesions, but more frequent and severe following left-sided lesions[8]

3. Spatial acalculia

Clinical Indicators

a. Incorrect vertical alignment of number columns on paper prior to attempting to solve a dictated or horizontally written calculation problem. For example, when shown or dictated the problem "4582.64 + 17.9126 = ," the patient writes:

    4582.64
    + 17.9126

b. Horizontal or vertical rotation of individual digits when copying, transcribing, or writing numbers on demand
c. Incorrect spacing between digits in multidigit numbers when copying, transcribing, or writing numbers upon demand (e.g., "one thousand sixty-six" written as "10 66")
d. Transposition of digits in multidigit numbers (e.g., "sixty-one" written as "16")

Associated Features

a. Calculations that are incorrectly done on paper as a result of the previously described errors possibly done correctly orally
b. Impaired ability to draw or construct two- and three-dimensional puzzles (see Constructional disability)
c. Confusion of the right and left sides of the body, of space, or both (see Right-left disorientation)
d. Loss of acuity in one (usually the right) visual half-field (homonymous hemianopsia)
e. Failure to detect portions of visual stimuli as a result of stimulus neglect (see Chap. 4)
f. Impaired matching and discrimination of visual stimuli (see Visual form imperception)

g. Inaccurate judgment of the orientation in space of visual stimuli (see Spatial disorientation)
h. Failure to dress one side of the body (see Dressing apraxia)
i. Decreased global intellectual functioning (see Global intellectual decline)
j. Impaired oral language, particularly Wernicke's aphasia (see Chap. 12)
k. Impaired written language (see Chap. 13)
l. Impaired recognition of the fingers (see Finger agnosia)
NOTE: When acalculia, impaired written language (agraphia), right-left disorientation, and finger agnosia occur together in the same patient, the entire complex is referred to as Gerstmann's syndrome.

Factors to Rule Out

a. Inability to write recognizable numbers as a result of any of the following disorders:
    1) Agraphic acalculia
    2) Weakness of the muscles of the arm or hand
    3) Impaired coordination of the muscles of the arm or hand
    4) Impaired ability to initiate arm or hand movements (see Akinesia)
    5) Impaired ability to persist with ongoing arm or hand movements (see Motor impersistence)
    6) Impaired ability to terminate ongoing arm or hand movements (see Motor perseveration)
    7) Impaired ability to perform movements involved in writing on demand (see Apraxic agraphia)
    8) Oral language impairment (see Aphasic alexia-agraphia)
b. Incorrect vertical alignment of number columns as a result of a failure to detect portions of multidigit numbers (see Stimulus neglect)
c. Failure to learn the correct vertical alignment, orientation, spacing, or column position (e.g., tens column, hundreds column) of numbers as a result of limited education or learning disability

Lesion Locations

a. Parietal lobe[10]
b. Thalamus[11]

Lesion Lateralization

a. May follow left- or right-hemisphere lesions, but more frequent and severe following right-sided lesions[8]

4. Anarithmetria

Clinical Indicators

a. Inaccurate solution of oral addition, subtraction, multiplication, or division problems
b. Inaccurate solution of written addition, subtraction, multiplication, or division problems

Associated Features

a. Combined deficits in written and oral calculation, although the severity of deficits in each modality may differ
b. Impaired oral language (see Chap. 12)

c. Impaired written language (see Chap. 13)
d. Loss of acuity in one (usually the right) visual half-field (homonymous hemianopsia)
e. Decreased tactile sensation on one (usually the right) side of the body, of space, or both
f. Impaired ability to draw or construct two- and three-dimensional puzzles (see Constructional disability)
g. Confusion of the right and left sides of the body, of space, or both (see Right-left disorientation)
h. Impaired recognition of the fingers (see Finger agnosia)
   NOTE: When acalculia, impaired written language (agraphia), right-left disorientation, and finger agnosia occur together in the same patient, the entire complex is referred to as Gerstmann's syndrome.
i. Decreased global intellectual functioning (see Global intellectual decline)

Factors to Rule Out

a. Impaired ability to read numbers and arithmetic signs (see Alexic acalculia) during written calculation
b. Incorrect vertical alignment, orientation, spacing, or column positioning of numbers (see Spatial acalculia) during written calculation
c. Impaired ability to sustain concentration sufficient to account for the deficit in calculation (see Chap. 3 for assessment techniques)
d. A reduction in the amount of information that can be concentrated on sufficient to account for the deficit in calculation (see Chap. 3 for assessment techniques)
e. A reduction in the ability to divide concentration between two or more tasks (see Chap. 3 for assessment techniques)
f. The presence of oral language impairment (see Chap. 12) sufficient to impede performance of calculations
g. Impaired speech articulation as a result of weakness or poor coordination of the speech muscles (dysarthria or anarthria) sufficient to preclude intelligible responses during oral calculation
h. Impaired ability to perform skilled movements of the mouth and speech muscles on demand (see Buccofacial apraxia) sufficient to preclude intelligible responses during oral calculation
i. Loss of visual acuity so severe that numbers and arithmetic signs cannot be perceived regardless of where they are presented in the visual field during written calculation
j. Failure to detect portions of written stimuli as a result of stimulus neglect (see Chap. 4), which may manifest itself during written calculation as a failure to perceive number columns or as a failure to carry or borrow numbers to or from adjacent columns
k. Inability to write recognizable numbers during written calculation as a result of any of the following disorders:
   1) Agraphic acalculia
   2) Weakness of the muscles of the arm or hand
   3) Impaired coordination of the muscles of the arm or hand

4) Impaired ability to initiate arm or hand movements (see Akinesia)
5) Impaired ability to persist with ongoing arm or hand movements (see Motor impersistence)
6) Impaired ability to terminate ongoing arm or hand movements (see Motor perseveration)
7) Impaired ability to perform movements involved in writing on demand (see Apraxic agraphia)
8) Oral language impairment (see Aphasic alexia-agraphia)

l. Premorbid failure to learn the principles of addition, subtraction, multiplication, division, or all of these as a result of limited education or learning disability

Lesion Locations

a. Parietal lobe, alone or with extension to the frontal, temporal, and occipital lobes[5,6,12–16]
b. Combined basal ganglia (caudate, putamen, or lenticular nucleus) and anterior limb of external capsule, with frequent extension to periventricular white matter and external capsule[9,17]
c. Periventricular white matter[17]
d. Thalamus, alone or with the anterior or posterior limb of the internal capsule, with frequent extension to the periventricular white matter[11,17]
e. Insula, with frequent extension to external capsule, basal ganglia (lenticular nucleus), and periventricular white matter[17]

Lesion Lateralization

a. May follow left- or right-hemisphere lesions, but more frequent and severe following left-sided lesions[8]

ETIOLOGY

Acalculia can appear in any neurological condition capable of producing hemispheric damage. Cerebrovascular disease, particularly that involving the middle cerebral artery, and traumatic brain injury are the most common causes. Neoplasm, demyelinating disease, and degenerative disease can also result in acalculia.

DISABLING CONSEQUENCES

The ability to read and write numbers is as important in daily life as the ability to read and write words. Patients with alexic and agraphic acalculia have difficulty telling time from digital clocks, locating addresses, finding a particular office in a building, looking up a phone number, reading a bus schedule, and performing a myriad of other daily tasks. All forms of acalculia can impair a person's ability to manage finances independently. Pricing merchandise, summing the prices of items before purchase, calculating change, writing checks, balancing a checking account, and filling out or verifying information on tax forms may all be compromised.

Functioning in Western society requires frequent interaction with technology, and an important means of interacting with technology is through numbers. The automatic teller machine, the oven, the telephone, thermostat, the speedometer, the television set, and the computer all require reading, interpreting, and selecting numbers. These skills become even more critical for individuals in occupations that emphasize the use of numbers and mathematics; the number of such occupations is staggering. From the landscaper who must measure the size of flower beds before deciding what to plant to the anesthesiologist whose calculations may determine life or death, few people are able to function in the workplace without coming in contact with numbers.

ASSESSMENT INSTRUMENTS

Boston Spatial-Quantitative Battery, Calculation Subtest

The Boston Spatial-Quantitative Battery (BSQB; formerly the Boston Parietal Lobe Battery)[18] is *not commercially available.*

The test can be constructed from information provided in the test manual.[18] Patients are asked to solve progressively more difficult problems in addition, subtraction, multiplication, and division. They are also asked to draw hour and minute hands set to specified times on blank and prenumbered clock face drawings. Reliability coefficients are not reported for the BSQB. Normative data are available on 147 neurologically normal men stratified by age (25 to 85 years) and education.[19] Factor analysis of the BSQB revealed that the calculation subtest loaded on a spatial-quantitative factor.[18]

Careful qualitative analysis of calculation subtest results is required to determine what specific subtypes of acalculia are present in a given patient. Consequently, the test should be interpreted only by neuropsychologists, behavioral neurologists, and speech pathologists experienced in the diagnosis of acalculia. The subtest is most easily administered in office and laboratory settings, although bedside administration is possible.

Western Aphasia Battery

See discussion of this test in Chapter 12.

Halstead-Reitan Battery Aphasia Screening Test

See discussion of this test in Chapter 12.

Wechsler Adult Intelligence Scale–Revised, Arithmetic Subtest

See discussion of this test in Chapter 19.

Wechsler Adult Intelligence Scale–Revised as a Neuropsychological Instrument, Arithmetic Subtest

See discussion of this test in Chapter 19.

NEUROPSYCHOLOGICAL TREATMENT

Retraining patients to read numbers is largely a function of practice and repetition. If reading of words is preserved, then the number symbol can be paired with its written name to facilitate recognition of the symbol. The patient should be able to perform without error when the written name accompanies the number. At this point, the written name can be reduced one letter at a time, beginning with the final letter in the name. Thus, the patient would be presented with "1 – on_," and "2 – tw_." This should be a sufficient cue for the patient to continue to achieve a high level of accuracy. When the patient responds incorrectly, the missing letter can be shown. Once the patient is accurate in responding, an additional letter can be removed to provide a greater challenge. If errors occur, letters can be added to the name until the patient can again correctly identify the number symbol. In this manner, over a long series of trials, the patient may again come to recognize the number symbols without cues. The task is then to train the patient to recognize the same numbers in different contexts and situations.

Performance in patients with agraphic acalculia may be improved with practice in copying numbers. Again, lengthy repetition is likely to be required to produce any improvement in performance. Treatment of spatial acalculia can be approached in a similar manner, but if perceptual deficits also are present, the patient may make little progress. To perform successfully, the patient may need to trace directly over the target number. To increase the difficulty of the task, the end points of each line in the number symbol can be shown without the lines filled in. For example, "7" might be shown as:

•   •

•

The patient is then asked to connect the dots in the order pointed to by the examiner to produce the desired number.

Anarithmetria is most readily approached by encouraging the patient to use a calculator. "Fingermath,"[20] a technique for doing rapid calculations with the fingers, has been taught to some learning-disabled and mentally retarded populations, and may be of use in patients with acquired brain damage. All basic arithmetic operations can be done using fingermath, and the technique works even for long series of calculations involving multidigit numbers. I am not aware of any published accounts of the use of fingermath with adult patients with brain damage, but the technique deserves exploration.

The patient's attitude is an important factor in all of these treatments. Unfortunately, calculation tasks can evoke anxiety even in healthy, well-educated individuals. This reaction is likely to be even worse in neurological patients who are all too aware of their limitations with numbers. Getting the patient to relax, and perhaps to view the calculation exercises as a challenging game, can be critical preliminary steps in improving performance with numbers.

CASE ILLUSTRATIONS

CASE 15–1

W.B. was an 80-year-old woman with a doctorate in education who had worked as a professor of music at a university until her retirement at 65 years of age. At age 79 years, she suffered a left middle cerebral artery embolic cerebrovascular accident. A large left parietal lobe infarction was visible on her computed tomography scan. W.B. had a history of atrial fibrillation, which was the probable source of the embolus. Her initial neuropsychological examination, conducted 5 months after her infarction, revealed decreased intellectual functioning represented by a Full Scale IQ of 69 on the WAIS-R. Notably, W.B. scored two standard deviations below the average of people in the 70- to 74-year-old age group, the oldest group for which norms are available, on the arithmetic subtest of the WAIS-R.

The WAB was administered, with results consistent with the presence of a borderline-to-mild Wernicke's aphasia (see Chap. 12). On the calculation section of the WAB, the patient obtained 18 of a possible 24 points. All addition and subtraction problems were performed correctly. Her errors occurred on multiplication and division problems, in which she appeared to misinterpret the arithmetic symbol. For example, when presented with the following problems:

$$\begin{array}{r} 4 \\ \underline{\times\ 2} \end{array} \quad \text{and} \quad \begin{array}{r} 18 \\ \underline{\div\ 3} \end{array}$$

she chose "6" and "21" as the correct answers, suggesting that she added the numbers. She accurately interpreted the arithmetical symbols to multiply 6 by 7 and divide 64 by 8. Overall, W.B. was correct on only one half of the multiplication and division problems because of symbol misinterpretation.

When asked to write the numbers 0 through 20, W.B. wrote only "22." When writing numbers in response to dictation, she was correct on only two trials. All of her errors involved the substitution of incorrect digits for the numbers dictated (e.g., she wrote "300" when "700" was dictated). In no instance were her digits illegible, distorted, rotated, or poorly spaced. No errors were made on the WAB trials requiring W.B. to point to numbers spoken by the examiner.

DISCUSSION

The patient in Case 15–1 exhibited alexic acalculia confined to arithmetical symbols. She was able to read numbers well enough to select the number spoken by the examiner from a larger series of choices. Although some degree of language impairment was present, it is not so severe as to preclude testing of numerical ability. W.B. comprehended test instructions and was able to communicate her ideas through speech. She had no difficulty seeing the test stimuli and had progressed far enough in school to be familiar with arithmetical signs.

W.B. also showed agraphic acalculia when attempting to write numbers on command or to dictation. Lack of education is not a compelling explanation for these deficits, because the patient held a doctorate. She demonstrated that she had the motor capacity to write digits because her number agraphia manifested itself simply as the production of digits different from those dictated.

Despite problems with reading arithmetical signs and writing numbers, W.B. did well on oral calculation tasks. The few errors she made were attributable to incorrect interpretation of the arithmetical signs.

CASE 15–2

A.H. was a 68-year-old woman with a 10th-grade education who had worked as a nurse's aide until her retirement. Although she did not complete high school, she reported having been an average student who never failed any subjects. Her medical history was significant for diabetes, hypertension, and a left-hemisphere stroke 1 year before the current admission. She developed gangrene in a decubitus ulcer on her left leg, necessitating an above-knee amputation. She then underwent prosthesis training, which was complicated by her difficulty in learning new information.

A neuropsychological examination revealed that intellectual functioning was in the borderline range; she had a full scale IQ of 74 on the WAIS-R. A.H. was able to sustain concentration over long intervals without becoming distracted, but showed significant reductions in her forward and reversed digit span, suggesting the presence of concentration deficits. Portions of the Wechsler Memory Scale–Revised were administered and revealed moderate to severe dysmnesia (see Chap. 16). On the HRB-AST, the patient was impaired in her ability to do line drawings, to name pictures of geometric shapes, to read orally (including numbers), and to do computations. She failed all computation items regardless of whether they were performed mentally or with the aid of paper and pencil. A.H.'s speech was fluent and free of errors and she was able to comprehend and explain the sentence "He shouted the warning" from the AST.

To further assess calculation ability, sections of the WAB were administered. A.H. pointed to numbers named by the examiner without error. She was unable to write the numbers 0 to 20 on command, writing only "0" and then stopping, with no clear idea of what to do next. She was prompted to proceed with writing 1 to 20, but she produced no further numbers. She wrote correctly all but one number dictated by the examiner but was hesitant throughout. Her one error consisted of writing a "c" when "five" was dictated. The patient immediately recognized that this was incorrect, and with encouragement she was able to produce a "5."

When attempting the WAB calculation section, A.H. failed to interpret subtraction and multiplication signs correctly, although she correctly recited all the numbers presented. Whenever she made an error in reading the arithmetical sign, the patient was corrected to ensure that she understood what was to be done before attempting the calculation. A.H. obtained only 8 out of a possible 24 points, choosing an incorrect answer on virtually every subtraction, division, and multiplication problem.

The patient was questioned about how proficient she had been in mathematics during her life. She denied having difficulty with calculations in school. She reported that she had kept a checking account most of her adult life. A.H. reported having had trouble balancing her account since her stroke, and consequently no longer kept one. She denied having any trouble planning her finances or making change during grocery shopping when she was younger but reported that she now relied on family members to assist her in these areas.

DISCUSSION

Like the former patient, the patient in Case 15–2 also exhibited alexic acalculia confined to arithmetical symbols. She was able to read numbers well enough to select the number spoken by the examiner from a larger series of choices. Some inconsistency across tests was noted. She was unable to read correctly the stimulus "7 SIX 2" on the HRB-AST, but she did recite the numbers presented to her on the WAB calculation section. It is possible that the combination of numbers and words in the AST item confused her to the point that her performance declined.

Language impairment was again present, but it was not so severe as to preclude testing of numerical ability. The patient comprehended test instructions and was able to communicate her ideas through speech. A.H. had no difficulty seeing the test stimuli and had progressed far enough in school to be familiar with arithmetical signs.

A.H. also showed agraphic acalculia when attempting to write numbers on command. Unlike the patient in Case 15–1, she was able to write numbers specifically dictated to her. Lack of education is not a compelling explanation for these deficits, because A.H. had completed the 10th grade with no history of grade failure or problems specific to numbers. Motor problems cannot explain her deficit because she wrote well during dictation.

A.H. was significantly impaired in her calculations, suggesting an additional diagnosis of anarithmetria. The WAB calculation subtest does not require the patient to write or speak; therefore, motor problems, agraphic acalculia, and spatial acalculia do not complicate the interpretation of the test results. Lack of arithmetical knowledge does not appear to be a factor because of this patient's history of successfully managing her finances, making change when shopping, and balancing her checkbook. To mitigate the influence of her alexia for arithmetical signs, A.H. was asked to name the sign before beginning her calculation and was corrected when wrong. She did not show alexia for the numbers themselves. The fact that she correctly read each calculation problem aloud rules out the possibility that she failed to detect or attend to portions of the visual display.

Concentration deficits cannot be entirely eliminated as factors in A.H.'s performance on calculation tests. However, she was not distractible and was able to perform addition problems with fair accuracy. It seems unlikely that a concentration deficit would manifest itself solely on subtraction, multiplication, and division problems. Thus, a concentration disorder alone does not appear to account for her calculation problems. Anarithmetria is the most probable diagnosis.

REFERENCES

1. Hécaen, H, Angelergues, R, and Houillier, S: Les variétés cliniques des acalculies au cours des lésions rétrorolandiques: Approche statistique du probléme. Rev Neurol 105:85, 1961.
2. Levin, HS, and Spiers, PA: Acalculia. In Heilman, KM, and Valenstein, E (eds): Clinical Neuropsychology, Second Edition. Oxford University Press, New York, 1985, p 97.
3. American Psychiatric Association: Diagnostic and Statistical Manual of Mental Disorders, Fourth Edition. American Psychiatric Association, Washington, DC, 1994.
4. The International Classification of Diseases, Ninth Revision, Clinical Modification. Med-Index Publications, Salt Lake City, 1991.
5. Cipolotti, L, Butterworth, B, and Denes, G: A specific deficit for numbers in a case of dense acalculia. Brain 114:2619, 1991.
6. Dehaene, S, and Cohen, L: Two mental calculation systems: A case study of severe acalculia with preserved approximation. Neuropsychologia 29:1045, 1991.
7. Ferro, JM, and Silveira-Botelho, MA: Alexia for arithmetical signs. A cause of disturbed calculation. Cortex 16:175, 1980.
8. Roselli, M, and Ardila, A: Calculation deficits in patients with right and left hemisphere damage. Neuropsychologia 27:607, 1989.
9. Corbett, AJ, McCusker, EA, and Davidson, OR: Acalculia following a dominant-hemisphere subcortical infarct. Arch Neurol 43:964, 1986.
10. Chiarello, C, Knight, R, and Mandel, M: Aphasia in a prelingually deaf woman. Brain 105:29, 1982.
11. Bogousslavsky, J, Regli, F, and Assal, G: The syndrome of unilateral tuberothalamic artery territory infarction. Stroke 17:434, 1986.
12. Freedman, L, et al: Posterior cortical dementia with alexia: Neurobehavioural, MRI, and PET findings. J Neurol Neurosurg Psychiatry 54:443, 1991.
13. Matsuoka, H, et al: Impairment of parietal cortical functions associated with episodic prolonged spike-and-wave discharges. Epilepsia 27:432, 1986.
14. Marinkovic, SV, Kovacevic, MS, and Kostic, VS: The isolated occlusion of the angular gyri artery. A correlative neurological and anatomical study—case report. Stroke 15:366, 1984.
15. Miyazaki, S, et al: False aneurysm with subdural hematoma and symptomatic vasospasm following head injury. Surg Neurol 16:443, 1981.
16. Benson, DF, and Weir, WF: Acalculia: Acquired anarithmetria. Cortex 8:465, 1972.
17. Basso, A, Della-Sala, S, and Farabola, M: Aphasia arising from purely deep lesions. Cortex 23:29, 1987.
18. Goodglass, H, and Kaplan, E: The Assessment of Aphasia and Related Disorders, Second Edition. Lea & Febiger, Philadelphia, 1983.
19. Borod, J, Goodglass, H, and Kaplan, E: Normative data on the Boston Diagnostic Aphasia Examination, Parietal Lobe Battery and Boston Naming Test. J Clin Neuropsychol 2:209, 1980.
20. Lieberthal, EM: The Complete Book of Fingermath. McGraw-Hill, New York, 1979.

MEMORY DISORDERS (AMNESIA AND DYSMNESIA)

16

Amnesia is the inability to remember information that an individual can reasonably be expected to know. The information may be familiar and from the person's past, or it may be new information recently presented to the person. The memory deficit can be so severe that not only is the target information lost, but all recollection of having ever been exposed to the information is lost as well. In less severe cases, the patient's recollection may show only an absence of detail, which is recalled when a hint or cue is supplied. In these less severe cases, the term *dysmnesia* is used to describe the memory disorder.

Amnesia is highly variable in its presentation. The sources of this variability are described briefly.

1. **Age and education level.** In the absence of neurological disease, a decline in some aspects of memory occurs with advancing age. Age-related memory decline, often termed *benign senescent forgetfulness,* is easily confused with amnesia. The relationship between education and memory is opposite to the relationship between age and memory. Individuals with higher levels of education often perform better on memory tasks, and this can mask a mild degree of memory decline.

2. **Mood.** Depressed mood is associated with poorer memory performance and can be confused with amnesia. When depression and amnesia occur together, the amnesia can appear worse than it actually is.

3. **Information characteristics.** Patients may perform differently depending on the type of information they are asked to remember. This can occur even with seemingly similar types of information. For example, a list of unrelated words may not be remembered as well as a paragraph, despite the fact that both are verbal tasks and may contain the same number of words. This occurs because the meaningful relationship shared by words in a paragraph can make them easier to remember than an equivalent number of unrelated words in a list.

4. **Memory strategy.** The strategy taken by a patient can alter his or her memory performance. If a patient is better at remembering verbal information, he or she may approach nonverbal information with a verbal strategy. For example, abstract designs can be given a verbal label based on their similarity to concrete objects. The task for the patient then becomes one of remembering a verbal label rather than remembering an abstract design, and performance may improve correspondingly.

5. **Assessment methodology.** Patients have greater difficulty in recalling information than recognizing the information (i.e., distinguishing target from nontarget information) when it is again presented to them. Phonemic cues (e.g., the beginning sound of a target word) and semantic cues (e.g., the category in which a target word belongs) may aid recall. Allowing patients to rehearse information leads to better recall than when they are distracted or otherwise prevented from rehearsing. Assessing recall immediately after information presentation is likely to reveal less memory deficit than assessing recall after a delay of a few minutes or hours. Telling the patient in advance that memory of a piece of information will be tested can result in better recall than exposing the patient to the information without telling him or her that memory will be tested. Assessing changes in skill level as a result of practicing a task, regardless of whether the patient consciously recalls the practice,

may lead to a different conception of an amnesic patient's ability to learn. Skill level may advance even when conscious recall remains negligible.

6. **Underlying cognitive deficits.** Memory can fail for multiple reasons. Information may be learned incompletely because the patient failed to analyze the crucial features of the material. Some patients show an unusually rapid decay of information over time. In other patients, recall of older information may be impeded by more recently presented information. Alternatively, old information may interfere with learning new information in some patients. Memory may fail because the patient cannot generate a strategy for retrieving the target information. Controversy continues over which factor or factors underlie amnesia.

7. **Associated deficits.** The neurological diseases that lead to amnesia often lead simultaneously to other neuropsychological disorders. In some cases, these other disorders can additionally impede memory performance. For example, patients who simultaneously have mild Broca's aphasia (see Chap. 12) and amnesia are likely to perform worse on verbal memory tasks than patients who have amnesia alone. In other cases, memory functioning may be lowered not because the patient has amnesia but because another neuropsychological disorder is mimicking the effects of amnesia. For example, patients who are unable to draw because of constructional disability (see Chap. 7) do poorly on visuospatial memory tasks that require a graphic response. This may be misinterpreted as a visuospatial memory deficit. Assessing these patients' visuospatial memory with tasks that do not require drawing may lead to an entirely different conclusion about their memory capacity.

8. **Lesion location.** Lesions in different parts of the brain can produce different patterns of amnesia. The subtyping of amnesia in this text is based, in part, on these different patterns.

Amnesia and dysmnesia include various subtypes. *Retrograde amnesia* is an inability to remember information acquired prior to the onset of brain damage. *Anterograde amnesia* is a failure to remember information presented to the patient subsequent to the onset of brain damage. Some neuropsychologists do not consider these distinct phenomena because both types of memory loss are usually present in amnesic patients. However, stroke patients who do not lose consciousness during their stroke may show only anterograde dysmnesia, with no loss of information acquired before the onset of the brain lesion. Thus, at least in some stroke patients, anterograde and retrograde dysmnesia are dissociable.

In addition, anterograde and retrograde amnesia characteristically show different recovery patterns. Anterograde amnesia may be permanent, whereas a patient with retrograde amnesia that initially extends for weeks may recover to the point that only a few hours before the onset of the brain lesion are forgotten. The differences in presentation and recovery are the basis for separating anterograde and retrograde amnesia in this text.

Anterograde amnesia may be *global* in that it extends to virtually all types of information presented to the patient, or it may be specific to certain types of information. Neuropsychologists have principally been concerned with anterograde amnesia for *verbal* and *visuospatial* information. A few cases of anterograde *tactual-*

spatial and *nonverbal auditory amnesia* have also been reported; therefore, mention is made of these syndromes as putative memory disorders. Some neuropsychologists contend that anterograde and retrograde amnesia can be further divided into "bitemporal" and "diencephalic" subtypes.[1]

Bitemporal retrograde amnesia is limited to a few years preceding the lesion onset, whereas *diencephalic retrograde amnesia* may extend back for decades in a temporally graded fashion, such that older memories are better preserved than more recent memories. However, whether this extensive, temporally graded retrograde amnesia occurs depends on the etiology of the diencephalic lesion. The Wernicke-Korsakoff syndrome, which occurs in alcoholics and is associated with diencephalic and cortical lesions, produces an extensive, temporally graded retrograde amnesia. In contrast, one well-studied patient with trauma-induced unilateral diencephalic amnesia had only a limited retrograde amnesia.[2]

Bitemporal anterograde amnesia is characterized by a rapid rate of forgetting of new information. Patients with *diencephalic anterograde amnesia* show a normal rate of forgetting, but beyond this characteristic, the nature of their impairment is controversial. It has been suggested that their amnesia is produced by a failure to analyze information in sufficient detail. A variety of procedures have been used to test this hypothesis, with conflicting results.[3]

The diencephalic-bitemporal distinction is important. As the foregoing discussion suggests, however, a full understanding of the nature of the deficits produced by diencephalic and bitemporal lesions has yet to be achieved. Diencephalic and bitemporal amnesias are not listed as distinct subtypes in this text. The differences in deficits produced by lesions in these two areas, however, are noted in the lesion location sections of the retrograde and global anterograde amnesia subtypes.

Pseudoamnesia involves memory failure as a result of a psychological disorder (e.g., depression) or a deliberate attempt to fake or exaggerate memory deficits. Pseudoamnesia can coexist with amnesia as a result of brain damage or can occur alone. Pseudoamnesia should be ruled out whenever one of the other amnesias is suspected.

Reduplicative paramnesia is related to, and may accompany, amnesia. Patients with reduplicative paramnesia mislocate their surroundings. For example, they may be aware that they are in Detroit Receiving Hospital, but will nonetheless insist that Detroit Receiving Hospital is located somewhere other than Detroit. Although related to amnesia, reduplicative paramnesia has an element of delusional thinking. Consequently, reduplicative paramnesia is discussed with other ideational disorders in Chapter 18 (see Reduplication).

NOMENCLATURE

Memory and amnesia have long been a focus of psychological and neuroscientific research. The complex system of terminology that has grown from this research is far too extensive for review in this text. Appendix 16–1 lists and defines the major terms used by researchers and clinicians working in the area of memory and amnesia. As it is typically used, the term *amnesic syndrome* refers to severe and global memory impairment, which includes deficits in retrograde and anterograde memory. Verbal, visuospatial, tactual-spatial, and nonverbal auditory amnesias are sometimes collectively referred to as "material-specific," "modality-specific," or "sensory-specific" amnesias. Verbal anterograde amnesia is perhaps the least sensory specific, because verbal information can be presented aurally (e.g., reading the patient a list of words), visually (e.g., having the patient read a paragraph), or tactually (e.g., having the patient palpate a set of objects that can be identified by a verbal label). In most clinical examinations, however, verbal information is presented aurally.

DSM-IV[4] includes a single diagnostic label, "Amnestic Disorder Due to a General Medical Condition," for coding all subtypes of neurologically based amnesia. The additional label "Substance-Induced Persisting Amnestic Disorder" is provided for drug-induced amnesia that persists beyond the period of intoxication and withdrawal from the drug. Pseudoamnesia occurs in the context of the DSM-IV diagnoses of "Dissociative Amnesia," "Dissociative Identity Disorder," and as a part of "Dissociative Fugue." Cases of pseudoamnesia that involve deliberate feigning of memory loss to obtain a tangible goal can be classified as "Malingering" in DSM-IV. If the patient feigns amnesia for no reason other than to assume a sick role, then the amnesia can be coded as a "Factitious Disorder." The code for "Somatization Disorder" can be used if the amnesia is part of a broad spectrum of complaints having no apparent physiological basis.

ICD-9-CM[5] includes two additional diagnostic codes that allow for a slightly more precise differentiation of the amnesias. Retrograde amnesia is coded under "Other General Symptoms." This diagnostic code unfortunately includes many unrelated conditions such as chill and generalized pain. "Auditory Amnesia" is included under "Other Symbolic Dysfunction." However, in this context, "auditory amnesia" does not necessarily refer to a sensory-specific amnesia. Instead, the term *amnesia* is used as if it were synonymous with *agnosia*. In agnosia, stimulus recognition is impaired to such an extent that the patient can no longer determine the identity of certain classes of stimuli. When the term *amnesia* is restricted to auditory information, the problem lies not in recognizing the identity of stimuli, but in later remembering what specific stimuli were presented. Amnesia and agnosia are distinct in their clinical presentation and are listed separately in this text. It may one day be discovered, however, that these disorders are related and perhaps even belong on a continuum. Agnosia is discussed in Chapter 9.

VARIETY OF PRESENTATION

1. Retrograde amnesia

Clinical Indicators

a. Failure to remember information or events known or experienced before the presumed onset of a brain lesion
b. Absence of detail during remembrance of information or events known or experienced before the presumed onset of a brain lesion

RULES FOR DIAGNOSIS

Clinical Indicators: Each is independent (only one must be observed for the disorder to be suspected) *except* when subscripting is used. Subscripted numbers (a_1, a_2) denote an indicator with multiple parts that must be considered together.
Associated Features: These are listed to give a more complete picture of the disorder. The presence or absence of these features does not affect the diagnosis.
Factors to Rule Out: All must be taken into account. Failure to rule out even one of these factors makes a firm diagnosis impossible.
Lesion Locations: Each location stands alone; damage in only one of the listed areas is sufficient to produce the disorder.

c. Inaccuracy or distortion in memory of information or events known or experienced before the presumed onset of a brain lesion

Associated Features

a. Amnesia possibly extending back anywhere from minutes to decades
b. Memory of information or events learned or experienced closer to the onset of the brain lesion possibly worse than memory of information or events more remote in time
c. Memory of information or events may be progressively better the farther back in time they were learned or experienced (*temporally graded retrograde amnesia*)
d. Retrograde amnesia possibly extending to routes known before the onset of brain damage (*retrograde topographical amnesia*) (see Topographical agnosia)
e. Filling of gaps in memory by seemingly concocted events or by events that actually occurred at another time (see Confabulation)
f. Amnesia transient or permanent
g. Shrinkage of the time period of the amnesia with recovery from the brain lesion, so that only events immediately preceding the lesion onset are poorly remembered
h. Impaired memory for information and events presented or experienced since the presumed onset of the brain lesion (see the Anterograde amnesias)
i. Inaccurate knowledge of personal information, location, time, situation, or all of these (see Ideational disorientation or confusion)
j. Global intellectual decline (see Chap. 19)

Factors to Rule Out

a. Memory performance consistent with age and education
b. Normal decline in memory of previously learned or experienced information or events with the passing of time

c. Use of prescribed or recreational drugs that temporarily lower memory performance (drugs that the patient is taking should be checked for memory-related side effects in a current *Physician's Desk Reference*)[6]
d. Deliberate or psychologically motivated forgetting of previously known or experienced information or events (see Pseudoamnesia)
e. Depressed mood or major depressive disorder sufficient to account for the memory impairment (see Chap. 18 for assessment techniques)
f. Failure to have previously learned or experienced the information used to test memory

Lesion Locations

a. Medial and inferior temporal lobe,* particularly the hippocampus and parahippocampal gyrus[7–15]
b. Septal-hippocampal pathway, including the posterior cingulate bundle, the longitudinal striae, and the fornix, with extension to the corpus callosum, thalamus, and parietal lobe[10,16]
c. Basal forebrain, including the nuclei of the diagonal band of Broca, the septal nuclei, the nucleus accumbens, and the substantia innominata[17,18]
d. Diencephalon,† particularly the dorsomedial thalamic nucleus, mammillary bodies, and/or the mammilothalamic tract, with occasional extension to additional thalamic nuclei[19–27]
e. Retrosplenial cortex (i.e., the most posterior part of the cingulate gyrus), with extension to the subjacent white matter (cingulate bundle), the splenium of the corpus callosum, and possibly the fornix[28,29]
f. Parietal lobe[30]

Lesion Lateralization

a. Most commonly reported following bilateral or left-sided lesions, but this may be an artifact of the common use of verbal stimuli to assess retrograde amnesia

2. Global anterograde amnesia

Clinical Indicators

a_1. Impaired remembrance of information or events presented or experienced after the presumed onset of a brain lesion, as evidenced by any of the following signs:
   1) Failure to remember the information or events
   2) Absence of detail in the remembrance of the information or events
   3) Inaccuracy or distortion in memory of the information or events

a_2. Deficit extending to verbal and nonverbal (e.g., nonverbal auditory, visuospatial, tactual-spatial) information

---

*The retrograde amnesia that occurs following temporal lobe lesions typically extends back a maximum of a few years and is a component of the syndrome termed *bitemporal amnesia.*

†The retrograde amnesia seen following diencephalic lesions may extend back for decades in a temporally graded manner such that more remote events are recalled better than more recent events. Temporally graded retrograde amnesia is a component of the syndrome termed *diencephalic amnesia.*

Associated Features

a. Unaided, free recall of information usually worse than recognition of the information when it is presented again
b. Poorer performance when a delay is introduced between information presentation and memory testing
c. Poorer performance when rehearsal is prevented in the interval between information presentation and memory testing
d. Presence of a recency effect (see Appendix 16–1)
e. Presence of semantic intrusions (see Appendix 16–1) when attempting to remember verbal information
f. Unintended intrusion of incorrect but visually similar shapes when attempting to remember visuospatial information
g. Failure to spontaneously cluster, categorize, or otherwise make use of semantic meaning when attempting to learn or remember new verbal information
h. Failure to benefit from semantic cues (see cued recall in Appendix 16–1) provided to aid memory of verbal information
i. Greater than normal proactive interference (see Appendix 16–1)
j. Failure to release from proactive interference (see Appendix 16–1) during attempts to remember verbal information
k. Filling of gaps in memory by seemingly concocted events or events that actually occurred at another time (see Confabulation)
l. Relatively preserved procedural learning (see Appendix 16–1)
m. Presence of a normal priming effect (see Appendix 16–1)
n. Relatively preserved immediate recall of information sufficiently limited in amount that it does not exceed the span of concentration (see Appendix 16–1)
o. Transient or permanent amnesia
   NOTE: The term transient global amnesia is used to refer to global anterograde amnesia of brief duration (i.e., longer than 15 minutes, but shorter than 48 hours).
p. Impaired memory for information or events known or experienced before the presumed onset of a brain lesion (see Retrograde amnesia)
q. Inaccurate knowledge of personal information, location, time, situation, or all of these (see Ideational disorientation or confusion)
r. The belief that familiar people have been replaced by impostors (see Reduplication)
s. Mislocation of geographical surroundings (see Reduplication)
t. Global intellectual decline (see Chap. 19)

Factors to Rule Out

a. Memory performance appropriate for age and education
b. Normal decline in memory of previously learned or experienced events with the passing of time
c. Use of prescribed or recreational drugs that temporarily lower memory performance (drugs that the patient is taking should be checked for memory-related side effects in a current *Physician's Desk Reference*)[6]

d. Deliberate or psychologically motivated forgetting of information or events (see Pseudoamnesia)
e. Failure to concentrate when information is presented or events occur (see Chap. 3)
f. Oral or written language disorder (see Chaps. 12 and 13) sufficient to account for a deficit in remembrance of verbal information
g. Impaired perception of nonverbal stimuli (see Stimulus imperception) sufficient to account for a deficit in remembrance of nonverbal information
h. Impaired perception of spatial relations (see Spatial imperception) sufficient to account for a deficit in remembrance of nonverbal information
i. Unilateral failure to remember nonverbal information as a result of hemispatial neglect (see Chap. 4)
j. Impaired ability to draw (see Constructional disability) sufficient to account for impaired performance on nonverbal memory tasks that require a graphic response
k. Impaired sensation in the sensory modalities in which information is presented sufficient to account for the memory deficits

Lesion Locations

For transient global amnesia

a. Medial and inferior temporal lobe, particularly the hippocampus, the parahippocampal gyrus, or both[7,8,12–15,31–39]
b. Frontal lobe, including the combined superior frontal gyrus, inferior frontal gyrus, and gyrus rectus involvement disconnecting basal forebrain and hippocampus[40]
c. Occipital lobe, with occasional extension to the parietal lobe[39]
d. Thalamus[39,41]
e. Anterior corpus callosum[36]
f. Diffuse atrophy with focal involvement of the basal ganglia or internal capsule[36,41]

For chronic global anterograde amnesia

a. Medial and inferior temporal lobe,* particularly the amygdala, hippocampus, parahippocampal gyrus, the temporal stem, or a combination of these, sometimes with extension to the occipital lobe[13–15,42–48]
b. Basal forebrain, including the nuclei of the diagonal band of Broca, the septal nuclei, the nucleus accumbens, and the substantia innominata[12,17,18,49,50]
c. Diencephalon,† particularly the dorsomedial thalamic nucleus, mammillary bodies, the mammilothalamic tract, or a combination of these, with occa-

*The anterograde amnesia that follows unilateral and bilateral temporal lobe lesions (the latter is termed *bitemporal amnesia*) is characterized by a more rapid rate of forgetting compared to normal persons and compared to amnesic patients who have diencephalic lesions.

†The anterograde amnesia that follows unilateral and bilateral diencephalic lesions *(diencephalic amnesia)* is characterized by a tendency to encode information by superficial surface features rather than at a deeper semantic level, a rate of forgetting comparable to what is seen in healthy individuals, and a tendency to confabulate (see Confabulation).

sional extension to additional thalamic nuclei and the midbrain tegmentum[12,19,20,22–25,27,43,51–54]

d. Combined parietal and occipital lobes*[55]
e. Frontal lobe, possibly as a result of basal forebrain involvement in some cases[56,57]*
f. Fornix[58]

Lesion Lateralization

a. Most commonly follows bilateral lesions, but has been noted following unilateral (left hemisphere more often than right) lesions

3. Verbal anterograde amnesia

Clinical Indicators

a_1. Impaired remembrance of verbal information presented after the presumed onset of a brain lesion, as evidenced by any of the following signs:
   1) Failure to remember the information
   2) Absence of detail in the remembrance of the information
   3) Inaccuracy or distortion in memory of the information

a_2. Relatively preserved remembrance of nonverbal (e.g., visuospatial, tactual-spatial, nonverbal auditory) information

Associated Features

a. Unaided, free recall of information usually worse than recognition of the information when it is presented again
b. Poorer performance when a delay is introduced between information presentation and memory testing
c. Poorer performance when rehearsal is prevented in the interval between information presentation and memory testing
d. Presence of a recency effect (see Appendix 16–1)
e. Presence of semantic intrusion errors (see Appendix 16–1)
f. Failure to spontaneously cluster, categorize, or otherwise make use of semantic meaning when attempting to learn or remember new verbal information
g. Failure to benefit from semantic cues (see Cued recall in Appendix 16–1) provided to aid memory of verbal information
h. Greater than normal proactive interference (see Appendix 16–1)
i. Relatively preserved immediate recall of information sufficiently limited in amount that it does not exceed the span of concentration (see Appendix 16–1)
j. Transient or permanent amnesia
k. Impaired memory of information or events known or experienced before the presumed onset of a brain lesion (see Retrograde amnesia)
l. Inaccurate knowledge of personal information, location, time, situation, or all of these (see Ideational disorientation or confusion)

---

*Patients with lesions in this area are more likely to show a mild to moderate memory impairment (dysmnesia) rather than a full amnesic syndrome.

m. A degree of reduction of memory for nonverbal (e.g., visuospatial, tactual-spatial, nonverbal auditory) information, despite the relative preservation of memory in these areas

Factors to Rule Out

a. Memory performance appropriate for age and education
b. Normal decline in memory of verbal information with the passing of time
c. Use of prescribed or recreational drugs that temporarily lower memory performance, ruled out by documenting preserved nonverbal memory, because drugs generally do not selectively impair verbal memory
d. Deliberate or psychologically motivated forgetting of verbal information (see Pseudoamnesia)
e. Failure to concentrate when verbal information is presented (see Chap. 3)
f. Oral or written language disorder (see Chaps. 12 and 13) sufficient to account for a deficit in remembrance of verbal information
g. Impaired sensation in the sensory modalities in which verbal information is presented sufficient to account for a deficit in verbal memory

Lesion Locations

a. Medial and inferior temporal lobe,* particularly the amygdala, hippocampus, parahippocampal gyrus, the temporal stem, or a combination of these, or the convex surface of the temporal lobe[9,10,48,57,59]
b. Diencephalon,† particularly the dorsomedial thalamic nucleus, mammillary bodies, mammilothalamic tract, or a combination of these, with occasional extension to additional thalamic nuclei[10,21,23,26,60,61]
c. Septal-hippocampal pathway, including the posterior cingulate bundle, the longitudinal striae, and the fornix, with extension to the corpus callosum, thalamus, and parietal lobe[10,16]
d. Retrosplenial cortex (i.e., most posterior part of the cingulate gyrus), with extension to the subjacent white matter (cingulate bundle), the splenium of the corpus callosum, and possibly the fornix[28,29,62]
e. Dorsolateral, orbital, or medial (including the cingulate gyrus) frontal lobe‡[63]
f. Parietal lobe[30]

Lesion Lateralization

a. Left hemisphere

---

*Verbal anterograde amnesia following temporal lobe lesions is characterized by a more rapid rate of forgetting of verbal information compared to normal persons and compared to patients with amnesia who have diencephalic lesions.

†Verbal anterograde amnesia following diencephalic lesions is characterized by a tendency to encode verbal information by superficial surface features rather than at a deeper semantic level and a rate of forgetting comparable to that seen in healthy individuals.

‡Patients with lesions in this area are more likely to show a mild to moderate verbal memory impairment (i.e., verbal dysmnesia) rather than a full amnesic syndrome.

4. Visuospatial anterograde amnesia (also called "visual amnesia")

Clinical Indicators

a_1. Impaired remembrance of visuospatial information presented after the presumed onset of a brain lesion as evidenced by any of the following signs:

1) Failure to remember the information
2) Absence of detail in the remembrance of the information
3) Inaccuracy or distortion in memory of the information

a_2. Relatively preserved remembrance of verbal, tactual-spatial, and nonverbal auditory information

Associated Features

a. Unaided, free recall of information usually worse than recognition of the information when it is presented again
b. Poorer performance when a delay is introduced between information presentation and memory testing
c. Poorer performance when rehearsal is prevented in the interval between information presentation and memory testing
d. Unintended intrusion of incorrect but visually similar shapes when attempting to remember visuospatial information
e. Relatively preserved procedural learning (see Appendix 16–1)
f. Presence of a normal priming effect (see Appendix 16–1)
g. Relatively preserved immediate recall of information sufficiently limited in amount that it does not exceed the span of concentration (see Appendix 16–1)
h. The anterograde amnesia possibly extending to routes presented after the onset of brain damage (*anterograde topographical amnesia;* see Topographical agnosia)
i. Transient or permanent amnesia
j. Impaired memory for information or events known or experienced before the presumed onset of a brain lesion (see Retrograde amnesia)
k. Inaccurate knowledge of personal information, location, time, situation, or all of these (see Ideational disorientation or confusion)
l. A degree of reduction of memory for verbal, tactual-spatial, or nonverbal auditory information, despite the relative preservation of memory in these areas

Factors to Rule Out

a. Memory performance appropriate for age and education
b. Normal decline in memory of visuospatial information with the passing of time
c. Use of prescribed or recreational drugs that temporarily lower memory performance, ruled out by documenting preserved memory for verbal, tactual-spatial, and nonverbal auditory information because drugs generally do not selectively impair visuospatial memory
d. Deliberate or psychologically motivated forgetting of visuospatial information (see Pseudoamnesia)

e. Failure to concentrate when visuospatial information is presented (see Chap. 3)
f. Impaired perception of visual stimuli (see Visual form and facial imperception) sufficient to account for a deficit in remembrance of visuospatial information
g. Impaired perception of spatial relations (see Spatial imperception) sufficient to account for a deficit in remembrance of visuospatial information
h. Unilateral failure to remember visual information as a result of hemispatial neglect (see Chap. 4)
i. Impaired ability to draw (see Constructional disability) sufficient to account for impaired performance on visuospatial memory tasks that require a graphic response
j. Loss of visual acuity sufficient to account for a deficit in remembrance of visuospatial information

Lesion Locations

a. Medial and inferior temporal lobe,* particularly the amygdala, hippocampus, parahippocampal gyrus, the temporal stem, or a combination of these, or the convex surface of the temporal lobe[48,59]
b. Diencephalon,† particularly the dorsomedial thalamic nucleus, the mammillothalamic tract, or both, with occasional extension to additional thalamic nuclei[23]
c. Combined fornix and anterior commissure[64]
d. Medial occipital lobe, including the inferior longitudinal fasciculus, with occasional extension to the parietal lobe[57,65]

Lesion Lateralization

a. Left- or right-hemisphere lesions, but more common following right-sided lesions
b. When a result of occipital lobe involvement, the lesion is likely to be bilateral[65]

5. Tactual-spatial anterograde amnesia‡

Clinical Indicators

a_1. Impaired remembrance of tactual-spatial information presented after the presumed onset of a brain lesion as evidenced by any of the following signs:
  1) Failure to remember the information
  2) Absence of detail in the remembrance of the information
  3) Inaccuracy or distortion in memory of the information

a_2. Relatively preserved remembrance of verbal, visuospatial, and nonverbal auditory information

---

*Visuospatial anterograde amnesia following temporal lobe lesions is characterized by a more rapid rate of forgetting of visuospatial information compared to normal persons and compared to amnesic patients who have diencephalic lesions.

†Visual anterograde amnesia following diencephalic lesions is characterized by a rate of forgetting of visual information comparable to that seen in healthy individuals.

‡This disorder must be considered putative because there are few cases reported in the literature.

Associated Features

a. Unilateral or bilateral tactual memory impairment
b. Loss of acuity in one visual half-field (homonymous hemianopsia)
c. Impaired ability to draw or to construct two- and three-dimensional puzzles (see Constructional disability)
d. A degree of reduction in memory of verbal, visuospatial, or nonverbal auditory information, despite the relative preservation of memory in these areas

Factors to Rule Out

a. Memory performance appropriate for age and education
b. Normal decline in memory of tactual-spatial information with the passing of time
c. Use of prescribed or recreational drugs that temporarily lower memory performance, ruled out by documenting preserved memory for verbal, visuospatial, and nonverbal auditory information because drugs generally do not selectively impair tactual-spatial memory
d. Deliberate or psychologically motivated forgetting of tactual-spatial information (see Pseudoamnesia)
e. Failure to concentrate when tactual-spatial information is presented (see Chap. 3)
f. Impaired perception of tactual stimuli (see Tactual form imperception) sufficient to account for a deficit in remembrance of tactual-spatial information
g. Impaired perception of spatial relations (see Spatial disorientation and Spatial inflexibility) sufficient to account for a deficit in remembrance of tactual-spatial information
h. Unilateral failure to remember tactual-spatial information as a result of hemispatial neglect (see Chap. 4)
i. Impaired ability to draw (see Constructional disability) sufficient to account for impaired performance on tactual-spatial memory tasks that require a graphic response
j. Loss of tactual sensation sufficient to account for a deficit in remembrance of tactual-spatial information

Lesion Locations

a. Medial occipital, medial temporal, and inferior temporal lobes, with occasional extension to the parietal lobe[66]

Lesion Lateralization

a. Unilateral left or right hemisphere
b. Tactile memory deficit occurring on the side of the body contralateral to the lesion

6. Nonverbal auditory anterograde amnesia*

Clinical Indicators

a_1. Impaired remembrance of nonverbal auditory (e.g., tonal) information pre-

*This disorder must be considered putative because there are few cases reported in the literature.

sented after the presumed onset of a brain lesion as evidenced by any of the following signs:
   1) Failure to remember the information
   2) Absence of detail in the remembrance of the information
   3) Inaccuracy or distortion in memory of the information

a_2. Relatively preserved remembrance of verbal, visuospatial, and tactual-spatial information

Associated Features

No information currently available

Factors to Rule Out

a. Memory performance appropriate for age and education
b. Normal decline in memory of nonverbal auditory information with the passing of time
c. Use of prescribed or recreational drugs that temporarily lower memory performance, ruled out by documenting preserved memory for verbal, visuospatial, or tactual-spatial information because drugs generally do not selectively impair nonverbal auditory memory
d. Deliberate or psychologically motivated forgetting of nonverbal auditory information (see Pseudoamnesia)
e. Failure to concentrate when nonverbal auditory information is presented (see Chap. 3)
f. Impaired perception of auditory stimuli (see Auditory pattern imperception) sufficient to account for a deficit in remembrance of nonverbal auditory information
g. Unilateral failure to remember nonverbal auditory information as a result of auditory sensory extinction (see Chap. 4)
h. Loss of auditory sensation sufficient to account for a deficit in remembrance of nonverbal auditory information

Lesion Locations

No information currently available

Lesion Lateralization

No information currently available

7. Pseudoamnesia (also called "pseudodementia")

Clinical Indicators

a_1. Unaccountably excessive memory impairment as evidenced by any of the following signs:
   1) Remembrance of less information than expected by chance alone
   2) Failure to remember overlearned information (see Appendix 16–1)
   3) Failure to remember information that is high in associative value (see Appendix 16–1)

a_2. Atypical pattern or course of the memory disorder as evidenced by any of the following signs:
   1) Absence of a clear precipitating illness or brain lesion

2) An unaccountable lag between illness or lesion onset and the onset of memory impairment
3) Severity of memory impairment exceeding known extent of the illness or brain lesion
4) Recognition of information when it is repeated worse than unaided free recall of the information
5) Severe loss of memory for events that occurred in the remote past (e.g., during childhood); memory for recent events relatively preserved
6) Loss of all personal memories from the past, including knowledge of personal identity
7) Memory loss limited to specific painful or otherwise unpleasant events from the past

a_3. Motivational factors contribute to the presence of memory impairment as evidenced by any of the following signs:
1) Failure to exert the effort required to learn new information
2) Forgetting specific events or information permitting avoidance of unpleasant consequences or responsibilities
3) Memory loss leading to, or expected to soon produce, emotional benefits or material compensation

Associated Features

a. Some degree of impaired memory for information or events as a result of neurological illness or a brain lesion
b. Depressed mood or major depressive disorder
c. Psychogenic amnesia: A mental disorder that manifests itself as a sudden inability to recall important personal information and that is not explainable by normal forgetting, drug use, or neurological disease
d. Multiple personality disorder: A mental disorder that manifests itself in the presence of two or more "personality states" within the same person, which alternately take control of the person's behavior
e. Psychogenic fugue: A mental disorder that manifests itself in sudden, unexpected travel, inability to recall the past, and assumption of a new identity and that is not attributable to neurological disease
f. Malingering: Deliberate feigning of symptoms to obtain a goal
g. Factitious disorder: A mental disorder characterized by the intentional feigning of symptoms as a result of a need to assume a sick role
h. Somatization disorder: A mental disorder characterized by a history of multiple physical complaints of uncertain etiology
i. Hysterical conversion disorder: A mental disorder characterized by the unconscious expression of mental and emotional conflicts and stress via physical symptoms

Factors to Rule Out

a. Use of prescribed or recreational drugs that temporarily lower memory performance (drugs that the patient is taking should be checked for memory-related side effects in a current *Physician's Desk Reference*)[6]

b. Neurological illness or a brain lesion of sufficient extent to account for the memory impairment, ruled out by documenting unaccountably excessive memory impairment and an atypical pattern or course of impairment

Lesion Locations

Not directly attributable to brain damage

ETIOLOGY

Dysmnesia may follow any pathological process that compromises hemispheric function, including cerebrovascular disease, traumatic brain injury, neoplasm, degenerative disease, demyelinating disease, and exposure to substances toxic to the brain. Transient dysmnesia may occur during metabolic compromise of the brain or electrolyte imbalance. Dysmnesia may also follow central nervous system infection.

Retrograde and global anterograde amnesia follow pathological conditions that produce diffuse brain damage or that specifically damage hippocampal, diencephalic, or basal forebrain areas. Prolonged anoxia not only diffusely affects the brain, but also differentially compromises the hippocampi because their vascular supply is not sufficiently dense to permit neuronal survival under conditions of oxygen deprivation. Some infectious agents, particularly herpes simplex, have a predilection for damaging the hippocampi. Bilateral occlusion of the posterior cerebral arteries can result in a so-called "amnesic stroke" by causing inferior medial temporal lobe ischemic infarctions. These infarctions can involve the fornix, mammillary bodies, and hippocampi. Contrastingly, paramedian artery infarction produces severe amnesia as a result of thalamic damage. Traumatic brain injury produces a high frequency of bilateral frontal and temporal pole damage, resulting in potentially severe anterograde amnesia and some degree of retrograde amnesia.

Amnesia can also be iatrogenic. Severe temporal lobe epilepsy that fails to respond to anticonvulsant medication may be treated by surgical removal of portions of the temporal lobe. When this is done bilaterally, which has become a rarely chosen surgical option, the result is permanent and severe global anterograde amnesia and some degree of retrograde amnesia, with the degree of amnesia related to the extent of hippocampal removal. A material-specific (verbal or visuospatial) anterograde amnesia results when the less radical option of performing a unilateral temporal lobectomy is chosen. In many cases of intractable temporal lobe epilepsy, bilateral temporal lobe damage and a degree of global dysmnesia exist prior to surgery. Unilateral temporal lobectomy in these patients may produce global anterograde amnesia, because the spared temporal lobe is already dysfunctional.

Chronic alcoholics typically show a degree of dysmnesia and have degenerative changes in a number of brain areas, including the area surrounding the third ventricle. Alcoholic patients who have Wernicke-Korsakoff syndrome also show periventricular damage but have additional notable degeneration in diencephalic areas, particularly in the dorsomedial thalamic nucleus and the mammillary bodies. This syndrome includes a period of acute agitation and confusion during which hallucinations are frequent. The acute phase gradually subsides, leaving a temporally graded retrograde amnesia that can extend back for decades and a severe and permanent global anterograde amnesia with marked confabulation. This syndrome is thought to result from a thiamine deficiency attributable to poor nutritional intake. A genetic deficiency in the body's ability to incorporate thiamine may also be involved in some cases of Wernicke-Korsakoff syndrome.

Basal forebrain areas are vulnerable to hemorrhages from anterior communicating artery aneurysms. The severity of the amnesia varies, and some potential for recovery exists in less severe cases.

Most patients with transient global amnesia also recover completely. This disorder is typically seen in patients who have a history of migraine headaches, cerebrovascular disease (including transient ischemic attacks and vertebrobasilar insufficiency), or seizure disorder. These amnesic episodes are often triggered by physical exertion.

DISABLING CONSEQUENCES

Patients who have moderate to severe amnesic disorders experience significant, if not total, disability. Retrograde amnesia, if it extends back for decades, can rob a patient of precious memories of family, friends, and important personal experiences. This affects not only the patient but also people in the patient's life, who may no longer be remembered by the patient. A devoted father (see Case 16–1) who developed a retrograde amnesia of several years' duration following bleeding of an anterior communicating artery aneurysm lost all memory of his young son, including cherished memories of being present at his son's birth. Although the patient was able to re-establish a relationship with his son, the entire family was deeply affected by the patient's initial failure to recognize and respond to the child.

If the retrograde amnesia extends to job-related skills and academic knowledge acquired at a specific point in time, then vocational disability will occur. More typically, the retrograde amnesia is limited in its extent, and the forgotten time period will shrink with the passage of time so that it does not pose a lasting problem in the patient's functioning. In those unfortunate cases when the amnesia does persist, vocational skills may be lost and relationships irrevocably sundered.

Transient global amnesia is disturbing to the patient and impairs vocational functioning for the period of time for which it lasts. The patient also needs constant supervision at home. After the episode has ended, there is usually no permanent disability.

Persistent moderate to severe global anterograde amnesia carries the greatest potential for disability. The patient may be completely unable to work, even when job-related skills are preserved. A teacher with global anterograde amnesia whom I treated was unable to remember students' names, could not recall where he was in the course of lectures, could not remember which assignments had been given, and could not get from the classroom to the teachers' lounge unaided, despite having fully intact knowledge of the subject matter of his courses. Remembering to attend irregularly scheduled meetings, to grade papers in the evening, or to pass on information to the principal was completely beyond the patient's capacity. Writing notes to remind himself of what he had to do failed to improve his performance because he invariably lost the notes or forgot to look at them.

Because most jobs require people to remember details that fluctuate and change from one day to the next, memory-impaired patients have great difficulty functioning in occupational settings. Only jobs that involve repetitive, rote activities, and in which supervision is available, are easily performed by severely amnesic individuals.

The disability experienced by amnesic patients also extends to the home. Amnesic patients often require supervision at home to avoid leaving stoves and other appliances turned on. When left alone, these patients may be at significant risk for accidental injury as a result of their forgetfulness. They may also need assistance in remembering to pay bills, keep appointments, and perform chores. These patients are often unable to assume responsibility for others who need care and supervision, including small children and elderly relatives.

The material-specific anterograde amnesias can be as disabling as global amnesia, particularly if it is verbal information that the patient has difficulty in remembering. Western society places great emphasis on verbal information, and many individuals use verbal strategies to enhance memory, even when the information to be learned is nonverbal (e.g., using verbal directions to remember a route). It may be easier for the patient to compensate for anterograde amnesia for nonverbal information. Verbal strategies can be used to encode and retrieve information. In other cases, presenting the information in another or multiple sensory channels (e.g., listening to a description of a visual stimulus while simultaneously viewing it) may facilitate later recall.

ASSESSMENT INSTRUMENTS

Wechsler Memory Scale–Revised

The Wechsler Memory Scale–Revised (WMS-R)[67] can be obtained from *The Psychological Corporation, P.O. Box 9954, San Antonio, TX 78204-2498.*

The WMS-R is one of the most widely used batteries of memory tests. It incorporates tests of verbal and visual paired associate learning, prose recall, design recall, and recognition of previously presented visuospatial information. Memory is assessed using both an immediate and a delayed recall format. Norms extend from age 16 to age 74 years, and the normative sample was selected to be representative of the U.S. population based on 1980 census data in age, gender, race, geographic residence, and education. Scores obtained from the WMS-R include individual subtest scores and composite verbal, visual, delayed, and general memory indexes.

Test-retest and internal consistency reliability coefficients for the WMS-R subtest and composite indexes reported in the test manual range from .41 to .90. The average reliability coefficients for immediate and delayed recall of the prose passages (i.e., Logical Memory I and II) are fairly high (.74 and .75, respectively), but the average coefficients for the other memory subtests tend to be low, ranging from .41 to .60. The average reliability coefficients of the composite indexes are higher, ranging from .70 to .90. Factor analyses of the WMS-R revealed a two-factor structure, the first reflecting general memory and learning, and the second reflecting attention and concentration. Subsequent factor analysis in a neuropsychological population revealed a three-factor structure, consisting of verbal memory, nonverbal memory, and attention, when delayed-recall WMS-R scores were included in the analysis.[68]

Various WMS-R summary indexes are reported in the manual to differentiate at a statistically significant level between normal persons and patients who have alcoholism, dementia, Huntington's disease, Wernicke-Korsakoff syndrome, traumatic brain injury, stroke, brain neoplasm, epilepsy, and multiple sclerosis. A subsequent investigation, which analyzed subtest differences in patients with lateralized lesions, demonstrated differences on verbal and visual memory subtests in the expected directions.[69] The WMS-R composite indexes are reported in the manual to show modest but statistically significant correlations with ratings of everyday memory functioning; all correlations were below −.38.

The advantages of the WMS-R include its extensive normative database, its inclusion of standard error of measurements for the composite indexes, and its inclusion of a table permitting the examiner to determine significant differences between composite indexes at two levels of statistical confidence. A table showing the mean and standard deviation of the indexes for three levels of education is also included. It would be helpful if standard error of measurement, significant difference, and education norm tables were included for the individual subtests. This is a serious flaw because of the importance of the subtest scores to most neuropsychologists. Additionally, the WMS-R does not yield the rich "process" scores that can be obtained from the California Verbal Learning Test and the Memory Assessment Scale (discussed later). In practice, many neuropsychologists administer only selected WMS-R subtests, most frequently the prose passages and designs. The provision of percentile ranks for these subtests increases the flexibility of the battery; the WMS-R lends itself to both comprehensive assessment and screening of selected memory functions.

The WMS-R is suitable for bedside, office, or laboratory use and should be interpreted only by individuals trained in cognitive assessment who have extensive experience with neurological populations.

Memory Assessment Scales

The Memory Assessment Scale (MAS)[70] can be obtained from *Psychological Assessment Resources, Incorporated, P.O. Box 998, Odessa, FL 33556.*

The MAS is a comprehensive battery of tests assessing memory for lists, prose, names and faces, and designs. The word list is presented until all 12 words are recalled, up to a maximum of 6 list presentations. Scores reflecting the patient's acquisition of information with repetition, spontaneous clustering of words by semantic category, tendency to intrude nonlist words during attempts to recall target words, immediate and delayed free recall, cued recall, and recognition of previously presented information can be derived from the list subtest.

The other MAS subtests yield immediate and delayed free-recall scores with two exceptions; both free and cued (using probe questions) recall of prose are assessed, and both free recall and recognition of previously presented designs are assessed. Summary scores reflect immediate recall of lists and prose (verbal memory score), immediate recall and recognition of designs (visual memory score), and global memory performance. Delayed recall measures do not enter into the summary scores. All subtests can be directly compared to each other because their raw scores are converted to the same scale.

The norms for the MAS are based on a sample of 843 adults, 467 of whom were matched to the U.S. population using census data projections for 1995 in gender and education for each age level. The norms extend from age 18 to older than 70 years. Generalizability coefficients for the MAS subtests ranging from .70 to .95 are reported in the test manual for a sample of 30 subjects tested twice over an interval of 6 months.

Factor analysis of the MAS immediate-memory scores in a neurological sample yielded a nonverbal memory factor, a short-term memory and concentration factor, and a verbal memory factor. Factor analysis of the delayed memory scores yielded a similar factor structure. The test manual reports that all MAS subtest and summary scores differentiate normal and neurological subjects at a statistically significant level ($p < .05$). Patients with left- and right-hemisphere lesions differed at a statistically significant level ($p < .05$) in the expected direction on the verbal memory summary score. These groups of patients also differed in the expected direction on the visual memory summary score, but the difference did not achieve statistical significance.

The MAS includes separate normative tables by age and by education and age level. Tables are also included that help the examiner to determine the standard error of measurement for each subtest and summary score, the degree of discrepancy between MAS subtests that must be attained for the difference to be significant at the .05 level of statistical confidence, and the minimum difference between IQ and the MAS global memory score necessary for significance at the .05 level. This combination of features makes the MAS one of the best available composite memory batteries.

In some circumstances, however, an examiner may wish to administer only selected tests to measure specific memory abilities. The format of the MAS makes this difficult. The subtests are designed to be administered in a set sequence and serve as distractors for each other. When a comprehensive and exhaustive assessment of memory is desired, the MAS is the instrument of choice, but this test is not appropriate for brief screening of selected aspects of memory performance.

The MAS may be interpreted by individuals trained in cognitive assessment and experienced in working with neurological populations. It is most appropriate for office and laboratory use, but may be administered at bedside if a flat surface is available.

Rivermead Behavioural Memory Test

The Rivermead Behavioural Memory Test (RBMT)[71] can be obtained from *Thames Valley Test Company, 7-9 The Green, Flempton, Bury St. Edmunds, Suffolk, IP28 6EL, England.*

The RBMT is designed to provide an ecologically valid measure of memory (i.e., a measure that correlates with memory performance in the everyday environment). The RBMT includes items that assess memory for names, faces, an appointment, object pictures, the location of a belonging, prose, and a route. Four parallel forms of the RBMT are available. Cut-off scores for the RBMT are based on a sample of 118 normal controls ranging in age from 16 to 69 years.

Inter-rater reliability was established by having two raters score 40 subjects. Agreement between raters is reported in the manual to be 100%. Parallel-form reliability coefficients in the manual range from .67 to .88. Correlations computed between the RBMT and other measures of memory range from .20 to .63, suggesting that it has moderate convergent validity (i.e., it converges moderately with other measures of memory). Because the RBMT is designed to measure everyday memory, the question of ecological validity is of particular importance. The test manual reports a correlation between RBMT scores and therapist observations of patients' memory lapses of −.71 to −.75. Correlations with subjective self-ratings of memory problems are lower but still are statistically significant.

The advantages of the RBMT include its demonstrated ecological validity, its brevity, and the availability of parallel forms, which make repeat testing possible with less concern about practice effects. This is a particular advantage in patients who need to be serially assessed to monitor changes in their memory performance. The manual reports no significant impact of age or education on RBMT performance across the 16- to 70-year age span of the standardization sample, which is an unusual property for a memory test.

The RBMT is reported to discriminate normal control from neurological samples at a statistically significant level ($p < .001$).[72] This conclusion, however, is based on a standardization sample that showed a ceiling effect on the RBMT and a rather severely impaired neurological sample. How well the RBMT detects subtle deficits in mildly to moderately impaired patient samples needs to be investigated further.

The RBMT is appropriate for bedside, office, or laboratory use. It can be interpreted by individuals who possess training and experience in cognitive assessment.

California Verbal Learning Test

The California Verbal Learning Test (CVLT)[73] can be obtained from *The Psychological Corporation, P.O. Box 9954, San Antonio, TX 78204-2498.*

The CVLT consists of a list of 16 words, designated the "Monday shopping list." The words are drawn from four semantic categories and are presented five times, with free recall assessed after each presentation. A second list of 16 different words, designated the "Tuesday shopping list," is then presented. Tuesday-list words are also from four semantic categories, two of which are the same as the categories used on the Monday list and two of which are new. A single free-recall trial is obtained after presentation of the Tuesday list. Free and cued (using semantic category) recall are then obtained for the Monday list. Following a 20-minute delay filled with nonverbal testing, free and cued recall of the Monday list are again obtained. Finally, a recognition trial is presented which is composed of 44 words, 16 from the Monday list, 16 from the Tuesday list, and the remainder from neither list. The "neither-list" words are drawn from the same semantic categories as the Monday-list words, are phonemically similar to the Monday-list words, or have no semantic or phonemic relation to the Monday-list words.

Although simple and relatively quick to administer, the CVLT is a highly complex, process-oriented test that yields over 250 scores that reflect various aspects of a patient's learning and memory. Most of these scores are too cumbersome to be calculated manually (an optional computerized administration and scoring program is available), and in practice, most neuropsychologists use only a subset of the scores in their clinical interpretation. Fortunately the most useful scores are easy to calculate manually, and the entire protocol can be scored within 5 to 10 minutes. Experienced examiners are able to calculate many of the scores while administering the test.

The test manual describes the CVLT scores in detail. Only a few of the more important scores are mentioned in this section to illustrate the wealth of data provided by this test. The free-recall scores from the Monday list (trial 1, trial 5, and total of trials 1 through 5) provide global measures of learning capacity. A number of learning process scores are also computed. The semantic-clustering score reflects the extent to which the patient grouped words by semantic category during free recall. The serial-cluster score reflects attempts by the patient to recall words in their order of presentation—an ineffective recall strategy. Primacy and recency effects can be detected by looking at the regions of the list from which words are recalled. The slope of the patient's learning curve reflects the extent to which the patient benefited from repetition of the list. The types of errors made by patients (e.g., perseveratively recalling the same words, intruding nonlist words during a recall trial) also provide information regarding the nature of the patient's memory deficit.

Comparing initial Monday-list and Tuesday-list recall trials permits detection of proactive interference (see Appendix 16–1). A release-from-proactive-interference procedure (see Appendix 16–1) is built into the test because the Tuesday list contains words from two semantic categories that are the same as those used in the Monday list and two semantic categories that are not included in the Monday list. Retroactive interference can be detected by comparing Monday-list trial-5 recall with Monday-list recall after the administration of the Tuesday list. The CVLT also includes scores reflecting both immediate and delayed recall and the ability to recognize previously presented words. When even recognition memory is poor, the types of false-positive errors made by the patient give precise information on what factor accounts for the impaired recognition performance.

The CVLT ranks as one of the best-designed and most useful measures of verbal anterograde memory. The CVLT is available in a research edition with norms based on 273 neurologically intact individuals. Separate norms are provided for men and women ranging in age from 17 to 80 years. Further normative study is under way on a sample representative of the U.S. population. Several methods of estimating the internal consistency of the CVLT are reported in the manual, with the resulting reliability coefficients ranging from .69 to .92. Test-retest reliability coefficients for 18 CVLT scores are reported and range from .12 to .79, with 13 of the coefficients significant at acceptable levels of statistical confidence.

The results of several factor analyses, reported in the test manual, of 19 CVLT scores yielded a stable, six-factor solution, with factors reflecting general verbal learning, response discrimination, learning strategy, proactive effect, serial position effect, and acquisition rate. These results suggest that the main CVLT scores measure relatively independent and theoretically meaningful aspects of learning and memory. Various CVLT scores are able to distinguish normal controls from samples of patients with alcoholism, Parkinson's disease, multiple sclerosis, Huntington's disease, and Alzheimer's disease at statistically significant levels.

The CVLT is the test of choice for measuring verbal anterograde memory. It is psychometrically sound and is firmly rooted in cognitive theory. It does not, however, provide the comprehensive assessment offered by the WMS-R or MAS (discussed earlier). When a comprehensive assessment is needed, the CVLT should be supplemented with other tests of memory. The complexity of the data yielded by the CVLT requires that it be interpreted only by individuals trained in cognitive assessment who are also experienced in the diagnosis of amnesia. The test is appropriate for bedside, office, or laboratory use.

Taylor Complex Figure, Revised Administration

The Taylor Complex Figure, Revised Administration,[74] is *not commercially available.*

The Taylor Complex Figure is an abstract design composed of multiple geometric elements (i.e., circles, squares, rectangles, triangles, and ovals) in addition to arrows, dots, a wavy line, and an asterisk. In the original administration of this test,[75] the patient copied the figure without being told to memorize it, then after the model was removed, was asked to reproduce the figure from memory. A delayed recall was then often obtained after 20 or 45 minutes. Use of the Taylor Complex Figure as a memory test has been criticized on a number of grounds, including the lack of control over stimulus exposure time during the copy trial, the uncertain reliability of the scoring system, and the lack of adequate norms.[74] The revised administration remedies these weaknesses and greatly enhances the value of the test as a measure of visuospatial memory.

In the revised administration, the patient is told that he or she is to memorize the Taylor Complex Figure, changing the test from an incidental to an intentional learning task. The figure is exposed to the patient for 30 seconds and then removed, and the patient is given 2 minutes to draw whatever he or she remembers. This procedure is repeated for a total of four acquisition trials, permitting the examiner to measure learning as a function of repeated stimulus presentation. After a 15-minute delay (in the normative study,[74] the delay interval was filled with paired associate learning and digit-span tasks), recall is tested again without benefit of further stimulus exposure. The Taylor Complex Figure is again presented to the patient, and the patient is given 5 minutes to copy the figure from the model. The copy trial helps control for the effects of perceptual, constructional, and motor deficits on memory test performance.

The revised scoring system[74] divides the Taylor Complex Figure into 23 components and assigns points based on explicit criteria. Normative data are based on 480 healthy volunteers varying in age from 20 to 79 years.[76] Age-related declines in acquisition, retention, and copying were documented, and normative data are reported by age decade, permitting the examiner to control for this variable when interpreting test performance. Gender and education were judged to be sufficiently independent of Taylor Complex Figure performance so that no correction for these factors appeared necessary in the normative tables.

Normal persons show a ceiling effect by acquisition trial 3, and the authors of the revised administration recommend basing test interpretation on the scores for trial 1, total acquisition, delayed recall and retention, and the copy trial.[74] Test results should be interpreted in a stepwise fashion:

1. The presence of an overall memory deficit should be documented using age norms.
2. The copy trial should be examined to determine whether a constructional deficit is present.
3. If a constructional deficit is documented, memory test scores should be transformed to "percent of copy scores" and compared to the appropriate normative table to see if a significant memory impairment remains after the effect of the constructional deficit is removed.
4. Patterns among the memory scores should be examined (e.g., the trial 1 and total acquisition scores compared, the trial 4 and delayed recall and retention scores compared) to determine the specific nature of the memory impairment. A table is available to facilitate trial 4–delayed recall and retention comparisons.[76] Generally, a drop of more than seven points during the delay interval is considered clinically significant.[74]

Inter-rater reliability coefficients are exceptionally high (.98 to .99)[74] as a result of the refinement of the scoring system. Internal consistency coefficients are also quite high, varying from .92 to .94.[74] Data on the validity of the revised administration for measuring memory in brain-damaged populations are not available.

The Taylor Complex Figure is appropriate for office and laboratory administration. Bedside administration may impede drawing unless the patient can be placed in a sitting position and has a hard surface on which to draw. It is recommended that interpretation of the test be attempted only by psychologists experienced in memory assessment and diagnosis, because the revised administration has not been fully validated for use in neurological populations.

Benton Visual Retention Test

The Benton Visual Retention Test (BVRT)[77] can be obtained from *The Psychological Corporation, P.O. Box 9954, San Antonio, TX 78204-0954.*

The BVRT attempts to measure visuospatial memory using a set of designs. Five alternate forms (C, D, E, F, and G) and five administration formats (A, B, C, D, and M) are available. Under administration A, each design is displayed for 10 seconds and then withdrawn, and the patients are asked to draw what they remember. Administration B is identical to A except that designs are displayed for 5 seconds. Administration C tests constructional ability by having patients draw the designs while they are displayed. In administration D, patients view each design for 10 seconds, wait 15 seconds, and then draw what they remember. Administration M, which is used only with forms F and G, tests visual recognition memory. Each design is exposed for 10 seconds and then withdrawn; then patients are asked to pick the design from a set of four.

Age and level of intelligence are correlated with BVRT performance, and consequently, both of these factors are controlled for in the normative tables presented in the test manual. The norms for administration A are based on more than 600 non-brain-damaged patients ranging in age from 15 to 69 years. Research suggests that administration B yields scores that are slightly lower than those yielded by administration A, and the test manual recommends using the norms for administration A minus 1 point for individuals up to age 60 years. No data are available on how to interpret administration-B scores in individuals older than age 60 years. Administration C is discussed in Chapter 7 with other tests of constructional ability. Normative data for administration D are limited, and this administration is not recommended for clinical use unless it is in conjunction with administration A. The test manual also includes data from several studies using the BVRT in samples of healthy individuals up to the age of 89 years. These data can guide interpretation of BVRT performance in individuals of advanced age. Administration M is not covered in the test manual.

Inter-rater reliability coefficients for the various administrations and scores derived from the BVRT are high, varying from .90 to .98.[77] Factor-analytic studies of administration A have found that the test loads on both memory and visual perception factors.[77] Studies reviewed in the test manual support the contention that the BVRT successfully differentiates patients with cerebral disease from nonneurological patients. The test is also reported to be useful in the early detection of dementia.

The BVRT is unquestionably a useful and well-established instrument. Its chief disadvantage is that it assesses only immediate recall of information. Even administration D employs only a 15-second delay before recall is tested. The importance of assessing delayed recall in amnesic patients is accepted by most researchers in the field of memory and amnesia. The BVRT, at best, provides a limited assessment of the factors of interest in amnesic populations.

The BVRT can be administered at bedside, in the office, or in the laboratory. Interpretation should be attempted only by individuals trained in the use of psychometric instruments and experienced in working with neurological populations.

Comprehensive Ability Battery, Auditory Ability Subtest

See discussion of this test in Chapter 5.

Boston Remote Memory Battery

The Boston Remote Memory Battery (BRMB)[78] is *not commercially available.*

The BRMB includes four tests. The first, the Facial Recognition Test, consists of 180 photographs of famous people from the 1920s to the 1970s, divided into six decades of approximately 25 photographs each. People whose fame endured across several decades are assigned to the decade in which they first gained public attention.

Photographs of 28 people whose fame endured at least 25 years are used in the second BRMB test, the Young-Old Test. The young photographs of these enduringly famous people are drawn from the Facial Recognition Test and are presented in a counterbalanced order with photographs of the same people taken later in life. The third test, the Recall Test, consists of 132 short-answer questions about public events and people from 1920 to 1975, with 24 questions per decade, excluding the 1970s, for which 12 questions are available. The content of this test does not overlap with any of the other BRMB tests. The fourth test, the Recognition Test, consists of 132 multiple-choice questions covering the same range of years, again, with content not overlapping with any other BRMB test.

Items on all of the BRMB tests are presented in a pseudorandom order to avoid cuing patients as to the organization of the tests. Items on three of the tests are also divided into "easy" and "hard" items based on a pilot study in a normal control sample. Easy items cover people and incidents of enduring fame, whereas hard items focus on people and incidents that gained only transient public attention. All tests are designed to produce flat retention curves across the decades in normal populations.

Tests of remote memory that utilize public events have several weaknesses. They require revision at least every 5 years, and items have been added to the original BRMB to update it.[79,80] It can never be known for certain that a patient learned about a public event at the time when the event occurred. Also, much of what a person knows about public events may be acquired years after the event occurred, particularly if the event is of lasting significance. Memory for events that a person learns about subsequent to their occurrence may be stronger than those learned at the time of occurrence, because the subsequent information reinforces what was learned during the initial exposure.

A relationship may exist between educational level and BRMB performance; individuals with more years of education may have had their initial exposure to a public event bolstered by subsequent reading or course work. The inclusion of easy and hard items in the BRMB partially addresses this problem. The content of hard items is more time-locked and is less likely to have been learned through subsequent secondary exposure. These items may better measure remote memory loss in well-educated individuals.

The BRMB has not been normed or validated on large, representative samples and is most useful for within-person comparisons (e.g., comparing what the same person can recall across several decades). The BRMB detects temporally graded retrograde amnesia in Wernicke-Korsakoff patients[78] and distinguishes them from amnesic populations in which temporal gradients in remote memory loss are not expected.[79,80]

The BRMB is appropriate for bedside, office, or laboratory administration. It is recommended for interpretation only by clinicians with extensive experience in the diagnosis of amnesia, because adequate normative guidelines are not available.

Memory for Personally Significant Events

The Memory for Personally Significant Events test is *not commercially available.*

This test is an informal procedure that I use to assess retrograde amnesia. A relative or close friend of the patient is interviewed to obtain a list of five to eight significant events experienced by the patient in the past few years. Events are obtained to cover the years to which retrograde amnesia is believed to extend plus 1 to 2 years further back. The informant must be able to recall the event in detail for it to be included. Holidays are often good markers to use in soliciting memories from the informant. Questions requiring an open-ended but content-specific response are developed from the information supplied by the informant. These questions are then presented to the patient, using first a free-recall and then a cued-recall format.

This procedure can systematically document the extent of retrograde amnesia in individual patients. It is appropriate for use in cases in which the retrograde amnesia extends back only a few days, weeks, months, or years. It is not practical in patients who have decades-long retrograde amnesia. Because the content of questions varies from case to case, standardization and norming of the procedure are not possible. The test's clinical validity is based on the fact that the patient's memory is being compared to that of the informant, who was presumably exposed to the same information as the patient. When the examiner has reason to believe the patient and informant had grossly different memory capacities before the onset of the patient's brain lesion, the procedure should not be used.

The Memory for Personally Significant Events procedure can be administered at bedside, in the office, or in a laboratory. It should be interpreted only by clinicians experienced in the diagnosis of amnesic disorders because of the absence of normative guidelines.

Autobiographical Memory Interview

The Autobiographical Memory Interview (AMI)[81] can be obtained from *Thames Valley Test Company, 7-9 The Green, Flempton, Bury St. Edmunds, Suffolk, IP28 6EL, England.*

The AMI provides a standardized test of retrograde amnesia based on patient's remote personal memories. The AMI consists of two parts: a "personal semantic schedule," which requires recall of facts from childhood, early adult life, and more recent times, and an "autobiographical incident schedule," which assesses the descriptive richness of memories for incidents from the same three periods of time. Cut-off scores are available from a sample of 34 healthy controls.

The test manual reports that age and estimated IQ are "uncorrelated" with AMI scores. However, given the small standardization sample, such a conclusion cannot be considered definite. A major weakness of the AMI is the failure to include even a cursory demographic description of the standardization sample in the test manual. A prior published account of the AMI[82] included a sample of normal controls ranging in age from 20 to 78 years, but this sample consisted of only 16 subjects. It is uncertain whether the previous sample was included in the standardization group reported in the test manual. Inter-rater reliability of the AMI is reported in the manual to vary from .83 to .86. The AMI is also reported to distinguish amnesic from healthy control subjects ($p < .001$) and to detect temporally graded retrograde amnesia in Wernicke-Korsakoff patients.

The AMI is an advance over other standardized tests of remote memory in that it is not dependent on the patient's attention to public events during the course of his or her life and does not have to be updated because of the passage of time. The AMI does, however, require more extensive validation. The test shows great promise, and the outcome of establishing better norms for this test is likely to be well worth the effort.

The limited normative and validity data on the AMI make interpretation of its results potentially perilous. Although it is appropriate for use by a broad range of clinicians, valid interpretation of the results depends on the extent of the examiner's experience with amnesic populations. The AMI is recommended for clinical use only by individuals with a solid understanding of amnesic disorder. It is appropriate for bedside, office, or laboratory administration.

University of Florida Level of Processing Procedure

The University of Florida Level of Processing Procedure is *not commercially available*.

Level of processing procedures have not been incorporated into standardized and normed memory batteries. They are most appropriate for use in detecting specific patterns of performance (i.e., a failure to encode based on the semantic features of a stimulus) in patients already diagnosed as amnesic. Documentation of specific patterns of performance can aid in localizing brain lesions. The University of Florida Level of Processing Procedure measures the efficiency of memory for words encoded based on visual, auditory, or semantic features.

Table 16–1 presents a set of stimuli for use in measuring level of processing in amnesic patients. The words in the second column are printed on index cards (one word per card) as they appear in the table. The words are shown one at a time, and the associated question in the third column is asked. Questions direct the patient's attention to the visual features of the word (upper- or lower-case letters), to the auditory features of the word (whether it rhymes with a stated word), or to the meaning of the word. Within each of the above three categories, the correct answer to the examiner's question is "yes" an equal number of times that it is "no."

Following a 10-minute delay, index cards with the words from Table 16–2 are presented (four words per card). The patient is asked to identify the word he or she saw during the previous question-and-answer trials. The target word is italicized in Table 16–2, but does not appear italicized in the multiple-choice cards shown to the patient. Table 16–2 also indicates the category each target word belongs to, based

Table 16–1. **UNIVERSITY OF FLORIDA LEVEL OF PROCESSING PROCEDURE: ACQUISITION TRIALS**

Trial	Word	Cue Question
1	CHURCH	Is this printed in upper-case letters?
2	leg	Is this part of the body?
3	stone	Does this rhyme with match?
4	beet	Is this a type of furniture?
5	bell	Does this rhyme with sell?
6	ice	Is this printed in upper-case letters?
7	moon	Is this printed in upper-case letters?
8	waltz	Is this a type of dance?
9	maid	Does this rhyme with fall?
10	toy	Does this rhyme with boy?
11	fox	Is this a type of flower?
12	SMOKE	Is this printed in upper-case letters?
13	steel	Is this a type of metal?
14	chair	Is this a type of animal?
15	cot	Does this rhyme with pot?
16	gun	Is this printed in upper-case letters?
17	fence	Does this rhyme with hour?
18	BARN	Is this printed in upper-case letters?
19	JAIL	Is this printed in upper-case letters?
20	sack	Does this rhyme with board?
21	axe	Is this a type of tool?
22	fly	Does this rhyme with cry?
23	daisy	Is this a type of flower?
24	pipe	Is this printed in upper-case letters?
25	cloud	Is this printed in upper-case letters?
26	plum	Is this a type of fruit?
27	beach	Does this rhyme with rug?
28	lad	Does this rhyme with fad?
29	flute	Is this a type of sport?
30	SALT	Is this printed in upper-case letters?
31	wind	Is this printed in upper-case letters?
32	hat	Is this a type of furniture?
33	toe	Does this rhyme with cab?
34	bread	Is this printed in upper-case letters?
35	deer	Is this a type of animal?
36	tire	Does this rhyme with wire?

Table 16–2. **UNIVERSITY OF FLORIDA LEVEL OF PROCESSING PROCEDURE: MULTIPLE-CHOICE RECOGNITION TRIALS**

Trial				
Trial 1: Semantic Category/Negative Cue Question Response				
	chair	coin	grass	nail
Trial 2: Visual Category/Positive Cue Question Response				
	clip	wood	*jail*	fern
Trial 3: Auditory Category/Negative Cue Question Response				
	globe	*stone*	clamp	scar
Trial 4: Auditory Category/Positive Cue Question Response				
	rug	haze	gift	*tire*
Trial 5: Visual Category/Negative Cue Question Response				
	cloud	foot	mast	sheet
Trial 6: Semantic Category/Positive Cue Question Response				
	tear	*waltz*	page	horse
Trial 7: Auditory Category/Positive Cue Question Response				
	toy	cream	oak	fear
Trial 8: Semantic Category/Negative Cue Question Response				
	path	coal	*hat*	tent
Trial 9: Semantic Category/Positive Cue Question Response				
	daisy	bat	ghost	lap
Trial 10: Visual Category/Positive Cue Question Response				
	moss	*church*	bed	cart
Trial 11: Auditory Category/Negative Cue Question Response				
	trout	egg	doll	*beach*
Trial 12: Visual Category/Negative Cue Question Response				
	string	paste	*gun*	cup
Trial 13: Visual Category/Negative Cue Question Response				
	band	cord	*bread*	tune
Trial 14: Semantic Category/Positive Cue Question Response				
	fur	*leg*	twig	mate
Trial 15: Auditory Category/Positive Cue Question Response				
	roll	chin	pork	*fly*
Trial 16: Semantic Category/Negative Cue Question Response				
	flute	key	steak	purple
Trial 17: Visual Category/Negative Cue Question Response				
	plot	*moon*	weed	cage
Trial 18: Auditory Category/Negative Cue Question Response				
	crumb	limb	*fence*	ash
Trial 19: Semantic Category/Positive Cue Question Response				
	wheel	lie	spade	*deer*
Trial 20: Visual Category/Positive Cue Question Response				
	pear	leaf	*barn*	knob
Trial 21: Visual Category/Negative Cue Question Response				
	pipe	roam	spear	art
Trial 22: Auditory Category/Positive Cue Question Response				
	bullet	*bell*	cat	oar
Trial 23: Semantic Category/Negative Cue Question Response				
	bone	pack	rock	*fox*

Table 16–2. **UNIVERSITY OF FLORIDA LEVEL OF PROCESSING PROCEDURE: MULTIPLE-CHOICE RECOGNITION TRIALS (*Continued*)**

Trial 24: Auditory Category/Negative Cue Question Response			
sack	grass	book	mire
Trial 25: Semantic Category/Positive Cue Question Response			
juice	rope	*steel*	acre
Trial 26: Semantic Category/Positive Cue Question Response			
silk	*axe*	fog	brass
Trial 27: Auditory Category/Negative Cue Question Response			
dog	lamp	wave	*toe*
Trial 28: Visual Category/Negative Cue Question Response			
ice	fad	gear	tan
Trial 29: Visual Category/Positive Cue Question Response			
salt	cop	prey	camp
Trial 30: Auditory Category/Positive Cue Question Response			
soap	pen	*cot*	chart
Trial 31: Auditory Category/Negative Cue Question Response			
float	*maid*	film	ant
Trial 32: Visual Category/Positive Cue Question Response			
paint	hinge	mute	*smoke*
Trial 33: Semantic Category/Negative Cue Question Response			
beet	ditch	surf	ache
Trial 34: Visual Category/Negative Cue Question Response			
horse	seam	ramp	*wind*
Trial 35: Auditory Category/Positive Cue Question Response			
floor	hen	steam	*lad*
Trial 36: Semantic Category/Positive Cue Question Response			
spark	*plum*	grip	site

on the question asked during the acquisition trials and whether the correct answer was affirmative or negative. A separate tally of correctly recognized words is made for words in each of the three categories. These tallies can be further subdivided based on whether the answer to the cue question was affirmative or negative.

The University of Florida Level of Processing Procedure is appropriate only for within-patient comparisons. It should not be used alone to diagnose the presence of amnesia.

This procedure is recommended for use only by clinicians with extensive experience in the diagnosis of amnesia. It can be administered at bedside, in the office, or in laboratory settings.

Release from Proactive Inhibition Procedure

The Release from Proactive Inhibition Procedure (RPI) is *not commercially available.*

Table 16–3 presents the words used for an RPI procedure that I use. Words listed for each trial are read to the patient at a rate of one every 2 to 3 seconds. The number listed in the table is then read, and the patient is asked to count backward from that number for 18 seconds. Patients who appear to be severely impaired in their concentration or calculation ability can be asked to count backward by one digit; less impaired patients should count backward by threes. After 18 seconds have elapsed, recall of the three words is requested.

Four blocks of five trials each are included in the procedure. Words in blocks A and C are from one semantic category (nonshift blocks). On trial 5 of blocks B and D, semantic category is shifted. A 5-minute delay during which no memory testing occurs is inserted between trial blocks. The number of words recalled on corresponding trials in blocks A and C are summed. Words recalled on corresponding trials in blocks B and D are also summed. This permits a comparison of performance from trials 1 through 5 broken across shift and nonshift trials.

If a patient is encoding words semantically, memory will worsen from trial 1 to trial 5 because of interference from words in the preceding trials. When semantic category shifts in trial 5, performance should improve to a level commensurate with performance during trial 1. Additionally, trial-5 performance should be superior in blocks in which a shift occurs compared with trial-5 performance in nonshift blocks.

The RPI procedure is appropriate for within-person comparisons, and the ob-

Table 16–3. **RELEASE FROM PROACTIVE INHIBITION STIMULI**

Block A (Nonshift)	***Block C (Nonshift)***
Trial 1: horse lion tiger 91	Trial 1: shirt pants blouse 267
Trial 2: bear mouse deer 147	Trial 2: shoes coat dress 45
Trial 3: sheep goat zebra 42	Trial 3: skirt hat tie 69
Trial 4: wolf donkey rabbit 66	Trial 4: jacket slacks gloves 54
Trial 5: mule bull moose 150	Trial 5: belt scarf vest 90
Block B (Shift)	***Block D (Shift)***
Trial 1: hammer saw nails 78	Trial 1: carrot pea beets 82
Trial 2: chisel ruler wrench 135	Trial 2: potato lettuce corn 51
Trial 3: pliers drill screws 49	Trial 3: celery tomato onions 190
Trial 4: sander wedge axe 96	Trial 4: turnip beans squash 75
Trial 5: camel lamb monkey 70	Trial 5: robe boots apron 48

tained data can be useful in localizing lesions in amnesic patients. This procedure should not be used alone to diagnose memory disorders but can be used in conjunction with other data on memory performance.

The RPI procedure is recommended for use only by clinicians with extensive experience in the diagnosis of amnesia. It can be administered at bedside, in the office, or in laboratory settings.

Rate of Forgetting Procedure

The Rate of Forgetting Procedure[83] is *not commercially available.*

In this test, patients view and are asked to remember 130 line drawings of common objects, presented one at a time for 4 seconds each. The drawings are from the larger set of 260 Snodgrass and Vanderwart pictures, available in the public domain, with norms for name agreement, image agreement, familiarity, and visual complexity.[84] Following a 90-second delay, eight randomly selected, previously seen drawings and eight new drawings are presented to test recognition memory for the previously seen drawings. If more than three false-positive or false-negative errors are made in the set of 16 test drawings, the entire set of 130 drawings is presented a second time, and the recognition test is performed again with a different random set of eight previously seen drawings and eight drawings that were not previously seen. The procedure must be repeated until the patient makes no more than three errors. Once this criterion is reached, it is assumed that the patient has learned all 130 pictures well enough to recognize them with the same error rate as in the recognition test. The validity of this assumption lies in the random selection of pictures for the recognition test.

Rate of forgetting is assessed at intervals of 10 minutes, 2 hours, and 48 hours; other time intervals may be used depending upon the examiner's needs. Each recognition test consists of 36 drawings from the previously presented set of 130, and 36 drawings that were not previously seen drawn from the remaining pool of unused Snodgrass and Vanderwart pictures. Care must be taken to select previously unseen drawings that match the 36 previously presented drawings on the dimensions deemed relevant by the individual examiner (e.g., stimulus complexity and imagery agreement[83]). The score obtained in each test interval is percent correct recognition (true-positives plus true-negatives).

The critical feature of the Rate of Forgetting Procedure is the establishment of an initial criterion level of memory performance, which serves as a baseline to which subsequent performance can be compared. This distinguishes the procedure from the common practice of looking at the percentage of information lost from immediate to delayed recall on memory tests that do not set an initial criterion level for the patient to reach. The absence of a criterion means that a patient who remembers 2 items of information immediately and 1 item after 30 minutes will have the same "rate of forgetting" as a patient who remembers 30 items of information immediately and 15 items after the delay. Because it is much easier to remember 2 items of information for 30 minutes than it is to remember 30 items for 30 minutes, it is unfair to characterize these two patients as having an equivalent rate of forgetting.

Helping severely amnesic patients attain an initial criterion level can be difficult and in some cases is impossible. This, combined with the large number of stimuli and the time required for testing, has made the use of the Rate of Forgetting Procedure uncommon outside laboratory settings. Normal rate of forgetting curves have not been established on large, representative samples of healthy individuals. The Rate of Forgetting Procedure is recommended only for research use and is appropriate mainly for laboratory settings.

Dichotomous Forced-Choice Symptom Validity Testing of Memory

The Dichotomous Forced-Choice Symptom Validity Testing of Memory[85] is *not commercially available.*

In the test, one of two stimuli is displayed and then removed from view. The patient is asked to count to 20 and then to identify which of the two stimuli he or she was shown. The same procedure is repeated 100 times, varying the stimulus shown such that each stimulus is presented 50 times. By chance, a patient will be correct on 50 percent of the trials. Patients who are attempting to fake memory deficits often perform at a level worse than chance. Giving the patient positive feedback on selected trials (e.g., "very good, that was correct again") increases the tendency to respond deliberately with the wrong choice. The probability that the number of errors on this task will exceed chance can be determined using the normal approximation to the binomial distribution.[86] Fifty-nine errors (41 correct) is significantly different from chance at the .05 level of statistical confidence, and 63 errors (37 correct) is significant at the .01 level.

In the original version of the test, the stimuli consisted of a black pen and a yellow pencil.[85] More recent versions (e.g., the Portland Digit Recognition Test) have used five-digit numbers to make the task appear more difficult to the malingerer.[87,88] In reality, any pair of stimuli can be used as long as the basic procedure is followed.

The forced-choice method of testing provides a powerful tool for detecting deliberate faking of memory deficits. The precise probability of making a given number of errors can be calculated, and the large number of trials administered makes it virtually impossible for a patient to keep track of the number of errors he or she has made. The malingerer, consequently, errs in the direction of making too many incorrect responses. In one instance, a suspected malingerer made far more errors than my secretary did taking the test with her eyes closed.

The forced-choice method can be administered at bedside, in the office, or in a laboratory. It is recommended for use only by physicians and psychologists because of the serious consequences to the patient of being labeled a malingerer. In any diagnostic decision, the possibility of clinician error exists. The advantage of a probability-based decision is that the likelihood that the clinician is in error is known.

Rey 15-Item Memory Test

The Rey 15-Item Memory Test[75] is *not commercially available.*

This test was designed to detect deliberate attempts to fake memory deficits. I have also found it useful for detecting reduced memory as a result of psychological factors (e.g., depression). The examiner stresses to the patient the difficulty of remembering 15 items before presenting the stimuli for the patient to view. The stimuli are actually very easy to remember, because they are overlearned sequences (e.g., the digits 1, 2, and 3) and are partially redundant (e.g., the first three letters of the alphabet written in upper and lower case). Clinical lore has established a cutoff score of 9 (or three of the five rows of stimuli), which has been supported by subsequent empirical investigation.[89,90] Although patients with brain damage score 9 or better on the test, some severely amnesic patients fall below the cutoff score and may potentially be misdiagnosed as malingerers.[91] In addition, the Rey 15-Item Memory Test does not always succeed in detecting malingerers.[92]

This test provides only one source of data about the factors influencing a given patient's memory performance, and no conclusions should be based solely on this test. The Rey 15-Item Memory Test alone cannot provide all the information needed to make a diagnosis of pseudoamnesia.

This test can be interpreted by physicians and psychologists who are experienced in the diagnosis of amnesic disorders. Others are cautioned about attempting to interpret the Rey 15-Item Memory Test because of the consequences to patients of an incorrect diagnosis of malingering. The test can be administered at bedside, in the office, or in a laboratory setting.

NEUROPSYCHOLOGICAL TREATMENT

Retrograde amnesia is not usually a focus of rehabilitation. Patients often solicit information from relatives and friends to fill in gaps in their memory of past events. Families should be encouraged to provide the patient with cues to see if they trigger past memories and then to fill in whatever details are missing. Visiting the scenes of important past events may help to trigger recall. Patients whose retrograde amnesia extends backward in time from an accident often ask to read police reports, to see any wreckage that was involved, to visit the site of the accident, and to retrace their steps on the day of the accident. As long as the patient does not become upset in the course of reading police reports or visiting the scene of an accident, such requests should be honored. Seeing the twisted metal, blood, and traces of human tissue that are often a part of car wreckage can be traumatizing and is not advisable in most cases. Ultimately, what the patient recalls of the past is a combination of recaptured memories and details gleaned from outside sources.

Various approaches to treating anterograde amnesia are available. Some neuropsychologists and rehabilitation therapists use activities, exercises, and games that require patients to "exercise" their memory abilities in the hopes that memory will improve. My experience has been that minimal improvement occurs in memory ability simply because a patient exercises it. However, use of memory games and exercises may be important in maintaining performance at its current level, and such procedures may be tried with patients who are unlikely to achieve any major gains in their performance, either because their deficits are severe or because considerable time has passed since the onset of the brain damage without improvement having been noted.

Patients with mild dysmnesia may improve their memory performance by learning mnemonic strategies that make information easier to retrieve. Such strategies often employ rhyming or visual imagery. For example, the "peg system" consists of words that rhyme with the numbers 1 to 10 (or 12). The word-and-number pairs are easy to learn because they rhyme (e.g., one-bun, two-shoe, three-tree). The words are also concrete and easily pictured. After the peg system is acquired, it can be used to recall numbers, appointments, and lists. For example, appointments can be remembered by associating a mental image of the appointment with an image of the peg word that rhymes with the hour of the appointment (e.g., a tree pictured growing in the middle of a bank lobby may aid one in remembering to go to the bank at 3:00).

Use of mnemonics takes effort and practice, and even with considerable training, many dysmnesic patients fail to master the techniques or to use them outside the clinic. The techniques are of greatest benefit to patients with mild global anterograde dysmnesia or more severe memory impairment restricted to one sensory modality or one type of material.

Amnesic patients of all levels of severity benefit by learning to record information externally rather than depending on their memory. External recording devices can be as simple as a notepad and pencil or as complex as a portable computer that stores appointments and messages. Generally, the simpler the device, the more likely it is to be effective. The current computer message-keepers are complicated to operate and can be difficult for even a neuropsychologically intact person to use. Amnesic patients may never master these devices, and consequently they sometimes fare better with a pad and pencil.

In addition to recording new information, amnesic patients should be taught habits and routines that minimize their chances of forgetting. For example, habitually putting keys in one place and nowhere else minimizes the chance that they will be lost. Learning to put objects where they will be used or near similar objects can save the amnesic patient hours of frustrated searching.

Severely amnesic patients can sometimes use mnemonics to learn specific information. For example, the patient may learn a therapist's name by associating the sound of the name with some feature of the therapist's face or body. The patient is not likely to use this technique with other new names and faces spontaneously, but with considerable rehearsal he or she may learn the target person's name.

Severely amnesic patients can be taught fairly complex new skills because their procedural learning system (see Appendix 16–1) is usually preserved. This is easiest when the skill being taught is a simple, repetitive motor activity. Thus, the amnesic patient may learn to perform a specific task on a production or assembly line. However, even complex skills such as typing or computer data entry can be acquired when the task is divided into small, discrete steps, and each step is trained and rehearsed separately until a high degree of mastery is attained. Using these procedures, it is possible to train even densely amnesic patients to do fairly complex tasks, even when the patient has no conscious recollection of any of the training. This situation produces the paradox of a patient who denies knowing how to perform an activity but who nonetheless shows mastery of the activity in his or her behavior.

The limits of such rote training procedures are that they require extensive rehearsal and are highly sensitive to even minor changes in the task. Extensive cues are required during training; these cues can be reduced gradually as performance improves. Hundreds of trials may be necessary to achieve even a small improvement in performance. Training should take place in the actual work setting because a change in the type of equipment or tools that the patient is required to use can lead to failure of the skill to generalize to the task at hand.

CASE ILLUSTRATIONS

CASE 16–1

S.S. was a 33-year-old man who was employed as an industrial arts teacher in a high school while he was working to obtain a doctorate in education. He suffered a subarachnoid hemorrhage and hydrocephalus following rupture of an anterior communicating artery aneurysm. A shunt was placed to relieve the hydrocephalus. The aneurysm bled a second time before it was ligated at its base, leaving the branches of the anterior communicating artery unimpeded. Postoperatively, S.S. developed diabetes insipidus and pituitary dysfunction as a result of a drop in hypothalamic releasing hormone. The pituitary dysfunction necessitated hormone replacement, and the patient received testosterone, hydrocortisone, and levothyroxine. After his appetite returned, he was noted to eat voraciously and constantly and showed a marked weight gain. By the time of discharge, the patient's neurological examination was normal except for a severe memory impairment.

Neuropsychological examination was conducted 2 months following the initial hemorrhage. The patient was cooperative and highly motivated to perform during testing, which he likened to the standardized achievement testing done in the public schools. The patient denied depression and other psychiatric problems, and expressed optimism about his potential for recovery.

S.S. showed an average level of intelligence and fully intact performance on tests of concentration, perception, language, drawing, and problem solving. However, mild motor perseveration (see Chap. 11) was present. Events of personal significance to S.S. that occurred during the past 8 years were obtained from his wife. The patient had no recollection of events that had occurred within the 6 months preceding his injury. For example, he did not recall events on the day of his hemorrhage and could not remember a weekend trip to photograph mountain scenery that he took with a group of his students 6 months before injury. This had been a satisfying trip which he had often talked about in the months before his injury. His memory was also spotty for events that occurred as long as 3 years before his injury. For example, he did not recall the death of his father-in-law 2 years before his injury or the birth of his 3-year-old son, even though he had been present during the delivery. Other events that occurred during the preceding 3 years were, however, recalled with reasonable accuracy. Beyond this 3-year period, S.S. had no notable difficulty recalling personally significant events in detail.

Memory was assessed using the University of Florida Level of Processing Procedure. S.S. recognized an equivalent number of words regardless of whether his attention had previously been drawn to the orthography, phonology, or meaning of the words, and in no case did he recognize more than 4 of the 12 words in each condition.

The severity of the patient's memory deficit was evident in his daily behavior. After coming to the neuropsychologist's office twice a week for more than 1 month, he was still unable to find his way up from the lobby without assistance. Whenever he entered the office, he noticed a photograph of an infant on the bookshelf and inquired about the age of the little boy in the picture, despite being told at every session that it was a girl. The patient frequently misplaced his wallet and house keys when at home.

When given verbal instructions, S.S. remembered approximately 20 percent of what he had been told immediately, but nothing 10 minutes later. His worst performance occurred when he was asked to do tasks at a specified future date or time. He consistently failed to perform tasks as little as 10 minutes in the future. As he became used to his prospective memory deficits (see Appendix 16–1), he began wearing a jacket with notes pinned or pasted on the sleeves and breast reminding him to perform various activities.

DISCUSSION

Even without benefit of extensive memory testing, the severity of amnesia in the patient in Case 16–1 was clinically evident. He showed a retrograde amnesia of several years duration and a global anterograde amnesia. The amnesia was more striking considering the relative absence of other neuropsychological disorders. The results of the Levels of Processing Procedure suggested that this patient processed information superficially, failing to take advantage of more meaningful aspects of the verbal stimuli. The patient's pattern of memory deficit was consistent with either a diencephalic or basal forebrain lesion; the latter localization was also supported by the history of anterior communicating artery aneurysm and hypothalamic involvement.

CASE 16–2

E.B. was a 39-year-old man with a 3rd-grade education who had worked as a gas station attendant and cook. He developed a seizure disorder at age 2 years following a case of the measles and head trauma from a fall. E.B. began abusing alcohol in his teens and continued until age 26 years. At age 32 years, he was briefly hospitalized with a diagnosis of atypical psychosis arising after a series of seizures. E.B.'s seizures were only partially controlled by anticonvulsants, and he continued to have tonic-clonic and complex partial seizures. At age 36 years, he underwent a right temporal lobectomy, consisting of a 5.5-cm resection including part of the anterior hippocampus, to bring his seizures under better control. This procedure reduced his seizure frequency to approximately four per month, and he continued to be maintained on phenytoin and phenobarbital, in addition to amitriptyline at bedtime. The patient complained of a subjective worsening of memory following surgery. He was referred for neuropsychological evaluation and treatment.

E.B.'s neuropsychological examination revealed that he was of low-average intelligence with an IQ of 82, with no sensory or motor deficits. He readily detected stimuli on both sides of space; recognized colors, objects, and familiar faces; made detailed and accurate copies of line drawings; and was intact in his language abilities. E.B. concentrated well during testing and was able to repeat six digits in forward sequence and four in reverse order. The patient showed significant difficulty in discriminating complex visual forms (see Visual form imperception) and performed poorly on problem-solving tasks. His worst performance occurred on the WMS-R logical memory (paragraphs) and visual reproduction (designs) subtests. His immediate recall of the paragraphs was at the second percentile of people his age, and his delayed recall was at the first percentile. His immediate recall of the designs was at the 18th percentile, and his delayed recall was at the 1st percentile.

Using the date of the patient's surgery as a starting point, an attempt was made to document loss of memory for events preceding surgery. This attempt failed because the patient complained of having a poor memory before this date. His wife was unable to provide significant personal events for use in testing, and tests using public events were not attempted because of E.B.'s limited education.

A Minnesota Multiphasic Personality Inventory was administered orally because of E.B.'s limited education. A valid clinical profile was obtained which suggested the possible presence of a thought disorder, hallucinations, and poor reality testing. The profile suggested a diagnosis of schizophrenic reaction. Notably, no elevations were present on scales sensitive to depressive symptomatology.

DISCUSSION

Diagnosis in Case 16–2 was particularly difficult because of the many confounding factors present in this patient's background. His memory performance suggested global anterograde dysmnesia, although the severity was less than would be seen in a full amnesic syndrome. If right temporal lobectomy were the only etiologic factor in this patient's history, visuospatial anterograde amnesia might be expected. However, it should be noted that the patient abused alcohol and had a long history of severe seizure disorder, which undoubtedly contributed to the more global memory deficits identified. Diagnosis of dysmnesia was further complicated by the patient's limited education, his long-term use of anticonvulsant and antidepressant medication, and the presence of perceptual deficits that could account for the visuospatial memory impairment. Definitive diagnosis was not possible because all confounding factors cannot be ruled out. Dysmnesia nonetheless remains a highly probable diagnosis because of the etiologic factors operating in this patient.

CASE 16–3

C.S. was a 67-year-old man with a high school education. He had been a marine and later worked in the civil service until he retired because of alcohol-related disability at age 60 years. He abused alcohol during much of his adult life and had a history of myocardial infarction, liver cirrhosis, splenectomy, and reportedly a left-sided cerebrovascular accident 5 years before presentation. The current admission occurred following a right-hemisphere cerebrovascular accident. Computed tomography (CT) scans showed old, bilateral infarctions in the occipital region, with a recent infarction in the right temporal lobe. Medical examination revealed bilateral motor weakness and poor speech articulation.

Neuropsychological examination was performed to determine the extent of the patient's impairment. The patient was cooperative with testing, appeared to exert appropriate effort, and was stable in mood. His affect was flat. Neither distress nor humor was observed, and only a generally complacent attitude was seen. No evidence of psychiatric disorder was found other than the already mentioned history of substance abuse. The patient's family reported that he had not been allowed to drink in the 5 years since his first stroke.

Significant deficits were seen in the patient's ability to divide concentration between simultaneous tasks. The patient could, however, sustain concentration without becoming distracted by internal thoughts or external stimuli. His visual fields were full, and he detected visual and auditory stimuli on both sides of space. Although there was left-sided loss of tactile sensitivity, he showed right hemispatial neglect when bisecting lines (see Chap. 4). The patient was inaccurate in making detailed visual comparisons and discriminations, but his visual perception was sufficient to permit him to identify pictured objects and familiar faces. C.S. was intact in his speech comprehension, repetition, and naming, but was impaired in his oral reading and reading comprehension. Severe constructional disability (see Chap. 7) was evident in the patient's line drawings.

C.S. was severely impaired on the WMS-R logical memory and visual reproduction subtests and on the BVRT recognition administration. His poor memory performance was consistent with reports from nursing and rehabilitation staff that he failed to retain any information presented and showed virtually no carryover of skills from one day to the next.

Table 16–4 presents C.S.'s results when the Release from Proactive Inhibition Procedure was administered. On the nonshift trials, the patient performed poorly throughout the procedure. He performed somewhat better at the beginning of the shift trials, but did not benefit at all from the shift in semantic category on trial 5.

Table 16–4. **RELEASE FROM PROACTIVE INHIBITION PROCEDURE RESULTS IN CASE 16–3**

Trial	Nonshift Condition*	Shift Condition*
1	2	5
2	1	1
3	2	2
4	1	1
5	2	1

*Numbers represent total correct.

Results by decade from the Boston Remote Memory Battery Recognition Test (oral administration) are presented in Table 16–5. Not unexpectedly, C.S. remembered few public events from decades when he was a minor. As can be seen, his performance was best for information from the 1950s, during which he reached the age of 31 years. His memory is progressively worse for public events from subsequent decades covered by the test.

The multiple etiologic factors operating in this case prompted the examiner to seek assistance from family members in determining when the patient's memory impairment began. The family was quite aware of the patient's deficits and indicated that they had been present before the most recent stroke. They dated the onset of deficits to approximately the time of the initial stroke 5 years ago. When questioned about whether they were ever told the patient had the Wernicke-Korsakoff syndrome, the family was uncertain whether they had heard this term before. Hospital records from 5 years ago were not available, but the family described the patient as being highly confused and agitated during the period of his initial stroke.

Table 16–5. **BOSTON REMOTE MEMORY BATTERY RECOGNITION TEST RESULTS IN CASE 16–3**

Decade	Age at Mid-decade	Percent Correct
1920s	1	38
1930s	11	38
1940s	21	25
1950s	31	63
1960s	41	50
1970s	51	25

DISCUSSION

Global anterograde amnesia was suspected in Case 16–3, but definitive diagnosis was difficult. The patient was unable to remember paragraphs or draw designs from memory. Constructional disability (see Chap. 7) might explain the latter deficit, but the patient's performance remained impaired even when drawing was not required. Unfortunately, the presence of hemispatial neglect in this patient could explain the poor performance on visual recognition memory procedures. Although poor memory performance was evident to both health care professionals and family members, it was not possible to rule out all alternative explanations for this patient's level of memory performance. Global anterograde amnesia remains a probable, but not a proven, diagnosis.

A notable feature of this patient is a failure to release from proactive inhibition. He also showed a temporally graded retrograde amnesia. The fact that memory of public events was relatively poor for the first two decades of the patient's life does not detract from this diagnosis, because most people are not closely attentive to public events until they reach maturity. Age, education, or use of prescribed medications cannot explain temporally graded retrograde amnesia. Also, this pattern of forgetting is not seen in normal, healthy populations.

The patient lacked any psychological motive for forgetting past information, and none of the information used to test his remote memory had any personal emotional significance for him. The patient's affect was flat but not depressed; no known mechanism exists for a mood disorder to produce a graded pattern of forgetting. When public events questionnaires are used to test remote memory, failure to have learned the information is a potential confound. The present results are valid only to the extent that the BRMB can be trusted to reflect what the average person should and does know from the decades tested.

The pattern of retrograde amnesia and the failure of C.S. to show a normal release from proactive inhibition suggest Wernicke-Korsakoff syndrome. This would have occurred some years prior to the current examination. Unfortunately, the family could not verify that this diagnosis was made in the past, and hospital records were not available. It is conceivable that the syndrome was missed if it occurred close to the time of the patient's first stroke. Bilateral posterior strokes can produce an amnesia, and without careful neuropsychological examination, the memory impairment evident 5 years ago could have been attributed to the stroke without investigation of other causes.

CASE 16–4

E.Q. was a 46-year-old woman who held a doctorate in psychology. She worked as a research psychologist until suffering a right-hemisphere embolic cerebrovascular accident as a result of aortic valve disease. On examination, she showed left-sided numbness, left hemiparesis, and poor speech articulation. She sustained concentration well but was impaired in her ability to divide concentration between multiple tasks (see Divided concentration deficiency). She showed no evidence of stimulus neglect and performed within normal limits on tests of visual and spatial perception. Her drawings of geometric shapes from models were spatially distorted, and she was aware of the errors in her performance (see Constructional disability). There was no history of psychiatric disorder. E.Q. was impatient and short-tempered but had no evidence of depression or other psychiatric symptomatology.

E.Q. scored at the 47th and 53rd percentiles, respectively, in her immediate and delayed recall of the WMS-R logical memory paragraphs. In contrast, compared to people her age, she scored at the 4th percentile in her immediate recall of the WMS-R visual reproduction subtest designs and at the 8th percentile in her delayed recall. Visual inspection of her responses on the latter test suggested that the poor performance was the result of completely forgetting some designs and forgetting details of others. Spatial distortion was not notable in the drawings that she did produce from memory. However, because of her previously documented constructional disability, the BVRT recognition administration was also administered. The patient continued to show severe impairment under these conditions.

DISCUSSION

The patient in Case 16–4 was less of a diagnostic challenge. E.Q. had no retrograde amnesia, and her memory for verbal information was preserved regardless of the modality of presentation. She showed impaired memory for visuospatial information regardless of whether the tasks required drawing. Even on memory tests that required drawing, significant forgetting of information was evident; therefore, her low scores cannot be attributed solely to constructional disability. A diagnosis of visuospatial dysmnesia is probable.

No other neuropsychological or psychiatric disorders were present to confound interpretation of E.Q.'s memory performance. Her level of performance was inconsistent with her age and certainly is not expected in an individual with a doctoral degree. Normal forgetting would not have placed the patient so low in relation to other individuals her age. The preserved verbal memory performance makes it unlikely that the visuospatial memory deficits were related to medication.

CASE 11–2

H.M. was a right-handed 54-year-old woman who had obtained a bachelor's degree. During the previous 17 months, she had experienced a decline in her memory. She repeated herself in conversations with her husband and forgot people's names. The patient also experienced a decline in her motor functioning, which is discussed in Chapter 11. An initial neurological examination was obtained, including a CT scan, electroencephalogram (EEG), and serological analysis, all of which were normal. Neuropsychological examination at that time showed her verbal intelligence to be in the average range, whereas nonverbal intelligence was in the borderline range. Severe deficits were seen in memory, and the patient was noted to have high levels of anxiety and depression. A tentative diagnosis of dementia of the Alzheimer's type was made. The patient was placed on an antidepressant and began psychotherapy to address her anxiety and mood disorder.

A second, independent neurological consultation was sought 2 months after the first. A magnetic resonance imaging (MRI) scan was obtained, and the patient was examined for Lyme disease. Results of these tests were negative. The patient continued to show deficits in memory and high levels of depression and anxiety. In light of the generally negative laboratory studies, a diagnosis of pseudodementia was made. A third neurological consultation with a dementia "specialist" was sought. The patient had to fly across the United States for this third evaluation, which was also negative.

H.M. then sought a second neuropsychological examination. During this examination, the patient described her deteriorating condition with apparent emotional indifference. She identified two possible causes of her problems, whereas previously she had been unable to determine any precipitating events. She described a febrile illness that had occurred 2 years ago and also a fall sustained during a tennis match, during which she struck her head but did not lose consciousness. It is notable, however, that the symptoms did not begin immediately after either of these episodes. H.M. admitted to marital problems, describing her husband as perfectionistic and controlling. She also indicated that 1 month before the onset of her decline in functioning, she had been preparing to confront her husband about their problems.

Comparison of the first and second neuropsychological examinations failed to reveal a clear pattern of progressive decline. The patient showed notable improvement in some areas, but worsened in other respects. Memory and motor dysfunction continued to be her severest problems. It was noted that, despite her poor performance on memory testing and her great difficulty in recounting events that occurred during the last year, she remembered the dates of all medical examinations, described in detail all tests she had taken, remembered the results, and remembered the names of health care professionals who had evaluated or treated her since the beginning of her decline in functioning.

I was consulted for the third neuropsychological examination approximately 5 months after the second examination. Results from selected memory tests are listed in Table 16–6; the WMS-R results are from the second examination. As can be seen, H.M. showed severe impairment on every memory test and procedure administered, with the exception of the Factitious Memory Complaint Procedure.

Finally, a Minnesota Multiphasic Personality Inventory was administered, and a valid clinical profile resulted. This profile was consistent with the presence of anxiety, agitation, tension, and depression. Patients obtaining similar profiles usually present with multiple and unsubstantiated somatic complaints. They are also likely to be lacking in assertiveness and frequently do not express uncomfortable feelings directly. Feelings of despair and worthlessness are also correlates of H.M.'s personality profile.

The patient's memory and motor deficits prompted many changes in her household. The patient no longer did housework; a maid was hired to handle these responsibilities. Her husband's 12- to 15-hour workdays were interrupted because

Table 16–6. **MEMORY TEST RESULTS IN CASE 11–2**

Wechsler Memory Scale—Revised*	
Verbal Memory Index	79
Visual Memory Index	59
General Memory Index	65
Attention or Concentration Index	95
Delayed Recall Index	60
California Verbal Learning Test	
Trial-1 Recall	4
Trial-5 Recall	5
Tuesday-List Recall	5
Short-Delay Free Recall	1
Short-Delay Cued Recall	2
Long-Delay Free Recall	2
Long-Delay Cued Recall	1
Recognition—True Positives	8
Recognition—False Positives	9
Factitious Memory Complaint Procedure	100
Rey 15-Item Memory Procedure	3

*Administered during the patient's second neuropsychological examination. All other tests are from the third examination.

he had to take his wife for various medical treatments and examinations. This was a source of frustration for him and fueled the antagonism between him and his wife. When the examiner expressed doubts about a diagnosis of Alzheimer's disease, the husband was unhappy. The patient's reaction was difficult to gauge; she seemed both disturbed and relieved.

DISCUSSION

The patient in case 11–2 illustrates pseudoamnesia. Her performance was markedly impaired on a variety of memory tasks. Her preserved performance on the Factitious Memory Complaint Procedure argued against deliberate malingering. However, the patient performed far below expectation on the Rey 15-Item Memory Procedure. This test is comprised of overlearned material that is high in associative value (see Appendix 16–1), yet the patient remembered only three items. Even with a dementia, the patient would have been expected to remember most or even all of the 15 items. The severity of memory deficit seen in psychometric performance was inconsistent with the absence of any pathology detectable by EEG, radiologic scan, or serologic analysis. The severity of the deficit is also inconsistent with the patient's apparently accurate and detailed recall of medical procedures and personnel.

No clear precipitant of the memory impairment could be identified in this patient's history. Ample evidence exists, however, to implicate motivational factors in H.M.'s presentation. She was clinically depressed and may have failed to exert the required effort on memory tasks. Marital discord was evident, and the neurologic deficits may have permitted this unassertive patient to express her anger. Her deficits clearly interfered with her husband's preferred style of life and led to the removal of possibly unwanted domestic responsibilities. Although acutely aware of her deficits, the patient did not consistently appear distressed by them, nor was she relieved by the failure to verify the original diagnosis of dementia caused by Alzheimer's disease.

GENERAL DISCUSSION

Of the patients described, the patient in Case 16–1 showed the greatest eventual recovery of memory performance, which might not have been expected given the severity of his amnesia. This patient is distinguished by the relative absence of disorders other than amnesia. Even the patient in Case 16–4, who presented with less severe memory impairment, did not achieve the same degree of functional change. She failed to achieve her goal of returning to work, whereas the patient in Case 16–1 returned to teaching after 1 year of memory remediation. He continued to have severe memory deficits, but learned to compensate for them with a variety of mnemonic techniques. The relative success of this patient may be the result of the absence of neuropsychological disorders other than amnesia. My experience has been that this is a good prognostic sign, even in patients who have severe memory deficits.

The patient in Case 11–2 continued to remain in a bad marriage, although she considered divorce on several occasions. Even after extensive psychotherapy and pharmacological intervention, little remission of her cognitive and emotional symptoms occurred. Notably, however, none of her symptoms ever worsened.

REFERENCES

1. Squire, LR: The neuropsychology of human memory. Annu Rev Neurosci 5:241, 1982.
2. Cohen, NJ, and Squire, LR: Retrograde amnesia and remote memory impairment. Neuropsychologia 19:337, 1981.
3. Butters, N, and Miliotis, P: Amnesic disorders. In Heilman, KM, and Valenstein, E (eds): Clinical Neuropsychology, Second Edition. Oxford University Press, New York, 1985, p 403.
4. American Psychiatric Association: Diagnostic and Statistical Manual of Mental Disorders, Fourth Edition. American Psychiatric Association, Washington, DC, 1994.
5. The International Classification of Diseases, Ninth Revision, Clinical Modification. Med-Index Publications, Salt Lake City, 1991.
6. Physician's Desk Reference, Forty-Eighth Edition. Medical Economics Company, Inc., Montvale, NJ, 1994.
7. Stillhard, G, et al: Bitemporal hypoperfusion in transient global amnesia: 99m-Tc-HM-PAO SPECT and neuropsychological findings during and after an attack. J Neurol Neurosurg Psychiatry 53:339, 1990.
8. Fazio, F, et al: Metabolic impairment in human amnesia: A PET study of memory networks. J Cereb Blood Flow Metab 12:353, 1992.
9. Chalmers, J, et al: Severe amnesia after hypoglycemia. Clinical, psychometric, and magnetic resonance imaging correlations. Diabetes Care 14:922, 1991.
10. Gaffan, EA, Gaffan, D, and Hodges, JR: Amnesia following damage to the left fornix and to other sites. A comparative study. Brain 114:1297, 1991.

11. Kapur, N, et al: Focal retrograde amnesia: A long term clinical and neuropsychological follow-up. Cortex 25:387, 1989.
12. Mayes, AR, et al: Location of lesions in Korsakoff's syndrome: Neuropsychological and neuropathological data on two patients. Cortex 24:367, 1988.
13. Benson, DF, Marsden, CD, and Meadows, JC: The amnesic syndrome of posterior cerebral artery occlusion. Acta Neurol Scand 50:133, 1974.
14. Mohr, JP, et al: Right hemianopia with memory and color deficits in circumscribed left posterior cerebral artery territory infarction. Neurology 21:1104, 1971.
15. Victor, M, et al: Memory loss with lesions of hippocampal formation. Arch Neurol 5:244, 1961.
16. Von Cramon, DY, and Schuri, U: The septo-hippocampal pathways and their relevance to human memory: A case report. Cortex 28:411, 1992.
17. Morris, MK, et al: Amnesia following a discrete basal forebrain lesion. Brain 115:1827, 1992.
18. Damasio, AR, et al: Amnesia following basal forebrain lesions. Arch Neurol 42:263, 1985.
19. Tatemichi, TK, et al: Paramedian thalamopeduncular infarction: Clinical syndromes and magnetic resonance imaging. Ann Neurol 32:162, 1992.
20. Malamut, BL, et al: Memory in a case of bilateral thalamic infarction. Neurology 42:163, 1992.
21. Dusoir, H, et al: The role of diencephalic pathology in human memory disorder. Evidence from a penetrating paranasal brain injury. Brain 113:1695, 1990.
22. Graff-Radford, NR, et al: Diencephalic amnesia. Brain 113:1, 1990.
23. Stuss, DT, et al: The neuropsychology of paramedian thalamic infarction. Brain Cogn 8:348, 1988.
24. Katz, DI, Alexander, MP, and Mandell, AM: Dementia following strokes in the mesencephalon and diencephalon. Arch Neurol 44:1127, 1987.
25. Waxman, SG, Ricaurte, GA, and Tucker, SB: Thalamic hemorrhage with neglect and memory disorder. J Neurol Sci 75:105, 1986.
26. Goldenberg, G, Wimmer, A, and Maly, J: Amnesic syndrome with a unilateral thalamic lesion: A case report. J Neurol 229:79, 1983.
27. Mair, WG, Warrington, EK, and Weiskrantz, L: Memory disorder in Korsakoff's psychosis: A neuropathological and neuropsychological investigation of two cases. Brain 102:749, 1979.
28. Verfaellie, M, Bauer, RM, and Bowers, D: Autonomic and behavioral evidence of "implicit" memory in amnesia. Brain Cogn 15:10, 1991.
29. Valenstein, E, et al: Retrosplenial amnesia. Brain 110:1631, 1987.
30. Grossi, D, et al: Selective "semantic amnesia" after closed-head injury. A case report. Cortex 24:457, 1988.
31. Matsuda, H, et al: High resolution Tc-99m HMPAO SPECT in a patient with transient global amnesia. Clin Nucl Med 18:46, 1993.
32. Palmini, AL, Gloor, P, and Jones-Gotman, M: Pure amnestic seizures in temporal lobe epilepsy. Definition, clinical symptomatology and functional anatomical considerations. Brain 115:749, 1992.
33. Laloux, P, et al: Technetium-99m HM-PAO single photon emission computed tomography imaging in transient global amnesia. Arch Neurol 49:543, 1992.
34. Tanabe, H, et al: Memory loss due to transient hypoperfusion in the medial temporal lobes including hippocampus. Acta Neurol Scand 84:22, 1991.
35. Croisile, B and Trillet, M: Cerebral blood flow and transient global amnesia. J Neurol Neurosurg Psychiatry 53:361, 1990.
36. Matias-Guiu, J, et al: Cranial CT scan in transient global amnesia. Acta Neurol Scand 73:298, 1986.
37. Findler, G, et al: Transient global amnesia associated with a single metastasis in the non-dominant hemisphere. Case report. J Neurosurg 58:303, 1983.
38. Shuping, JR, Toole, JF, and Alexander, E, Jr: Transient global amnesia due to glioma in the dominant hemisphere. Neurology 30:88, 1980.
39. Ladurner, G, Skvarc, A, and Sager, WD: Computed tomography in transient global amnesia. Eur Neurol 21:34, 1982.
40. Jacome, DE, and Yanez, GF: Transient global amnesia and left frontal haemorrhage. Postgrad Med J 64:137, 1988.
41. Colombo, A, and Scarpa, M: Transient global amnesia: Pathogenesis and prognosis. Eur Neurol 28:111, 1988.
42. Onofrj, M, et al: P3 recordings in patients with bilateral temporal lobe lesions. Neurology 42:1762, 1992.
43. Shimamura, AP, Janowsky, JS, and Squire, LR: Memory for the temporal order of events in patients with frontal lobe lesions and amnesic patients. Neuropsychologia 28:803, 1990.

44. Shimauchi, M, Wakisaka, S, and Kinoshita, K: Amnesia due to bilateral hippocampal glioblastoma. MRI finding. Neuroradiology 31:430, 1989.
45. Zola-Morgan, S, Squire, LR, and Amaral, DG: Human amnesia and the medial temporal region: Enduring memory impairment following a bilateral lesion limited to field CA1 of the hippocampus. J Neurosci 6:2950, 1986.
46. Duyckaerts, C, et al: Bilateral and limited amygdalohippocampal lesions causing a pure amnesic syndrome. Ann Neurol 18:314, 1985.
47. Huppert, FA, and Piercy, M: Normal and abnormal forgetting in organic amnesia: Effect of locus of lesion. Cortex 15:385, 1979.
48. Horel, JA: The neuroanatomy of amnesia. A critique of the hippocampal memory hypothesis. Brain 101:403, 1978.
49. Berti, A, Arienta, C, and Papagno, C: A case of amnesia after excision of the septum pellucidum. J Neurol Neurosurg Psychiatry 53:922, 1990.
50. Phillips, S, Sangalang, V, and Sterns, G: Basal forebrain infarction. A clinicopathologic correlation. Arch Neurol 44:1134, 1987.
51. Mennemeier, M, et al: Contributions of the left intralaminar and medial thalamic nuclei to memory. Comparisons and report of a case. Arch Neurol 49:1050, 1992.
52. Bogousslavsky, J, et al: Unilateral left paramedian infarction of thalamus and midbrain: A clinico-pathological study. J Neurol Neurosurg Psychiatry 49:686, 1986.
53. Von Cramon, DY, Hebel, N, and Schuri, U: A contribution to the anatomical basis of thalamic amnesia. Brain 108:993, 1985.
54. Winocur, G, et al: Amnesia in a patient with bilateral lesions to the thalamus. Neuropsychologia 22:123, 1984.
55. Benke, T: Visual agnosia and amnesia from a left unilateral lesion. Eur Neurol 28:236, 1988.
56. Freedman, M, and Cermak, LS: Semantic encoding deficits in frontal lobe disease and amnesia. Brain Cogn 5:108, 1986.
57. Luria, AR: Memory disturbances in local brain lesions. Neuropsychologia 9:367, 1971.
58. Heilman, K, and Sypert, GW: Korsakoff's syndrome resulting from bilateral fornix lesions. Neurology 27:490, 1977.
59. Milner, B: Disorders of learning and memory after temporal lobe lesions in man. Clin Neurosurg 19:421, 1972.
60. Cole, M, et al: Thalamic amnesia: Korsakoff syndrome due to left thalamic infarction. J Neurol Sci 110:62, 1992.
61. Metter, EJ, et al: Comparison of metabolic rates, language, and memory in subcortical aphasias. Brain Lang 19:33, 1983.
62. Heilman, KM, et al: Frontal hypermetabolism and thalamic hypometabolism in a patient with abnormal orienting and retrosplenial amnesia. Neuropsychologia 28:161, 1990.
63. Janowsky, JS, et al: Cognitive impairment following frontal lobe damage and its relevance to human amnesia. Behav Neurosci 103:548, 1989.
64. Botez-Marquard, T, and Botez, MI: Visual memory deficits after damage to the anterior commissure and right fornix. Arch Neurol 49:321, 1992.
65. Ross, ED: Sensory specific and fractional disorders of recent memory in man: I. Isolated loss of visual recent memory. Arch Neurol 37:193, 1980.
66. Ross, ED: Sensory-specific fractional disorders of recent memory in man: II. Unilateral loss of tactile recent memory. Arch Neurol 37:267, 1980.
67. Wechsler, D: Wechsler Memory Scale—Revised Manual. The Psychological Corporation, San Antonio, 1987.
68. Bornstein, RA, and Chelune, GJ: Factor structure of the Wechsler Memory Scale—Revised. Clin Neuropsychol 2:107, 1988.
69. Chelune, GJ, and Bornstein, RA: WMS-R patterns among patients with unilateral brain lesions. Clin Neuropsychol 2:121, 1988.
70. Williams, JM: Memory Assessment Scales Professional Manual. Psychological Assessment Resources, Inc., Odessa, FL, 1991.
71. Wilson, B, Cockburn, J, and Baddeley, A: The Rivermead Behavioural Memory Test Manual. Thames Valley Test Company, Bury St. Edmunds, England, 1985.
72. Wilson, B, et al: The development and validation of a test battery for detecting and monitoring everyday memory problems. J Clin Exp Neuropsychol 11:855, 1989.
73. Delis, DC, et al: California Verbal Learning Test Adult Version Research Edition Manual. The Psychological Corporation, San Antonio, 1987.

74. Tombaugh, TN, Schmidt, JP, and Faulkner, P: A new procedure for administering the Taylor Complex Figure: Normative data over a 60-year age span. Clin Neuropsychol 6:63, 1992.
75. Lezak, MD: Neuropsychological Assessment, Second Edition. Oxford University Press, New York, 1983.
76. Tombaugh, T: Personal communication. Carleton University, Ottawa, Canada, 1992.
77. Sivian, AB: Benton Visual Retention Test, Fifth Edition. The Psychological Corporation, San Antonio, 1992.
78. Albert, MS, Butters, N, and Levin, J: Temporal gradients in the retrograde amnesia of patients with alcoholic Korsakoff's disease. Arch Neurol 36:211, 1979.
79. Albert, MS, Butters, N, and Brandt, J: Patterns of remote memory in amnesic and demented patients. Arch Neurol 38:495, 1981.
80. Albert, MS, Butters, N, and Brandt, J: Development of remote memory loss in patients with Huntington's disease. J Clin Neuropsychol 3:1, 1981.
81. Kopelman, M, Wilson, B, and Baddeley, A: The Autobiographical Memory Interview Manual. Thames Valley Test Company, Bury St. Edmunds, England, 1990.
82. Kopelman, MD, Wilson, BA, and Baddeley, AD: The Autobiographical Memory Interview: A new assessment of autobiographical and personal semantic memory in amnesic patients. J Clin Exp Neuropsychol 11:724, 1989.
83. Hart, RP, et al: Rate of forgetting in dementia and depression. J Consult Clin Psychol 55:101, 1987.
84. Snodgrass, JG, and Vanderwart, M: A standardized set of 260 pictures: Norms for name agreement, image agreement, familiarity, and visual complexity. J Exp Psychol Hum Learn Mem 6:174, 1980.
85. Binder, LM, and Pankratz, L: Neuropsychological evidence of a factitious memory complaint. J Clin Exp Neuropsychol 9:167, 1987.
86. Hays, WL: Statistics for the Social Sciences, Second Edition. Holt, Rinehart and Winston, New York, 1973.
87. Hiscock, M, and Hiscock, CK: Refining the forced-choice method for the detection of malingering. J Clin Exp Neuropsychol 11:967, 1989.
88. Binder, LM, and Willis, SC: Assessment of motivation after financially compensable minor head trauma. Psychological Assessment: A Journal of Consulting and Clinical Psychology 3:175, 1991.
89. Goldberg, JO, and Miller, HR: Performance of psychiatric inpatients and intellectually deficient individuals on a task that assesses the validity of memory complaints. J Clin Psychol 42:792, 1986.
90. Bernard, LC and Fowler, W: Assessing the validity of memory complaints: Performance of brain-damaged and normal individuals on Rey's task to detect malingering. J Clin Psychol 46:432, 1990.
91. Morgan, SF: Effect of true memory impairment on a test of memory complaint validity. Arch Clin Neuropsychol 6:327, 1991.
92. Bernard, LC: Prospects for faking believable memory deficits on neuropsychological tests and the use of incentives in simulation research. J Clin Exp Neuropsychol 12:715, 1990.

APPENDIX 16–1 MEMORY AND AMNESIA TERMINOLOGY

Anterograde Amnesia: Inability to remember information presented after the onset of a brain lesion.

Associative Value: The number and richness of associated memories evoked by a stimulus.

Consolidation: Hypothetical process by which memories are strengthened (i.e., are made easier to recall) over time, perhaps as a result of forming links or associations with other memories.

Cued Recall: Remembrance of information after a hint has been provided. Hints often consist of the semantic category to which a target piece of information belongs.

Declarative Memory: A hypothetical memory system for storing information that will later be retrieved consciously and intentionally (see Procedural Learning or Memory).

Delayed Recall: Recall of information after a specified period of time has passed since presentation of the information.

Distributed Practice or Rehearsal: Spacing the practice of skills or the rehearsal of information so that a defined period of time passes between successive practice or rehearsal sessions (see Massed Practice or Rehearsal).

Echoic Memory: See Sensory Buffer.

Encoding: To convert external information into a form or code suitable for storage in the brain's memory system.

Episodic Memory: Hypothetical memory system for storing information gleaned during specific events or episodes in personal life (see Semantic Memory).

Explicit Memory: Conscious remembrance of previously presented information.

Free Recall: Remembrance of information without the benefit of externally provided cues and without regard to the order in which the information was presented.

Iconic Memory: See Sensory buffer.

Immediate Recall: Recall of information that exceeds a person's span (see Span) immediately after it has been presented.

Implicit Memory: Remembrance of information or skills without conscious awareness or deliberate effort. Remembrance is inferred by changes in task performance as a result of prior stimulus exposure or task practice.

Incidental Learning or Memory: Unintentional acquisition and later conscious remembrance of information as a by-product of being exposed to the information (see Intentional Learning or Memory).

Intentional Learning or Memory: Deliberate acquisition of information for the purpose of later recalling it (see Incidental Learning or Memory).

Level or Depth of Processing: Degree to which all meaningful aspects of a stimulus are perceived and processed. Varies from "superficial" processing of elementary visual or acoustic features to "deeper" processing of a stimulus's semantic features. The deeper the processing, the more likely the information will be remembered later.

Long-Term Memory: A hypothetical "store" or "state" that information enters for extended storage.

Massed Practice or Rehearsal: Practice of skills or rehearsal of information in one continuous block with no period of time interspersed between practice or rehearsal sessions (see Distributed Practice or Rehearsal).

Mnemonics: Strategies for encoding and remembering information.

Overlearning: Mastery of a skill or acquisition of information with extended practice, to the point that recall of the skill or information is virtually automatic and relatively impervious to the effects of brain damage.

Posttraumatic Amnesia (PTA): A period of extensive anterograde amnesia following the onset of brain trauma. PTA of more than 1 day in duration indicates severe brain dysfunction.

Primacy Effect: Better recall of information in early serial positions (e.g., the initial words in a list) than for information in middle positions (see Recency Effect).

Priming Effect: A change in task performance as a result of previous exposure to target information. Considered to be an aspect of procedural learning (see Procedural Learning or Memory).

Proactive Interference or Inhibition: Interference from previously learned information when attempting to learn new information (see also Release from Proactive Interference).

Procedural Learning or Memory: Improvement in performance on specific tasks as a result of repetition and practice, irrespective of whether there is conscious awareness of new information having been acquired or intentional retrieval of the information. Also a hypothetical memory system for storing rules and procedures that govern how tasks are performed (see Declarative Memory).

Prospective Memory: Remembering to perform tasks at specified times in the future.

Rate of Forgetting: The speed with which learned information is lost or forgotten over time.

Recency Effect: Better recall of information in late serial positions (e.g., the final words in a list) than for information in middle positions.

Recognition: Awareness that one has previously been exposed to a stimulus, often based on a subjective feeling of familiarity.

Release from Proactive Interference: A rebound in memory performance as a result of a shift in the nature of stimuli being presented (see Proactive Interference or Inhibition). The shift in the nature of the stimuli is along some salient dimension, such as the category the stimuli belong to (e.g., shifting from animals to fruits).

Retrieval: The process of accessing a memory and returning it to the focus of attention.

Retroactive Interference or Inhibition: Interference from newly learned information when attempting to recall previously learned information.

Retrograde Amnesia: Inability to remember information acquired prior to the onset of a brain lesion.

Semantic Intrusion: Intrusion of incorrect but meaningfully related items or concepts during attempts to remember target information.

Semantic Memory: Hypothetical memory system for storing facts and knowledge that do not correspond to any specific episode or event in one's personal life (see Episodic Memory).

Sensory Buffer: A hypothetical set of sensory-specific storage systems that preserve sensory impressions for 1 to 5 seconds. The iconic buffer stores visual sensations (iconic memory) and the echoic buffer stores auditory sensations (echoic memory). Tactile and other sensory buffers are also presumed to exist.

Short-Term Memory: A hypothetical "store" or "state" that information enters for temporary storage.

Span (of Attention, Concentration, or Memory): The amount of information that can be concentrated on simultaneously or maintained in working memory (see Working Memory).

Supraspan: Exceeding span of attention, concentration, or working memory (see Working Memory).

Topographical Amnesia: Impaired memory for routes.

Transfer Effect: Facilitation of performance of a new task by knowledge or skills obtained while performing a previous task.

Working Memory: A hypothetical temporary memory storage system of limited capacity used to hold information that is currently being processed (see Span).

ILLUSION (METAMORPHOPSIA) AND HALLUCINATION (HALLUCINOSIS)

17

Illusions or metamorphopsias involve an alteration in the perception of environmental stimuli. The alteration may occur as soon as the stimulus appears or after the stimulus has been present for some time. In hallucinosis, no actual environmental stimulus is necessary to trigger the abnormal perception. Instead, the perception is generated internally by the patient and perceived as if it is occurring in the environment.

Metamorphopsias and hallucinosis can occur in any sensory modality; this chapter is restricted to visual, auditory, and somesthetic illusions and hallucinations. Occasionally, the illusion or hallucination involves multiple senses simultaneously. In most cases, illusions and hallucinations are transient and episodic, but occasional patients have illusions and hallucinations that persist for extended periods. Accurate perception of environmental stimuli may be impeded while the hallucination or illusion is present. Unless they have another perceptual disorder (e.g., stimulus neglect, stimulus imperception, spatial imperception), patients' perception of the environment is unimpeded at other times.

The examiner cannot predict, control, or reliably elicit illusions or hallucinations. In addition, the examiner can never objectively document that an illusion or hallucination has occurred. The patient's subjective report provides the only evidence. In some cases, the examiner can infer from the patient's behavior that an illusion or hallucination is occurring. For example, the patient may speak to, reach out for, or strike at something that is clearly not present in the environment. Even in these instances, the examiner can only surmise that an illusion or hallucination is occurring; such behaviors do not constitute objective proof of the phenomenon.

Illusions and hallucinations are categorized in this text by the sensory modality in which they occur. This approach is consistent with previous reviews[1] and makes sense on clinical grounds, because somewhat different lesions lead to illusions and hallucinations in different senses. Thus, the variety of presentation includes the six subtypes listed in the chapter outline.

NOMENCLATURE

A variety of terms are used in the clinical literature to refer to various types of illusions and hallucinations. These terms are listed and defined in Appendix 17–1. In this text, the term *metamorphopsia* is used to refer to all forms of visual, auditory, and somesthetic illusions. Similarly, the term *hallucinosis* is used to refer to all visual, auditory, and somesthetic hallucination syndromes described in this text. Both of these terms are used in the clinical neurology literature. *Paresthesia* refers to abnormal and often painful somesthetic sensations. This condition, which may occur following nerve damage, is not included in the somesthetic metamorphopsias.

RULES FOR DIAGNOSIS

Clinical Indicators: Each is independent (only one must be observed for the disorder to be suspected) *except* when subscripting is used. Subscripted numbers (a_1, a_2) denote an indicator with multiple parts that must be considered together.
Associated Features: These are listed to give a more complete picture of the disorder. The presence or absence of these features does not affect the diagnosis.
Factors to Rule Out: All must be taken into account. Failure to rule out even one of these factors makes a firm diagnosis impossible.
Lesion Locations: Each location stands alone; damage in only one of the listed areas is sufficient to produce the disorder.

DSM-IV[2] does not have a distinct diagnostic code for metamorphopsia. Hallucinations as a result of brain damage can be coded under "Psychotic Disorder Due to a General Medical Condition." ICD-9-CM[3] includes "Organic Hallucinosis" and several related diagnostic labels, including "Hallucinations," which covers auditory and tactile hallucinations, and "Psychophysical Visual Disturbance," which covers visual hallucinations. Hallucinosis is also listed under "Unspecified Psychosis."

ICD-9-CM also includes "Oneirophrenia" under the diagnostic code for acute schizophrenic episode. Oneirophrenia is similar to oneirism (see Appendix 17–1), with the exception that acquired brain damage is not the presumed cause in oneirophrenia. Metamorphopsia is included in ICD-9-CM under the diagnosis "Visual Distortions of Shape and Size." Megalopsia, macropsia, and micropsia are also listed under this ICD-9-CM code. ICD-9-CM includes a separate diagnostic code, "Diplopia," for doubling of visual images, and it also lists polyopia under this code.

VARIETY OF PRESENTATION

1. Visual metamorphopsia

Clinical Indicators

a. Visual stimuli appearing larger or smaller than their actual size
b. Visual stimuli appearing farther away (as if seen through the wrong end of a telescope) than they actually are
c. Visual stimuli appearing closer (as if magnified) than they actually are
d. Visual stimuli appearing physically deformed (e.g., stretched, flattened, bent, curved)
e. The borders of visual stimuli appearing blurred and indistinct
f. Separate visual stimuli appearing to intersect and penetrate each other
g. Visual stimuli appearing inverted or partially rotated in the horizontal, vertical, or oblique planes
h. Stationary visual stimuli appearing in motion (e.g., rotating, jumping, moving away without becoming smaller)
i. Moving visual stimuli appearing to be traveling faster or slower than they actually are
j. Individual parts of continuous visual stimuli appearing fragmented and separated by space
k. Multiple copies of a visual image appearing in the environment

Associated Features

a. Illusions possibly confined to a particular type of stimulus (e.g., may involve only faces)
b. Illusions transient and episodic
c. A history of decreased visual acuity or the loss of vision in one half of the visual field (homonymous hemianopsia)
d. Impaired perception of color (see Achromatopsia)
e. Impaired localization of visual stimuli (see Stimulus mislocalization)
f. Impaired perception of visual stimuli while visual illusions are occurring

Factors to Rule Out

a. Use of prescribed or recreational drugs with hallucinogenic properties [drugs that the patient is taking should be checked in a current *Physician's Desk Reference* (PDR[4])].
b. Prolonged absence of environmental visual stimulation as a result of external causes.
c. Peripheral ocular damage (ophthalmological consultation required)
d. Depth perception disorders (see Local and global astereopsia) in patients who have visual illusions of closeness or distance. Assessment must be done when illusions are not occurring.
e. Migraine headache, ruled out by documenting visual illusions in the absence of other migraine symptoms.

Lesion Locations

a. Occipital lobe, with occasional extension to temporal lobe, parietal lobe, or both[5–10]
b. Retrosplenial area, including the posterior cingulate gyrus and the corpus callosum, with extension to the putamen[11]
c. Parietal lobe[12]

Lesion Lateralization

a. Most frequently following right-hemisphere or bilateral lesions
b. Unilateral illusions following contralateral lesions

2. Auditory metamorphopsia (also called paracusia)

Clinical Indicators

a. Auditory stimuli seeming louder or softer than they actually are
b. Auditory stimuli seeming closer or farther than they actually are
c. The tone, timbre, pitch, or rhythm of musical sounds seeming distorted

Associated Features

a. Transient and episodic illusions
b. Visual illusions (see Visual metamorphopsia)
c. Visual hallucinations (see Visual hallucinosis)
d. Impaired perception of auditory stimuli while auditory illusions are occurring
e. A history of hearing loss

Factors to Rule Out

a. Use of prescribed or recreational drugs with hallucinogenic properties (drugs that the patient is taking should be checked in a current PDR[4]).
b. Prolonged absence of environmental auditory stimulation as a result of external causes.
c. Severe bilateral hearing loss as a result of middle ear disease. Otolaryngological consultation is required.
d. Impaired localization of auditory stimuli (see Stimulus mislocalization) in patients who have illusions involving the distance of auditory stimuli. Assessment must be done when illusions are not occurring.

e. Impaired perception of music (see Auditory pattern imperception) in patients who have illusions involving the tone, timbre, pitch, or rhythm of musical sounds. Assessment must be done when illusions are not occurring.

Lesion Locations

Insufficient information available

Lesion Lateralization

Insufficient information available

3. Somesthetic metamorphopsia

Clinical Indicators

a. Objects palpated in the hand appearing deformed
b. All or a portion of the body feeling lighter or heavier
c. All or a portion of the body feeling bigger or smaller
d. Feeling taller or shorter than actual height
e. Feeling of floating

Associated Features

a. Illusions are transient and episodic
b. Visual illusions (see Visual metamorphopsia)
c. Visual hallucinations (see Visual hallucinosis)
d. Impaired perception of tactile stimuli while somesthetic illusions are occurring

Factors to Rule Out

a. Use of prescribed or recreational drugs with hallucinogenic properties (drugs that the patient is taking should be checked in a current PDR[4])
b. Prolonged absence of environmental somesthetic stimulation as a result of external causes
c. Peripheral somesthetic sensory organ damage
d. Impaired perception of tactile objects (see Tactile form imperception) in patients with illusions involving the perception of object shapes (assessment must be done when illusions are not occurring)

Lesion Locations

a. Parietal lobe, particularly the posterior area[1]

Lesion Lateralization

a. More common after right-hemisphere lesions, but occasionally occurs after left-sided lesions[1]
b. Unilateral illusions following contralateral lesions

4. Visual hallucinosis

Clinical Indicators

a. Perception of light flashes, colors, stars, or floating objects where none exist
b. Perception of stationary forms, shapes, objects, or people where none exist
c. Perception of moving forms, shapes, objects, or people where none exist
d. Perception of self in the environment as if looking into a mirror

Associated Features

a. Hallucinations possibly unilateral or bilateral
b. Hallucinated figures possibly small in size
c. Scintillation of the hallucinated images
d. Hallucinations possibly disappearing after saccadic but not slow-pursuit eye movements
e. When hallucinations move, direction typically from the center to the periphery of the visual field
f. Elements of past personal experiences possibly contained in the hallucinations
g. Hallucinations may be transient and episodic or persistent
h. Hallucinations more frequent at night or when patient is drowsy
i. Firm belief in the reality of hallucinations
j. Impaired perception of visual stimuli while hallucinations are occurring
k. Attempts to interact with the hallucinated images
l. Hallucinations possibly provoking strong emotional reactions (e.g., anxiety, distress, disgust)
m. Feelings of unreality or strangeness during the hallucinations (e.g., feeling that a past experience is being relived, feeling as if one is in a dream)
n. Confused ideation (see Ideational disorientation or confusion)
o. Reduction in alertness (see Chap. 2)
p. Hallucinations recalled or not recalled later
q. Auditory hallucinations (see Auditory hallucinosis)
r. Somesthetic hallucinations (see Somesthetic hallucinosis)
s. Visual illusions (see Visual metamorphopsia)
t. Partial or total blindness following a cortical lesion (i.e., cortical blindness)
u. Sudden and rapid episodes of sleep onset during periods of wakefulness (narcolepsy), accompanied by sudden temporary muscle paralysis (catalepsy)

Factors to Rule Out

a. Psychotic and other mental disorders that include visual hallucinations as a component (e.g., schizophrenia, bipolar affective disorder, post-traumatic stress disorder; see Chap. 18 for assessment techniques)
b. Use of prescribed or recreational drugs with hallucinogenic properties (drugs that the patient is taking should be checked in a current PDR[4])
c. Prolonged absence of environmental visual stimulation as a result of external causes
d. Peripheral ocular damage; ophthalmological consultation required

Lesion Locations

a. Occipital lobe, particularly the striate cortex and lingual and fusiform gyri, with frequent extension to temporal lobe, particularly the parahippocampal gyrus and posterior hippocampus, and parietal lobe and occasional extension to the basal ganglia (caudate)[7–10,13–27]
b. Parietal lobe, with occasional extension to the frontal lobe[10,20,28,29]
c. Temporal lobe, including the sylvian fissure and amygdala, with frequent extension to frontal lobe[30–34]

d. Frontal lobe, particularly the deep orbital-frontal[30–35]*
e. Diencephalon, particularly the ascending reticular activating system, substantia nigra, thalamus, hypothalamus, and subthalamus, with frequent extension to the basal ganglia, internal capsule, hippocampus, and deep white matter[36–41]†
f. Pons (tegmentum)[42,43]†
g. Optic nerve[44–46]

Lesion Lateralization

a. Following right, left, or bilateral lesions
b. Unilateral hallucinations following contralateral lesions

5. Auditory hallucinosis

Clinical Indicators

a. Hearing indistinct noises (e.g., wind, trickling water, buzzing, humming, whispering) for which no environmental source is present
b. Hearing distinct sounds (e.g., footsteps, clapping) for which no environmental source is present
c. Hearing isolated or conversing voices for which no environmental source is present
d. Hearing music or singing for which no environmental source is present

Associated Features

a. Hallucinated sounds possibly rhythmic and repetitive
b. Intensity of hallucinated sounds varying over time
c. Hallucinated sounds appearing either close or far away
d. Hallucinated voices possibly issuing orders
e. Elements of past personal experiences possibly contained in the hallucinations
f. Hallucinations transient and episodic or persistent
g. Firm belief in the reality of the hallucinations
h. Impaired perception of auditory stimuli while the hallucinations are occurring
i. Hallucinations possibly provoking strong emotional reactions (e.g., anxiety, distress, disgust)
j. Feelings of unreality or strangeness during the hallucinations (e.g., feeling that a past experience is being relived, feeling as if one is in a dream)
k. Oral language impairment, particularly pure word deafness (see Chap. 12)
l. Auditory illusions (see Auditory metamorphopsia)
m. Impaired matching and discrimination of auditory sounds (see Auditory pattern imperception), even when hallucinations are not occurring
n. Visual hallucinations (see Visual hallucinosis)

---

*Frontal lobe lesions may produce hallucinations with aggressive content.
†Termed *peduncular hallucinosis*.

Factors to Rule Out

a. Psychotic and other mental disorders that include auditory hallucinations as a component (e.g., schizophrenia, bipolar affective disorder, posttraumatic stress disorder; see Chap. 18 for assessment techniques)
b. Use of prescribed or recreational drugs with hallucinogenic properties (drugs that the patient is taking should be checked in a current PDR[4])
c. Prolonged absence of environmental auditory stimulation as a result of external causes
d. Severe bilateral hearing loss as a result of middle ear disease; otolaryngological consultation required

Lesion Locations

a. Temporal lobe, particularly the sylvian fissure area or the superior temporal, anterior temporal, and/or midtemporal gyri, with frequent extension to the frontal, parietal, and occipital lobes and basal ganglia (caudate)[16,30,31,34,47–50]
b. Deep orbital frontal lobe[35]
c. Insula[51]
d. Medial surface of the superior parietal gyrus, with compression of the superior parietal lobule and precuneus[52]
e. Diencephalon, particularly the thalamus, hypothalamus, and subthalamus, with frequent extension to the basal ganglia, hippocampus, and deep white matter[36,38,39]*
f. Pons (tegmentum)[43,53]*

Lesion Lateralization

a. Following left, right, or bilateral lesions, but more common after right-hemisphere lesions[54]
b. Unilateral hallucinations typically following contralateral lesions
c. Pontine lesions possibly causing ipsilateral hallucinations[53]
d. Content of hallucination does not aid determination of lesion lateralization[47]

6. Somesthetic hallucinosis

Clinical Indicators

a. Feeling of having an extra (supernumerary) limb
b. Feeling that a part of the body is absent (e.g., missing limb, missing an entire side of the body)
c. Feeling of floating in air
d. Feeling of being outside of one's body
e. Presence of a somesthetic sensation, including postural sensations, in the absence of an environmental stimulus

Associated Features

a. Hallucinations transient and episodic
b. Recent history of paresthesia, or abnormal tactile sensations (e.g., tingling, numbness, burning, tickling)

---

*Termed *peduncular hallucinosis.*

c. Hallucinations possibly provoking strong emotional reactions (e.g., anxiety, distress, disgust)
d. Belief that a part of one's body belongs to someone else (see Somatoparaphrenia)

Factors to Rule Out

a. Psychotic mental disorders that include bizarre ideation, hallucinations, or both as a component (e.g., schizophrenia, bipolar affective disorder; see Chap. 18 for assessment techniques)
b. Prolonged absence of environmental somesthetic stimulation as a result of external causes
c. Peripheral somesthetic sensory-organ damage

Lesion Locations

a. Parietal lobe, with extension to occipital lobe[24,55]
b. Occipital lobe, with occasional extension to pons[16]
c. Combined frontal and temporal lobes[30]
d. Medial substantia nigra pars reticulata[41]*
e. Posterior column of the spinal cord[56]

Lesion Lateralization

a. May follow left, right, or bilateral lesions

ETIOLOGY

Metamorphopsia and hallucinosis can be difficult diagnoses to make because of the non-neuropsychological factors that can cause illusions and hallucinations. As indicated previously, care must be taken to rule out the use of hallucinogenic drugs. Drugs prescribed to treat legitimate medical or psychiatric disorders (e.g., trazodone hydrochloride[57]) can produce hallucinations as an unintended side effect. Care must also be taken to rule out the possibility that the patient has been deprived of environmental stimulation, which can readily happen in some hospital settings. The presence of psychotic and other mental disorders and peripheral sensory-organ damage must be carefully evaluated because either could account for the occurrence of hallucinations. When some or all of these factors cannot be ruled out, the diagnosis of metamorphopsia or hallucinosis remains equivocal. However, once the diagnosis is made, a number of neurological diseases and conditions can then be considered as causes.

Seizure disorder is one of the most common causes of metamorphopsia and hallucinosis. Illusions or hallucinations may occur as part of a seizure that has many other motor and behavioral manifestations, or they may be its only outward manifestation. Illusions and hallucinations also may be seen in patients who have migraine headaches, either during the headache or as part of the aura that precedes and warns of an impending attack.

---

*Termed *peduncular hallucinosis*.

Hallucinations are seen in alcoholic patients as part of the syndrome of delirium tremens. In general, prolonged disturbance of central nervous system metabolism can lead to metamorphopsia and hallucinosis. Metabolic dysfunction is often the result of toxicity or the failure of vital body organs. Conditions such as hyperglycemia can produce hallucinations in patients who lack other neurological signs,[58] creating the potential for misdiagnosis.

Infections of the central nervous system, cerebrovascular disease, demyelinating disease, and neoplasm are also known precursors of metamorphopsia and hallucinosis. Traumatic brain injury can produce behavioral changes that mimic psychiatric disorders, a fact that complicates the testimony of physicians and psychologists during personal injury litigation. Hallucinations and illusions may be among the behavioral changes seen in brain trauma patients, particularly when a secondary seizure disorder is present.

DISABLING CONSEQUENCES

When an illusion or hallucination occurs, ongoing activities are likely to be interrupted. Consequently, the patient may be at risk when driving and may experience work interruptions. If the disorder is transient and infrequent, the interruption may be minimal. However, even a brief and infrequent hallucination or illusion can have devastating consequences if it occurs at the wrong time. No one would wish to begin hallucinating while changing lanes at 65 miles per hour on a freeway.

Considerable subjective distress is likely to accompany frequent hallucinations. The patient may feel that he or she is going crazy. Feelings of being out of control and unable to trust oneself are also common. Loss of self-confidence may follow.

Just as the patient may fear that he or she is going crazy, others may have a similar reaction. Pity, derision, and even rejection may follow. People tend to think of hallucinations as aspects of mental illness rather than physical illness. Employers, colleagues, and even family members are apt to doubt the patient's stability and to lose confidence in the patient's ability to handle the demands of the workplace or the home.

ASSESSMENT INSTRUMENTS

Psychiatric Diagnostic Interview–Revised

See discussion of this test in Chapter 18.

Minnesota Multiphasic Personality Inventory 2

See discussion of this test in Chapter 18.

Neuroemotional-Neuroideational-Neurobehavioral Symptom Survey

See discussion of this survey in Chapter 18.

Behavioral Monitoring Procedure

The Behavioral Monitoring Procedure is *not commercially available*. Also see discussion of this procedure in Chapter 3.

Hallucinations and illusions occur intermittently and are not readily elicited by specific tasks or activities. When considerable confusion is also present, the patient may not be able to provide a lucid description of the hallucinations and illusions. The Behavioral Monitoring Procedure, described in detail in Chapter 3, can be used to document the occurrence of hallucinations and illusions, provided they are described in specific, objective terms that can be easily identified by all monitoring staff members. This may not be possible when the patient shows no outward signs of having an hallucination or illusion.

Patients who respond to their hallucinations and illusions verbally, behaviorally, or emotionally are easier for staff to monitor. Staff members focus on detecting the specific outward changes in speech, behavior, or affect and infer that a hallucination or illusion is occurring. Lucid and cognitively intact patients can cue staff when hallucinations or illusions occur and may even be able to monitor these disorders themselves.

NEUROPSYCHOLOGICAL TREATMENT

The treatment of metamorphopsia and hallucinosis is medical rather than neuropsychological. The underlying medical etiology must be identified and appropriate remedies applied. In patients whose illusions and hallucinations result from seizures, anticonvulsant medication is often the optimal treatment and can lead to full cessation of the problem. When efforts to identify and treat the cause of illusions and hallucinations fail, the physician may begin to carefully consider use of neuroleptic medication.

The neuropsychologist functions as educator in the treatment of illusions and hallucinations. Patients and family need to understand that illusions and hallucinations can be a consequence of brain damage, just as motor weakness or speech difficulty are. Illusions and hallucinations in a patient with brain damage and no prior history of psychotic mental disorder should not be viewed as a sign that the patient is going crazy. A better understanding of the cause of and treatment options for the illusions and hallucinations may help to alleviate anxiety in patients and family members.

Behavioral strategies and environmental modifications that help the patient cope with his or her hallucinations or illusions can be implemented. The patient should be advised to terminate any activity that could lead to injury when the illusion or hallucination begins. Closing the eyes, attempting to relax, and concentrating on something else may hasten the end of the disturbance. Family members should be involved in providing comfort and verbal reassurance to the patient during illusions and hallucinations. Patients who experience these disturbances only at night may be aided by a dim light in the bedroom. Although these behavioral and environmental changes are useful in helping the patient to cope with the disorder, they should never be presented as substitutes for medical intervention. However, behavioral and environmental interventions may, by default, become the only treatment options in patients who fail to respond to medical intervention or who cannot tolerate certain medications.

CASE ILLUSTRATIONS

CASE 17–1

L.B. was a 35-year-old man who had completed high school and worked as an automobile and diesel-engine mechanic. He had a chronic history of epilepsy that was controlled with low doses of anticonvulsants. Two months before the current examination, the patient showed an increase in irritability and aggressive outbursts. He also began to have seizures more frequently. Anticonvulsant blood levels were found to be in the therapeutic, nontoxic range. The patient's neurologist obtained computed tomographic (CT) scans and an angiogram, which revealed a left temporal arteriovenous malformation fed by both the posterior and middle cerebral arteries.

The patient reported a number of cognitive changes since the increase in his seizure frequency. These included word-finding problems, difficulty in recalling names and faces, forgetting to turn off appliances, and clumsiness. Most disturbing were episodes when L.B. reportedly saw objects that were not visible to others. At other times, he complained of seeing objects in an inverted position.

Neuropsychological examination revealed visual acuity of 20/20 in each eye, full visual fields, a full range of eye movements, accurate bisection of lines, no consistent suppressions to bilateral simultaneous stimulation, preserved object and color recognition, and inaccurate reaching for targets in space (see Optic ataxia). The most striking perceptual error noted in this patient was a tendency to invert stimuli when he was asked to draw or write what he saw in a model. For example, when copying letters and numbers, he inverted the letters D, G, M, Z, A, T, C, S, F, and J. He also reversed the number 3 in the horizontal plane. When queried about this, he responded that he had copied what he had seen.

DISCUSSION

The patient in Case 17–1 presented with visual metamorphopsia. The deficit consisted of inversions of stimuli. L.B. had no optic or oculomotor abnormalities that could account for his symptoms. Sensory deprivation and use of hallucinogenic drugs were not factors in this case. The patient was taking anticonvulsants, but nontoxic blood levels of his seizure medications had recently been verified.

CASE 17–2

M.B. was a 66-year-old woman with a 10th-grade education who had retired from a cashier position. She was hospitalized following rupture of an anterior communicating artery aneurysm. CT scans revealed a right frontal lobe infarction, right basal ganglia infarcts, and hydrocephalus. The patient underwent shunting to relieve the hydrocephalus, and the aneurysm was ligated. There was no premorbid history of psychiatric disorder or visual impairment.

When her condition was stable, M.B. was admitted to a rehabilitation hospital for treatment of a left hemiparesis. She showed significantly reduced alertness that varied from lethargy to stupor (see Chap. 2). M.B. was more alert in the morning and could maintain concentration on tasks for up to 20 minutes. However, during such times, she would periodically turn and speak to people who were not present. When queried, she identified the people as being various family members and friends. It could not be determined whether she heard the people speak to her, and she had no explanation for why she saw them and the examiner did not.

DISCUSSION

Visual hallucinosis was evident in this patient. No premorbid psychiatric or ophthalmological history was present. Sensory deprivation and use of hallucinogenic drugs were not factors in this case.

CASE 6–5

A.S. was a 76-year-old retired teacher with no premorbid psychiatric history. She suffered a right cerebral infarction following atrial fibrillation and was admitted to a rehabilitation hospital for treatment of a left hemiparesis. The patient was alert and attentive during neuropsychological examination. She had full visual fields and was accurate in her recognition of colors, objects, and faces of recent presidents. She was also accurate in her line bisection, but showed significant spatial misestimation (see Chap. 6). The patient complained of seeing multiple plates and cups on her food tray at meals. When reading, she reported seeing multiple images of each word, to the point where she was forced to discontinue. This distressed her because reading had been a major source of pleasure before her illness. A.S. denied having experienced anything resembling her current problem before her illness. The visual illusions were also evident during testing; the patient complained of seeing multiple copies of test stimuli in front of her. Testing was discontinued because the multiple images made her feel nauseous.

DISCUSSION

The patient in Case 6–5 presented with visual metamorphopsia. In this instance, the disorder manifested itself as polyopia. Full examination was not possible, but the fact that the symptoms arose only after the infarction suggests that they were not the result of any peripheral visual problem. Sensory deprivation and use of hallucinogenic drugs were not factors in this case.

REFERENCES

1. Hecaen, H, and Albert, ML: Human Neuropsychology. John Wiley & Sons, New York, 1978.
2. American Psychiatric Association: Diagnostic and Statistical Manual of Mental Disorders, Fourth Edition, Revised. American Psychiatric Association, Washington, DC, 1994.

3. The International Classification of Diseases, Ninth Revision, Clinical Modification. Med-Index Publications, Salt Lake City, 1991.
4. Physician's Desk Reference, Forty-Eighth Edition. Medical Economics Company, Montvale, NJ, 1994.
5. Ardila, A, Botero, M, and Gomez, J: Palinopsia and visual allesthesia. Int J Neurosci 32:775, 1987.
6. Brau, RH, et al: Metamorphopsia and permanent cortical blindness after a posterior fossa tumor. Neurosurgery 19:263, 1986.
7. Safran, AB, et al: Television-induced formed visual hallucinations and cerebral diplopia. Br J Ophthalmol 65:707, 1981.
8. Taguchi, K, et al: Subjective visual symptoms and electroencephalographic analysis before and after removal of occipital falx meningioma. Electroencephalogr Clin Neurophysiol 49:162, 1980.
9. Brust, JC, and Behrens, MM: "Release hallucinations" as the major symptom of posterior cerebral artery occlusion: A report of 2 cases. Ann Neurol 2:432, 1977.
10. Lance, JW: Simple formed hallucinations confined to the area of a specific visual field defect. Brain 99:719, 1976.
11. Ebata, S, et al: Apparent reduction in the size of one side of the face associated with a small retrosplenial hemorrhage. J Neurol Neurosurg Psychiatry 54:68, 1991.
12. Young, WB, et al: Metamorphopsia and palinopsia. Association with periodic lateralized epileptiform discharges in a patient with malignant astrocytoma. Arch Neurol 46:820, 1989.
13. Salanova, V, et al: Occipital lobe epilepsy: Electroclinical manifestations, electrocorticography, cortical stimulation and outcome in 42 patients treated between 1930 and 1991. Surgery of occipital lobe epilepsy. Brain 115:1655, 1992.
14. Williamson, PD, et al: Occipital lobe epilepsy: Clinical characteristics, seizure spread patterns, and results of surgery. Ann Neurol 31:3, 1992.
15. Vanroose, E, et al: Altitudinal hemianopia; A clinical and anatomical entity or a mere coincidence? Case report and review of literature. Acta Neurol Belg 90:254, 1990.
16. Breitner, JC, et al: Cerebral white matter disease in late-onset psychosis. Biol Psychiatry 28:266, 1990.
17. Lefebre, C, and Kolmel, HW: Palinopsia as an epileptic phenomenon. Eur Neurol 29:323, 1989.
18. Gates, TJ, Stagno, SJ, and Gulledge, AD: Palinopsia posing as a psychotic depression. Br J Psychiatry 153:391, 1988.
19. Bosley, TM, et al: Recovery of vision after ischemic lesions: Positron emission tomography. Ann Neurol 21:444, 1987.
20. Landis, T, et al: Loss of topographic familiarity. An environmental agnosia. Arch Neurol 43:132, 1986.
21. Kolmel, HW: Complex visual hallucinations in the hemianopic field. J Neurol Neurosurg Psychiatry 48:29, 1985.
22. Newman, RP, Kinkel, WR, and Jacobs, L: Altitudinal hemianopia caused by occipital infarctions. Clinical and computerized tomographic correlations. Arch Neurol 41:413, 1984.
23. Lazaro, RP: Palinopsia: Rare but ominous symptom of cerebral dysfunction. Neurosurgery 13:310, 1983.
24. Cummings, JL, et al: Palinopsia reconsidered. Neurology 32:444, 1982.
25. Kattah, JC, et al: Removal of occipital arteriovenous malformations with sparing of visual fields. Arch Neurol 38:307, 1981.
26. Michel, EM, and Troost, BT: Palinopsia: Cerebral localization with computed tomography. Neurology 30:887, 1980.
27. Meadows, JC, and Munro, SS: Palinopsia. J Neurol Neurosurg Psychiatry 40:5, 1977.
28. King, PH, and Bragdon, AC: MRI reveals multiple reversible cerebral lesions in an attack of acute intermittent porphyria. Neurology 41:1300, 1991.
29. Young, WB, et al: Metamorphopsia and palinopsia. Association with periodic lateralized epileptiform discharges in a patient with malignant astrocytoma. Arch Neurol 46:820, 1989.
30. Devinsky, O, et al: Autoscopic phenomena with seizures. Arch Neurol 46:1080, 1989.
31. Price, BH, and Mesulam, M: Psychiatric manifestations of right hemisphere infarctions. J Nerv Ment Dis 173:610, 1985.
32. Swash, M: Visual perseveration in temporal lobe epilepsy. J Neurol Neurosurg Psychiatry 42:569, 1979.
33. Julien, J, et al: Epilepsy and agitated delirium caused by an astrocytoma of the amygdala. Eur Neurol 18:387, 1979.
34. Dyck, P: Sylvian lipoma causing auditory hallucinations: Case report. Neurosurgery 16:64, 1985.

35. Fornazzari, L, et al: Violent visual hallucinations and aggression in frontal lobe dysfunction: Clinical manifestations of deep orbitofrontal foci. J Neuropsychiatry Clin Neurosci 4:42, 1992.
36. Schmidbauer, M, et al: Subacute diencephalic angioencephalopathy: An entity similar to angiodysgenetic necrotizing encephalopathy and Foix-Alajouanine disease. J Neurol 239:379, 1992.
37. Serra-Catafau, J, Rubio, F, and Peres-Serra, J: Peduncular hallucinosis associated with posterior thalamic infarction. J Neurol 239:89, 1992.
38. Kolmel, HW: Peduncular hallucinations. J Neurol 238:457, 1991.
39. Reeves, A, and Plum, F: Hyperphagia, rage, and dementia accompanying a ventromedial hypothalamic neoplasm. Arch Neurol 20:616, 1969.
40. Feinberg, WM, and Rapcsack, S: Peduncular hallucinosis following paramedian thalamic infarction. Neurology 39:1535, 1989.
41. McKee, A, et al: Peduncular hallucinosis associated with isolated infarction of the substantia nigra pars reticulata. Ann Neurol 27:500, 1990.
42. Hattori, T, et al: Pontine lesion in opsoclonus-myoclonus syndrome shown by MRI. J Neurol Neurosurg Psychiatry 51:1572, 1988.
43. Cambier, J, Decroix, JP, and Masson, C: Hallucinose auditive dans les lesions du tronc cerebral. Rev Neurol 143:255, 1987.
44. Ram, Z, et al: Visual hallucinations associated with pituitary adenoma. Neurosurgery 20:292, 1987.
45. Jacome, DE: Palinopsia and bitemporal visual extinction on fixation. Ann Ophthalmol 17:251, 1985.
46. Jacobs, L, et al: Auditory-visual synesthesia: Sound-induced photisms. Arch Neurol 38:211, 1981.
47. Paquier, P, et al: Transient musical hallucinosis of central origin: A review and clinical study. J Neurol Neurosurg Psychiatry 55:1069, 1992.
48. Tanabe, H, et al: Lateralization phenomenon of complex auditory hallucinations. Acta Psychiatr Scand 74:178, 1986.
49. Mackworth-Young, CG: Sequential musical symptoms in a professional musician with presumed encephalitis. Cortex 19:413, 1983.
50. Schneider, RC, Calhoun, HD, and Crosby, EC: Vertigo and rotational movement in cortical and subcortical lesions. J Neurol Sci 6:493, 1968.
51. De Reuck, J, et al: Positron emission tomography studies of changes in cerebral blood flow and oxygen metabolism in arteriovenous malformation of the brain. Eur Neurol 29:294, 1989.
52. Scott, M: Musical hallucinations from meningioma. JAMA 241:1683, 1979.
53. Cascino, GD, and Adams, RD: Brainstem auditory hallucinosis. Neurology 36:1042, 1986.
54. Berrios, GE: Musical hallucinations: A statistical analysis of 46 cases. Psychopathology 24:356, 1991.
55. Stacy, CB: Complex haptic hallucinations and palinaptia. Cortex 23:337, 1987.
56. Nathan, PW, Smith, MC, and Cook, AW: Sensory effects in man of lesions of the posterior columns and of some other afferent pathways. Brain 109:1003, 1986.
57. Hughes, MS, and Lessell, S: Trazodone-induced palinopsia. Arch Ophthalmol 108:399, 1990.
58. Johnson, SF, and Loge, RV: Palinopsia due to nonketotic hyperglycemia. West J Med 148:331, 1988.

APPENDIX 17–1 ILLUSIONS AND HALLUCINATIONS: CLINICAL NOMENCLATURE

Visual Illusions

Macropsia: (see Megalopsia)
Megalopsia: Object appearing larger than it is
Micropsia: Object appearing smaller than it is
Pelopsia: Objects appearing closer than they are
Polyopia: Visual images duplicated multiple times (doubling of the image is referred to as *diplopia,* tripling of the image is *triplopia,* quadrupling of the image is *quadriplopia,* and so on)
Teleopsia: Objects appearing farther away than they are

Visual Hallucinations

Autoscopic hallucination: Seeing oneself as if in a mirror
Heautoscopia: Seeing an image of oneself, usually at a younger age than at present
Lilliputianism: Hallucinations of smaller-than-normal people or objects
Oneirism: An extremely vivid, dreamlike hallucination in which alertness is reduced and the patient is confused and emotionally distressed, often involving other sensory modalities in addition to vision
Palinopsia: A previously perceived image returning as a hallucination
Visual synesthesia: Visual sensation produced by a nonvisual stimulus (e.g., a sound)

Auditory Hallucinations

Paliacousia: Previously heard words returning again as a hallucination

Somesthetic Illusions

Macrosomatognosia: All or a portion of the body feeling larger than it is
Metamorphotaxis: Objects feeling deformed in shape when they are palpated
Microsomatognosia: All or a portion of the body feeling smaller than it is

Somesthetic Hallucinations

Palinaptia: A previously felt tactile sensation returning as a hallucination

NEUROPSYCHOLOGICAL DISORDERS OF EMOTION, IDEATION, AND BEHAVIOR

18

It has long been known that brain damage could produce disturbances of emotion, ideation, and behavior. Harlow's[1] description of the "fitful," "irreverent," "pertinaciously obstinate," and "capricious" behavior of the patient Phineas Gage after damage to his frontal lobes is only one early example of clinicians' awareness of the association between brain damage and behavioral disorder. It is sometimes argued that emotional disorders are a reaction to brain damage rather than a result of the damage itself. Something more than a "reaction" occurs, however, in cases in which the emotion shown by the patient is out of proportion to its stimulus (e.g., a fit of crying after watching a television commercial), or the emotion is incompatible with its stimulus (e.g., indifference to hemiparesis).

Emotional reactions do occur that are quite understandable in light of what the patients are enduring, and sometimes these reactions become problematic and require psychological or psychiatric intervention. A group of emotional, ideational, and behavioral disorders nonetheless exist that are a direct result of brain damage or neurological disease and that are distinguishable from the expected emotional reactions of disabled patients. The subtypes of these disorders are listed under "Variety of Presentation" in the chapter outline.

Psychiatric mental disorders thought to have biological components (e.g., schizophrenia) and problematic emotional reactions to disability (e.g, depression) are beyond the scope of this chapter. Assessment procedures sensitive to these mental disorders and problematic emotional reactions are discussed later in this chapter because these procedures may be useful when attempting to diagnose the neuropsychological disorders covered in this chapter.

Despite the assertion that the disorders included in this chapter result from brain damage, it must be acknowledged that highly similar patterns of behavior can occur in individuals who lack a history of neurological illness or brain trauma. For example, individuals who have antisocial personality disorder may show much the same degree of impulse disinhibition that can be seen following frontal lobe brain damage. Neurological and psychosocial factors may lead to the same behavior, and in some cases, both sets of factors may be operating, greatly complicating the process of neuropsychological diagnosis.

To decrease the likelihood of misdiagnosis of a psychosocial behavior pattern as a neuropsychological disorder, the clinical indicators, when appropriate, require that the patient's current behavior be demonstrably different from his or her premorbid behavior. This requirement is unnecessary for disorders such as anosognosia (unawareness of disability) because the behaviors that constitute the disorder do not occur in healthy individuals (i.e., a patient cannot be unaware of his or her disability before the time he or she acquired the disability). This requirement does not preclude current behavior from being an exaggeration of premorbid behavior.

To minimize the chances of misdiagnosis even further, the clinical indicators for all of the disorders in this chapter require the presence of illness or trauma that is capable of causing brain damage. This is analogous to the requirement in DSM-IV[2] that there be evidence from the patient history, physical examination, or laboratory findings that certain mental disorders are a direct consequence of a medical condition before those disorders can be diagnosed. An unfortunate consequence of the inclusion of this condition is that diagnosis of one or more of the disorders in this chapter by itself does not prove the existence of brain damage. To conclude that brain damage has occurred based on the diagnosis of the disorders in this chapter would involve circular reasoning because the disorders require that neurological illness or trauma be present before they can be diagnosed. However, the presence of these disorders can support a suspicion of brain damage that arises from other data. In addition, diagnosis of these disorders can, in some cases, aid in localizing the damage to a particular brain area.

NOMENCLATURE

Many of the disorders included in this chapter are considered part of the "frontal lobe syndrome." Unfortunately, this term fails to account for the fact that many of the components of the "syndrome" occur alone as distinct clinical entities. In addition, these disorders do not invariably occur in patients who have frontal lobe lesions. Finally, components of the frontal lobe syndrome may be seen in patients with damage in other brain areas. The term *dysexecutive syndrome* sometimes replaces *frontal lobe syndrome* and has the advantage of not implying an invariant distribution of brain damage. However, this term fares no better when considering the frequency with which syndrome components are missing from the clinical profile of a given patient and the frequency with which syndrome components occur alone.

Anosodiaphoria, pathological laughing and crying, anosognosia, reduplication, perseveration, and *confabulation* are commonly used terms familiar to experienced neuropsychologists and neurologists. The terms *abulia, moria,* and *somatoparaphrenia* are less common. *Abulia* refers to a diminution of motivation that can present in a manner very similar to depression. *Moria* refers to a euphoric mood akin to mania that is sometimes seen after brain damage. Patients who have *somatoparaphrenia* suffer from certain delusions concerning the ownership of their limbs.

In this text, a distinction is made between motor perseveration (see Chap. 11) and behavioral perseveration, which is discussed in this chapter. I often see patients who perseverate on simple motor tasks (e.g., when copying triple loops) but who show no other signs of perseveration in their behavior. Conversely, patients may fail to shift cognitive set on complex problem-solving tasks (a more subtle and complex type of perseveration) but show no perseveration on simple motor tasks. This clinical distinction is preserved in this text by separately listing the two types of perseveration. The two disorders may, nonetheless, occur together in some patients and may share some common underlying property that future research may elucidate.

I selected the terms *ideational constriction, ideational disorientation or confusion,* and *impulse disinhibition,* and their use requires some explanation. Lesions in several brain areas cause a reduction in the ability to think abstractly, to approach tasks and problems flexibly, to reason, to plan, and to organize time or resources. The term *ideational constriction* is used in this text to identify this pattern of impaired performance.

The term *disorientation* is typically used to describe patients who are unaware of basic personal information (e.g., their age and occupation), time (e.g., the month or year), location (e.g., the name of the hospital or city they are in), or their current situation (e.g., that they have had a stroke and are undergoing rehabilitation). Disorientation can progress further to gross confusion and sometimes to the point that the patient's speech is entirely incoherent and meaningless despite the absence of any basic impairment in oral language. For example, one patient, when asked to identify her location, responded to me that she was in "an underwater school for fish."

Patients such as this are said to be in a *confusional state* when they also evidence a major reduction in the capacity to concentrate. Concentration deficits may occur in patients who are not disoriented or confused (see Chap. 3), but few confused patients manage to sustain concentration for long periods. Because concentration disorders and confusion are at least partially dissociable, they are treated separately in this text, with the term *ideational disorientation or confusion* referring to the latter component of the syndrome.

Impulse disinhibition is used to refer to patients who are unable to inhibit impulses and consequently behave in socially inappropriate ways. Such patients are often thought to exemplify the effects of frontal lobe lesions. As is often the case in neuropsychology, however, patients can be found with no evidence of frontal lobe involvement who are every bit as disinhibited as patients with verified frontal lesions.

DSM-IV[2] provides several options for coding neuropsychological disorders of emotion, ideation, and behavior. Delusional thinking is prominent in somatoparaphrenia and reduplication, and these disorders can be viewed as exemplars of the DSM-IV diagnosis "Psychotic Disorder Due to a General Medical Condition." This diagnostic code can also be used for anosognosia if the lack of awareness seen in anosognosic patients is viewed as a type of delusional thinking. Ideational disorientation or confusion is a part of the DSM-IV diagnosis of delirium, but delirium can be diagnosed only if a prominent deficit in concentration is also present.

The DSM-IV diagnosis "Personality Change Due to a General Medical Condition" comes closest to capturing the presentation of patients who show abulia and anosodiaphoria. The DSM-IV diagnosis "Mood Disorder Due to a General Medical Condition" captures some aspects of abulia and moria, but these disorders are defined in this text in a manner that clearly distinguishes them from depression and mania. The mood of patients diagnosed as having "Mood Disorder Due to a General Medical Condition" may not be qualitatively different from the mood of manic or depressed patients. Consequently, the conceptual overlap with abulia and moria is only partial.

Like the previous disorders, impulse disinhibition can also be coded under "Personality Change Due to a General Medical Condition." Alternatively, a DSM-IV diagnosis of "Impulse-Control Disorder Not Otherwise Specified" can be used; however, this diagnosis is not as closely tied to a physiological cause and therefore may not be as useful. Confabulation is not included as a disorder in DSM-IV. Similarly, no diagnostic code is provided for ideational constriction, although abstract-thinking deficits are included as criteria for a DSM-IV diagnosis of dementia. No coding options are available in DSM-IV for behavioral perseveration and pathological laughing and crying.

ICD-9-CM[3] presents some additional options for diagnostic coding. Abulia is included under the code for "Other Ill-Defined Conditions," and moria is listed as an "Unspecified Psychosis." Anosognosia and reduplication are listed under "Other General Symptoms." The wording of these labels unfortunately implies that these disorders cannot be defined in precise and objective terms, a contention I hope to dispel, at least partially.

Ideational disorientation or confusion can be coded as "Acute or Subacute Delirium" in ICD-9-CM if it is accompanied by other features of delirium. Alternatively, disorientation or confusion may be coded as a "Confused Mental State" under the ICD-9-CM diagnosis of "Unspecified Psychosis." No distinction exists in ICD-9-CM between motor and behavioral perseveration. Both can be coded under the diagnosis "Other Symbolic Dysfunction." A code exists for confabulation in ICD-9-CM, but it is linked with amnesia under the label "Amnestic Confabulatory Syndrome." In practice, virtually all cases of confabulation occur in the context of an amnestic disorder, although the amnesia often persists after the confabulation has waned.

Ideational constriction and impulse disinhibition may be coded in ICD-9-CM as "Frontal Lobe Syndromes" if this in fact is the locus of damage in the patient. No good coding options exist for these disorders arising in association with damage in other parts of the brain. Impulse disinhibition that manifests itself mainly as aggressiveness can be coded under "Disturbance of Conduct Not Elsewhere Classified." If facetious remarks dominate the patient's presentation, then "Witzelsucht" (see p. 426) can be diagnosed and coded under "Unspecified Personality Disorder." The neurological etiology of the disorder is unfortunately obscured when this code is used, making it a less desirable option for the neurologist or neuropsychologist. No unique coding options exist in ICD-9-CM for anosodiaphoria, pathological laughing and crying, or somatoparaphrenia.

RULES FOR DIAGNOSIS

Clinical Indicators: Each is independent (only one must be observed for the disorder to be suspected) *except* when subscripting is used. Subscripted numbers (a_1, a_2) denote an indicator with multiple parts that must be considered together.

Associated Features: These are listed to give a more complete picture of the disorder. The presence or absence of these features does not affect the diagnosis.

Factors to Rule Out: All must be taken into account. Failure to rule out even one of these factors makes a firm diagnosis impossible.

Lesion Locations: Each location stands alone; damage in only one of the listed areas is sufficient to produce the disorder.

VARIETY OF PRESENTATION

1. Abulia (also called pseudodepression)

Clinical Indicators

a_1. A decline in intrinsic motivation to perform activities as evidenced by any of the following signs:
   1) Loss of initiative
   2) Torpor and inertia
   3) Loss of spontaneity
   4) Absence of effort
   5) Placidity

a_2. A decline in interest (e.g., apathy, indifference) and time spent engaged in previously pleasurable activities

NOTE: A decline in sexual interest and activity is termed hyposexuality.

a_3. Absence of each of the following correlates of depression:
   1) Subjective reports of persistent and severe dysphoric affect
   2) Hopelessness about the future
   3) Negative interpretation of neutral or innocuous events
   4) Self-reproachful feelings of guilt and worthlessness
   5) Current suicidal ideation or intent

a_4. A decline in motivation and interest that arose following the onset of illness or trauma capable of causing brain damage

a_5. No premorbid history of similar declines in motivation and interest in the absence of depression

Associated Features

a. Current behavior a possible exaggeration of premorbid tendencies
b. May alternate with periods of euphoria (see Moria)
c. A recent history of absent speech output (see Mutism)
d. A recent history of impaired initiation of movement (see Akinesia)
e. Impaired ability to persist with ongoing movements (see Motor impersistence)
f. Impaired termination of ongoing movements (see Motor perseveration)
g. Absence of spontaneous vocal and facial expressions of emotion (see Aprosodia)
h. Impaired recognition of familiar faces, visually or tactually presented objects, or sounds (see Agnosia)
i. Altered sexual activity, including increases or decreases in activity and changes in sexual orientation
j. Continuous manual exploration of the environment (termed *hypermetamorphosis*)
k. Continuously putting objects in the mouth, oral exploration of the environment (termed *hyperorality*)
l. Altered dietary habits, including bulimia and the consumption of nonfood items

NOTE: When agnosia, placidity and apathy, altered sexual activity, hypermetamorphosis, hyperorality, and altered dietary habits occur simultaneously, the entire complex is referred to as the Klüver-Bucy syndrome.

Factors to Rule Out

a. Depression sufficient to account for the decline in motivation and interest ruled out by documenting the absence of depression correlates (i.e., dysphoric affect, hopelessness, negative interpretation of neutral events, self-reproach, and suicidal ideation)
b. Use of prescribed or recreational drugs that reduce motivation, interest, and activity [the properties of drugs that the patient is taking should be checked in a current *Physician's Desk Reference* (PDR[4])]

Lesion Locations

a. Cerebral hemisphere[5]
b. Frontal lobe[6–9]
c. Temporal lobe, particularly the medial, inferior, and anterior temporal cortex, amygdala, and temporal white matter tracts[10]*
d. Combined parietal and occipital lobes[11]
e. Internal capsule (anterior limb and inferior genu), often with extension to the corona radiata and caudate nucleus[12,13]
f. Dorsolateral caudate nucleus, with or without extension to the internal capsule[14,15]
g. Thalamus[7,16–18]
h. Hypothalamus[19,20]†
i. Corpus callosum[7]
j. Midbrain[7]
k. Pons[7]
l. Periventricular white matter[21]

Lesion Lateralization

a. More common after left- than right-sided lesions

2. Anosodiaphoria (also called the indifference reaction)

Clinical Indicators

a_1. Indifference or lack of expected concern about medical or disability status
a_2. Relatively preserved awareness of medical and disability status
a_3. Indifference that arose following the onset of illness or trauma capable of causing brain damage
a_4. Current lack of concern varying from typical premorbid reaction to stress and personal misfortune

Associated Features

a. Current behavior a possible exaggeration of premorbid tendencies
b. Failure to notice stimuli on one or both sides of space (see Stimulus neglect)

---

*Lesions in these areas produce a full or partial Klüver-Bucy syndrome.

†Hypothalamic lesions have been associated with hyposexuality but not necessarily with the other features of abulia.

c. Impaired oral language, particularly Wernicke's aphasia (see Chap. 12)
d. Loss of vision following a cortical lesion (termed *cortical blindness*)
e. Lack of concern about unilateral motor weakness (hemiplegia) associated with mislocalization of tactual stimuli (see Stimulus mislocalization)

Factors to Rule Out

a. Denial or lack of awareness of illness or disability sufficient to account for the lack of concern (see Anosognosia), ruled out by documenting preserved awareness of medical and disability status
b. Stoical attempt to cope by remaining unaffected by personal misfortune, ruled out by documenting a discrepancy between current reaction and typical premorbid reactions to personal misfortune
c. Use of prescribed or recreational drugs that tranquilize or blunt emotional reactions (the properties of drugs that the patient is taking should be checked in a current PDR[4])

Lesion Locations

a. Cerebral hemisphere[22]
b. Inferior frontal gyrus[23]
c. Combined parietal and temporal lobes[23]
d. Combined internal capsule and putamen[24]

Lesion Lateralization

a. More common following right-sided lesions[22]

3. Moria

Clinical Indicators

a_1. An excited and euphoric mood despite the presence of significant illness or disability
a_2. Euphoria that arose following the onset of illness or trauma capable of causing brain damage
a_3. No premorbid history of euphoric reactions to stress or personal misfortune
a_4. No premorbid history of manic episodes during which all or a majority of the following signs were present:
  1) Expansive, elevated, or irritable mood
  2) Increased activity level
  3) Increased rate or amount of speech (i.e., pressured speech)
  4) Subjective experience of thoughts racing (i.e., flight of ideas)
  5) Delusional grandiosity
  6) Involvement in multiple ill-advised or high-risk activities

Associated Features

a. Current behavior a possible exaggeration of premorbid tendencies
b. May alternate with periods of decreased motivation and interest (see Abulia)
c. Irritability
d. Frequent caustic or facetious remarks (see Impulse disinhibition)
e. Increased verbal output (termed *hyperverbosity*)

Factors to Rule Out

a. Manic episode or the manic phase of bipolar affective disorder, ruled out by documenting the absence of premorbid manic episodes and the presence of illness or trauma capable of causing brain damage
b. Use of prescribed or recreational drugs that stimulate or elevate mood (the properties of drugs that the patient is taking should be checked in a current PDR[4])

Lesion Locations

a. Frontal lobe[9]
b. Ventromedial caudate nucleus[15]

Lesion Lateralization

a. More common following right-sided lesions[9]

4. Pathological laughing and crying

Clinical Indicators

a_1. Sudden involuntary laughter
a_2. Absence of a subjective feeling of mirth during the laughing episode
a_3. Involuntary laughter that arose following the onset of illness or trauma capable of causing brain damage
b_1. Sudden involuntary crying
b_2. Absence of a subjective feeling of sadness during the crying episode
b_3. Involuntary crying that arose following the onset of illness or trauma capable of causing brain damage

Associated Features

a. Attempts to explain the laughter or tearfulness by relating it, after the fact, to some event or thought that preceded the episode
b. Weakness of the facial muscles during voluntary movement but not during reflexive or automatic movement (termed *pseudobulbar palsy*)

Factors to Rule Out

a. Feelings or emotional reactions that are inappropriate or out of proportion to their stimulus (see Impulse disinhibition), ruled out by documenting the absence of subjective feelings of mirth or sadness during the laughing or crying episode
b. Use of prescribed or recreational drugs that have emotional side effects (the properties of drugs that the patient is taking should be checked in a current PDR[4])
c. Psychotic mental disorders, including schizophrenia, in which inappropriate affect may appear

Lesion Locations

a. Corticobulbar tract, typically in the pons, but also ventral to the pons[25–30]
b. Cerebral hemisphere[31–33]
c. Inferior frontal lobe, with frequent extension to the parietal lobe, temporal lobe, or basal ganglia[34,35]
d. Temporal lobe, particularly the middle and inferior temporal gyri[36,37]

Lesion Lateralization

a. Typically following bilateral lesions.

b. Pathological laughing more common following right-sided lesions; pathological crying associated with left-sided lesions[32]

5. Anosognosia

Clinical Indicators

a_1. Unawareness of obvious disability

a_2. Denial of disability even after it is demonstrated

a_3. Denial not caused by fear of and an attempt to avoid the consequences of a disability

a_4. Denial that arose following the onset of illness or trauma capable of causing brain damage

Associated Features

a. Invention of excuses to explain or minimize demonstrated disabilities (see Somatoparaphrenia)

b. Anger when confronted about disability

c. Blindness in all or a portion of the visual field

NOTE: Blindness and subsequent denial of the blindness is known as Anton's syndrome.

d. Failure to notice stimuli on one or both sides of space (see Stimulus neglect)

e. Impaired memory (see Amnesia) in patients who have Anton's syndrome

f. Visual hallucinations (see Visual hallucinosis) in patients who have Anton's syndrome

g. Confused ideation (see Ideational disorientation or confusion) in patients who have Anton's syndrome

h. Inaccurate localization of visual, auditory, or tactual stimuli (see Stimulus mislocalization) in patients who deny unilateral weakness (hemiparesis)

i. Oral language disorders that leave speech fluent, including Wernicke's aphasia and transcortical sensory aphasia

Factors to Rule Out

a. Failure to have been informed about own neurological and disability status

b. Minimization of the severity or frank denial of disability as a result of fear of the consequences of being disabled (e.g., loss of a job, loss of independence)

Lesion Locations

a. Cerebral hemisphere[38]

b. Cortical or subcortical frontal lobe, particularly the dorsolateral cortex, supplementary motor area, and cingulate gyrus, sometimes with extension to the area adjacent to the genu of the corpus callosum, the anterior limb of the internal capsule, and the caudate nucleus[9,39–41]

c. Parietal lobe, with frequent extension to temporal lobe and occasional extension to occipital lobe[40,42–44]

d. Temporal lobe[45]
e. Occipital lobe[40]
f. Insula[40]
g. Thalamus[40,43,46]
h. Basal ganglia (lenticular nucleus, head of the caudate nucleus, and/or putamen), with frequent extension to the internal capsule (anterior limb, genu, and/or superior aspect of posterior limb) and external capsule[40,43,47,48]
i. Posterior internal capsule[40]
j. Corona radiata[40]

Anton's syndrome

a. Occipital lobe, with occasional extension to the pons, midbrain, and thalamus[49,50]
b. Combined optic nerve and frontal lobe[51]

Lesion Lateralization

a. More common following right-sided lesions[40,52]
b. Anton's syndrome typically following bilateral lesions

6. Somatoparaphrenia

Clinical Indicators

a_1. Denial of ownership of a body part, usually a limb
a_2. Persistence of the denial despite being shown that the body part is attached to the rest of the body
a_3. Denial that arose following the onset of illness or trauma capable of causing brain damage

Associated Features

a. Assertion that the body part belongs to someone else
b. Referring to or treating the body part as if it were an impersonal object
c. Weakness in the limb for which ownership is denied
d. Denial of disability (see Anosognosia) because the impaired part of the body is believed to be foreign
e. Failure to notice stimuli on one or both sides of space (see Stimulus neglect)
f. Inaccurate localization of visual, auditory, or tactual stimuli (see Stimulus mislocalization)

Factors to Rule Out

a. Psychotic mental disorders, including schizophrenia, in which somatic delusions can occur

Lesion Locations

a. Cerebral hemisphere, simultaneously involving the frontal, parietal, and temporal lobes or the temporal, parietal, and occipital lobes[53,54]
b. Combined posterior corona radiata and supramarginal gyrus, with extension to larger areas within cerebral hemisphere[55]

Lesion Lateralization

a. Right hemisphere

7. **Ideational constriction**

Clinical Indicators

a_1. Reduced ability to think flexibly and abstractly, as indicated by any of the following signs:
   1) Concrete, literal interpretation of abstract concepts
   2) Rigid, inflexible approach to problems, tasks, or situations
   3) Failure to generate or perceive alternative approaches to problems, tasks, or situations

a_2. Current capacity for abstract thinking below what would be expected from education and occupation

a_3. Reduction in abstract thinking that arose following the onset of illness or trauma capable of causing brain damage

b_1. Reduced ability to reason (i.e., to draw conclusions or inferences) from known information

b_2. Current capacity for reasoning below what would be expected from education and occupation

b_3. Reduction in reasoning that arose following the onset of illness or trauma capable of causing brain damage

c_1. Reduced ability to plan ahead and organize time and activity

c_2. Current capacity for planning and organization below what would be expected from education and occupation

c_3. Reduction in planning and organization that arose following the onset of illness or trauma capable of causing brain damage

Associated Features

a. Current behavior a possible exaggeration of premorbid tendencies
b. Reduced word fluency (i.e., the ability to generate words starting with a specified letter or belonging to a specified category)
c. Failure to terminate movements (see Motor perseveration) or more complex behaviors (see Behavioral perseveration) at the required or specified time
d. Inability to inhibit impulses (see Impulse disinhibition)

Factors to Rule Out

a. Poor abstract thinking, reasoning, planning, or organization prior to the onset of illness or trauma

Lesion Locations

a. Frontal lobe, particularly the dorsolateral, medial, and supplementary motor* areas[56–64]
b. Temporal lobe,* alone or with extension to the parietal and occipital lobes[62]
c. Parietal lobe,* alone or with extension to the temporal and occipital lobes[62]

Lesion Lateralization

a. No documented consistent laterality effect[57–65]
b. Verbal or visuospatial nature of the reasoning task not consistently predicting the side on which the lesion has occurred

---

*A less severe form of this disorder results from lesions in this area.

8. **Ideational disorientation or confusion (see also Reduplication and Confabulation)**

Clinical Indicators

a_1. Confused ideation as indicated by one or more of the following signs:
   1) Inaccurate information or absence of information concerning the immediate situation or circumstances
   2) Inaccurate information or absence of information concerning the immediate environment
   3) Inaccurate information or absence of information concerning the general time of day (i.e., morning, afternoon, evening, night) or approximate date (i.e., year, month, day of the week, or season)
   4) Inaccurate information or absence of information concerning oneself (e.g., name, age, date of birth, occupation)
   5) Confusion of people, facts, and events
   6) Intelligible but incoherent speech

a_2. Confusion may include, but is not limited to, any of the following signs:
   1) Belief that familiar people have been replaced by impostors (see Reduplication)
   2) Belief that the current environment is in a different location than where it objectively is (see Reduplication)
   3) Belief that people have interchanged their physical appearances and personal identities (see Reduplication)
   4) Belief that a familiar person is recognized in someone having no physical resemblance to that person (see Reduplication)
   5) Unintentional filling of gaps in memory by seemingly concocted events (see Confabulation)

a_3. Confusion that persists or returns despite attempts to provide correct information

a_4. Confusion that arose following the onset of illness or trauma capable of causing brain damage

a_5. Confusion not present before the onset of illness or trauma

Associated Features

a. Degree of confusion that may fluctuate over time
b. Confusion that may be worse at night
c. Confusion that may prevent the performance of goal-directed activities
d. Impaired memory (see Amnesia)
e. Illusions and hallucinations (see Chap. 17)
f. Reduced alertness (see Chap. 2)
g. Decreased concentration (see Chap. 3)

NOTE: Decreased ability to concentrate in combination with ideational disorientation or confusion is referred to as a confusional state.

h. Inability to inhibit impulses (see Impulse disinhibition)
i. A decline in intrinsic motivation and interest (see Abulia)
j. Euphoric episodes (see Moria)

k. Failure to sustain ongoing movements (see Motor impersistence)
l. Failure to terminate movements at the required time (see Motor perseveration)
m. Impaired ability to find words to express ideas (see Anomic aphasia)
n. Written language disorder (see Chap. 13)
o. Impaired calculation ability (see Acalculia)
p. Impaired ability to draw or to construct puzzles (see Constructional disability)

Factors to Rule Out

a. Normal inaccuracy in response to questions about person, place, time, or situation
b. Psychotic mental disorders, including schizophrenia, that reduce contact with reality
c. Depressed mood or major depressive disorder sufficiently severe to lessen concern about and attention to the environment and ongoing events
d. Psychogenic amnesia: a mental disorder that manifests itself as a sudden inability to recall important personal information and is not explainable by normal forgetting, drug use, or neurological disease
e. Multiple personality disorder: a mental disorder that manifests itself in the presence of two or more "personality states" within the same person that alternately take control of the person's behavior
f. Psychogenic fugue: a mental disorder that manifests itself in sudden, unexpected travel, inability to recall the past, and assumption of a new identity and is not attributable to neurological disease
g. Acute or recent prolonged intoxication by alcohol or other drugs that reduce alertness and attention to the environment and ongoing events (drugs the patient has recently taken should be checked for intoxicating effects in a current PDR[4])
h. Loss of contact with the environment or ongoing events as a result of prolonged unconsciousness, isolation (as can occur in intensive care units), or confinement (including prolonged hospitalization)

Lesion Locations

a. Frontal lobe, particularly the inferior and middle frontal gyri, with occasional extension to the parietal lobe or basal ganglia[8,23,66–70]
b. Temporal lobe, including the amygdala and hippocampus, with occasional extension to the parietal or occipital lobes[23,71–75]
c. Medial occipital lobe, particularly the calcarine cortex and the lingual gyrus, alone or with extension to the temporal lobe, particularly the hippocampus and the fusiform and parahippocampal gyri, or the parietal lobe[11,23,72,73,76,77]
d. Basal ganglia, particularly the caudate nucleus[15,69,78]
e. Thalamus, particularly the dorsomedial nucleus, the mammillary bodies, and the mamillothalamic tract[11,18,79,80]
f. Pons[81]

g. Dura and choroid plexus[82]
h. Diffuse cerebral hemisphere[83]

Lesion Lateralization

a. May follow left, right, or bilateral lesions

9. Reduplication (including *reduplicative paramnesia, intermetamorphosis,* and *Capgras' and Frégoli's syndromes;* see also Ideational disorientation or confusion and Confabulation)

Clinical Indicators

a_1. Belief that the current environment is in a different location from where it objectively is
a_2. Relatively preserved awareness of the identity or nature of the current environment (e.g., patient is aware that he or she is in a hospital)
a_3. Persistence of the erroneous belief despite contrary evidence or the physical impossibility of the believed location
a_4. Erroneous belief that arose following the onset of illness or trauma capable of causing brain damage

NOTE: The previously described pattern of behavior is known as reduplicative paramnesia.

b_1. The belief that familiar people have been replaced by similar-looking or identical impostors
b_2. Relatively preserved visual recognition of people despite the belief that they are impostors
b_3. Persistence of the erroneous belief despite contrary evidence and its implausibility
b_4. Erroneous belief that arose following the onset of illness or trauma capable of causing brain damage

NOTE: The previously described pattern of behavior is known as Capgras' syndrome.

c_1. Belief that people have interchanged their physical appearances and personal identities
c_2. Persistence of the erroneous belief despite contrary evidence and its implausibility
c_3. Erroneous belief that arose following the onset of illness or trauma capable of causing brain damage

NOTE: The previously described pattern of behavior is known as intermetamorphosis.

d_1. Belief that one recognizes a familiar person in someone having no physical resemblance to that person
d_2. Persistence of the erroneous belief despite contrary evidence and its implausibility
d_3. Erroneous belief that arose following the onset of illness or trauma capable of causing brain damage

NOTE: The previously described pattern of behavior is known as Frégoli's syndrome.

Associated Features

a. Current environment possibly believed to be located in places of past or current personal significance
b. A decline in intrinsic motivation and interest (see Abulia)
c. Euphoric episodes (see Moria)
d. Impaired memory (see Amnesia)

Factors to Rule Out

a. Psychotic mental disorders, including schizophrenia, that lessen contact with reality and that are characterized by delusional thinking

Lesion Locations

a. Frontal lobe, with frequent extension to occipital and temporal lobes or the entire cerebral hemisphere[84–90]
b. Temporal lobe, including the hippocampus, with occasional extension to the parietal and frontal lobes and possible interruption of occipital-temporal fibers[91–94]
c. Medial parietal lobe[95]
d. Diffuse cerebral cortex[96]

Lesion Lateralization

a. Right-sided or bilateral lesions

10. Confabulation (see also Ideational confusion or disorientation and Reduplication)

Clinical Indicators

a_1. Unintentional filling of gaps in memory by seemingly concocted events, as indicated by any of the following signs:
   1) Reported events distortions or embellishments of actual events
   2) Reported events out of time frame (actually occurred at other times)
   3) Reported events fabricated

a_2. Tendency to confabulate that arose following the onset of illness or trauma capable of causing brain damage

Associated Features

a. Impaired memory (see Amnesia)
b. Impaired ability to place recently experienced stimuli in temporal order or to otherwise judge the relative recency of stimuli

NOTE: Impaired temporal ordering and judgment of recency are thought to reflect, and are often referred to as, deficits in time-tagging stimuli.

c. A decline in intrinsic motivation and interest (see Abulia)

Factors to Rule Out

a. Deliberate and inaccurate guessing about past events as a strategy to compensate for failing memory
b. Psychotic mental disorders, including schizophrenia, that lessen contact with reality

Lesion Locations

a. Frontal lobe, particularly the medial frontal lobe, with frequent extension to the temporal and parietal lobes and basal ganglia[8,97–100]

b. Basal forebrain[8,97,101,102]
c. Temporal lobe, with frequent extension to the parietal and occipital lobes[97,103,104]
d. Occipital lobe[97]
e. Thalamus, particularly the dorsomedial nucleus and the mammillothalamic tract[18,79,97]
f. Diffuse cerebral cortex[105]

Lesion Lateralization

a. May follow left, right, or bilateral lesions, but most frequent after right-sided lesions[106]

11. Behavioral perseveration (see also Motor perseveration)

Clinical Indicators

a_1. Failure to terminate behaviors at the required or specified time, as indicated by any of the following signs:
   1) Failure to shift from one set of behaviors to another
   2) Failure to abandon a previously established pattern of behavior or response
   3) Interference of a previous behavior on a current task

a_2. Perseveration that may include, but is not limited to, elementary movements (see Motor perseveration)

a_3. Perseveration that continues or recurs despite corrective feedback

a_4. Perseveration that arose following the onset of illness or trauma capable of causing brain damage

a_5. Perseveration not present before the onset of illness or trauma

Associated Features

a. Failure to terminate movements at the required or specified time (see Motor perseveration)
b. Reduced ability to think abstractly, reason, plan, and organize (see Ideational constriction)
c. Inability to inhibit impulses (see Impulse disinhibition)

Factors to Rule Out

a. Failure to generate or perceive alternative approaches to problems, tasks, or situations (see Ideational constriction) sufficient to account for the behavioral perseveration, ruled out by documenting continued or recurrent perseveration despite corrective feedback
b. Failure to comprehend the specified point at which a behavior should be terminated, ruled out by documenting continued or recurrent perseveration despite corrective feedback

Lesion Locations

a. Frontal lobe[66,85,98,107–112]
b. Retro-Rolandic* areas, without further localization[108]

---

*Although clinical lore suggests that perseveration is most often associated with anterior lesions, clinical reports vary as to whether greater frequency is seen after anterior or posterior lesions, and some clinical samples show no anterior-posterior difference.

c. Temporal lobe, with frequent extension to the parietal lobe[109–112]
d. Parietal lobe[110]
e. Occipital lobe[113]
f. Thalamus[112,114–116]
g. Hypothalamus[112]
h. Basal ganglia (caudate and putamen), with extension to the thalamus (anterior nucleus) and internal capsule[117]

Lesion Lateralization

a. May follow right, left, or bilateral lesions
b. Verbal tasks more likely to elicit perseveration after left-sided lesions and visuospatial tasks after right-sided lesions

12. Impulse disinhibition (also called pseudopsychopathy)

Clinical Indicators

a_1. Loss of impulse control and self-restraint, as evidenced by any of the following signs:
1) Outbursts of irritation, aggression, or rage in response to no or minimal provocation
2) Destruction of property with no motive or minimal provocation
3) Theft of objects of minimal or no personal use or monetary value
4) Disrobing in public places or in the presence of people with whom an intimate relationship is not shared
5) Erotic, lewd, or sexually exhibitionistic behavior in public places or in the presence of people with whom an intimate relationship is not shared

NOTE: Public disrobing and erotic, lewd, or sexually exhibitionistic behavior are sometimes referred to as hypersexuality.

6) Performance of personal bodily functions (e.g., relieving the bowel or bladder, picking the nose) in public places or inappropriate social contexts
7) Socially inappropriate facetious, caustic, or sexual remarks

NOTE: Inappropriate facetious and caustic remarks are termed Witzelsucht.

8) Feelings and emotional reactions that are inappropriate or out of proportion to their stimulus (termed *emotional lability*)

a_2. Failure to use past experience or feedback to guide current or future behavior, as evidenced by any of the following signs:
1) Failure to persist with behaviors that have previously led to desirable outcomes
2) Failure to inhibit or avoid behaviors that have previously led to undesirable outcomes
3) Failure to use credible feedback and advice to alter current or future behavior

a_3. Failure to anticipate and be influenced by negative or undesirable consequences (i.e., lack of foresight and judgment)
a_4. Inability to tolerate frustration or delays in gratification

a_5. Disinhibition that arose following the onset of illness or trauma capable of causing brain damage

a_6. Current degree and frequency of disinhibition differing from typical premorbid behavior

a_7. No premorbid history of any of the following mental disorders in which impulse disinhibition can occur:

1) Paraphilia: a group of mental disorders characterized by the use of unusual objects or activities to achieve sexual excitement and expression
2) Kleptomania: inability to inhibit impulses to steal objects, even if they are of little use or monetary value
3) Pyromania: inability to inhibit urges to set fires
4) Explosive disorder: intermittent loss of control of aggressive impulses
5) Antisocial personality disorder: persistence into adult life of a pattern of behavior in which the rights of others are violated
6) Borderline personality disorder: a personality disorder characterized by impulsive and self-damaging acts, intense but unstable relationships, lack of control over anger, rapid shifts in mood, and uncertainty about personal identity and direction
7) Schizophrenia and related psychotic mental disorders in which inappropriate behavior may occur

Associated Features

a. Current behavior a possible exaggeration of premorbid tendencies
b. Partial presentation of the disorder (e.g., showing some but not all clinical indicators) or presentation of different indicators over time
c. Increased verbal output (termed *hyperverbosity*)
d. Euphoric episodes (see Moria)
e. Failure to terminate behaviors at the required or specified time (see Behavioral perseveration)
f. Confused ideation (see Ideational disorientation or confusion)
g. Failure to generate or perceive alternative approaches to problems, tasks, or situations (see Ideational constriction)

Factors to Rule Out

a. Deliberate and premeditated violation of societal rules to achieve an objective (i.e., intentional criminal behavior)
b. Mental disorders in which impulse disinhibition can occur (see disorders listed under "Clinical Indicators") ruled out by documenting the absence of impulse disinhibition before the onset of illness or trauma
c. Acute or recent prolonged intoxication by alcohol or other drugs that reduce inhibitions and impair judgment (the properties of drugs that the patient is taking should be checked in a current PDR[4])

Lesion Locations

a. Frontal lobe, particularly the inferior frontal gyrus and the orbital and medial frontal cortex)[23,51,69,118–120]

b. Basal forebrain, particularly the septal nuclei, with frequent extension to orbital or medial frontal cortex[101,120,121]
c. Temporal lobe, including the amygdala and other parts of the limbic system, with occasional extension to parietal and occipital lobes, particularly the lingual gyrus[77,119,122–127]
d. Basal ganglia, particularly ventromedial caudate nucleus[15,69]
e. Pons[81]

Lesion Lateralization

a. Most common after bilateral lesions, but may follow unilateral left- or right-sided lesions

ETIOLOGY

Many of the disorders discussed previously are associated with frontal and anterior temporal lobe lesions. A common cause of such lesions is traumatic brain injury. The inner surface of the skull is relatively smooth posteriorly, but it contains bony protrusions over the frontal and anterior temporal lobes. More extensive damage occurs when the force of an impact drives the brain into these bony protrusions than when the brain is forced against the smoother posterior surface. Even when the initial impact site is in the rear of the skull, the contrecoup damage in the anterior brain regions may be more severe because of the differences in the topography of the inner skull surface. Most brain trauma cases involve closed-head injuries, although skull fracture is common. A smaller percentage of these cases involve penetrating brain wounds, most of which are injuries resulting from industrial accidents or gunshot.

Cerebrovascular accident (stroke) is also a common cause of neuropsychological disorders of emotion, ideation, and behavior. Strokes in the distribution of the anterior branches of the middle cerebral artery, the anterior cerebral artery, the anterior choroidal artery, or the basilar artery can lead to these disorders. Anterior communicating artery aneurysms are also associated with disorders of emotion, ideation, and behavior.

Compromise of the brain's electrolyte balance and metabolism is perhaps the commonest cause of ideational disorientation or confusion and is also associated with reduplication. The causes of electrolyte imbalance and compromised brain metabolism, which were discussed at length in Chapter 2, include conditions related to organ failure, nutritional deficiency, and exposure to toxic substances (e.g., mercury poisoning). Bronchial carcinoma without metastasis is a rare cause of disorientation caused by metabolic compromise.[71] Disorientation and confusion dominate the early clinical presentation of patients with Wernicke-Korsakoff syndrome. Confabulation is common in the chronic phase of this syndrome, in which amnesia dominates the clinical presentation.

Additional causes of the neuropsychological disorders of emotion, ideation, and behavior include hydrocephalus, neoplasm, degenerative disease (e.g., Alzheimer's disease, Pick's disease), demyelinating disease (e.g., multiple sclerosis), and central nervous system infection. Infections by herpes simplex, syphilis, and rabies, in particular, have been associated with behavioral changes. Diseases of the basal ganglia, such as Parkinson's and Huntington's diseases, have known behavioral correlates. Parkinsonism patients often present with abulia, whereas impulse disinhibition may be seen in patients with Huntington's disease. Pathological laughing and crying most often follow stroke but may also be seen as a consequence of carbon dioxide poisoning or amyotrophic lateral sclerosis.

Emotional, ideational, and behavioral disorders may be seen in epileptic populations. Ideational disorientation or confusion is common following seizures. In rare cases, pathological laughing (termed *gelastic epilepsy*), pathological crying (termed *dacrystic epilepsy*), and features of impulse disinhibition (e.g., aggression and inappropriate sexual behavior) may be seen during seizures. Impulse disinhibition during seizures remains a controversial phenomenon because of both its rare occurrence and its social implications. Proving that an act of aggression was the result of a seizure is very difficult and raises problems in the legal system, in which the act of aggression leads to adjudication. Less controversial are the behavioral disorders seen between seizures in patients with temporal lobe epilepsy. These include features of abulia (hyposexuality) and impulse disinhibition (aggression), as well as symptoms of depression, anxiety, and psychosis.

The disorders of emotion, ideation, and behavior are all too often iatrogenic. As noted previously, substance use and medication side effects should be ruled out before diagnosing many of the disorders listed in this chapter. Careful attention should be paid to use of barbiturates, opioids, analgesics, hypnotics, sedatives, tranquilizers, antihypertensives, anticholinergics, antidepressants, and any other neuroleptic substance that the patient may be taking. Surgical interventions, such as frontal lobectomy to remove necrotic or otherwise diseased tissue, may have unfortunate behavioral effects. So-called "psychosurgery" for the treatment of psychiatric disorders (e.g., frontal lobotomy, leukotomy) is also associated with neuropsychological disorders, although such cases are rare because these procedures have fallen out of favor. Abulia has been reported to occur as a consequence of thalamotomy, prophylactic cranial irradiation, and chemotherapy in cases of nonmetastasized small-cell lung cancer.

DISABLING CONSEQUENCES

Anosognosia and anosodiaphoria do not produce disability by themselves but rather add to the disability caused by other neuropsychological conditions. Patients who have one or both of these disorders are often poorly motivated for treatment of their other deficits. In extreme cases, they may refuse treatment even when their refusal leads to loss of jobs and relationships. Their disability is compounded by their unwillingness to consider therapy or their failure to give their best effort to the therapies they do receive.

Pathological laughing and crying can be socially embarrassing and personally perplexing. Occupational disability occurs when the patient has a career in which social communication and poise are essential to advancement and success. Individuals in the performing arts are impacted by this disability, because their work demands that they have control over their demeanor and emotional expression.

Moria and abulia can both produce severe disability. If these disorders manifest themselves intermittently, the disability may be somewhat less than that occurring when the disorders are virtually continuous. The abulic patient may lack motivation for therapy, school, or work. The motivation even to get out of bed and attend to daily grooming and hygiene may be lacking. If they fail to care for their personal needs, these patients may become dependent on others, even in their home environment. Family and friends who perceive an otherwise capable individual may blame the patient for his or her lack of motivation and eventually reject and abandon the patient as a hopeless loafer.

Patients who have moria can create an even greater degree of disturbance in work and home settings. Their exaggerated mood and behavior makes them socially inappropriate and creates a not-unfounded impression of unreliability. Such individuals are unlikely to function successfully in any work setting without a high degree of structure and close supervision.

Severe disability accompanies the ideational disorders. Patients who show confabulation or disorientation/confusion are unable to work, even with supervision. Their distorted thought processes can make them argumentative and disruptive, particularly in situations involving cooperation with others. Their decisions are inevitably poor because they are based on faulty or totally erroneous information. Their behavior can be dangerous to themselves and others, depending on the degree of confusion. They cannot assume responsibility for others, and usually cannot be trusted to tend to their own needs. Such patients are likely to be unsafe without continuous supervision. They are also unlikely to be competent to manage their own personal and financial affairs; family members often have to assume guardianship for the patient's protection. These patients cannot be considered competent to make decisions about their medical care or to give their consent to treatment. In many cases, the confusion is only transitory; if this is the case, the issue of guardianship can be avoided.

The faulty thinking that occurs in patients who have somatoparaphrenia or reduplication is less disabling. Nonetheless, these patients suffer great social stigma and may be regarded as less capable than they are. Society has little tolerance for those with strange ideas, and it is often assumed (many times rightly) that even an isolated delusion is sufficient to make an individual untrustworthy and unreliable. Ideational constriction is disabling mainly to individuals in occupations that require innovation, creativity, or the solution of problems. This disorder can effectively end the career of a scientist or artist. It can also greatly limit the careers of people in such widespread fields as law, machine repair, systems analysis, medical diagnosis, office management, and any supervisory or organizational occupation.

The defective planning seen in patients with ideational constriction may also produce a high degree of inefficiency in handling routine domestic chores. The patient may be unable to plan his or her leisure time or the time spent handling chores and errands. Planning meals for a week, or even a day, may be beyond the patient. The problem is compounded when others (e.g., child, spouse) depend on the patient.

Individuals who suffer from impulse disinhibition are likely to be in frequent or constant conflict with societal rules and expectations. They may be able to work, but only with a high degree of structure and supervision. Their safety in the home environment is uncertain, and in most cases they require constant supervision. These patients are unable to engage in any activity, including driving, in which the potential exists for causing injury to themselves or others. Domestic chores such as cooking often have to be avoided entirely or performed under maximum supervision. Impulsive patients are typically unable to manage their own affairs and can do themselves great financial harm if family members do not assume responsibility for them. Guardianship is almost always required, although in some cases the need for it can be difficult to demonstrate to the judicial system until the patient has squandered a portion of his or her finances. These patients are also often not competent to make decisions about their medical care or even to give their consent for treatment.

Similar limitations can occur in patients who show behavioral perseveration, although in many of these cases, the greatest disability is social. These patients' behavior makes them act inappropriately and often disruptively in social situations. This is particularly true if the patient fails to notice and respond to the social cues that normally guide behavior. When their failure to shift to alternative strategies compromises problem solving, significant occupational disability can occur. This is particularly true if the patient has a job that involves evaluation of alternatives, conflict resolution, or decision making. Interpersonal relationships also involve considerable compromise and flexibility and can suffer following the onset of behavioral perseveration.

ASSESSMENT INSTRUMENTS

Wisconsin Card-Sorting Test

The Wisconsin Card-Sorting Test (WCST)[128] can be obtained from *Psychological Assessment Resources, Incorporated, P.O. Box 98, Odessa, FL 33556-0998.*

The WCST consists of 4 stimulus cards and 128 response cards. The four stimulus cards depict one red triangle, two green stars, three yellow crosses, and four blue circles, respectively. The stimulus cards are arranged in a row in front of the patient in the previously listed order. The response cards are given to the patient in 2 decks of 64 cards each. Each response card depicts one of four possible shapes (i.e., triangles, stars, crosses, or circles) in one of four possible colors (i.e., red, green, yellow, or blue). The number of shapes on each card also varies from one to four.

In the standard administration, the patient is given a deck of response cards and is asked to match each consecutive card to one of the stimulus cards. The task is complicated by the fact that the "rule" for matching the cards is known only by the examiner. The patient must discover the target rule by choosing a potential match and noting whether the examiner responds with "correct" or "incorrect." The target rule specifies the attribute (i.e., color, form, or number) on which cards are to be matched. After the rule is discovered and the patient responds correctly for 10 consecutive trials, the rule is changed without any announcement to the patient. The patient must realize that he or she is now matching incorrectly, surmise that the rule has changed, and attempt to discover the new attribute that should guide matching. The process of discovery is further complicated by the fact that a response card may share more than one attribute with a particular stimulus card. For example, if the patient matches a response card showing three red triangles to the stimulus card showing one red triangle and the examiner responds "correct," the patient has no way of determining whether color or form is the correct sorting attribute for that trial.

Standard administration requires that 2 decks of cards be used, for a total of 128 trials. The test can be discontinued after all cards are used or the patient has successfully completed six sorts. The WCST can be frustrating and exhaustingly long for patients. Several shortened versions of the WCST have been proposed, including discontinuing after 64 cards or after 30 to 40 consecutive errors have been made.[129]

In the Nelson[62] modification of the WCST, all response cards sharing multiple attributes with the stimulus cards are removed from the deck, leaving 24 cards. Two decks are used for a total of 48 trials. Patients are told in advance what the possible matching rules are and are cued when the rule shifts. The smaller number of trials requires that the rule be shifted after every sixth consecutive correct match. The final modification consists of accepting as correct whatever matching rule the patient employs on the first trial. The Nelson modification decreases the length of the WCST and makes it less frustrating for patients to take. However, the WCST becomes a substantially easier test, which may lower its sensitivity to subtle problem-solving deficits.

I favor an approach to the WCST that combines features of the standard administration and the Nelson modification. The Nelson deck of cards is used, but the patient is not informed of the possible matching rules and is left to discover them based on trial-by-trial feedback, as in the standard administration. After the stimulus cards are placed on the table, the examiner asks the patient to list all the ways in which he or she thinks the response cards can be matched. The same request is made again after trial 24 and at the end of the test. The patient's initial choice of matching rules is accepted as correct, and shifts are made after every sixth consecutive correct response, but shifts in the target-matching rule are not announced.

A variety of scores can be obtained from the WCST. Many of the scores are calculated differently, depending on the version of the test being used. I calculate the following scores:

1. The number of completed sorts (6 consecutive correct responses) in 48 trials.
2. The total number of errors (incorrect matches).
3. The number of perseverative errors (i.e., responses that employ the same attribute as the immediately preceding incorrect response). By definition, tallying of this error can begin only after the second consecutive incorrect response. The first incorrect response is not included in the tally. This definition of the perseverative error score is derived from the Nelson modifica-

tion and differs from the perseverative error score calculated in the standard WCST administration.

4. The percentage of total errors that are perseverative in nature.
5. Failure-to-maintain-set errors (i.e., the number of trials on which the patient interrupts a sequence of three or more correct matches by suddenly matching based on another attribute).
6. The number of matching options identified by the patient before trial 1, after trial 24, and after trial 48.

Normative data are available for the WCST standard administration and scoring system for individuals aged 6.5 to 89 years.[128] The adult norms are derived from samples of 49 southwestern U.S. college students and their friends, 150 control subjects recruited in Texas and Colorado for a pesticide poisoning study, 50 subjects recruited in Colorado for a normative study, 124 commercial airline pilots recruited in Colorado and Washington, DC, and 73 healthy adults recruited in the metropolitan Detroit area. A subsample of 384 subjects over age 20 years was selected to reflect the age distribution of the U.S. population based on census data. Subjects in the younger age ranges are slightly underrepresented, whereas older subjects are slightly overrepresented in the WCST normative sample. The mean education level of the sample is 3 years higher than that of the U.S. population as of 1987.

Age and education are correlated significantly with performance on the standard version of the WCST.[128] Proficiency on the WCST increases to age 19 years, remains fairly stable to age 60 years, and begins to decline from age 60 years on. Education and WCST are linearly related, such that proficiency increases with years of education. Gender differences are reported to be not significant.[128] The test manual provides normative tables that enable the examiner to correct for age alone or age and education together. A table presenting normative data for the U.S. census–matched subsample is also available in the manual and is particularly useful for determining a patient's functional problem-solving capacity. The test manual also includes tables documenting the base rate of various levels of performance on the WCST in normal and clinical samples.

In one study, inter-scorer reliability coefficients for various WCST scores varied from .91 to .93 when experienced clinicians scored the test.[130] Reliability coefficients varied somewhat more (.75 to .97) for novice scorers. The sensitivity of the WCST standard administration to brain damage has been documented across multiple studies and patient samples.[128,131,132]

The WCST may be administered in the office, in the laboratory, or at bedside if a flat surface is available. A computerized administration is also available from the test's publisher. The WCST should be interpreted only by an experienced neuropsychologist.

Halstead-Reitan Battery, Category Test

The Halstead-Reitan Battery (HRB), Category Test,[133] manual version, can be obtained from *Reitan Neuropsychology Laboratory, 1338 Edison Street, Tucson,*

AZ 85719. The booklet and computerized versions can be obtained from *Psychological Assessment Resources, Incorporated, P.O. Box 998, Odessa, FL 33556.*

The HRB Category Test includes seven subtests, six of which have one underlying principle that the patient must discover. On each trial, the patient is shown stimuli that he or she is told suggest a number from 1 to 4. The target number is based on the principle underlying the subtest (e.g., the number of objects shown, the ordinal position of an odd or missing object). The patient selects a number and receives feedback about the correctness of his or her response. After the underlying principle is discovered, consistent application of it will yield all correct responses on the remainder of trials within the subtest. At the end of each subtest, the patient is told that the same principle may or may not apply to the next subtest. The final subtest consists of items drawn from the previous six subtests. The patient must attempt to recall the principles that applied to the items.

The HRB Category Test can be frustrating and exhausting for moderately to severely impaired patients, and several shortened versions have been developed.[134–136] Extensive normative data and corrections for the effects of age, gender, and education are available for the long form of the test.[137] Test-retest reliability coefficients for the HRB Category Test vary from .60 to .96 across normal, psychiatric, and neurological patient samples.[138,139] Internal consistency coefficients as high as .97 and .98 have been reported.[140,141] The HRB Category Test discriminates brain-damaged from non-brain-damaged patients better than the WCST, although the WCST is more accurate in specifically detecting frontal lobe damage.[142,143]

The HRB Category Test is a complex instrument that measures many cognitive abilities, including reasoning, problem solving, visual perception, concentration, and endurance. The complexity of the HRB Category Test probably accounts for both its high sensitivity and its lower specificity.

The manual version of the HRB Category Test is suitable only for office or laboratory administration because of the bulky stimulus presentation and response feedback equipment required. The booklet version can be administered at bedside, in the office, or in the laboratory. The HRB Category Test should be interpreted only by neuropsychologists trained and experienced in its use.

Wechsler Memory Scale–Revised, Information and Orientation Questions

The Wechsler Memory Scale–Revised (WMS-R), Information and Orientation Questions,[144] can be obtained from *The Psychological Corporation, P.O. Box 9954, San Antonio, TX 78204-2498.*

Questions in this test cover personal information (e.g., name, age), time, location, and to a limited degree, current events. Only the assessments of personal information, time, and place are sufficiently comprehensive for inclusion in most neuropsychological examinations. Awareness of one's current situation is virtually neglected, with the exception of three questions about hearing, visual acuity, and color blindness.

Like other WMS-R subtests (see Chaps. 3 and 16), the orientation section has the advantage of a normative database that extends from age 16 to 74 years and is representative of the U.S. population based on 1980 census data in age, gender, race, geographic residence, and education. Test-retest reliability coefficients reported in the manual for the orientation section vary from .24 to .72 across the three age groups that were tested twice. The orientation section differentiated patients with dementia, Huntington's disease, Wernicke-Korsakoff syndrome, traumatic brain injury, stroke, brain neoplasm, or seizure disorder from normal individuals at a statistically significant level.[144] In many instances, however, the difference between patients and normal control groups was one point or less, bringing into doubt the clinical significance of the statistical results.

The WMS-R information and orientation questions are a useful beginning for clinicians who wish to evaluate patients' ideational status, but the examiner will need to extend the assessment beyond the data gathered by these questions. The information and orientation section can be administered at bedside, in the office, or in the laboratory and is appropriate for use by a wide range of clinicians, including physicians, psychologists, and speech pathologists.

Benton Temporal Orientation Test

The Benton Temporal Orientation Test[145] can be obtained from *Oxford University Press, Incorporated, 200 Madison Avenue, New York, NY 10016.*

Awareness of the day of the week, the day of the month, the month, the year, and the time of day are assessed. Data are reported in the manual for 434 normal controls. Most control subjects obtained perfect scores, with the most frequent error being misidentification of the day of the month. Education appears to have a slight relationship to test performance (subjects with less than 12 years of education performed slightly worse than subjects with more education), but no effects of age, gender, or verbal intelligence on temporal orientation have been documented.[145] The Temporal Orientation Test appears to be sensitive to disorientation, particularly in patients who have bilateral cerebral disease.[145] Reliability data are not reported for the test.

The Temporal Orientation Test is brief and can be administered at bedside, in the office, or in the laboratory. It is appropriate for use by virtually any health care professional. Unfortunately, the test provides only a limited assessment of orientation, failing to measure domains such as awareness of personal information, awareness of location, and appreciation of one's situation. The test has few advantages over other orientation procedures that incorporate a more comprehensive assessment of the relevant domains of patient knowledge and awareness.

Minnesota Multiphasic Personality Inventory 2

The Minnesota Multiphasic Personality Inventory 2 (MMPI-2)[146] can be obtained from *National Computer Systems, Incorporated, P.O. Box 1416, Minneapolis, MN 55440.*

Since its inception about 50 years ago, the MMPI has become the most commonly used objective measure of personality and emotional disorder. The MMPI-2 is a restandardization of the original test that incorporates a national normative database more representative of the current U.S. population. It also features uniform T-score conversions, which produce an equivalent range and distribution of scores for the basic clinical (excluding scales 5 and 0) and content scales. The item content of the MMPI was edited to eliminate ambiguity, sexist wording, and dated or objectionable content. Several new scales are included in the MMPI-2 that require further investigation before their utility can be known. Overall, however, the MMPI and MMPI-2 yield very similar profiles.[147] The MMPI-2 is extensively discussed elsewhere.[146,148]

The role of the MMPI-2 in neuropsychological diagnosis lies in its ability to detect emotional and personality disorders that accompany or mimic neuropsychological disorders and that can affect cognitive test performance. A problem with using the MMPI-2 in this capacity is that many MMPI-2 items reflect symptoms that are actually a part of some neuropsychological disorders. This has led to the development of "neurocorrective factors" in an attempt to remove or lessen the impact of items that tap neuropsychological domains.

MMPI-2 neurocorrective factors have been developed for patients with traumatic brain injury[149] and cerebrovascular disease[150] that may increase the validity of the MMPI-2 results in these populations. It is recommended that MMPI-2 responses obtained from patients with brain injury or stroke be scored twice (with and without the neurocorrection factors)[150] and that the resulting profiles be compared to evaluate their relative fit for the patient. The applicability of these neurocorrective factors to patients with other neurological disorders is unknown.

The MMPI-2 can be administered at bedside, in the office, or in laboratory settings. Interpretation of results in neurological populations should be attempted only by clinical psychologists or neuropsychologists who are specifically trained in the use of the MMPI-2 and who have extensive experience with neurological patients.

Psychiatric Diagnostic Interview–Revised

The Psychiatric Diagnostic Interview–Revised (PDI-R)[151] can be obtained from *Western Psychological Services, 12031 Wilshire Boulevard, Los Angeles, CA 90025.*

The PDI-R is a structured interview, administered manually or by computer, consisting of predominantly yes-no questions that lead to a DSM-IV-R[2] diagnosis. The PDI-R covers 17 basic and 4 derived psychiatric syndromes, including depression, mania, schizophrenia, antisocial personality disorder, and somatization disorder. Questions for each of the basic disorders are arranged in four sections:

1. Cardinal questions, which review the critical symptoms of the disorder
2. Social significance questions, which measure the degree of disruption caused by the symptoms
3. Auxiliary questions, which elicit more information about how the disorder manifests itself in the person being interviewed
4. Time profile questions, which identify the age of onset and duration of the disorder

Each section of questions is contingent on the previous section. The examiner proceeds beyond the cardinal section only when a specified number of questions are answered in the affirmative. In this manner, the PDI-R can be administered rapidly, with the examiner concentrating only on the disorders present in the individual patient.

The PDI-R incorporates a hierarchical model of differential diagnosis, dividing the syndromes into "masking," "ordinal," and "additional" categories. A patient's current diagnosis is the disorder highest in the hierarchy that has been active during the last 2 years. For example, patients meeting criteria for both polydrug abuse and antisocial personality disorder in the last 2 years would receive a diagnosis of polydrug abuse because it falls higher in the hierarchy. Procedures are detailed in the PDI-R manual for determining a longitudinal diagnosis that best characterizes the psychiatric symptoms experienced by the patient over the course of his or her lifetime.

The reliability and validity of the original version of the PDI were extensively investigated and are reviewed in the PDI-R manual.[151] The reliability and validity of the PDI-R are based on its similarity to the previous version of the instrument. Both versions were administered to 53 psychiatric patients by independent examiners. When all disorders that met criteria for being "positive" were entered into the analysis, agreement between the two instruments ranged from 81 to 100 percent (median, 96.2 percent).[151] The current diagnoses derived from each version of the instrument were in agreement 85 percent of the time, and the longitudinal diagnoses agreed 87 percent of the time. Diagnoses were considered to be in agreement when they were the same or similar (e.g., schizophrenia and schizoaffective disorder). Overall, the two versions of the instrument appear to lead to similar diagnoses. Further specific investigation of the reliability and validity of the PDI-R is desirable.

The PDI-R has been criticized for the limited scope of its questions covering the diagnosis of organic brain syndrome and for its failure to include other sources of information about patients (e.g., mental status examination results). Although it is not always possible to arrive at a diagnosis based on interview and history, the PDI-R nonetheless structures and standardizes an important part of the diagnostic process. The principal use of the PDI-R in neuropsychological diagnosis is as an aid in ruling out psychiatric disorders that mimic neuropsychological disorders or that may alter the interpretation of cognitive test results.

Interpretation of the PDI-R should be attempted only by experienced psychiatrists, clinical psychologists, or neuropsychologists. The instrument is appropriate for bedside, office, or laboratory administration.

Adult Neuropsychological History Protocol

The Adult Neuropsychological History Protocol (ANH)[152] can be obtained from *International Diagnostic Systems, Incorporated, P.O. Box 389, Worthington, OH 43085.*

The ANH can be administered either as a questionnaire or as part of a structured diagnostic interview. Items cover the patient's early history (prenatal, perinatal, postnatal, and developmental problems), medical history (accidents and illnesses), family history, personal history (educational achievement and school-related problems, marital history, occupational history, and recreational interests), drug use, current symptomatology, and previous medical testing. The survey of current symptoms is comprehensive and includes an assessment of problem-solving, language-related, perceptual, concentration, memory, sensory, motor, behavioral, and physical problems.

The ANH is not a substitute for neurological or neuropsychological examination, and the data obtained cannot be considered proof of the presence or absence of any particular disorder or syndrome. Instead, the ANH furnishes subjective data that can be used to guide or plan an objective examination. Compared to unstructured preliminary interviews, the ANH is efficient, organized, and thorough, reducing the likelihood that pertinent information will be overlooked. The ANH has not been subjected to empirical validation. Documentation of its test-retest reliability and factor structure would be highly desirable, as would a systematic investigation of how closely ANH results parallel objective test findings.

The ANH is appropriate for bedside, office, or laboratory administration and can also be sent home with the patient to be filled out as a questionnaire. The ANH can be administered directly to patients or can be filled out by a family member or other person familiar with the patient's past and current problems. As long as the ANH symptom responses are viewed as a source of subjective data that may or may not coincide with objective test findings, the protocol can be used by a broad range of clinicians, including physicians, psychologists, speech pathologists, social workers, and nurses.

Neuroemotional-Neuroideational-Neurobehavioral Symptom Survey

The Neuroemotional-Neuroideational-Neurobehavioral Symptom Survey is *not commercially available.*

The Symptom Survey is presented in Appendix 18–1. This survey was designed to elicit and organize data that aid in the diagnosis of neuropsychological disorders of emotion, ideation, and behavior. Items also cover illusions and hallucinations associated with brain dysfunction (see Chap. 17). The first section of the survey establishes the patient's level of orientation and includes items covering personal information, time, location, and situation. Items are also included that elicit information about reduplication.

The second section of the survey addresses the patient's awareness of and concern about perceptual, motor, communication, concentration, memory, calculation, thinking-skill, and emotional-behavioral deficits. The questions listed for assessing the patient's reaction to his or her deficits can be used interchangeably or paraphrased to fit the patient's circumstances. It is important to solicit specific examples from the patient of any deficit that he or she acknowledges to fully evaluate the degree to which the patient is actually aware of the problem. Patients who are unable to give specific examples may not genuinely understand their deficits.

The next two sections of the survey attempt to solicit subjective data that may indicate the presence of illusions and hallucinations. When making these inquiries, it is important to stress that such experiences are a part of the illness or condition and do not mean that the patient is "going crazy." This may alleviate concerns the patient has about his or her experiences and also may make the patient more willing to report them. The final two sections solicit information about somatoparaphrenia, diagonistic apraxia (see Chap. 10), motivation, and pathological laughing and crying.

Two sets of qualitative observations are also included in the Symptom Survey. The Post-survey Observations section should be completed immediately after the interview. This section addresses the quality and content of the patient's answers. The Post-examination Observations section is completed after the entire neuropsychological examination has been performed. Items in this section cover the patient's motivation, affect, and behavior. Additionally, the examiner is asked to indicate the validity of the examination.

The Symptom Survey includes several tallies of responses, which are provided for summary purposes only. The most useful data are not the number of items checked but rather the specific items checked, the subjective information obtained from the patient, and the examiner's observations. Reliability and validity data are not available for the Symptom Survey. Its function is not to provide an objective assessment, but rather to guide and structure the examiner's interview so that information pertinent to establishing a diagnosis is obtained.

The Symptom Survey can be administered at bedside, in the office, or in laboratory settings. I use it in conjunction with sections of the PDI-R and the ANH. Data obtained from the Symptom Survey should be interpreted only by an experienced neuropsychologist, neurologist, psychiatrist, or physiatrist.

Behavioral Monitoring Procedure

The Behavioral Monitoring Procedure is *not commercially available.* See discussion in Chap. 3.

Intermittent emotional, ideational, and behavioral disorders (e.g., behavioral perseveration, pathological laughing and crying, impulse disinhibition) sometimes cannot be elicited by direct testing or questioning. In these instances, diagnosis may depend on sustained observation of the patient and assessment when the disorder happens to manifest itself. A behavioral monitoring procedure was presented in Chap. 3 for use in detecting concentration deficits. The same procedure and forms can be adapted for use with intermittent emotional, ideational, and behavioral disorders.

NEUROPSYCHOLOGICAL TREATMENT

Many treatment approaches are available for neuropsychological disorders of emotion, ideation, and behavior. These approaches are based on techniques developed for use with similar psychological problems arising in neurologically healthy individuals. The efficacy of such treatments in neurological populations is a subject of ongoing investigation. A review of this area is beyond the scope of this text, but a brief summary of some available treatment options is provided.

Educating Patients and Families

Of primary concern in the treatment of the disorders in this chapter is the education of the family and patient. In many cases, the patient's disorder prevents him or her from developing a clear understanding of the nature and causes of the behavior problem, but family members can comprehend and benefit from this information. I have found it useful to use diagrams or models of the brain to map the location of the patient's lesion for the patient and family members. A visual model of what has happened to the patient often lends credibility and gravity to the explanations offered by the neuropsychologist. Once the area of damage is known, the nature of the resulting disorders can be discussed. It is important to help the family distinguish neuropsychological disorders from the psychiatric mental disorders that they may resemble. Finally, recommendations about how to cope with the problem can be made.

Treatment of Disorders of Emotion

Patients suffering from abulia are often the most difficult to treat successfully. Psychologists may approach depression by getting the patient to discuss his or her feelings and offering support and advice on how to eliminate the causes of the dysphoric mood, by attempting to get the patient reinvolved in rewarding and enjoyable activities, or by challenging the erroneous ideas and interpretations that are presumed to precede depressed affect. The abulic patient, unfortunately, may have nothing to discuss. The patient does not feel depressed or, for that matter, may not feel much of anything. There are no evident erroneous ideas to challenge. The patient often leaves the therapist with little material on which to focus.

In general, the abulic patient can best be approached from the standpoint of providing external motivation to make up for the lack of internal motivation. The patient typically must be given a schedule of activities that are themselves intrinsically rewarding. Providing tangible and immediate external rewards for performing scheduled activities is essential. Abulic patients may require a "coach" who cajoles, pushes, demands, praises, prods, and structures the patient throughout the day. Graphic monitoring procedures and charts that the patient can review on a daily basis to note progress should also be incorporated. Such procedures may never return the patient's internal capacity for motivated behavior, but they may make the patient more active, functional, and independent.

If the psychological treatment of mania is used to obtain ideas on how to treat moria, there will be little to draw on. Effective psychological treatments of mania are not available; manic patients typically are treated pharmacologically. The neuropsychologist can try fostering behaviors incompatible with the excitement seen in patients suffering from moria. Progressive deep muscle relaxation and relaxation via imagined scenes can be tried with these patients, although the likelihood of success is questionable.

Many cases of anosognosia are transient, but when the disorder persists, it can greatly impede treatment. I have observed patients who remained oblivious to obvious disabilities for longer than 1 year despite experiencing failures in virtually all aspects of their lives. Anosognosic patients require gentle confrontation about their deficits. Forceful confrontation may engender anger and rejection of the therapist. Often, the best approach is to let the patient test his or her abilities in realistic and meaningful settings. Care must be taken to ensure the patient's safety, and situations in which a real potential for injury exists must be avoided. Care must also be taken to minimize the long-term consequences of the patient's failure. Allowing the patient to return to work and then fail may lead to loss of the job, a price that is too high to pay for the sake of proving a point.

With these cautions in mind, the therapist can allow the patient to try various activities and fail. It is helpful to have the patient state in advance how he or she expects to perform. The failure to live up to his or her own expectations can have a powerful impact on the patient's awareness of deficits. In other cases, a family member or coworker can be recruited to perform activities just before the patient tries them. Failure to do as well as a spouse or peer can also be an eye-opening experience for the patient.

Patients can sometimes accept that they have deficits if the therapist allows them the possibility of overcoming the deficits in the future. American culture mythologizes the person who overcomes impossible odds or great personal obstacles. The print and film industries constantly reinforce this myth to the point where the average person often believes that recovery from brain damage is just a matter of willpower. For the patient to admit a permanent disability is tantamount to giving up and being a loser. Patients must be allowed to keep their hopes. Challenging deeply held personal myths is rarely appreciated and rarely successful. A more fruitful approach involves tapping into the patient's personal mythology to increase motivation for treatment. Declaring that recovery, as well as adjustment to disability, is more likely the harder the patient works in therapy can give a resistant patient a reason to participate in his or her own treatment.

Somatoparaphrenia can be approached in a manner similar to that used for anosognosia. The patient can be exposed carefully to situations in which his or her disability is apparent. In this instance, the objective is not to overcome a lack of disability awareness but rather to instill an appropriate degree of concern about the disability to foster a desire for rehabilitation.

Neuropsychological approaches to pathological laughing and crying are not available. Intervention is usually limited to educating the patient and family about the nature of the disorder so that it does not become a source of unnecessary concern. Family members often misinterpret pathological crying as depression. The mother of an adolescent with brain injury who was one of my patients was convinced that her son's pathological laughing was a deliberate attempt on his part to be rude, silly, and obnoxious. Correcting these misconceptions is an important step in getting family members to respond in appropriate ways. Often the distress and attention caused by the behaviors exacerbates the problem. Calm inattention in many cases is the preferred response, unless the patient becomes embarrassed and distressed by this reaction. Once they understand the nature of the disorder, the family can offer support and reassurance, reminding the patient of the cause of the problem and that each episode of laughing and crying is likely to be brief. Showing the patient that family members can accept and adjust to the behavior may make it easier for the patient to accept the behavior as well.

Treatment of Disorders of Ideation

Somatoparaphrenia usually responds to repeated demonstrations of the impossibility of the delusion. Showing the patient clearly that the disowned body part is attached to the rest of the body eventually dispels the delusion. Use of mirrors and having the patient touch the affected body part may facilitate his or her acceptance of reality. Often, some remnants of the delusion remain, but at least on an abstract level, the patient conforms to that which is undeniably real.

Medical intervention is essential in severe cases of ideational disorientation or confusion. The cause of the confusion is often treatable, and every effort should be made to identify the cause and intervene as appropriate. Nevertheless, confusion may persist for days or weeks after the cause is treated. It is during this phase that neuropsychological intervention is of value. Patients should be provided with accurate information to help orient them to time and location. Correction of erroneous ideas in a gentle but firm manner is also of value. All staff members involved in the patient's care should participate in reorienting the confused patient. Corrective information provided by multiple sources throughout the day is more effective than a 5- or 10-minute orientation session each morning by one staff person. Involvement of family and other visitors is also helpful. Displaying calendars, a written schedule, and a chart with other orienting information can facilitate clearing of confusion. Television, in contrast, may exacerbate a patient's confusion because of its intermingling of reality and fiction. Room changes, variations in schedule, staff changes, and changes in roommates should be kept to a minimum because they can further disturb a patient's sense of reality and stability.

When patients are adamant about their erroneous or confused notions, argument is of no use. Staff members should calmly state accurate information and then reduce stimulation (e.g., remaining quietly beside the patient or taking a few steps away) until the patient calms down, stops making erroneous assertions, and is again ready to listen to what the staff person has to say. It is advisable to ignore the patient's arguments and protestations and not to try to reason with the patient or prove a point of view. Instead, the staff person should present information to the patient in a calm and nonconfrontational manner. Similar procedures are appropriate for patients who confabulate or who evidence reduplication.

Techniques for the treatment of ideational constriction may be found in procedures used to teach students problem solving and creative thinking. Although patients usually cannot learn or apply multistep problem-solving methods, they may be able to learn simplified techniques and may benefit from practice in working out solutions to problems. Patients can be taught to write down their goals and their current position with respect to their goals when confronted with a problem. The task then becomes one of "brainstorming": figuring out as many ways as possible to bridge the gap between the current position and the goal. No concern is given to the practicality of the solutions during brainstorming; the goal is simply to think of as many alternatives as possible. Patients who have difficulty in thinking of alternatives should be encouraged to consult other individuals for possible ways of reaching the goal. Once the patient has several alternative solutions to choose from, the task becomes one of sifting through the alternatives until the best solution is found. As is the case with normal, healthy individuals, the process of arriving at the right solution is often one of trial and error.

Patients who lack the ability to brainstorm and evaluate alternatives may benefit from simply learning to ask for and follow the guidance of others. When a problem is repeatedly presented to the patient in various guises, and the same solution works each time, the patient may eventually learn to generate and carry out the solution independently.

The temptation when treating problem-solving deficits is to use exercises that are as abstract and far removed from life as the procedures used in the clinic to test problem-solving, reasoning, abstract thinking, and organization. This approach should be avoided. Problems and exercises should be drawn from the patient's home and work environments. In many cases, the patient performs better with realistic and familiar problems than with mock problems. In all cases, the patient's motivation to work on problem solving is higher when the problems are familiar and seem relevant to daily life.

Treatment of Behavioral Disorders

In most clinical settings, behavioral perseveration is managed rather than treated. Patients are redirected by staff away from ideas and behaviors they are fixated on. Similar techniques can be taught to family members for use at home or in social situations. It may also be of benefit to work with patients on recognizing the social cues that signal the unwanted persistence of a behavior. In some rare cases, patients may succeed in responding to these cues and spontaneously shift away from the perseverative behavior without more overt external intervention.

Neuropsychologists have a rich repertoire for addressing the behaviors that make up impulse disinhibition. The goal of the procedures used is never the total elimination of impulsive and undesirable behaviors. Such a goal would not be realistic in any setting. Instead, the objective of the various behavioral techniques is to produce a tangible reduction in the frequency of undesirable behaviors and a corresponding increase in the frequency of desirable behaviors. This is an important point for treatment teams to keep in mind when they work with impulsive patients. Total elimination of the impulsivity is unlikely, but reduction of impulsivity is a reasonable objective.

Time-out, a procedure that can be as easy as reducing environmental stimulation or that can involve removing the patient to a location of quiet and solitude, is effective in reducing aggression and many other socially inappropriate acts. The rationale for this procedure is that unwanted behaviors can be reduced by taking the patient out of the environment that reinforces these behaviors. In many cases, however, the procedure works simply by giving the patient time to cool off and regain his or her composure and self-control. It often helps to tell the patient that he or she is out of control and that time-out is being used to give him or her an opportunity to calm down and regain control. Time-out should be brief (5 to 10 minutes) and delivered in a nonpunitive and unemotional manner. Time-out is not meant to be a punishment. When used correctly, patients may even ask for a time-out period when they perceive themselves as being out of control.

Social disapproval can also be effective in correcting inappropriate behaviors. Patients need feedback, both positive and negative, about the effect their behavior has on others. Such feedback should be delivered in a calm, impersonal manner. Communicating disapproval without communicating anger is particularly difficult for family members because of their emotional involvement with the patient. It can also be difficult for staff when they are angry about something the patient has done. Social disapproval is not an opportunity for staff to retaliate against the patient. In all cases, as much or more time should be spent in communicating approval for appropriate behaviors as is spent in communicating disapproval.

Modeling socially appropriate behaviors and having patients rehearse these behaviors in mock situations may help the patient actually to exhibit these behaviors in realistic situations. Rehearsal can also occur covertly. In this approach, the therapist guides the patient in imagining how he or she will cope and behave in various problem situations. Such procedures can help inoculate the patient against situations in which loss of control is likely. When a patient begins to lose control in an actual situation, staff members can intervene by redirecting the patient to some other situation or topic. The success of this technique depends on its use before the patient has gotten so far out of control that he or she can no longer respond to social and verbal cues.

Patients who impulsively destroy property or abuse the rights of others can be required to make restitution.[153] Restitution involves immediately restoring the disrupted environment to better than its original condition. Similarly, restitution can be made to offended or injured individuals, by requiring the patient to apologize and perform some service to the person, for example. This procedure repairs the damage done by the patient, prevents the patient from enjoying the results of his or her impulsive behavior, and has face validity in that it matches an appropriate and natural consequence with the patient's inappropriate behavior.

Other techniques, familiar to most behavioral psychologists, are also available. These include traditional techniques such as extinction, which involves removing the reinforcers for an unwanted behavior. Often, this involves ignoring inappropriate behaviors (depriving the patient of attention) while reinforcing desirable behaviors that are incompatible with impulsive acting out. Contracts can be negotiated with patients who are sufficiently intact to understand and remember the contingencies specified in the contract. Behavioral contracts define desirable and undesirable behaviors and specify the consequences of each behavior.

Contracts have the advantage of making the patient a partner in his or her treatment. Once they agree to and sign a contract, the patient and therapist can work together toward the same goal rather than working at cross purposes. Having staff members monitor the patient's behavior and sometimes having the patient monitor his or her own behavior, using a tally sheet, help to ensure compliance with contracts and allows all parties to see the changes occurring in the patient's behavior. With or without a contract, behavioral monitoring can have a potent effect. In many instances, the act of monitoring itself is sufficient to greatly reduce the frequency of problem behaviors.

CASE ILLUSTRATIONS

CASE 4–5

R.M. was a 50-year-old man with a high school education. Following triple coronary artery bypass grafting, he developed atrial fibrillation and an anoxic encephalopathy. Magnetic resonance imaging (MRI) scans revealed bilateral watershed area infarctions (i.e., C-shaped infarctions extending from the frontal to the occipital poles), with greater damage evident in the right hemisphere. R.M.'s history was negative for any psychiatric hospitalization or treatment. At the time of examination, R.M. showed no loosening of associations, hallucinations, delusions, or any other symptoms of psychiatric disorder. The patient did present with a number of visual deficits, including an inability to simultaneously perceive multiple stimuli (see Simultanagnosia) and an additional tendency to neglect visual information on his left side (see Hemispatial neglect).

R.M. had bilateral motor weakness that was mild in the right upper extremity but severe in the left to the point that the left arm and hand could not be used for purposeful and coordinated movements. R.M. was unable to point accurately to positions on the left side of his body, pointing instead to the corresponding locations on his right side. When the mislocated body parts were touched by the examiner while the patient's vision was occluded, R.M. indicated having perceived the touch at locations to the right of where the touch had actually been.

When asked what the effect of his stroke had been, R.M. readily indicated that he was weak on both sides and pointed out that he could, however, move his right arm fairly well. When asked to indicate his left arm, R.M. raised the right arm. When the left arm was moved by the examiner to a position in front of the patient, R.M. identified it as belonging to his wife. The examiner asked R.M. to move his right hand along the left arm up to the shoulder and asked him how his wife's arm could be attached to his body. R.M. shrugged and made no reply. Some time later, the examiner again moved the left arm into view and queried the patient as to what it was. R.M. replied that it was "R's arm." After lowering the arm to the patient's side, the examiner asked R.M. to point to his left arm, and R.M. again raised his right arm instead.

DISCUSSION

The patient in Case 4–5 presented with somatoparaphrenia associated with simultanagnosia and left hemispatial neglect (see Chap. 4), bilateral weakness that was worse in the left arm, and mislocalization of tactual stimuli (see Chap. 8).

Although anosognosia is typical in such cases, this patient was able to describe his bilateral weakness while believing that his left arm belonged to his wife. It is possible that he had only an abstract notion of what his deficits were based on what his physicians had told him, which he was able to repeat when queried.

A similar phenomenon may have occurred when it was demonstrated to R.M. that what he believed was his wife's arm was attached to his body. He seemed initially confused by this demonstration, but later referred to his arm as "R's arm." This remark does not clearly indicate acceptance of ownership because the arm is referred to in the third person. R.M. appears to acknowledge intellectually that the arm belongs to him while continuing to view the arm from an impersonal perspective.

CASE 18–1

H.S. was a 63-year-old man who had worked as a bank courier until retiring as a result of poor health. He suffered from hypertension and recurrent pulmonary edema. His medical history was positive for double coronary artery bypass grafts and a right carotid endarterectomy. He suffered an apparent left cerebrovascular accident while hospitalized for treatment of pulmonary edema and cardiac arrhythmia. Computed tomographic (CT) scans revealed left cerebellar and left occipital lobe embolic infarctions, and left temporal slowing was documented by electroencephalogram.

The examiner met the patient 1 day prior to his scheduled neuropsychological examination to explain the purpose of the upcoming procedures. At that time, the patient denied having had a stroke, although he was aware of being in the hospital. The examiner asked H.S. directly if he had any weakness in his limbs, and the patient responded that he did not. The examiner insisted that he, the patient, was indeed weak on one side of his body and further queried the patient as to which side was the weaker, cautioning the patient to try to move both sides of his body before answering. Yielding to the examiner's arguments about his weakness, H.S. reported that the left side of his body was weak. At the time, H.S. had a severe right hemiparesis.

To verify that H.S. had not confused the sides of his body, the examiner placed his hand on the patient's left shoulder and queried as to whether this was the side he was referring to. H.S. again indicated the left side was the weaker. When asked how he felt about having weakness, the patient had no immediate response, but finally stated, "I guess it's okay, I guess they'll help me." He denied any specific concerns about his future, indicating that he expected to go home with his wife after he got well.

DISCUSSION

H.S. presented with anosognosia for his hemiparesis. The examiner's insistence that H.S. had weakness resulted in an abstract acceptance without genuine personal acknowledgment of the disability. Even when asked to move his limbs to compare their relative strength, H.S. still had no clear perception of his deficit. Although he was not totally indifferent to having weakness, H.S. did not show any great emotional distress, nor could the examiner detect any specific concerns or fears for the future that might have motivated the patient's denial.

CASE 18–2

A.P. was an 89-year-old woman with a bachelor's degree in education who had worked as a teacher until her retirement. She suffered two right cerebrovascular accidents, 1.5 years apart. The first produced an area of infarction in the right occipital lobe, and the second resulted in areas of infarction in the posterior right frontal and right temporal lobes. A small anterior meningioma, along with widespread brain atrophy consistent with the patient's age, was noted in CT and MRI scans. Neuropsychological examination revealed a left hemiparesis, a left visual field cut, and severe neglect of left-sided visual stimuli. Performance on all tests of visual perception was impaired as a result of the neglect. The patient showed severe motor perseveration and impaired ability to execute alternating series of movements rapidly. Memory for verbal information and problem solving were intact relative to people her age.

The patient was tearful at several points in the examination. When asked if she was distressed by her performance, she denied that she was. She did report occasional bouts of depressed affect and self-pity but denied that this accounted for her crying. She expressed embarrassment and apologized for the tearful episodes, stating that she felt fine and did not know why she cried. She specifically denied that the crying episodes were related to her mood. The patient denied any history of psychiatric disorder, nor were any current symptoms of psychiatric disorder present other than the reported episodes of sad affect and the tearfulness. At the time of examination, A.P.'s medications included digoxin, propranolol hydrochloride, nifedipine, and diphenhydramine hydrochloride.

DISCUSSION

A.P. presented with pathological crying. Although she had a degree of depression, she did not subjectively associate her mood with the tearful episodes. The episodes were experienced as being inexplicable and beyond her control. Propranolol is associated with emotional lability but not specifically with pathological crying episodes.

CASE 18–3

D.A. was a 29-year-old woman with a 10th-grade education who worked at a convenience store. She suffered a traumatic brain injury when struck by a car while walking across a parking lot. In addition to suffering multiple fractures (including a skull fracture), the patient had bilateral frontal lobe contusions and a left temporal-parietal hematoma. Following an initial inpatient rehabilitation stay, the patient resumed work at the convenience store. Her performance was notably worse than before. D.A. was unable to remember where items were located in the store and on several occasions consumed liquor that was sold in the store. This continued despite being told by her physician not to drink and despite threats by the store manager to fire her. The patient was eventually fired and entered the state vocational rehabilitation system, which arranged for a comprehensive day rehabilitation program.

The current neuropsychological examination was conducted 1 year after her accident. The patient was intact in her concentration, stimulus and spatial perception, and oral language. She showed no decrease in strength or motor speed, but was notably clumsy on fine motor coordination tasks. No other movement problems were present. D.A. was severely impaired in her memory for new verbal and visuospatial information, and she complained of being unable to clearly remember events that occurred several weeks before her accident. The most severe impairment was seen on the WCST. The patient attained only a single sort, despite being aware of all three possible sorting principles. Although most of her errors were perseverative (60 percent), she also frequently interrupted sequences of correct responses with sudden changes in strategy.

In social situations, the patient often made inappropriate comments that embarrassed others (e.g., she began talking about sexual orgasm in a group of elderly patients she had just met). Additionally, the patient was given to bouts of prolonged and excessively loud laughter in response to comments made by herself or others that struck her as humorous. Although some of these comments drew laughter from others, D.A.'s laughter was always the loudest and persisted long after everyone else had stopped laughing.

When playing board games with other patients, D.A. got into frequent disputes about the rules of the games, and she had daily incidents during which she lost her temper. She was particularly frustrated when playing with older patients who were slow to take their turns or who made mistakes during the game. At these times, she would angrily give them orders to speed their play or would attempt to take their turns for them (e.g., taking cards from other players and deciding for them what card to play). Her anger was always expressed verbally, but because of the frequency with which she lost her temper, other patients avoided her and staff members noted her anger as being a problem.

Consultation with the patient's husband revealed that he also noted a decrease in her ability to control her anger. She got into frequent arguments with her mother, which had not been characteristic of her before the accident. Her husband also noted the increase in socially inappropriate comments and the exuberance of her laughter, but was not as concerned about these latter problems. The patient and her husband confirmed the absence of any history of mental or personality disorder before the onset of brain damage.

DISCUSSION

A diagnosis of pathological laughing might be considered in this case, but the fact that the laughter was associated with subjective feelings of humor ruled out this possibility. The laughter was part of a larger set of problems attributable to impulse disinhibition. The patient showed temper outbursts, made socially inappropriate remarks that were sexual or facetious in content, had emotional responses that were out of proportion to their stimulus (e.g., loud and persistent laughter), and had poor tolerance for frustration during board games. She failed to use feedback to modify her behavior and was not always affected by the potential consequences of her behavior. This was particularly evident in her behavior at the convenience store. The patient also failed to persist with successful strategies on problem-solving tasks. The patient, her husband, and her former employer all attested to the fact that her current behavior was quite different from her premorbid behavior. Although she was consuming alcohol before entering the day rehabilitation program, the patient did not have access to alcohol or any other drugs during the time of her treatment, ruling out acute intoxication as a confounding factor.

An additional diagnosis of behavioral perseveration can be made in this case in light of the high number of perseverative errors that occurred despite corrective feedback during performance of the WCST. It is notable that motor perseveration is not present in this patient.

CASE 18–4

N.L. was a 65-year-old man who served as a criminal court judge until suffering a right middle cerebral artery cerebrovascular accident. CT scans revealed an area of infarction in the right parietal lobe. Examination revealed a left hemiparesis, decreased tactile sensitivity on the left, left-sided extinction to visual and auditory stimuli, and left hemispatial neglect (see Chap. 4). Despite the left hemispatial neglect, performance was preserved on tests of visual form and spatial perception. Severe motor perseveration was evident when the patient attempted to copy triple loops, with more than 30 extra loops produced.

N.L. successfully completed two sorts on the WCST, with 71 percent of his errors being perseverative in nature. The patient was, however, able to identify all three possible strategies for sorting the WCST cards. Despite his poor problem-solving performance, N.L. was above average in intellectual functioning on the Wechsler Adult Intelligence Scale–Revised and was notably intact in his ability to identify abstract similarities in superficially different objects and concepts.

CASE 18–5

W.W. was a 67-year-old man who was employed as a shipping clerk until he suffered a left-hemisphere cerebrovascular accident. CT scans revealed multiple areas of infarction in the left parietal lobe and a possible additional infarction in the right parietal lobe. Neuropsychological examination revealed a mild right hemiparesis but no other movement disorders. Notably, the patient was free of perseveration when copying triple loops. Visual fields were full, and there were no indications of stimulus neglect (see Chap. 4). Performance on tests of visual form and spatial perception was intact. Memory for verbal information was preserved, but a moderate reduction in ability to recall visuospatial information was documented.

W.W.'s intellectual functioning was in the average range, with notably preserved ability to identify abstract similarities in superficially different objects and concepts. Although the patient verbally identified all possible strategies for sorting on the Nelson administration of the WCST, he used only form. Despite very directive feedback to shift his approach and try something new, W.W. persisted in sorting by form, eventually resulting in a perseverative error score of 98 percent.

DISCUSSION

Cases 18–4 and 18–5 are discussed together because of the high similarity of their presentation. Both had behavioral perseveration. The patient in Case 18–4 additionally presented with severe motor perseveration, whereas motor perseveration was not evident in the patient in Case 18–5. An additional notable feature of these patients was that they had parietal lesions, underscoring the importance of not automatically viewing behavioral perseveration as a feature of frontal lobe damage and not automatically viewing the WCST as a "frontal lobe test." The presence of motor weakness in both patients may, however, suggest some anterior extension of the lesions, perhaps as far as the motor strip. Nonetheless, it would be an error to conclude from the test data that the frontal lobe was the principal area of the brain compromised in these two patients.

CASE 18–6

C.D. was a 72-year-old man who worked part-time as an accountant. He showed a nonhemorrhagic left parietal lobe lesion on CT scans. The patient also had an old right occipital infarct detected by CT scans. His medical history was positive for mild renal insufficiency and hypertension. Current medications included warfarin sodium and nifedipine. Neurological examination revealed poor coordination and weakness on the right side, decreased right-sided tactile sensation, a right visual field cut, and possible right hemispatial neglect (see Chap. 4). Neglect was not detected in a subsequent neuropsychological examination, but the patient did show a mild Wernicke's aphasia characterized by decreased comprehension and repetition of oral language with fluent speech (see Chap. 12).

Staff members noted euphoric episodes since the beginning of C.D.'s admission. During these episodes, C.D. appeared to be bursting with energy. He had no worries or concerns and greeted everyone in sight with expansive exuberance, as if everyone were a long-lost friend. He was motivated to try anything and would move so rapidly that staff had to race to keep up with him. At such times he was notably unsafe in transferring from wheelchair to bed and required constant supervision to prevent him from attempting activities that were beyond his capacity. His speech was rapid and he joked constantly. C.D.'s wife became highly distressed by his behavior when she took him home for a day. A subsequent interview with her confirmed the absence of a premorbid history of psychiatric disorder and no prior instances that even remotely resembled C.D.'s current behavior.

DISCUSSION

The patient in case 18–6 presented with moria. The patient's wife clearly attested to the change in his behavior since his stroke and the absence of any premorbid signs of mania. The two medications he was taking do not have elation or mania as side effects.

CASE 18–7

L.S. was a 65-year-old man with a law degree who worked as a small-business consultant. He developed a basilar artery occlusion that produced bilateral posterior infarctions. Computed tomographic scans showed large left occipital and temporal infarctions, a small right occipital infarction, and a possible left cerebellar infarction. Examination revealed an ataxic gait, dysmetric movements of the hands toward targets, and a right visual field cut. L.S.'s mood was jovial and stable, and no symptoms of psychiatric disorder other than those reported here were present. The only medication the patient was taking at the time of admission was nifedipine. Severe impairment was seen in L.S.'s recall of verbal and visuospatial information. On the WMS-R Paragraphs and Designs subtests, the patient could recall no information after the 30-minute delay interval.

L.S.'s immediate recall of the WMS-R paragraphs was also poor, but this was not so much the result of a loss of information as it was the result of intrusion of erroneous information from his personal and professional life. For example, in the first paragraph, L.S. reported that the main character was an employee of the YMCA (the patient had at one time been administratively involved in a YMCA). The second paragraph, which deals with a delivery truck driver's highway accident, was even more distorted in L.S.'s memory. He lost sight of the fact that the examiner had simply read a paragraph to him and began to recall the story as if it personally involved the examiner. The driver was described as being "near your [the examiner's] office in southwest Atlanta." L.S. added that the driver was entitled to restitution and stated that he thought the examiner was providing express service.

Confusion was also evident in the patient's response to general orientation questions. Although he was aware of his own identity, he did not know where he was, believing he was in the "Augusta headquarters for the YMCA." He identified the city as Atlanta, but reported that the state was Virginia. Other locations were reported when inquiries were made on other occasions. He was incorrect about the season, the month (variously reporting it was April or May, neither of which was correct), and the year (he variously reported the year as being 1950, 1983, 1987, 1990, and 1982, all of which were incorrect).

The patient had no concept of his current situation. He insisted that the examiner, whom he in fact had never met before, was an old friend from Boston. He would not abandon this belief despite the examiner's repeated attempts to dissuade him, and he showed signs of clear irritation at the examiner's denial of a prior relationship. When asked what had happened for him to be in his current environment, the patient gave the almost incomprehensible answer, "I don't know without any intervening convention. [I] just split."

The confusion and disorientation persisted during several weeks of inpatient hospitalization and were not greatly affected by the attempts of staff members to reorient him. He gradually reached a point at which he would respond and behave as if cognizant of his environment and situation, but then he would suddenly make a comment or exhibit a behavior clearly indicative of continued confusion and disorientation. An interview with a relative indicated that the patient had been eccentric premorbidly (e.g., he insisted on bathing three times daily) but had shown no behaviors remotely resembling his current behavior. He had no prior history of psychiatric disorder or treatment and had worked successfully as an attorney, community activist, and business consultant.

DISCUSSION

Diagnosis in Case 18–7 was fairly straightforward. L.S. presented with confabulation that was particularly notable during structured memory tasks. The content of his confabulation related to past personal and business experiences and resulted in his losing his perspective on the test situation and responding as if a story that was read to him were actually true and involved the examiner. His tendency to confabulate was not a deliberate strategy to fill gaps in his memory, as was evident from his minimal confabulation during delayed recall of paragraphs when he in fact was unable to recall any information at all. His confabulation was prominent only during immediate recall, when he in fact still held onto much of the content that was read to him. Rather than filling gaps in his memory with guesses during the delayed recall, the patient was content with stating that he could recall nothing.

Ideational disorientation or confusion was also quite evident in this patient. The confusion was most notable with regard to time, place, and situation, whereas awareness of personal identity remained clear. The confusion was resistant to correction, and the patient became argumentative and adamant when staff members tried to correct him. His responses to questions about location were also suggestive of reduplication (e.g., locating Atlanta in the state of Virginia), but he did not maintain this belief with enough consistency to warrant this additional diagnosis. The patient's one medication does not produce side effects that could account for his prolonged confusion and confabulation, and no additional confounding factors were present to alter interpretation of the examination results.

REFERENCES

1. Harlow, JM: Recovery after severe injury to the head. Publ Mass Med Soc 2:327, 1868.
2. American Psychiatric Association: Diagnostic and Statistical Manual of Mental Disorders, Fourth Edition. American Psychiatric Association, Washington, DC, 1994.
3. The International Classification of Diseases, Ninth Revision, Clinical Modification. Med-Index Publications, Salt Lake City, 1991.

4. Physician's Desk Reference, Forty-Eighth Edition. Medical Economics Company, Montvale, NJ, 1994.
5. Calvanio, R, Levine, D, and Petrone, P: Elements of cognitive rehabilitation after right hemisphere stroke. Neurol Clin 11:25, 1993.
6. Gautier, JC, Awada, A, and Loron, P: A cerebrovascular accident with unusual features. Stroke 14:808, 1983.
7. Fisher, CM: Honored guest presentation: Abulia minor vs. agitated behavior. Clin Neurosurg 31:9, 1983.
8. Vilkki, J: Amnesic syndromes after surgery of anterior communicating artery aneurysms. Cortex 21:431, 1985.
9. Belyi, BI: Mental impairment in unilateral frontal tumours: Role of the laterality of the lesion. Int J Neurosci 32:799, 1987.
10. Lilly, R, et al: The human Kluver-Bucy syndrome. Neurology 33:1141, 1983.
11. Fisher, CM: Disorientation for place. Arch Neurol 39:33, 1982.
12. Tatemichi, TK, et al: Confusion and memory loss from capsular genu infarction: A thalamocortical disconnection syndrome? Neurology 42:1966, 1992.
13. Barrett, K: Treating organic abulia with bromocriptine and lisuride: Four cases studies. J Neurol Neurosurg Psychiatry 54:718, 1991.
14. Caplan, LR, et al: Caudate infarcts. Arch Neurol 47:`133, 1990.
15. Mendez, MF, Adams, NL, and Lewandowski, KS: Neurobehavioral changes associated with caudate lesions. Neurology 39:349, 1989.
16. Fox, MW, Ahlskog, JE, and Kelly, PJ: Stereotactic ventrolateralis thalamotomy for medically refractory tremor in post-levodopa era Parkinson's disease patients. J Neurosurg 75:723, 1991.
17. Haley, EC, Jr, et al: Deep cerebral venous thrombosis. Clinical, neuroradiological, and neuropsychological correlates. Arch Neurol 46:337, 1989.
18. Waxman, SG, Ricaurte, GA, and Tucker, SB: Thalamic hemorrhage with neglect and memory disorder. J Neurol Sci 75:105, 1986.
19. Meyers, R: Evidence of a locus of the neural mechanisms for libido and penile potency in the septo-fornico-hypothalamic region of the human brain. Trans Am Neurol Assoc 86:81, 1961.
20. Dusoir, H, et al: The role of diencephalic pathology in human memory disorder. Evidence from a penetrating paranasal brain injury. Brain 113:1695, 1990.
21. So, NK, et al: Delayed leukoencephalopathy in survivors with small cell lung cancer. Neurology 37:1198, 1987.
22. Stone, SP, Halligan, PW, and Greenwood, RJ: The incidence of neglect phenomena and related disorders in patients with an acute right or left hemisphere stroke. Age Ageing 22:46, 1993.
23. Mesulam, MM, et al: Acute confusional states with right middle cerebral artery infarctions. J Neurol Neurosurg Psychiatry 39:84, 1976.
24. Ortiz, N, and Barraquer-Bordas, L: Place disorientation as a clinical feature of a right capsulo-putaminal hematoma. Contribution to the understanding of neuropsychologic symptomatology in subcortical lesions of the right hemisphere. Neurologia 6:103, 1991.
25. Asfora, WT, et al: Is the syndrome of pathological laughing and crying a manifestation of pseudobulbar palsy? J Neurol Neurosurg Psychiatry 52:523, 1989.
26. Van Hilten, JJ, et al: Pathologic crying as a prominent behavioral manifestation of central pontine myelinolysis. Arch Neurol 45:936, 1988.
27. Bouvier, A, Chevalier, JF, and Brion, S: Pathological laughing and posterior fossa tumours. Encephale 7:83, 1981.
28. Bauer, G, Gerstenbrand, F, and Hengl, W: Involuntary motor phenomena in the locked-in syndrome. J Neurol 223:191, 1980.
29. Cantu, RC, and Drew, JH: Pathological laughing and crying associated with a tumor ventral to the pons. Case report. J Neurosurg 24:1024, 1966.
30. Green, RL, McAllister, TW, and Bernat, JL: A study of crying in medically and surgically hospitalized patients. Am J Psychiatry 144:442, 1987.
31. Robinson, RG, et al: Pathological laughing and crying following stroke: Validation of a measurement scale and a double-blind treatment study. Am J Psychiatry 150:286, 1993.
32. Sackeim, HA, et al: Hemispheric asymmetry in the expression of positive and negative emotions. Neurologic evidence. Arch Neurol 39:210, 1982.
33. Pilleri, G: A case of pathological crying. Confinia Neurologica 27:367, 1966.
34. Ross, ED, and Stewart, RS: Pathological display of affect in patients with depression and right frontal brain damage. An alternative mechanism. J Nerv Ment Dis 175:165, 1987.
35. Ross, ED: The aprosodias. Functional-anatomic organization of the affective components of language in the right hemisphere. Arch Neurol 38:561, 1981.

36. Sethi, PK, and Rao, TS: Gelastic, quiritarian and cursive epilepsy: A clinicopathological appraisal. J Neurol Neurosurg Psychiatry 39:823, 1976.
37. Gascon, GG, and Lombroso, CT: Epileptic (gelastic) laughter. Epilepsia 12:63, 1971.
38. Cutting, J: Study of anosognosia. J Neurol Neurosurg Psychiatry 41:548, 1978.
39. Starkstein, SE, et al: Anosognosia and major depression in 2 patients with cerebrovascular lesions. Neurology 40:1380, 1990.
40. Starkstein, SE, et al: Anosognosia in patients with cerebrovascular lesions. A study of causative factors. Stroke 23:1446, 1992.
41. Dronkers, NF, and Knight, RT: Right-sided neglect in a left-hander: Evidence for reversed hemispheric specialization of attention capacity. Neuropsychologia 27:729, 1989.
42. Grand Maison, F, et al: Transient anosognosia for episodic hemiparesis: A singular manifestation of TIAs and epileptic seizures. Can J Neurol Sci 16:203, 1989.
43. Bisiach, E, et al: Unawareness of disease following lesions of the right hemisphere: Anosognosia for hemiplegia and anosognosia for hemianopia. Neuropsychologia 24:471, 1986.
44. Hier, DB, Mondlock, J, and Caplan, LR: Behavioral abnormalities after right hemisphere stroke. Neurology 33:337, 1983.
45. Welman, AJ: Right-sided unilateral visual spatial agnosia, asomatognosia and anosognosia with left hemisphere lesions. Brain 92:571, 1969.
46. Watson, RT, and Heilman, KM: Thalamic neglect. Neurology 29:690, 1979.
47. Jacome, DE: Subcortical prosopagnosia and anosognosia. Am J Med Sci 292:386, 1986.
48. Healton, EB, et al: Subcortical neglect. Neurology 32:776, 1982.
49. Cusumano, JV, Fletcher, JW, and Patel, BK: Scintigraphic appearance of Anton's syndrome. JAMA 245:1248, 1981.
50. Lantos, G: Cortical blindness due to osmotic disruption of the blood brain barrier by angiographic contrast material: CT and MRI studies. Neurology 39:567, 1989.
51. McDaniel, KD, and McDaniel, LD: Anton's syndrome in a patient with posttraumatic optic neuropathy and bifrontal contusions. Arch Neurol 48:101, 1991.
52. Gilmore, RL, et al: Anosognosia during Wada testing. Neurology 42:925, 1992.
53. Bogousslavsky, J, and Regli, F: Response-to-next-patient stimulation: A right-hemisphere syndrome. Neurology 38:1225, 1988.
54. Richardson, JK: Psychotic behavior after right hemisphere cerebrovascular accident: A case report. Arch Phys Med Rehabil 73:381, 1992.
55. Feinberg, TE, Haber, LD, and Leeds, NE: Verbal asomatognosia. Neurology 40:1391, 1990.
56. Goldstein, LH, et al: Unilateral frontal lobectomy can produce strategy application disorder. J Neurol Neurosurg Psychiatry 56:274, 1993.
57. Owen, AM, et al: Planning and spatial working memory following frontal lobe lesions in man. Neuropsychologia 28:1021, 1990.
58. Glosser, G, and Goodglass, H: Disorders in executive control functions among aphasic and other brain-damaged patients. J Clin Exp Neuropsychol 12:485, 1990.
59. Wallesch, CW, et al: Language and cognitive deficits resulting from medial and dorsolateral frontal lobe lesions. Archiv fur Psychiatrie und Newenkrankheiten 233:279, 1983.
60. Petrides, M, and Milner, B: Deficits on subject-ordered tasks after frontal- and temporal-lobe lesions in man. Neuropsychologia 20:249, 1982.
61. Shallice, T, and Evans, ME: The involvement of the frontal lobes in cognitive estimation. Cortex 14:294, 1978.
62. Nelson, HE: A modified card-sorting test sensitive to frontal lobe defects. Cortex 12:313, 1976.
63. Drewe, EA: The effect of type and area of brain lesion on Wisconsin Card Sorting Test performance. Cortex 10:159, 1974.
64. Milner, B: Some effects of different brain lesions on card sorting: The role of the frontal lobes. Arch Neurol 9:90, 1963.
65. Caramazza, A, et al: Right-hemispheric damage and verbal problem solving behavior. Brain Lang 3:41, 1976.
66. Konow, A, and Pribram, K: Error recognition and utilization produced by injury to the frontal cortex in man. Neuropsychologia 8:489, 1970.
67. Mori, E, and Yamadori, A: Acute confusional state and acute agitated delirium. Occurrence after infarction in the right middle cerebral artery territory. Arch Neurol 44:1139, 1987.
68. Packer, RJ, et al: Focal encephalopathy following methotrexate therapy. Administration via a misplaced intraventricular catheter. Arch Neurol 38:450, 1981.
69. Yudofsky, S, Williams, D, and Gorman, J: Propranolol in the treatment of rage and violent behavior in patients with chronic brain syndromes. Am J Psychiatry 138:218, 1981.

70. Van Zandycke, M, Orban, LC, and Vander-Eecken, H: Acute prolonged ictal confusion (resembling petit mal status) presenting "de novo" in later life. Acta Neurol Belg 80:174, 1980.
71. Delsedime, M, et al: A syndrome resembling limbic encephalitis, associated with bronchial carcinoma, but without neuropathological abnormality: A case report. J Neurol 231:165, 1984.
72. Devinsky, O, Bear, D, and Volpe, BT: Confusional states following posterior cerebral artery infarction. Arch Neurol 45:160, 1988.
73. Terzano, MG, et al: Confusional states with periodic lateralized epileptiform discharges (PLEDs): A peculiar epileptic syndrome in the elderly. Epilepsia 27:446, 1986.
74. Schlitt, M, Lakeman, FD, and Whitley, RJ: Psychosis and herpes simplex encephalitis. South Med J 78:1347, 1985.
75. Duyckaerts, C, et al: Bilateral and limited amygdalohippocampal lesions causing a pure amnesic syndrome. Ann Neurol 18:314, 1985.
76. Horenstein, S, Chamberlin, W, and Conomy, Y: Infarction of the fusiform and calcarine regions: Agitated delirium and hemianopia. Trans Am Neurol Assoc 92:85, 1967.
77. Medina, JL, Rubino, FA, and Ross, A: Agitated delirium caused by infarction of the hippocampal formation and fusiform and lingual gyri: A case report. Neurology 24:1181, 1974.
78. Waga, S, Shimosaka, S, and Kojima, T: Arteriovenous malformations of the lateral ventricle. J Neurosurg 63:185, 1985.
79. Tatemichi, TK, et al: Paramedian thalamopeduncular infarction: Clinical syndromes and magnetic resonance imaging. Ann Neurol 32:162, 1992.
80. Mair, WG, Warrington, EK, and Weiskrantz, L: Memory disorder in Korsakoff's psychosis: A neuropathological and neuropsychological investigation of two cases. Brain 102:749, 1979.
81. Marra, TR: Hemiparesis apparently due to central pontine myelinolysis following hyponatremia. Ann Neurol 14:687, 1983.
82. Kim, RC: Rheumatoid disease with encephalopathy. Ann Neurol 7:86, 1980.
83. Vliegenthart, WE, et al: An unusual CT-scan appearance in multiple sclerosis. J Neurol Sci 71:129, 1985.
84. Forstl, H, et al: Neuroanatomical correlates of clinical misidentification and misperception in senile dementia of the Alzheimer type. J Clin Psychiatry 52:268, 1991.
85. Kapur, N, Turner, A, and King, C: Reduplicative paramnesia: Possible anatomical and neuropsychological mechanisms. J Neurol Neurosurg Psychiatry 51:579, 1988.
86. Hakim, H, Verma, NP, and Greiffenstein, MF: Pathogenesis of reduplicative paramnesia. J Neurol Neurosurg Psychiatry 51:839, 1988.
87. Lewis, SW: Brain imaging in a case of Capgras' syndrome. Br J Psychiatry 150:117, 1987.
88. Filley, CM, and Jarvis, PE: Delayed reduplicative paramnesia. Neurology 37:701, 1987.
89. Alexander, MP, Stuss, DT, and Benson, DF: Capgras syndrome: A reduplicative phenomenon. Neurology 29:334, 1979.
90. Benson, DF, Gardner, H, and Meadows, JC: Reduplicative paramnesia. Neurology 26:147, 1976.
91. Forstl, H, et al: Psychiatric, neurological and medical aspects of misidentification syndromes: A review of 260 cases. Psychol Med 21:905, 1991.
92. Cummings, JL: Organic delusions: Phenomenology, anatomical correlations, and review. Br J Psychiatry 146:184, 1985.
93. Joseph, AB: Bitemporal atrophy in a patient with Fregoli syndrome, syndrome of intermetamorphosis, and reduplicative paramnesia. Am J Psychiatry 142:146, 1985.
94. Staton, RD, Brumback, RA, and Wilson, H: Reduplicative paramnesia: A disconnection syndrome of memory. Cortex 18:23, 1982.
95. Crichton, P, and Lewis, S: Delusional misidentification, AIDS and the right hemisphere. Br J Psychiatry 157:608, 1990.
96. Quinn, D: The Capgras syndrome: Two case reports and a review. Can J Psychiatry 26:126, 1981.
97. DeLuca, J and Cicerone, KD: Confabulation following aneurysm of the anterior communicating artery. Cortex 27:417, 1991.
98. Baddeley, A, and Wilson, B: Frontal amnesia and the dysexecutive syndrome. Brain Cogn 7:212, 1988.
99. Shapiro, BE, et al: Mechanisms of confabulation. Neurology 31:1070, 1981.
100. Stuss, DT, et al: An extraordinary form of confabulation. Neurology 28:1166, 1978.
101. Morris, MK, et al: Amnesia following a discrete basal forebrain lesion. Brain 115:1827, 1992.
102. Damasio, AR, et al: Amnesia following basal forebrain lesions. Arch Neurol 42:263, 1985.
103. Sandson, J, Albert, ML, and Alexander, MP: Confabulation in aphasia. Cortex 22:621, 1986.
104. Kertesz, A: Visual agnosia: The dual deficit of perception and recognition. Cortex 15:403, 1979.
105. Dall Ora, P, Della-Sala, S, and Spinnler, H: Autobiographical memory. Its impairment in amnesic syndromes. Cortex 25:197, 1989.

106. Hough, MS: Narrative comprehension in adults with right and left hemisphere brain damage: Theme organization. Brain Lang 38:253, 1990.
107. Vilkki, J: Perseveration in memory for figures after frontal lobe lesion. Neuropsychologia 27:1101, 1989.
108. Vilkki, J: Differential perseverations in verbal retrieval related to anterior and posterior left hemisphere lesions. Brain Lang 36:543, 1989.
109. Santo-Pietro, MJ, and Rigrodsky, S: Patterns of oral-verbal perseveration in adult aphasics. Brain Lang 29:1, 1986.
110. Albert, ML, and Sandson, J: Perseveration in aphasia. Cortex 22:103, 1986.
111. Jones-Gotmann, M, and Milner, B: Design fluency: The invention of nonsense drawings after focal cortical lesions. Neuropsychologia 15:653, 1977.
112. Hudson, A: Perseveration. Brain 91:571, 1968.
113. Denes, G, et al: An unusual case of perseveration sparing body-related tasks. Cortex 26:269, 1990.
114. Fensore, C, et al: Language and memory disturbances from mesencephalothalamic infarcts. A clinical and computed tomography study. Eur Neurol 28:51, 1988.
115. Mazaux, JM, and Orgogozo, JM: Analysis and quantitative study of language disorders in lesions of the left thalamus: Thalamic aphasia. Cortex 18:403, 1982.
116. Elghozi, D, et al: Quasi-aphasia associated with thalamic lesions: Relation between the language disorder and elective activation of the left hemisphere in 4 cases of left and right thalamic lesions. Rev Neurol 134:557, 1978.
117. Barat, M, et al: Aphasic-type language disorders associated with lesions of the putamen and caudate nucleus: Clinicopathological findings in one case. Rev Neurol 137:343, 1981.
118. Miller, LA: Impulsivity, risk-taking, and the ability to synthesize fragmented information after frontal lobectomy. Neuropsychologia 30:69, 1992.
119. Gautier-Smith, PC: Cerebral dysfunction and disorders of sexual behavior. Rev Neurol 136:311, 1980.
120. Eslinger, PJ, and Damasio, AR: Severe disturbance of higher cognition after bilateral frontal lobe ablation: Patient EVR. Neurology 35:1731, 1985.
121. Gorman, DG, and Cummings, JL: Hypersexuality following septal injury. Arch Neurol 49:308, 1992.
122. Besser, R, et al: Acute trimethyltin limbic-cerebellar syndrome. Neurology 37:945, 1987.
123. Freemon, FR, and Nevis, AH: Temporal lobe sexual seizures. Neurology 19:87, 1969.
124. Hooshmand, H, and Brawley, BW: Temporal lobe seizures and exhibitionism. Neurology 19:1119, 1960.
125. Terzian, H, and Dalle Ore, G: Syndrome of Kluver and Bucy reproduced in man by bilateral removal of the temporal lobes. Neurology 5:373, 1955.
126. Blumer, D, and Walker, AE: Sexual behavior in temporal lobe epilepsy. Arch Neurol 16:37, 1967.
127. Currier, RD, et al: Sexual seizures. Arch Neurol 25:260, 1971.
128. Heaton, RK, et al: Wisconsin Card Sorting Test Manual. Revised and Expanded. Psychological Assessment Resources, Odessa, FL, 1993.
129. Lezak, MD: Neuropsychological Assessment, Second Edition. Oxford University Press, New York, 1983.
130. Axelrod, BN, Goldman, BS, and Woodard, JL: Interrater reliability in scoring the Wisconsin Card Sorting Test. The Clinical Neuropsychologist 6:143, 1992.
131. Drewe, EA: The effect of type and area of brain lesion on Wisconsin Card Sorting Test Performance. Cortex 10:159, 1974.
132. Tarter, RE, and Parsons, OA: Conceptual shifting in chronic alcoholics. J Abnorm Psychol 77:71, 1971.
133. Reitan, RM, and Davison, LA: Clinical Neuropsychology: Current Status and Applications. H.V. Winston, Washington, DC, 1974.
134. Boyle, GL: Clinical neuropsychological assessment: Abbreviating the Halstead Category Test of brain dysfunction. J Clin Psychol 42:615, 1986.
135. Caslyn, DA, O'Leary, MR, and Chaney, EF: Shortening the Category Test. J Consult Clin Psychol 48:788, 1980.
136. Russell, EW, and Levy, M: Revision of the Halstead Category Test. J Consult Clin Psychol 55:898, 1987.
137. Heaton, RK, Grant, I, and Matthews, CG: Comprehensive Norms for an Expanded Halstead-Reitan Battery. Demographic Corrections, Research Findings, and Clinical Applications. Psychological Assessment Resources, Odessa, FL, 1991.
138. Matarazzo, JD, et al: Psychometric and clinical test-retest reliability of the Halstead Impairment Index in a sample of healthy, young, normal men. J Nerv Mental Dis 158:37, 1974.

139. Goldstein, G, and Watson, JR: Test-retest reliability of the Halstead-Reitan battery and the WAIS in a neuropsychiatric population. Clin Neuropsychol 3:265, 1989.
140. Charter, RA, et al: Reliability of the WAIS, WMS, and Reitan Battery: Raw scores and standardization scores corrected for age and education. Int J Clin Neuropsychol 9:28, 1987.
141. Shaw, DJ: The reliability and validity of the Halstead Category Test. J Clin Psychol 37:847, 1966.
142. King, MC, and Snow, WG: Problem-solving task performance in brain damaged subjects. J Clin Psychol 37:400, 1981.
143. Pendleton, MG, and Heaton, RK: A comparison of the Wisconsin Card Sorting Test and the Category Test. J Clin Psychol 38:392, 1982.
144. Wechsler, D: Wechsler Memory Scale-Revised Manual. The Psychological Corporation, San Antonio, 1987.
145. Benton, AL, et al: Contributions to Neuropsychological Assessment. A Clinical Manual. Oxford University Press, New York, 1983.
146. Hathaway, SR, and McKinley, JC: Minnesota Multiphasic Personality Inventory—2. Manual for Administration and Scoring. University of Minnesota Press, Minneapolis, 1989.
147. Ben-Porath, YS, and Butcher, JN: The comparability of the MMPI and MMPI-2 scales and profiles. J Consult Clin Psychol 1:345, 1989.
148. Butcher, JN: MMPI-2 in Psychological Treatment. Oxford University Press, New York, 1990.
149. Gass, CS: MMPI-2 interpretation of closed-head-trauma: A correction factor. J Consult Clin Psychol 3:27, 1991.
150. Gass, CS: MMPI-2 interpretation of patients with cerebrovascular disease: A correction factor. Arch Clin Neuropsychol 7:17, 1992.
151. Other, E, et al: Psychiatric Diagnostic Interview, Revised (PDI-R) Manual. Western Psychological Services, Los Angeles, 1989.
152. Greenberg, GD: Guide to the Adult and Child Neuropsychological History Protocols. International Diagnostic Systems, Philadelphia, 1990.
153. Foxx, RM, and Azrin, NH: Restitution: A method of eliminating aggressive-disruptive behavior of retarded and brain-damaged patients. Behav Res Ther 10:15, 1972.

APPENDIX 18–1 NEUROEMOTIONAL-NEUROIDEATIONAL-NEUROBEHAVIORAL SYMPTOM SURVEY

Orientation and Clarity

1. What is your full name? + −
2. What is your date of birth? + −
3. How old are you? + −

4a. What type of work do/did you do? + −

Orientation to Person: ________ /4

4b. Have you noticed anything unusual or upsetting about your friends and family? If so, what?

4c. Has it seemed to you that the people around you are impostors? If so, in what way are they impostors?

Reduplication of Person Indicators: *Absent* *Present*

5. Where are you right now?

6a. Where is this place located?

6b. [If the answer to 5 is correct, but 6a is incorrect, ask:] How can [answer given to question 5] be located in [answer given to question 6a]?

Reduplication of Place Indicators: *Absent* *Present*

[Score correct and omit any of the following questions if their correct answers were given above.]

7. What is the name of the place we are in? + –
8. What type of place is it? + –
9. What city are we in? + –
10. What state are we in? + –

Orientation to Place: ________/4

11. What season is it? + –
12. What month is it? + –
13. What year is it? + –
14. What day of the week is it? + –

Orientation to Time: ________/4

15. What illness, condition, or problem, if any, led to your coming here? + –
16. Tell me one physical or mental ability that you think has been affected by your illness or condition. + –
17. Tell me one thing that you could not do well at home/work the way you are right now. + –
18. What are you here in the hospital/my office to accomplish? + –

Orientation to Situation: ________/4

Awareness and Concern

Since the start of your illness/condition, have you noticed: [For any item checked, ask one of the following: How has this change affected the way you feel? Are you worried or concerned about this change? Does it matter that you've changed in this way?]

______ Any decrease in your ability to see or to understand what you are seeing?

Example: Reaction:

______ Any decrease in your ability to hear or to understand what you are hearing?

Example: Reaction:

______ Any change or decrease in your sense of touch?

Example: Reaction:

______ Any change or decrease in your ability to use your arms or legs?

Example: Reaction:

______ Any change or decrease in your ability to talk?

Example: Reaction:

______ Any change or decrease in your ability to understand what other people say to you?

Example: Reaction:

______ Any change or decrease in your ability to read or write?

Example: Reaction:

______ Any decrease in your ability to concentrate?

Example: Reaction:

______ Any decrease in your ability to remember new things?

Example: Reaction:

______ Any decrease in your ability to add, subtract, multiply, or divide?

Example: Reaction:

______ Any decrease in your ability to think and reason clearly?

Example: Reaction:

______ Any decrease in your ability to solve problems or to plan ahead?

Example: Reaction:

______ Any change in your feelings about yourself, people, or things in general?

Example: Reaction:

______ Any change or decrease in your ability to express what you feel?

Example: Reaction:

______ Any change in the way you act toward people or act in different situations?

Example: Reaction:

Total Items Checked: ________ */15*

Illusions and Hallucinations

People who have your illness/condition often find that their senses play tricks on them. I'm going to ask you some questions about things you may have seen, heard, or felt.

1. Since the start of your illness/condition, when you look at a solid object, does it ever seem to:

______ Be larger or smaller than you know it is?

Example: Initial Onset: Frequency: Duration:

______ Be farther away or closer than you know it is?

Example: Initial Onset: Frequency: Duration:

______ Be stretched out, flattened, bent, curved, or otherwise changed from its normal shape?

Example: Initial Onset: Frequency: Duration:

______ Have blurred borders so that you can't tell where it begins and ends?

Example: Initial Onset: Frequency: Duration:

______ Penetrate, intersect, or cut through other objects around it?

Example: Initial Onset: Frequency: Duration:

______ Be turned upside down or rotated from its actual position?

Example: Initial Onset: Frequency: Duration:

______ Be moving when you know it must be standing still?

Example: Initial Onset: Frequency: Duration:

______ Be moving faster or slower than normal?

Example: Initial Onset: Frequency: Duration:

______ Have parts or fragments that are separate and away (like the handle of a cup being separated from the body of the cup)?

Example: Initial Onset: Frequency: Duration:

______ Be duplicated one or more times (e.g., double or triple images of objects)?

Example: Initial Onset: Frequency: Duration:

Visual Metamorphopsia: ________ */10*

2. Since the start of your illness/condition, does sound or music seem:

______ Louder or softer than it should be?

Example: Initial Onset: Frequency: Duration:

______ Closer or farther than it should be?

Example: Initial Onset: Frequency: Duration:

______ Distorted or changed in any way?

Example: Initial Onset: Frequency: Duration:

Auditory Metamorphopsia: ________ */3*

3. Since the start of your illness/condition, when you touch an object in either of your hands, does it:

______ Seem deformed in any way?

Example: Initial Onset: Frequency: Duration:

______ Feel lighter or heavier than it should?

Example: Initial Onset: Frequency: Duration:

______ Feel bigger or smaller than it should?

Example: Initial Onset: Frequency: Duration:

______ Feel taller or shorter than it should?

Example: Initial Onset: Frequency: Duration:

______ Seem to be floating in space rather than in your hand?

Example: Initial Onset: Frequency: Duration:

Somesthetic Metamorphopsia: __________/5

4. Since the start of your illness/condition, have you seen any of the following when nothing was really there?

______ Flashes of light, color, or stars

Example: Initial Onset: Frequency: Duration:

______ Any object, form, shape, or person

Example: Initial Onset: Frequency: Duration:

______ Yourself standing in front of you as if you were looking in a mirror

Example: Initial Onset: Frequency: Duration:

Visual Hallucinosis: __________/3

5. Since the start of your illness/condition, have you heard any of the following sounds when nothing was really there?

______ Indistinct noises like wind, trickling water, hissing, humming, or whispering

Example: Initial Onset: Frequency: Duration:

______ Any distinct sound

Example: Initial Onset: Frequency: Duration:

______ One or more voices

Example: Initial Onset: Frequency: Duration:

______ Music or singing

Example: Initial Onset: Frequency: Duration:

Auditory Hallucinosis: __________/4

6. Since the start of your illness/condition, have you felt like:

______ You have an extra arm or leg?

Example: Initial Onset: Frequency: Duration:

______ A part of your body is missing?

Example: Initial Onset: Frequency: Duration:

Somesthetic Hallucinosis: __________/2

Somatoparaphrenia and Diagonistic Apraxia

1. Since the start of your condition, have you felt like:

______ An arm or leg doesn't actually belong to you?

Example: Initial Onset: Frequency: Duration:

______ Someone else's body has been left with you?

Example: Initial Onset: Frequency: Duration:

______ A part of your body is foreign or strange?

Example: Initial Onset: Frequency: Duration:

Somatoparaphrenia: __________ */3*

2. Does one of your hands:

______ Carry out activities that you do not control or do not want it to do?

Example: Initial Onset: Frequency: Duration:

______ Seem to have a mind of its own?

Example: Initial Onset: Frequency: Duration:

______ Try to change or undo what the other hand has done?

Example: Initial Onset: Frequency: Duration:

______ Fight with the other hand?

Example: Initial Onset: Frequency: Duration:

Diagonistic Apraxia: __________ */4*

Motivation and Pathological Emotional Expression

1. What did you enjoy doing before the start of your illness/condition?
2. Are you still interested in these things?
3. Do you have any trouble getting yourself going in therapy, work, or leisure tasks? If so, please give an example.

Decreased Motivation: Absent Present

4. Since the start of your illness/condition, have you had times when you laugh or cry for no apparent reason? If so, how often does this happen? How long do these episodes last?
5. Do these episodes seem out of your control, and to just come on their own?
6. What are you usually thinking about or feeling just before these episodes occur?
7. What do you feel when the episodes occur?

Pathological Laughing Indicators: Absent Present

Pathological Crying Indicators: Absent Present

POST-SURVEY OBSERVATIONS

Answers were:
_____ relevant to questions asked
_____ occasionally rambling and tangential
_____ frequently rambling and tangential

Reported past incidents were:
_____ accurate in content and temporal context
_____ accurate in content but out of temporal context
_____ distorted or embellished
_____ completely fabricated

People, facts, and events were:
_____ discussed accurately
_____ occasionally confused
_____ frequently confused

Speech content was:
_____ coherent
_____ occasionally incoherent
_____ frequently incoherent

POST-EXAMINATION OBSERVATIONS

Patient Motivation

If A is checked, do not check B through F.
_____ A. Good intrinsic motivation and effort throughout

Check all that apply.
_____ B. Did little without being told
_____ C. Poor or absent effort
_____ D. Placid, inert, or lacking spontaneity
_____ E. Deliberately uncooperative
_____ F. Tired, fatigued, or nonalert

Examination Validity

If A is checked, do not check B or C.

_____ A. Valid and complete examination.

Check one.

_____ B. Because of one or more of the previous factors, the examination is partially invalid.

Specify invalid portions:

_____ C. Because of one or more of the previous factors, the examination is completely invalid.

Affect and Behavior

If A is checked, do not check B through L.

_____ A. Fully appropriate in affect and behavior

Check all that apply.

_____ B. Excessively excited, happy, or energetic

_____ C. Sudden episodes of laughter

_____ D. Sudden episodes of crying

_____ E. Got stuck on topics or tasks and would not shift away

Examples:

_____ F. Inappropriate repetition of previous responses on new tasks

Examples:

_____ G. Frequent facetious or caustic remarks

Examples:

_____ H. Sexually explicit remarks or behavior

Examples:

_____ I. Excessive or inappropriate emotional reactions and behavior (e.g., tearfulness, anger)

Examples:

_____ J. Destruction or damage of materials

Examples:

_____ K. Stealing

Examples:

_____ L. Volitionally performed private bodily functions

Examples:

INTELLECTUAL DECLINE

19

The concept of intelligence, despite its importance in psychological theory and research, has defied precise definition. It is variously defined as the ability to learn from experience, the ability to adapt to new situations, or the ability to reason, among others. Modern psychology focuses less on defining intelligence than on describing its various attributes, which include both cognitive and personality factors. Intelligence is also increasingly viewed as a dynamic human attribute, a product of both individual heredity and personal experience, that is capable of development and change. The term *intellectual functioning* is often used in place of *intelligence* to emphasize the dynamic nature of the concept.

Debate continues on whether intelligence is a unitary ability or is actually made up of various subabilities. Neuropsychology, with its tradition of careful analysis of patients with discrete focal lesions, has tended toward a view of intellectual functioning as consisting of many dissociable components.[1] Such dissociations are not always apparent in normal populations but become evident in selected clinical patients. Researchers and theoreticians have postulated as many as 120 distinct intellectual abilities.[2] In practice, few clinicians attempt so comprehensive a measurement of intellectual functioning. Although acknowledging the many dissociable components of intelligence, neuropsychology tends to focus on two clusters of intellectual ability: verbal skills and perceptual skills.

In keeping with this approach, intellectual decline is conceptualized in this text as consisting of three subtypes:

1. Verbal intellectual decline
2. Perceptual intellectual decline
3. Global intellectual decline (a combination of subtypes 1 and 2)

It is acknowledged that the subtyping of intellectual decline will change drastically with new theoretical developments in the understanding of human intelligence and its biological substrate.

NOMENCLATURE

Below-average intellectual functioning is the essential feature of mental retardation as defined in DSM-IV.[3] However, this diagnostic code is inappropriate for adult-onset intellectual decline as a result of brain trauma or disease. Deficits in aspects of intellectual functioning are an essential feature of "Dementia" in DSM-IV, and this is an acceptable diagnostic code to use for cases of intellectual decline that also show memory impairment and compromise of work or social activities. If the decline in functioning is relatively mild, a DSM-IV diagnosis of "Borderline Intellectual Functioning" may be considered. Adult-onset intellectual decline is similarly coded in ICD-9-CM[4] as "Dementia."

RULES FOR DIAGNOSIS

Clinical Indicators: Each is independent (only one must be observed for the disorder to be suspected) *except* when subscripting is used. Subscripted numbers (a_1, a_2) denote an indicator with multiple parts that must be considered together.
Associated Features: These are listed to give a more complete picture of the disorder. The presence or absence of these features does not affect the diagnosis.
Factors to Rule Out: All must be taken into account. Failure to rule out even one of these factors makes a firm diagnosis impossible.
Lesion Locations: Each location stands alone; damage in only one of the listed areas is sufficient to produce the disorder.

VARIETY OF PRESENTATION

1. Verbal intellectual decline

Clinical Indicators

a_1. Verbally based intellectual functioning below expectation

a_2. Relatively preserved perceptually based intellectual functioning

a_3. Evidence of a previously higher level of verbally based intellectual functioning

a_4. Decline in verbally based intellectual functioning that arose following the onset of illness or trauma capable of causing brain damage

Associated Features

a. A static, steadily progressive, or stepwise (i.e., repeated episodes of decline followed by partial recovery) course, depending on cause
b. Full or partial recovery, depending on cause
c. Unilateral (usually right-sided) motor weakness
d. Reduced fine motor coordination
e. Loss of visual acuity in one (usually the right) visual half-field (termed *homonymous hemianopsia*)
f. Persistent closing of the eyes in response to a repeated light tap between the eyebrows (termed a *positive glabella reflex*)
g. Excessive facial grimacing in response to tapping the nose (termed a *positive snout reflex*)
h. Sucking movements in response to a light stroke on the lips (termed a *positive suck reflex*)
i. Grasping in response to a stroke across the palm (termed a *positive grasp reflex*)
j. Disorders of concentration (see Chap. 3)
k. Impaired ability to learn and retain new verbal information (see Verbal anterograde amnesia)
l. Disorders of stimulus recognition (see Chap. 9)
m. Disorders of voluntary cognitive control of movement (see Chap. 11)
n. Disorders of oral language (see Chap. 12)
o. Disorders of written language (see Chap. 13)
p. Calculation disorders (see Chap. 15)
q. Illusions or hallucinations (see Chap. 17)
r. Emotional, ideational, or behavioral disorders (see Chap. 18)

Factors to Rule Out

a. Reduced concentration sufficient to account for the decline in verbally based intellectual functioning
b. Oral language impairment sufficient to account for the decline in verbally based intellectual functioning
c. Major depressive episode of sufficient severity to account for the intellectual decline
d. Limited or poor quality of educational or occupational experiences
e. Normal decline in verbally based intellectual functions with age

f. Insufficient prior exposure to the body of information from which the intelligence test is drawn as a result of differing cultural background

Lesion Location

a. Cerebral hemisphere, particularly the combined frontal, anterior temporal, and parietal lobes[5–8]

Lesion Lateralization

a. Left hemisphere more commonly than right

2. Perceptual intellectual decline

Clinical Indicators

a_1. Perceptually based intellectual functioning below expectation
a_2. Relatively preserved verbally based intellectual functioning
a_3. Evidence of a previously higher level of perceptually based intellectual functioning
a_4. Decline in perceptually based intellectual functioning that arose following the onset of illness or trauma capable of causing brain damage

Associated Features

a. A static, steadily progressive, or stepwise (i.e., repeated episodes of decline followed by partial recovery) course, depending on cause
b. Full or partial recovery, depending on cause
c. Unilateral (usually left-sided) motor weakness
d. Reduced fine motor coordination
e. Loss of visual acuity in one (usually the left) visual half-field (termed *homonymous hemianopsia*)
f. Persistent closing of the eyes in response to a repeated light tap between the eyebrows (termed a *positive glabella reflex*)
g. Excessive facial grimacing in response to tapping the nose (termed a *positive snout reflex*)
h. Sucking movements in response to a light stroke on the lips (termed a *positive suck reflex*)
i. Grasping in response to a stroke across the palm (termed a *positive grasp reflex*)
j. Disorders of concentration (see Chap. 3)
k. Impaired ability to learn and retain new visuospatial information (see Visuospatial anterograde amnesia)
l. Impaired ability to notice or detect stimuli on one (usually the left) side of space (see Stimulus neglect)
m. Inaccurate perception of visual, auditory, or tactile stimuli (see Stimulus imperception)
n. Impaired ability to determine the position, orientation, or direction of stimuli in space (see Spatial imperception)
o. Disorders of stimulus localization (see Chap. 8)
p. Disorders of visual-motor integration (see Chap. 7)
q. Disorders of emotional communication (see Chap. 14)

r. Illusions or hallucinations (see Chap. 17)
s. Emotional, ideational, or behavioral disorders (see Chap. 18)

Factors to Rule Out

a. Reduced concentration sufficient to account for the decline in perceptually based intellectual functioning
b. Stimulus neglect sufficient to account for the decline in perceptually based intellectual functioning
c. Major depressive episode of sufficient severity to account for the intellectual decline
d. Limited or poor quality of educational or occupational experiences
e. Normal decline in perceptually based intellectual functions with age
f. Insufficient prior exposure to the body of information from which the intelligence test is drawn as a result of differing cultural background

Lesion Locations

a. Cerebral hemisphere, particularly the frontal and temporal lobes, including the amygdala, parahippocampal gyrus, and basal forebrain, with extension to the basal ganglia[5,6,9]
b. Basal ganglia (caudate and putamen), sometimes with extension to cerebral hemisphere[9,10]

Lesion Lateralization

a. Right hemisphere more commonly than left, although some studies report no laterality effect[7]

3. Global intellectual decline

Clinical Indicators

a_1. Verbally based intellectual functioning below expectation
a_2. Perceptually based intellectual functioning below expectation
a_3. Evidence of a previously higher level of intellectual functioning
a_4. Decline in intellectual functioning that arose following the onset of illness or trauma capable of causing brain damage

Associated Features

a. A static, steadily progressive, or stepwise (i.e., repeated episodes of decline followed by partial recovery) course, depending on cause
b. Full or partial recovery, depending on cause
c. Motor weakness
d. Reduced fine motor coordination
e. Persistent closing of the eyes in response to a repeated light tap between the eyebrows (termed a *positive glabella reflex*)
f. Excessive facial grimacing in response to tapping the nose (termed a *positive snout reflex*)
g. Sucking movements in response to a light stroke on the lips (termed a *positive suck reflex*)
h. Grasping in response to a stroke across the palm (termed a *positive grasp reflex*)

i. Disorders of concentration (see Chap. 3)
j. Impaired ability to learn and retain new information (see Global anterograde amnesia)
k. Impaired ability to notice or detect stimuli (see Stimulus neglect)
l. Inaccurate perception of visual, auditory, or tactile stimuli (see Stimulus imperception)
m. Impaired ability to determine the position, orientation, or direction of stimuli in space (see Spatial imperception)
n. Disorders of visual-motor integration (see Chap. 7)
o. Disorders of stimulus localization (see Chap. 8)
p. Disorders of stimulus recognition (see Chap. 9)
q. Disorders of voluntary cognitive control of movement (see Chap. 11)
r. Disorders of oral language (see Chap. 12)
s. Disorders of written language (see Chap. 13)
t. Disorders of emotional communication (see Chap. 14)
u. Calculation disorders (see Chap. 15)
v. Illusions or hallucinations (see Chap. 17)
w. Emotional, ideational, or behavioral disorders (see Chap. 18)

Factors to Rule Out

a. Reduced concentration sufficient to account for the decline in intellectual functioning
b. Oral language impairment sufficient to account for the decline in intellectual functioning
c. Stimulus neglect sufficient to account for the decline in intellectual functioning
d. Major depressive episode of sufficient severity to account for the intellectual decline
e. Limited or poor quality of educational or occupational experiences
f. Normal decline in intellectual functions with age
g. Insufficient prior exposure to the body of information from which the intelligence test is drawn as a result of a differing cultural background

Lesion Location

a. Cerebral hemisphere, including the parietal, temporal, and/or frontal lobes[7,11–13]

Lesion Lateralization

a. Left-sided or bilateral lesions

ETIOLOGY

Intellectual decline and the neurological conditions that cause it can be divided into three categories: reversible, static, and progressive. Recovery can be hoped for in patients whose intellectual decline is the result of a reversible condition. There is potential for rehabilitation of some patients whose intellectual decline arises from static conditions. Patients with progressive intellectual decline cannot be expected

Table 19–1. **MAJOR CAUSES OF THE INTELLECTUAL-DECLINE SUBTYPES**

Verbal Intellectual Decline	
Cerebrovascular disease	Traumatic brain injury
Neoplasm	
Perceptual Intellectual Decline	
Alzheimer's disease	Renal failure[43]
Cerebrovascular disease	Traumatic brain injury
Huntington's disease[9,42]	Wilson's disease[10]
Neoplasm	
Global Intellectual Decline	
Alcoholism	Multiple sclerosis
Alzheimer's disease	Neoplasm
Anoxia	Neurosyphilis
Autoimmune disease	Nutritional deficiency
Binswanger's disease	Parkinson's disease
Cerebral lipidosis	Pick's disease
Cerebrovascular disease	Polyarteritis nodosa
Demyelinating disease	Progressive supranuclear palsy
Endocrine disease	Renal dialysis
Huntington's disease	Renal failure
Hydrocephalus	Toxicity
Hypoglycemia	Traumatic brain injury
Infection	Wernicke-Korsakoff syndromes
Jakob-Creutzfeldt disease	Wilson's disease
Liver failure	
Metabolic abnormality	

to respond to medical treatment or rehabilitation therapy, and the efforts of health care professionals and family should be directed toward maintaining the patient for as long as possible in a safe and supportive environment. A comprehensive list of conditions giving rise to the intellectual decline subtypes is presented in Table 19–1. A discussion of the more common causes of reversible, static, and progressive intellectual decline follows.

Conditions Giving Rise to Reversible or Static Intellectual Decline

Depression can produce a pattern of performance that resembles intellectual decline as defined in this text. Depression can also increase the severity of intellectual decline resulting from neurological conditions. Consequently, all patients suspected of having intellectual decline should be evaluated for depression. If their presentation is even partially accounted for by depression, some remission of the intellectual decline may follow successful treatment of the depression.

Central nervous system toxicity, nutritional deficiency, endocrine disorder, and metabolic dysfunction can also produce intellectual decline from which recovery is possible in many instances once the underlying cause has been diagnosed and treated. Intellectual decline resulting from neoplasms can also remit if the tumor is diagnosed early and appropriately treated. Patients who develop hydrocephalus following a cerebrovascular accident or traumatic brain injury may show improved functioning once they undergo surgical shunting. The possibility of hydrocephalus should immediately be investigated in patients with brain injury who show a sudden decline in performance after a period of recovery.

Additional reversible causes of intellectual decline include hypoglycemia, alcoholism, central nervous system infection, and autoimmune diseases. In each case, the intellectual decline may remit when the underlying cause is diagnosed and treated. Failure to treat patients with these conditions can result in irreversible brain dysfunction. Not all central nervous system infections and autoimmune diseases respond to treatment, however, and relapse rates are always high in alcoholic populations. For these patients, the prognosis is not as optimistic.

Central nervous system infections that fail to respond to treatment before damaging critical brain regions can produce a static intellectual decline. A similar outcome can occur when neoplasms are detected late or when they are positioned in such a way that total extirpation is impossible without damaging surrounding brain tissue. Alcoholics who develop Wernicke-Korsakoff syndrome are also left with a static pattern of deficits. Toxic exposure to chemicals can also produce permanent deficits. In all of these cases, the intellectual decline neither worsens nor improves. Additional conditions that may lead to static intellectual decline include severe traumatic brain injury, anoxia, and cerebrovascular disease.

Conditions Giving Rise to Progressive Intellectual Decline

Alzheimer's disease, which is associated with extensive cortical atrophy and some additional white-matter degeneration, accounts for the greatest number of cases of progressive intellectual decline. In these patients, the intellectual decline worsens over a period of months or years until the patient can no longer be maintained in his or her home without constant supervision. Institutionalization often becomes necessary. Death ultimately ensues, typically from other medical conditions that are exacerbated by the intellectual decline. Additional causes of progressive intellectual decline include the following conditions:

1. Pick's disease: a condition that is clinically similar to Alzheimer's disease and that is characterized by frontal and anterior temporal atrophy.
2. Wilson's disease: a condition arising from an hereditary disturbance in copper metabolism that can be treated in some cases but leads to progressive mental deterioration in others.

3. Parkinson's disease: a condition associated with loss of dopaminergic cells in the substantia nigra and ventral tegmentum.
4. Huntington's disease: a condition associated with neuronal loss in the frontal cortex and the head of the caudate nucleus.
5. Multiple infarction: a stepwise decline in cognitive functioning is seen in patients who suffer multiple cerebrovascular accidents. In some cases, the individual strokes can be so mild that they are unnoticed. When questioned, the family will report past periods of unexplained decline in functioning from which the patient spontaneously recovered. However, the cumulative effect of the strokes eventually becomes evident in a permanent diminution of functioning. The intellectual decline progresses as strokes continue to occur. Patients who have intellectual decline following multiple infarctions are typically hypertensive and have extensive atherosclerosis. Their radiologic scans may show multiple small infarcts (lacunae). In Binswanger's disease, demyelination and scattered white-matter lacunae are found.
6. Progressive supranuclear palsy: a condition associated with basal ganglia, brainstem, and cerebellar degeneration producing impairment of eye and limb movement in addition to intellectual decline.
7. Jakob-Creutzfeldt disease: a disease thought to be transmitted by a slow-acting virus. Patients show an intellectual decline associated with widespread cortical and subcortical atrophy.
8. Demyelinating diseases (e.g., multiple sclerosis).
9. Autoimmune diseases (e.g., systemic lupus erythematosus).

DISABLING CONSEQUENCES

Whether or not disability is permanent in patients with intellectual decline depends largely on the cause of the impairment. If the intellectual decline arises from a treatable cause, permanent disability need not occur. Even if the neurological illness produces a static intellectual decline, some degree of rehabilitation may be possible. Prognosis is obviously poorest in cases of progressive intellectual decline.

The extent of the disability depends on the severity of intellectual decline. Table 19–2 presents the traditional classification of intelligence test scores. Intelligence test scores tend to correlate with school grades, and patients who have intellectual functioning in the low average range are likely to experience difficulty in undergraduate college courses. Graduate-level courses may be unrealistic for these individuals. Patients in the borderline range are unlikely to succeed at any college-level course work but may function in vocational training programs that are slow paced and involve extensive hands-on demonstration and practice. Severe academic disability is a virtual certainty below the borderline range, and the lower the level of intellectual functioning, the more limited are the training options.

Intelligence test scores tend to be less closely related to job performance than to school performance. Nonetheless, intellectual decline leads to significant disability for individuals in occupations that require continuous updating of knowledge,

Table 19–2. **CLASSIFICATION OF LEVEL OF INTELLECTUAL FUNCTIONING**

IQ Score	Classification
130 and above	Very superior
120–129	Superior
110–119	High average
90–109	Average
80–89	Low average
70–79	Borderline
51–69	Mild retardation
26–50	Moderate-severe retardation
25 and below	Profound retardation

flexible thinking, and active generalization and application of knowledge and concepts derived from one situation to novel situations. Fields such as medicine, law, basic and applied science, engineering, and the liberal arts require above-average intellectual functioning. A drop in intellectual functioning that leaves a patient in the average range may still totally disable the patient in these and other intellectually demanding occupations. In such cases, a career change must be contemplated, and certainly the vast majority of occupations available in modern society require at least average intelligence. Unfortunately, for the individual who was initially above average and in an intellectually demanding occupation, such a downward career shift can mean a loss in income and personal esteem.

Vocational options become restricted at the lower ranges of intellectual functioning. Borderline-range patients are trainable and may become employable at an unskilled or semiskilled level. Individuals in the mild retardation range may function in manual labor or sheltered workshop settings. Individuals below this range are rarely employable, and when they are, they can perform only jobs that involve simple, repetitive tasks performed under continuous supervision.

Social and domestic functions are compromised in individuals functioning in the moderate to profound retardation ranges. These individuals cannot function independently, may be dangerous to themselves or others, and typically require an institutional setting. They can be maintained at home only with constant close supervision at a level beyond what most families can provide. Individuals in the borderline to mild retardation ranges may not always understand their legal and moral obligations and may be vulnerable to unscrupulous individuals. For this reason, they often require some supervision of their activities. A family member must often assume guardianship to protect the patient, but typically the patient can assume many independent responsibilities. Money and time management are often a problem, and this is the area in which help is needed. Significant deficits in social and domestic behavior are not expected in patients above the borderline range unless other neuropsychological disorders are present.

ASSESSMENT INSTRUMENTS

Three types of assessment instruments are listed below:

1. Instruments that were designed to measure intellectual functioning (e.g., the Wechsler Adult Intelligence Scale–Revised)
2. Instruments that tend to correlate with measures of intellectual functioning (e.g., the Halstead-Reitan Battery)
3. Instruments that measure a broad range of cognitive functions (e.g., the Dementia Rating Scale)

The instruments share a broad-based approach to cognitive assessment and yield summary scores that reflect the overall functional status of the central nervous system.

Dementia Rating Scale

The Dementia Rating Scale (DRS)[14] can be obtained from *Psychological Assessment Resources, Incorporated, P.O. Box 998, Odessa, FL 33556.*

The DRS provides a brief measure of attention, initiation, perseveration, constructional ability, abstract conceptualization, and memory, employing 36 tasks. This test is suitable for patients with severe impairment who might otherwise be untestable or who would show a "floor effect" on other measures of cognitive ability. Studies reviewed in the DRS manual suggest that normal individuals consistently show a ceiling effect on the DRS, although slight decreases in performance are found in some normal elderly persons. Cut-off scores are provided in the test manual for individuals aged 65 to 81 years.

One-week-interval test-retest reliability coefficients included in the manual range from .61 to .97, and split-half reliability is reported to be .90.[14] One study reviewed in the manual found that only one DRS subscale differentiated normal from mildly demented subjects; another study reported that three subscales successfully differentiated these groups.[14] Both studies found that all DRS subscales differentiate mildly and moderately demented patients. The DRS total score reportedly correlates .70 with the Wechsler Adult Intelligence Scale Full Scale IQ, .67 with the Wechsler Memory Scale Memory Quotient, and .59 with cerebral glucose metabolism.[14]

The DRS appears to be a useful measure of cognitive status in moderately to severely demented patients. It does not appear to be as useful in detecting mild intellectual decline, and like most psychometric instruments, it does not provide information on cause or reversibility of the intellectual decline.

The DRS can be administered at bedside, in the office, or in laboratory settings and is appropriate for interpretation by neuropsychologists, neurologists, neurosurgeons, physiatrists, psychiatrists, and clinical psychologists.

Wechsler Adult Intelligence Scale–Revised

The Wechsler Adult Intelligence Scale–Revised (WAIS-R)[15] can be obtained from *The Psychological Corporation, P.O. Box 839954, San Antonio, TX 78204-0954.*

The WAIS-R, which is familiar to all mental health professionals, is the most commonly used measure of adult intellectual functioning. The WAIS-R consists of Verbal and Performance Scales that respectively measure verbal and perceptually based cognitive abilities, although verbal ability and motor speed also play a large role in many of the Performance Scale subtests. The six Verbal Scale subtests measure the patient's fund of general information, knowledge of social rules and customs, concentration, vocabulary, numerical reasoning and mental calculation, and ability to identify abstract similarities in superficially dissimilar objects or concepts. The five Performance Scale subtests require the identification of missing details from pictures, arrangement of pictures by thematic content, construction of abstract designs using multicolored blocks (the Block Design subtest), puzzle construction, and rapid copying of coded symbols.

Verbal subtest scores are combined and transformed by using age-stratified normative tables into a Verbal Intelligence Quotient (VIQ) with a mean of 100 and standard deviation of 15. The Performance subtest scores are similarly combined to yield a Performance Intelligence Quotient (PIQ), again with a mean of 100 and standard deviation of 15. A Full-Scale Intelligence Quotient (FSIQ), which is reflective of global intellectual functioning, is derived from the sum of all the WAIS-R subtests. Standard scores with a mean of 10 and standard deviation of 3 are calculated for the individual WAIS-R subtests. The IQ scores indicate a patient's standing relative to others his or her age. The subtest standard scores reflect a person's performance relative to a reference group of individuals between the ages of 20 and 34 years. Age-corrected subtest standard scores can also be obtained.

Normative data are based on a sample of 1880 neurologically normal individuals stratified to match the U.S. population in age, race, gender, education, occupation, and geographic residence, based mainly on 1970 census data. Extensive reviews of the reliability and validity of the WAIS-R are available[15–18] and are not duplicated here. The WAIS-R has been used in neuropsychological examinations to detect the presence of lateralized brain dysfunction, to detect decline in intellectual functioning from presumed premorbid levels, to determine the degree of patient disability, and to identify cognitive strengths and weaknesses.

Several abbreviated versions of the WAIS-R have been developed, because the full test can take up to 90 minutes to administer in neurological populations. The Kaufman[19] short form of the WAIS-R estimates the full-form IQ from four subtests and takes under 20 minutes to administer. The original Kaufman short form underestimated FSIQ, but this problem was corrected in a recent revision of the Kaufman IQ table,[20] resulting in a .963 correlation between the Kaufman estimated FSIQ and the WAIS-R FSIQ. Few subtest comparisons are possible when the Kaufman short form is administered, because only four subtests are included.

The Satz-Mogel short form of the WAIS-R estimates IQ based on the administration of selected items within each of the WAIS-R subtests.[21] Correlations between the Satz-Mogel IQ scores and the full WAIS-R IQs are reported as .90 and above in various studies,[21–23] but correlations between the shortened versions of the subtests and the full versions are much more variable. Users of the Satz-Mogel short form must also contend with the poor test-retest reliability of the PIQ.[24]

Regardless of which version of the WAIS-R is used, a discrepancy of 15 or more points between VIQ and PIQ is statistically significant[15] and has been interpreted as reflecting lateralized brain dysfunction (i.e., VIQ is lower following left-hemisphere damage, and PIQ is lower following right-hemisphere damage). Unfortunately, an average of 10 percent of individuals in each age group of the WAIS-R normative sample show VIQ-PIQ discrepancies of 18 points or more.[25] Groups of patients with right- and left-hemisphere damage generally show VIQ-PIQ discrepancies in the expected direction,[26] but clinicians are concerned with individuals rather than groups of patients. In my experience, patients with lateralized brain damage may lack VIQ-PIQ discrepancies or may have discrepancies in the wrong direction with regard to the side of their lesion (see Case 14–1). In general, it is inadvisable to attempt to lateralize brain dysfunction based on VIQ-PIQ discrepancy alone.

The main difficulty in using the WAIS-R to measure decline from premorbid intellectual functioning is in determining the patient's premorbid status. The earliest approach to this problem involved comparing performance on subtests thought to be resistant to the effects of aging and brain damage (the so-called "hold" subtests) with subtests sensitive to age and organicity (the "don't-hold" subtests). None of the WAIS-R subtests can truly be said to be impervious to all forms of brain damage, however, and the "hold" versus "don't-hold" approach has met with little success.[16]

A more recent approach attempts to establish a premorbid level of intellectual functioning using demographic data. In the Barona regression equations,[27,28] values are assigned to patients based on their age, gender, race, education, occupation, residence (urban or rural), and geographic region (e.g., southern, western). These values are multiplied by regression coefficients and are summed along with a constant value to yield estimates of premorbid VIQ, PIQ, and FSIQ.

The demographic-regression approach to estimating premorbid IQ has the advantage of using historical factors that do not change simply because the patient has a brain lesion. This approach is not, however, without limitations. In general, the equations estimate FSIQ more accurately than PIQ or VIQ.[29] In addition, the Barona equations underestimate IQ in individuals who are above average in intelligence.[29] It is recommended that the Barona equations be used mainly to estimate premorbid FSIQ and that clinicians also consider other sources of information (e.g., premorbid school grades, premorbid work evaluations, reports from objective observers who knew the patient before the onset of the lesion) when determining whether intellectual deterioration has occurred.

The WAIS-R subtest scaled scores permit the examiner to compare individual patients with neurologically normal people in the 20- to 34-year-old age range. This age range was chosen as a reference group because peak performance on the WAIS-R occurs in this group. This group serves as a standard to which individual patients can be compared to determine their degree of disability. However, documenting that a patient performs poorly with respect to the reference group does not prove that a patient has brain damage. Poor performance can be the result of a number of factors, including limited education and aging. The effects of aging can, however, be examined using tables supplied in the WAIS-R manual to correct for age-related decline in WAIS-R subtest performance.

Perhaps the most common use of the WAIS-R by neuropsychologists is to document intellectual strengths and weaknesses. This is accomplished by comparison of individual subtests. What constitutes a significant difference between subtests remains controversial. A difference of 3 scaled score points is significant at the .15 level of statistical confidence and is recommended in the test manual as the minimum interpretable subtest discrepancy.[15] Lezak,[16] however, recommends basing interpretations on a more conservative minimum difference of 4 (borderline significant) or 5 (significant) scaled score points. Such differences in scaled scores should not be attributed automatically to brain damage because average scaled score discrepancies of 7 points have been documented in normal adult samples.[30] Scaled score comparison and interpretation based on the administration of only a portion of the items within the WAIS-R subtests, as in the Satz-Mogel short form, are of uncertain validity and is not recommended.

The interpretation of scaled scores in brain-damaged patients is rarely straightforward. All of the WAIS-R subtests measure multiple abilities, any one of which can be responsible for a patient's poor performance on a given subtest. The subtests that are most sensitive to brain damage are also sensitive to the effects of aging, limited education, fatigue, and other factors. The WAIS-R was not designed to be a neuropsychological instrument, and its subtests lack the specificity needed for precise neuropsychological interpretation.

The WAIS-R is appropriate for office or laboratory administration. Bedside administration is inadvisable because of the materials that must be manipulated by the patient and the deleterious effects of background noise and interruptions. The WAIS-R has long been restricted to use by psychologists because of the many factors that must be considered in its interpretation and the sometimes excessive emphasis placed on IQ scores in academic and occupational settings.

Wechsler Adult Intelligence Scale–Revised as a Neuropsychological Instrument

The Wechsler Adult Intelligence Scale–Revised as a Neuropsychological Instrument (WAIS-R NI)[31] can be obtained from *The Psychological Corporation, P.O. Box 839954, San Antonio, TX 78204-0954.*

The WAIS-R NI is an attempt to overcome the weaknesses of the WAIS-R when used as a part of neuropsychological examinations. In the WAIS-R NI, the "process approach" to testing is adopted, so that WAIS-R subtests are restructured to yield information on the factors that account for a patient's level of performance. Many modifications in procedure are incorporated in the WAIS-R NI. In most cases, the modifications do not invalidate the WAIS-R administration, because they occur after the standard procedures have been completed or involve changes only in the way responses are recorded and scored. The WAIS-R NI modifications do, however, alter the standard administration of the Block Design subtest; therefore a scaled score cannot be computed.

The WAIS-R NI modifications are briefly described. Standard WAIS-R administration calls for discontinuation of the subtests after a specified number of consecutive incorrect responses. The WAIS-R NI eliminates the discontinuation rules on most subtests and requires administration of all items. Standard time limits are abandoned on the Picture Completion, Picture Arrangement, Block Design, Object Assembly, and Arithmetic subtests in the WAIS-R NI; responses obtained within time limits are used for calculation of standard scaled scores. Multiple-choice options are incorporated for missed items on the Information, Vocabulary, Comprehension, and Similarities subtests.

On the Picture Arrangement subtest, patients must not only arrange sequences of pictures according to their theme but must also explain the progression of the theme from one picture to the next. Additional items are included on the Block Design subtest, and patients are asked to judge the correctness of their block constructions. A segmented (via a grid) version of each failed design is presented to see if this improves Block Design performance. Failed Arithmetic subtest items are presented again in written story-problem form, and if they are still failed, they can be presented a third time in computational form. Paper-and-pencil calculation is also permitted if written story problems cannot be solved otherwise.

Two methods are included for administering the Object Assembly subtest, one of which requires the patient to verbally identify the object being constructed as soon as he or she recognizes it. Additional items are included in the WAIS-R NI version of the Object Assembly subtest. Recall of symbols and digit-symbol correspondence is tested after completion of the Digit Symbol subtest.

In addition to modifying existing WAIS-R subtests, the WAIS-R NI includes several new subtests. The Sentence Arrangement subtest requires patients to organize words into sentences, providing a verbal analogue to the Picture Arrangement subtest. The Spatial Span subtest (see Chap. 3) provides a visual analogue of the Digit Span subtest. The Symbol Copy subtest requires patients to copy symbols into boxes that are immediately below the symbols. This subtest assesses many of the same perceptual and motor skills as the Digit Symbol subtest without having a major visual scanning component.

The WAIS-R NI manual includes instructions for recording and scoring qualitative and quantitative data obtained during test administration. One of the most innovative instructions is a procedure for deriving a "scatter score" that reflects the degree of intra-subtest variability in the adequacy of response to individual items. The manual incorporates cumulative-frequency tables derived from the WAIS-R standardization sample. These tables permit the examiner to determine the frequency of an obtained difference between subtest scores (highest minus lowest subtest score). Additional frequency tables for intra-subtest scatter scores are also provided to aid interpretation of within-subtest performance. The manual includes a wealth of interpretative hypotheses for various patterns of WAIS-R NI performance.

The WAIS-R NI greatly increases the usefulness of the WAIS-R in neuropsychological examinations. Use of the WAIS-R NI permits the examiner to ferret out the reasons patients fail certain items or perform poorly in certain areas of intellectual functioning. The WAIS-R NI does have the unfortunate effect of increasing the length of time necessary for administration of the WAIS-R; therefore it may not be possible to finish the test in one session. The WAIS-R NI grew out of the extensive clinical experience of one of the most distinguished contemporary neuropsychologists and her interns and colleagues. However, as the test authors themselves point out, this is not a substitute for empirical demonstration of the WAIS-R NI's reliability and validity. Empirical study of the instrument and of the interpretative hypotheses that grow out of it is essential if the WAIS-R NI is to fulfill its potential.

The WAIS-R NI is appropriate for office or laboratory administration. Interpretation should be attempted only by trained and highly experienced neuropsychologists because of the absence of empirical guidelines for its interpretation.

Halstead-Reitan Battery

The Halstead-Reitan Battery (HRB)[32] can be obtained from *Reitan Neuropsychology Laboratory, 1338 Edison Street, Tucson, AZ 85719.*

The HRB consists of the Category Test, the Tactual Performance Test, the Rhythm Test, the Speech Sounds Perception Test, the Finger-Tapping Test, and a number of supplemental tests, including the Aphasia Screening Test, Sensory Perceptual Examination, Grooved Pegboard, the Hand Dynamometer, and the Trail-Making Test Parts A and B. All but the latter test are described elsewhere in this text. The Trail-Making Test requires patients to draw a continuous line from one circle to another based on a numeric (Part A) or alternating numeric-alphabetic (Part B) sequence.

Age, education, and gender corrections and extensive normative data are available for the HRB.[33] Scores from the first five tests listed yield an "impairment index" that represents the proportion of scores falling in the impaired range. The impairment index summarizes the results of the HRB and is employed as a general indicator of the presence of brain dysfunction.

As a global measure of neuropsychological functioning, the basic HRB is lacking in comprehensiveness. In practice, however, the battery is virtually always supplemented by the WAIS-R and the Wechsler Memory Scale–Revised. Measures of emotional and personality functioning are also typically incorporated. With the addition of these instruments, the HRB provides a more thorough coverage of brain-related cognitive and behavioral functions.

The HRB was designed to detect the presence of brain damage; the focus of the subsequent modifications of the battery has been on refining its ability to detect and localize lesions. The HRB was not designed to indicate a precise neuropsychological diagnosis. The complex tests comprising the HRB have high sensitivity but rather low diagnostic specificity. Extensive testing of limits and use of more specific supplemental diagnostic measures are required before HRB data will yield a neuropsychological diagnosis consistent with the disorders included in this text.

The HRB is appropriate for office and laboratory administration. Interpretation should be attempted only by neuropsychologists who have specific training and experience in the HRB.

Luria's Neuropsychological Investigation

Luria's Neuropsychological Investigation (LNI)[34] can be obtained from *Spectrum Publications, Incorporated, 86-19 Sancho Street, Holliswood, NY 11423.*

The LNI is a compilation of techniques and procedures based on the work of the Russian neuropsychologist Aleksandr Luria. The procedures are divided into 11 sections and include the following:

1. A preliminary conversation in which information is obtained about orientation to person, place, and time. The patient's education, work history, and interests also are reviewed. The patient is additionally asked to describe his or her illness or condition (Section B).
2. An examination of motor deficits (Section D).
3. An assessment of nonverbal sound perception and the ability to reproduce rhythms (Section E).
4. An assessment of somesthetic perception (Section F).
5. An assessment of visual and spatial perception (Section G).
6. An examination of oral language comprehension and repetition (Section H).
7. An examination of oral language expression (Section J).
8. An examination of reading and writing that incorporates procedures to test oral and written spelling, copying, writing to dictation, reading of letters, pronounceable syllables, words, ideograms (e.g., "USA," "USSR"), low-frequency words (e.g., "astrocytoma"), sentences, and paragraphs (Section K).
9. An assessment of number reading, writing, and calculation (Section L).
10. An assessment of learning and memory (Section M).
11. An examination of "intellectual processes" such as picture and story comprehension, concept formation, abstracting, and reasoning (Section N).

The LNI is neither a standardized nor a normed set of procedures. It is meant to be a flexible and modifiable approach that can be adapted to the circumstances of each individual case. Neither reliability nor validity studies are possible on procedures that are so malleable. However, the reliability and validity of the diagnostic decisions arising from the LNI can and should be studied, although to date this work has progressed little beyond Luria's own clinical studies.[35] The strength of the LNI lies in its systematic and careful analysis of the patient and in its emphasis on understanding what produces a particular deficit in a given patient.

The Luria-Nebraska Neuropsychological Battery (LNNB)[36] is an attempt to standardize and validate the LNI. Procedures from the LNI were incorporated (sometimes in modified form) into the LNNB based on their ability to differentiate groups with brain damage from control groups. The result was a battery consisting of 11 basic scales and 3 additional scales (i.e., Pathognomonic, Right Sensorimotor, and Left Sensorimotor) made up of items selected from the basic scales. Two additional scales provide information regarding recency and severity of injury and the degree of compensation that can be expected.

The rationale for developing the LNNB has been questioned because the core of Luria's approach to neuropsychology is a method of assessment and analysis rather than a specific set of tests. The LNNB has also been criticized on psychometric and methodological grounds. The problems noted by test reviewers[16,17] include the following:

1. The inclusion of items within scales that are inconsistent with what the scale is meant to measure
2. Excessive penalizing of patients who are slow to respond
3. Underestimation and overestimation of pathology in individual cases
4. Misidentification of neuropsychological disorders and lesion locations
5. Inability to measure fine gradations of performance because all items are scored on a three-point scale
6. The inappropriate use of multiple t-tests during scale development

The proponents of the LNNB have attempted to counter these and other criticisms through a series of studies documenting the battery's test-retest (.77 to .96)[37] and split-half reliability (.89 to .95).[38] The LNNB was reported to discriminate neurological from normal subjects at acceptable levels of statistical significance[39] and subsequently was reported to have a 74 to 89 percent correct localization rate.[40]

The debate over the LNNB has been acrimonious and is likely to continue with the publication of Form II of the LNNB.[41] Regardless of the final verdict on the validity and usefulness of LNNB, the original LNI remains a viable means of assessing a broad range of neuropsychological functions.

The LNI is readily administered at bedside, in the office, or in the laboratory. Interpretation should be attempted only by experienced neuropsychologists and behavioral neurologists who have specific training in Luria's methods and theories. It is recommended that users of the LNI supplement this test with additional standardized tests of language, memory, concentration, perception, and problem solving.

NEUROPSYCHOLOGICAL TREATMENT

Treatment for intellectual decline depends on its cause. When the cause is progressive, limited neuropsychological treatment options are available. In these cases, therapeutic intervention centers on providing the patient with appropriate stimulation and maintaining the patient's comfort and happiness. These patients can profitably participate in orientation groups in which information such as the date, location, and current news events is discussed. Social gatherings centered around a structured activity can be helpful in occupying patients and in providing stimulation. Formal cognitive remediation is not warranted, but more informal practice of motor skills, memory, perceptual skills, and basic reasoning can be useful, particularly if done in the context of a game.

Cognitive remediation is recommended in cases of intellectual decline resulting from a static cause. By their nature, intelligence measures are nonspecific and tend to tap a variety of cognitive functions within one subtest. The summary scores from intelligence measures provide little guidance for cognitive remediation. The therapist must determine the various functions measured by the test and isolate those functions that are impaired. In the process of doing this, a more precise neuropsychological diagnosis will be achieved. This diagnosis then becomes the focus of cognitive remediation.

For example, a patient may show poor WAIS-R Digit Symbol performance because of poor visual perception, impaired ability to learn the digit-symbol associations, impaired ability to read numbers, impaired ability to write numbers, slowing of eye or hand movements, or failure to detect numbers or symbols on one side of the page, among other causes. In other words, poor Digit Symbol performance could result from stimulus imperception, dysmnesia, alexic acalculia, agraphic acalculia, akinesia, stimulus neglect, or some other neuropsychological disorder. After the specific disorders that are responsible for the patient's poor Digit Symbol performance are identified, they become the focus of rehabilitation therapy.

The critical factor in treating intellectual decline of reversible cause is identification of the cause. Once the cause has been identified and treated, full recovery should be possible in many cases. The physician plays the key role in diagnosis and treatment of reversible intellectual decline, and it is recommended that all cases of intellectual decline be referred for medical consultation.

Regardless of whether the intellectual decline is reversible, static, or progressive, attention must be directed to providing the family with information and support. Families often harbor false hopes, even in cases of progressive intellectual decline. These illusions must be set aside as gently as possible and family members given a more realistic appraisal of the patient's situation. The family will bear the burden of caring for many of these patients and will need information and training in how to handle the disabled patient. The needs of family members should not be overlooked or sacrificed in favor of the patient's needs.

Some families do not have the resources to cope with a disabled patient; these families must be supported as they explore alternative care options. Guilt is often engendered by the decision to institutionalize a disabled family member, and the rest of the family will need support while such decisions are being made. No matter how motivated and resourceful, all families will need respite from caregiving, even if only temporarily. Letting families know that this need will arise and helping them make appropriate arrangements should be a priority for any physician, psychologist, or other health care professional involved in the care of intellectually declining patients.

CASE ILLUSTRATIONS

CASE 19–1

P.P. was a 68-year-old man who had completed a year of college. He was retired from a lumber business. He suffered a left intracerebral and intraventricular hematoma at age 61 years and a left-hemisphere stroke at age 64 years. He was reported to have made a good recovery in the months following each incident. At age 67 years, the patient's family noted increased irritability, emotional lability, and the development of unfounded jealous suspicions concerning his wife, which led to violent threats when other family members tried to defend her. The jealousy was based on the patient's belief that while listening from another extension, he heard his wife talking on the phone to someone with whom she was romantically involved. Neuropsychological testing was requested to help clarify this patient's situation.

The Satz-Mogel short form of the WAIS-R was administered and showed a VIQ of 85, a PIQ of 101, and an FSIQ of 90. Assessment of the patient's language skills revealed an anomic aphasia (see Chap. 12) characterized by difficulty in naming drawings of objects, with preserved oral comprehension, preserved phrase repetition, and fluent and grammatical speech production. Despite the difficulty with naming, P.P. was normal in his ability to generate words according to a specified rule (e.g., words beginning with a specific letter, words belonging to a specific semantic category). P.P. was additionally diagnosed as having pure alexia; see Chapter 13 for a discussion of P.P.'s written language deficits.

Compared to individuals of the same age, P.P. was severely impaired in his ability to recall word lists, paragraphs, and visuospatial stimuli. A Wechsler Memory Scale–Revised General Memory Quotient of 76 was obtained, which is far below what would be expected with history of P.P.'s 1 year of college. After delays of 20 to 30 minutes, the patient's recall of verbal and visuospatial information was essentially negligible. Repetition of information resulted in only marginal improvement in performance (e.g., after five repetitions of a word list, P.P. recalled only three more words than he had after the first list repetition). Perceptual abilities appeared to be preserved, with the exception of a possible right hemispatial neglect (see Chap. 4). The patient also had a severe bilateral hearing impairment. No deficits in motor performance or problem solving were evident.

DISCUSSION

The patient in Case 19–1 presented with verbal intellectual decline characterized by decreased verbal intellectual functioning with preserved perceptually based intelligence. Anomic aphasia, pure alexia, and global anterograde dysmnesia were also evident. Of the multiple deficits seen in this patient, anomic aphasia was the only deficit that might account for some of his reduction in intellectual and memory performance. However, the patient was able to speak in fluent and grammatical sentences and could generate words according to a specified rule or category. The naming difficulty is unlikely to account for the full deficit seen in this patient's intelligence and memory. The intellectual decline was most likely to have been caused by his multiple cerebrovascular events.

This patient's functioning appeared to have worsened recently, as evidenced by his unfounded jealousy. The jealousy was based on his listening to one of his wife's phone conversations. If it is assumed that the patient's hearing impairment led him to misinterpret what was said on the phone, it is possible that the "worsening" in his functioning was the result of the combined effects of deafness and static cognitive impairment. Audiologic examination was recommended in the hope that the patient might benefit from the use of hearing aids.

CASE 19–2

E.M. was a 73-year-old man who had worked at a variety of manual labor jobs before retiring. He was a poor personal historian and did not know how far he had gone in school. He indicated that he had never learned to read or write. E.M.'s medical history was positive for chronic diabetes, peripheral neuropathy, and kidney failure, for which he underwent renal dialysis. He was admitted to a rehabilitation hospital after suffering a left thalamic cerebrovascular accident. On examination, the patient was alert but became lethargic when fatigued. He was able to maintain alertness long enough for neuropsychological testing to be completed.

When asked to signal in response to hearing an odd number, E.M. was unable to maintain concentration on the task. He showed a severe reduction in both forward and reversed digit span. The patient made random errors in response to unilateral and bilateral simultaneous stimulation in the visual, auditory, and tactile sensory modalities as a result of his distractibility. He bisected lines to the right of center, and failed to notice several lines on the left side of the page. Performance was severely impaired on tests requiring detailed visual comparisons and discriminations. Severe constructional deficits were evident in the patient's attempts to copy line drawings, and the patient could not clearly describe or indicate his errors. E.M. was normal in his execution of skilled movements of the mouth and limbs on demand but was unable to rapidly sequence a series of three novel movements, although he could demonstrate each of the individual movements. His attempts to copy triple loops resulted in his making more than 50 perseverative errors.

E.M. was able to follow most commands but made occasional errors with multistep commands. He repeated phrases accurately and could express himself in grammatical sentences. The content of what he said, however, was sometimes confused and nonsensical. He was severely impaired in oral reading, reading comprehension, and oral and written spelling. E.M. was confused about the date, his location, and why he was hospitalized. Memory for verbal and visuospatial information was impaired compared with that of individuals of his age; he performed at or below the 5th percentile in his immediate and delayed recall of paragraphs and designs.

Overall intellectual functioning was in the mentally retarded range, with no significant discrepancy noted in WAIS-R VIQ and PIQ. Questioning of the patient's daughter, with whom he had lived before entering the hospital, revealed that he had functioned independently within her home, cooking and cleaning for himself, and showing none of the disorientation, distractibility, and severe memory impairment that was currently evident. The daughter tearfully indicated that she would be unable to take her father back to her home with his current level of functioning.

DISCUSSION

The patient in Case 19–2 presented with possible global intellectual decline. The diagnosis is complicated by the fact that the patient appears to have had a learning disability and his level of education is uncertain. The presence of concentration deficits and confused ideation further decreased the certainty of the diagnosis. The daughter's acute awareness of the change in her father bolstered the impression that his intellectual functions had declined from a previously higher level.

Two possible causes present themselves. The intellectual decline followed a thalamic stroke, so it is possible that this was responsible for the decline in functioning. However, this extensive decline in functioning is surprising after such a focal lesion. The other possibility is that the patient was metabolically compromised as a result of kidney failure, long-term renal dialysis, or both. Because the latter cause is treatable, it was investigated further. Questioning of the patient's rehabilitation team revealed an association between return from dialysis and a transient worsening in cognitive functioning. A new dialysis schedule was tried, and the patient began to make more consistent gains in his rehabilitation therapies. By the time of discharge, he had improved sufficiently for the daughter to take him home again, with arrangements made for supervision during his waking hours.

CASE 15–1

W.B. was an 80-year-old woman with a doctorate in education who had worked as a professor of music at a university until her retirement at 65 years of age. She lived independently until age 79 years, when she suffered a left middle cerebral artery embolic cerebrovascular accident with a large left parietal lobe infarction visible on computed tomographic scan. W.B. had a history of atrial fibrillation, which was the probable source of the embolus. An initial neuropsychological examination was conducted 5 months after the stroke. The results of W.B.'s WAIS-R are presented in Table 19–3. W.B.'s level of intellectual functioning was far below that which would be expected in an individual with a doctorate. No significant discrepancy between verbally and perceptually based measures of intelligence was evident.

A General Memory Index of 60 was obtained on the Wechsler Memory Scale–Revised, and a Verbal Memory Index of 60 and Visual Memory Index of 76 was obtained. W.B.'s Delayed Recall Index was 69. All memory test scores were below what would be expected in individuals falling in the 70-to-74-year-old age range (norms are not available for older individuals) and were inconsistent with the patient's level of education. Language testing revealed a mild Wernicke's

Table 19–3. **W.B.'S WAIS-R PERFORMANCE (CASE 15–1)**

Verbal Scale*		Performance Scale*	
Information	8	Picture Completion	5
Digit Span	2	Picture Arrangement	7
Vocabulary	7	Block Design	5
Arithmetic	3	Object Assembly	4
Comprehension	4	Digit Symbol	3
Similarities	6		
Verbal IQ: 69	Performance IQ: 73		Full Scale IQ: 69

*Age-corrected scaled scores (ages 70–74 years).

aphasia (see Chap. 12). The patient's comprehension deficit was restricted to complex, multistep commands. She made no errors when responding to yes-or-no questions and only one error when matching words to pictures. Her speech repetition and spontaneous speech contained many paraphasic errors. She monitored what she was saying, however, and would make multiple attempts to correct her speech until she succeeded in communicating the intended message. Oral and written spelling were impaired, as was reading comprehension. W.B. additionally showed alexic and agraphic acalculia. (Her calculation deficits are discussed in Chap. 15.)

W.B. accurately judged the orientation of lines in space but showed severe deficits in discriminating visual and facial stimuli. She was unable to rapidly sequence a series of movements, despite being able to demonstrate each of the individual movements and to state verbally the correct order of the movements. Motor perseveration (see Chap. 11) was notable when she copied triple loops. Severe problem-solving deficits were present. Although she was able to verbalize alternative approaches to the problem, the patient showed a tendency to persist with ineffective strategies despite contrary feedback.

DISCUSSION

The patient in Case 15–1 presented with a global intellectual decline. The diagnosis was easier to make than in Case 19–2 because of this patient's relatively uncomplicated premorbid history. The intellectual decline followed a static lesion. Some improvement in the patient's condition may be possible with the passage of time and with rehabilitation.

REFERENCES

1. Gardner, H: Frames of Mind. The Theory of Multiple Intelligences. Basic Books, New York, 1983.
2. Guilford, JP: Intelligence has three facets. Science 160:615, 1968.
3. American Psychiatric Association: Diagnostic and Statistical Manual of Mental Disorders, Fourth Edition. American Psychiatric Association, Washington, DC, 1994.
4. The International Classification of Diseases, Ninth Revision, Clinical Modification. Med-Index Publications, Salt Lake City, 1991.
5. Reitan, RM: Relationships between measures of brain functions and general intelligence. J Clin Psychol 41:245, 1985.
6. Bornstein, RA: Verbal IQ–performance IQ discrepancies on the Wechsler Adult Intelligence Scale—Revised in patients with unilateral or bilateral cerebral dysfunction. J Consult Clin Psychol 51:779, 1983.
7. Sundet, K: Sex differences in cognitive impairment following unilateral brain damage. J Clin Exp Neuropsychol 8:51, 1986.
8. Wszolek, ZK, et al: Comparison of EEG background frequency analysis, psychologic test scores, short test of mental status, and quantitative SPECT in dementia. J Geriatr Psychiatry Neurol 5:22, 1992.
9. Moss, RJ, Mastri, AR, and Schut, LJ: The coexistence and differentiation of late onset Huntington's disease and Alzheimer's disease. A case report and review of the literature. J Am Geriatr Soc 36:237, 1988.
10. Medalia, A, Isaacs-Glaberman, K, and Scheinberg, IH: Neuropsychological impairment in Wilson's disease. Arch Neurol 45:502, 1988.

11. Meguro, K, et al: Decreased cerebral glucose metabolism associated with mental deterioration in multi-infarct dementia. Neuroradiology 33:305, 1991.
12. Duara, R, et al: Positron emission tomography in Alzheimer's disease. Neurology 36:879, 1986.
13. Bigler, ED, et al: Intellectual and memory impairment in dementia. Computerized axial tomography volume correlations. J Nerv Ment Dis 173:347, 1985.
14. Mattis, S: Dementia Rating Scale Professional Manual. Psychological Assessment Resources, Odessa, FL, 1988.
15. Wechsler, D: Wechsler Adult Intelligence Scale—Revised Manual. The Psychological Corporation, New York, 1981.
16. Lezak, MD: Neuropsychological Assessment, Second Edition. Oxford University Press, New York, 1983.
17. Franzen, MD: Reliability and Validity in Neuropsychological Assessment. Plenum Press, New York, 1989.
18. Spreen, O, and Strauss, E: A Compendium of Neuropsychological Tests. Administration, Norms, and Commentary. Oxford University Press, New York, 1991.
19. Kaufman, AS: Assessing Adolescent and Adult Intelligence. Allyn and Bacon, New York, 1990.
20. Randolph, C, Mohr, E, and Chase, TN: Assessment of intellectual function in dementing disorders: Validity of WAIS-R short forms for patients with Alzheimer's, Huntington's, and Parkinson's disease. J Clin Exp Neuropsychol 15:743, 1993.
21. Dinning, WD, and Kraft, WA: Validation of the Satz-Mogel short form for the WAIS-R with psychiatric inpatients. J Consult Clin Psychol 51:781, 1983.
22. Evans, RG: Accuracy of the Satz-Mogel procedure in estimating WAIS-R IQs that are in the normal range. J Clin Psychol 41:100, 1985.
23. Silverstein, AB: Validity of the Satz-Mogel-Yudin-type short forms. J Consult Clin Psychol 50:20, 1982.
24. Paolo, AM, and Ryan, JJ: Test-retest stability of the Satz-Mogel WAIS-R short form in a sample of normal persons 75 to 87 years of age. Arch Clin Neuropsychol 8:397, 1993.
25. Grossman, FM: Percentage of WAIS-R standardization sample obtaining verbal-performance discrepancies. J Consult Clin Psychol 50:641, 1983.
26. Bornstein, RA: Unilateral lesions and Wechsler Adult Intelligence Scale—Revised in patients with unilateral or bilateral cerebral dysfunction. J Consult Clin Psychol 51:779, 1983.
27. Barona, A, Reynolds, CR, and Chastain, R: A demographically based index of premorbid intelligence for the WAIS-R. J Consult Clin Psychol 5:885, 1984.
28. Barona, A, and Chastain, RL: An improved estimate of premorbid IQ for blacks and whites on the WAIS-R. Int J Clin Neuropsychol 8:169, 1986.
29. Paolo, AM, and Ryan, JJ: Generalizability of two methods of estimating premorbid intelligence in the elderly. Arch Clin Neuropsychol 7:135, 1992.
30. Matarazzo, JD, and Prifitera, A: Subtest scatter and premorbid intelligence: Lessons from the WAIS-R standardization sample. Psychological Assessment 1:186, 1989.
31. Kaplan, E, et al: WAIS-R NI Manual. WAIS-R as a Neuropsychological Instrument. The Psychological Corporation, San Antonio, 1991.
32. Reitan, RM, and Wolfson, D: The Halstead-Reitan Neuropsychological Test Battery: Theory and Clinical Interpretation. Neuropsychology Press, Tucson, 1985.
33. Heaton, RK, Grant, I, and Matthews, CG: Comprehensive Norms for an Expanded Halstead-Reitan Battery. Demographic Corrections, Research Findings, and Clinical Applications. Psychological Assessment Resources, Odessa, FL, 1991.
34. Christensen, AL: Luria's Neuropsychological Investigation Manual. Spectrum Publications, New York, 1975.
35. Luria, AR: Higher Cortical Functions in Man, Second Edition, Revised and Expanded. Basic Books, New York, 1980.
36. Golden, CJ, Hammeke, TA, and Purish, AD: Manual for the Luria-Nebraska Neuropsychological Battery. Western Psychological Services, Los Angeles, 1980.
37. Golden, CJ, Berg, RA, and Braber, B: Test-retest reliability of the Luria-Nebraska Neuropsychological Battery in stable, chronically impaired patients. J Consult Clin Psychol 50:452, 1982.
38. Golden, CJ, Fross, KH, and Graber, B: Split-half reliability of the Luria-Nebraska Neuropsychological Battery. J Consult Clin Psychol 49:304, 1981.
39. Hammeke, TA, Golden, CJ, and Purisch, AD: A standardized, short and comprehensive neuropsychological test battery based on the Luria neuropsychological evaluation. Int J Neurosci 8:135, 1978.
40. Golden, CJ, et al: Cross-validation of the Luria-Nebraska Neuropsychological Battery of the presence, lateralization, and localization of brain damage. J Consult Clin Psychol 49:491, 1981.

41. Golden, CJ, Purish, AD, and Hammeke, TA: Luria-Nebraska Neuropsychological Battery: Forms I and II. Western Psychological Services, Los Angeles, 1985.
42. Taylor, HG, and Hansotia, P: Neuropsychological testing of Huntington's patients. Clues to progression. J Nerv Ment Dis 171:492, 1983.
43. Ryan, JJ, Souheaver, GT, and DeWolfe, AS: Intellectual deficit in chronic renal failure. A comparison with neurological and medical-psychiatric patients. J Nerv Ment Dis 168:763, 1980.

ANATOMICAL INDEX

ETIOLOGICAL INDEX

TEST INDEX

BEHAVIORAL INDEX